Genetics of Hearing Impairment

Genetics of Hearing Impairment

Editors
Ignacio del Castillo
Hannie Kremer

MDPI • Basel • Beijing • Wuhan • Barcelona • Belgrade • Manchester • Tokyo • Cluj • Tianjin

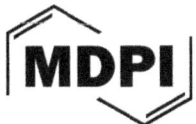

Editors
Ignacio del Castillo
Hospital Universitario
Ramón y Cajal, IRYCIS
Spain

Hannie Kremer
Radboud University Medical
Center
The Netherlands

Editorial Office
MDPI
St. Alban-Anlage 66
4052 Basel, Switzerland

This is a reprint of articles from the Special Issue published online in the open access journal *Genes* (ISSN 2073-4425) (available at: https://www.mdpi.com/journal/genes/special_issues/Hearing_Impairment).

For citation purposes, cite each article independently as indicated on the article page online and as indicated below:

LastName, A.A.; LastName, B.B.; LastName, C.C. Article Title. *Journal Name* **Year**, *Volume Number*, Page Range.

ISBN 978-3-0365-5223-1 (Hbk)
ISBN 978-3-0365-5224-8 (PDF)

© 2022 by the authors. Articles in this book are Open Access and distributed under the Creative Commons Attribution (CC BY) license, which allows users to download, copy and build upon published articles, as long as the author and publisher are properly credited, which ensures maximum dissemination and a wider impact of our publications.
The book as a whole is distributed by MDPI under the terms and conditions of the Creative Commons license CC BY-NC-ND.

Contents

About the Editors ix

Hannie Kremer and Ignacio del Castillo
Genetics of Hearing Impairment
Reprinted from: *Genes* **2022**, *13*, 852, doi:10.3390/genes13050852 1

Barbara Vona, Aboulfazl Rad and Ellen Reisinger
The Many Faces of DFNB9: Relating *OTOF* Variants to Hearing Impairment
Reprinted from: *Genes* **2020**, *11*, 1411, doi:10.3390/genes11121411 7

Edmond Wonkam-Tingang, Isabelle Schrauwen, Kevin K. Esoh, Thashi Bharadwaj, Liz M. Nouel-Saied, Anushree Acharya, Abdul Nasir, Samuel M. Adadey, Shaheen Mowla, Suzanne M. Leal and Ambroise Wonkam
Bi-Allelic Novel Variants in *CLIC5* Identified in a Cameroonian Multiplex Family with Non-Syndromic Hearing Impairment
Reprinted from: *Genes* **2020**, *11*, 1249, doi:10.3390/genes11111249 29

María Lachgar, Matías Morín, Manuela Villamar, Ignacio del Castillo and Miguel Ángel Moreno-Pelayo
A Novel Truncating Mutation in HOMER2 Causes Nonsyndromic Progressive DFNA68 Hearing Loss in a Spanish Family
Reprinted from: *Genes* **2021**, *12*, 411, doi:10.3390/genes12030411 41

María Domínguez-Ruiz, Montserrat Rodríguez-Ballesteros, Marta Gandía, Elena Gómez-Rosas, Manuela Villamar, Pietro Scimemi, Patrizia Mancini, Nanna D. Rendtorff, Miguel A. Moreno-Pelayo, Lisbeth Tranebjaerg, Carme Medà, Rosamaria Santarelli and Ignacio del Castillo
Novel Pathogenic Variants in *PJVK*, the Gene Encoding Pejvakin, in Subjects with Autosomal Recessive Non-Syndromic Hearing Impairment and Auditory Neuropathy Spectrum Disorder
Reprinted from: *Genes* **2022**, *13*, 149, doi:10.3390/genes13010149 51

Khushnooda Ramzan, Nouf S. Al-Numair, Sarah Al-Ageel, Lina Elbaik, Nadia Sakati, Selwa A. F. Al-Hazzaa, Mohammed Al-Owain and Faiqa Imtiaz
Identification of Novel *CDH23* Variants Causing Moderate to Profound Progressive Nonsyndromic Hearing Loss
Reprinted from: *Genes* **2020**, *11*, 1474, doi:10.3390/genes11121474 63

Saba Zafar, Mohsin Shahzad, Rafaqat Ishaq, Ayesha Yousaf, Rehan S. Shaikh, Javed Akram, Zubair M. Ahmed and Saima Riazuddin
Novel Mutations in *CLPP*, *LARS2*, *CDH23*, and *COL4A5* Identified in Familial Cases of Prelingual Hearing Loss
Reprinted from: *Genes* **2020**, *11*, 978, doi:10.3390/genes11090978 79

Isabelle Schrauwen, Khurram Liaqat, Isabelle Schatteman, Thashi Bharadwaj, Abdul Nasir, Anushree Acharya, Wasim Ahmad, Guy Van Camp and Suzanne M. Leal
Autosomal Dominantly Inherited GREB1L Variants in Individuals with Profound Sensorineural Hearing Impairment
Reprinted from: *Genes* **2020**, *11*, 687, doi:10.3390/genes11060687 89

Dominika Oziębło, Joanna Pazik, Iwona Stępniak, Henryk Skarżyński and Monika Ołdak
Two Novel Pathogenic Variants Confirm *RMND1* Causative Role in Perrault Syndrome with Renal Involvement
Reprinted from: *Genes* **2020**, *11*, 1060, doi:10.3390/genes11111060 107

Irina Resmerita, Romica Sebastian Cozma, Roxana Popescu, Luminita Mihaela Radulescu, Monica Cristina Panzaru, Lacramioara Ionela Butnariu, Lavinia Caba, Ovidiu-Dumitru Ilie, Eva-Cristiana Gavril, Eusebiu Vlad Gorduza and Cristina Rusu
Genetics of Hearing Impairment in North-Eastern Romania—A Cost-Effective Improved Diagnosis and Literature Review
Reprinted from: *Genes* **2020**, *11*, 1506, doi:10.3390/genes11121506 . . . . **121**

Paula Buonfiglio, Carlos D. Bruque, Leonela Luce, Florencia Giliberto, Vanesa Lotersztein, Sebastián Menazzi, Bibiana Paoli, Ana Belén Elgoyhen and Viviana Dalamón
*GJB*2 and *GJB*6 Genetic Variant Curation in an Argentinean Non-Syndromic Hearing-Impaired Cohort
Reprinted from: *Genes* **2020**, *11*, 1233, doi:10.3390/genes11101233 . . . . **135**

Marina V. Zytsar, Marita S. Bady-Khoo, Valeriia Yu. Danilchenko, Ekaterina A. Maslova, Nikolay A. Barashkov, Igor V. Morozov, Alexander A. Bondar and Olga L. Posukh
High Rates of Three Common *GJB2* Mutations c.516G>C, c.-23+1G>A, c.235delC in Deaf Patients from Southern Siberia Are Due to the Founder Effect
Reprinted from: *Genes* **2020**, *11*, 833, doi:10.3390/genes11070833 . . . . **153**

Anna Morgan, Stefania Lenarduzzi, Beatrice Spedicati, Elisabetta Cattaruzzi, Flora Maria Murru, Giulia Pelliccione, Daniela Mazzà, Marcella Zollino, Claudio Graziano, Umberto Ambrosetti, Marco Seri, Flavio Faletra and Giorgia Girotto
Lights and Shadows in the Genetics of Syndromic and Non-Syndromic Hearing Loss in the Italian Population
Reprinted from: *Genes* **2020**, *11*, 1237, doi:10.3390/genes1111237 . . . . **171**

Gema García-García, Alba Berzal-Serrano, Piedad García-Díaz, Rebeca Villanova-Aparisi, Sara Juárez-Rodríguez, Carlos de Paula-Vernetta, Laura Cavallé-Garrido, Teresa Jaijo, Miguel Armengot-Carceller, José M Millán and Elena Aller
Improving the Management of Patients with Hearing Loss by the Implementation of an NGS Panel in Clinical Practice
Reprinted from: *Genes* **2020**, *11*, 1467, doi:10.3390/genes11121467 . . . . **187**

Julia Doll, Barbara Vona, Linda Schnapp, Franz Rüschendorf, Imran Khan, Saadullah Khan, Noor Muhammad, Sher Alam Khan, Hamed Nawaz, Ajmal Khan, Naseer Ahmad, Susanne M. Kolb, Laura Kühlewein, Jonathan D. J. Labonne, Lawrence C. Layman, Michaela A. H. Hofrichter, Tabea Röder, Marcus Dittrich, Tobias Müller, Tyler D. Graves, Il-Keun Kong, Indrajit Nanda, Hyung-Goo Kim and Thomas Haaf
Genetic Spectrum of Syndromic and Non-Syndromic Hearing Loss in Pakistani Families
Reprinted from: *Genes* **2020**, *11*, 1329, doi:10.3390/genes11111329 . . . . **213**

Alba Escalera-Balsera, Pablo Roman-Naranjo and Jose Antonio Lopez-Escamez
Systematic Review of Sequencing Studies and Gene Expression Profiling in Familial Meniere Disease
Reprinted from: *Genes* **2020**, *11*, 1414, doi:10.3390/genes11121414 . . . . **229**

Risa Tona, Ivan A. Lopez, Cristina Fenollar-Ferrer, Rabia Faridi, Claudio Anselmi, Asma A. Khan, Mohsin Shahzad, Robert J. Morell, Shoujun Gu, Michael Hoa, Lijin Dong, Akira Ishiyama, Inna A. Belyantseva, Sheikh Riazuddin and Thomas B. Friedman
Mouse Models of Human Pathogenic Variants of *TBC1D24* Associated with Non-Syndromic Deafness DFNB86 and DFNA65 and Syndromes Involving Deafness
Reprinted from: *Genes* **2020**, *11*, 1122, doi:10.3390/genes11101122 . . . . **247**

Ken Hayashi, Yuna Suzuki, Chisato Fujimoto and Sho Kanzaki
Molecular Mechanisms and Biological Functions of Autophagy for Genetics of Hearing Impairment
Reprinted from: *Genes* **2020**, *11*, 1331, doi:10.3390/genes11111331 273

Peter A. Perrino, Dianne F. Newbury and R. Holly Fitch
Peripheral Anomalies in USH2A Cause Central Auditory Anomalies in a Mouse Model of Usher Syndrome and CAPD
Reprinted from: *Genes* **2021**, *12*, 151, doi:10.3390/genes12020151 291

About the Editors

Ignacio del Castillo

Servicio de Genética, Hospital Universitario Ramón y Cajal, Instituto Ramón y Cajal de Investigación Sanitaria (IRYCIS), and Centro de Investigación Biomédica en Red de Enfermedades Raras (CIBERER), Madrid, Spain.

Molecular biologist with experience in the field of inherited hearing impairment. He leads a research group focused on finding the genes that are involved in the different hearing disorders, identifying novel mutations, investigating the pathophysiological mechanisms of their effects and their genotype–phenotype correlations, and developing novel tools for genetic diagnosis. In recent years, his group has been using gene editing technologies to generate new murine models for specific types of non-syndromic hearing impairment.

Hannie Kremer

Hearing & Genes, Department of Otorhinolaryngology and Department of Human Genetics, Radboud University Medical Center, Nijmegen, The Netherlands.

Molecular geneticist with a research focus on hearing impairment. Research is primarily focused on the identification of novel causes of hereditary hearing loss, leading to studies on genotype–phenotype correlations, disease mechanisms, gene function, and the preclinical development of therapeutic strategies. Currently, genetic studies address defects of the noncoding region of the genome as a cause of hearing loss.

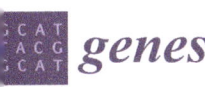

Editorial

Genetics of Hearing Impairment

Hannie Kremer [1,2,3] and Ignacio del Castillo [4,5,*]

1 Hearing and Genes, Department of Otorhinolaryngology, Radboud University Medical Center, 6525 GA Nijmegen, The Netherlands; hannie.kremer@radboudumc.nl
2 Department of Human Genetics, Radboud University Medical Center, 6525 GA Nijmegen, The Netherlands
3 Donders Institute for Brain, Cognition and Behaviour, Radboud University Medical Center, 6525 GA Nijmegen, The Netherlands
4 Servicio de Genética, Hospital Universitario Ramón y Cajal, Instituto Ramón y Cajal de Investigación Sanitaria (IRYCIS), 28034 Madrid, Spain
5 Centro de Investigación Biomédica en Red de Enfermedades Raras (CIBERER), 28034 Madrid, Spain
* Correspondence: ignacio.castillo@salud.madrid.org

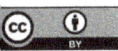

The inner ear is a complex structure at the cellular and molecular levels. Many different genes and proteins play roles in the development and maintenance of the structure and its function through participating in diverse molecular networks. A defect in any of these components can result in hearing impairment. Consequently, hearing impairment encompasses a wide variety of disorders that are clinically and genetically heterogeneous. Understanding their genetic causes and their pathophysiological mechanisms and characterizing the resulting phenotypes are essential for developing novel therapies that target the specific defects. This Special Issue consists of 15 original research articles and 3 reviews that address different issues in the field of the genetics and molecular biology of hearing impairment, including genetic epidemiology, diagnostic strategies, genotype–phenotype correlations, pathophysiological mechanisms and murine models.

The importance of describing known as well as novel variants and the associated phenotypes in genes previously reported to be associated with hearing loss is often underestimated. In medical genetic practice, however, confirmation of disease association for genes and knowledge of genotype–phenotype correlations are highly relevant in the process of variant interpretation for the counseling of families and for patient management. In this Special Issue, Lachgar et al. report a truncating variant in *HOMER2*, which is only the third variant associated with hearing loss (DFNA68) [1]. All three variants affect the coiled-coil region of the HOMER2 protein and the phenotype in the corresponding families is similar, although variant-dependent variation in the severity of hearing loss might occur, but this needs to be confirmed. In Wonkam-Tingang et al., the second family is reported with hearing loss associated with compound heterozygous variants in *CLIC5* (DFNB103) [2]. In addition to supporting the association of *CLIC5* with hearing loss, the phenotype is also shown to be similar to that in the first family with non-syndromic prelingual sensorineural hearing loss, progressing to profound [3]. Vona et al. review the pathogenic genetic variants of *OTOF*, the gene encoding otoferlin, and their phenotypic consequences [4]. Otoferlin is located at the auditory ribbon synapse, where it plays a dual role as a calcium sensor in the exocytosis of synaptic vesicles and as a priming factor for fast vesicle replenishment. Consequently, otoferlin defects lead to an auditory synaptopathy. Over 200 pathogenic variants have been reported in *OTOF*, and most of them result in a prelingual, profound hearing impairment (HI). However, the phenotypic spectrum is broader than initially expected. Vona et al. pay special attention to reviewing less-common phenotypes, such as milder or progressive hearing losses, and the intriguing temperature-sensitive auditory synaptopathy. Challenges for clinical and genetic diagnosis are discussed, as well as their relevance for newborn hearing screening protocols and for the development of gene therapy clinical trials. In addition, *PJVK* defects have been described to underlie auditory neuropathy spectrum disorder (ANSD), but the gene has been associated with cochlear hearing loss as well. Domínguez-Ruiz et al. identified novel *PJVK* variants in a case with ANSD and both known and novel variants of the gene in cochlear hearing loss [5]. The authors provided an overview of all *PJVK* variants reported to underlie ANSD and/or cochlear hearing loss, which revealed that ANSD cases have at least one allele with a missense variant. Although this suggests that specific missense variants lead to ASND, the genotype–phenotype correlations are more complicated. This is further discussed in the article, as are insights into *PJVK* expression and function and the outcome of cochlear implants in patients with *PJVK* defects.

For genes that can cause syndromic as well as non-syndromic hearing loss when defective, it is even more important to understand the genotype–phenotype correlations. Two articles in this issue report families with non-syndromic hearing loss caused by missense variants in *CDH23* [6,7]. Three (novel) missense variants in this gene underlie non-syndromic hearing loss (DFNB12). All three affect the extracellular cadherin domains, and two of the variants are in the highly conserved Ca^{2+}-binding domains. This confirms the previously observed association of bi-allelic missense variants with DFNB12 and not Usher syndrome type Id. The interpretation, and thus reporting, of variants in *CDH23* and other genes that are underlying both non-syndromic as well as Usher syndrome is a challenge in medical genetic practice and can lead to insecurity with parents about the future vision of their child. Also for defects of *GREB1L*, the phenotypic variability is high, as is typical for neurocristopathies. Schrauwen et al. describe two *GREB1L* variants in families with non-syndromic profound hearing loss [8]. In one of these families, temporal bone imaging revealed aplasia of the cochlea and of the cochlear nerve. A review of the literature, performed by the authors, indicated that in 14% of cases/families, dominantly inherited *GREB1L* disease is associated with an ear phenotype.

Two articles in this issue report novel cases with pathogenic variants in genes involved in Perrault syndrome, a disorder associating hearing loss with ovarian dysgenesis. Additionally, some patients develop neurological manifestations. Perrault syndrome is genetically heterogeneous, as eight genes are known to be involved. Zafar et al. report homozygous pathogenic variants in two of them, *CLPP* and *LARS2* [7]. These variants were found, respectively, in two Pakistani consanguineous familial cases with apparently non-syndromic HI. This is a common feature that illustrates the challenge of diagnosing this syndrome clinically. Indeed, male affected subjects, in the absence of neurological signs, only show HI. Moreover, ovarian dysgenesis cannot be detected in pre-pubertal affected females, and later, it is usually diagnosed after the second decade of life. Meanwhile, HI remains the only clinical sign. Also in this Special Issue, Oziębło et al. report two sisters with two novel compound heterozygous pathogenic variants, which confirm the involvement of *RMND1* in Perrault syndrome [9]. In addition to the classical features of the syndrome, a mild chronic kidney disease was observed in both sisters. Previously, mutations in *RMND1* had been reported to cause a more severe multiorgan phenotype, which includes neonatal lactic acidosis, encephalopathy, hearing loss and infantile-onset renal failure. Interestingly, a genotype–phenotype correlation is starting to emerge, so that missense variants (such as those reported by Oziębło et al.) would result in Perrault syndrome with mild kidney disease, whereas truncating variants may lead to the more severe phenotype. Identification and characterization of additional cases and mutations will show whether this hypothesis holds true.

Epidemiological studies provide useful data on which genes and causative genetic variants are more frequently involved in HI in each population. Accordingly, strategies for genetic diagnosis can be adapted to those particularities and to the resources and facilities of the different Services of Genetics. Three articles in this Special Issue report on epidemiological data for DFNB1, the most frequent type of non-syndromic HI. Resmerita et al. screened a cohort of 291 patients with congenital non-syndromic HI from Northeastern Romania, by using Multiplex-Ligation-dependent Probe Amplification (MLPA) followed by Sanger sequencing of the *GJB2* coding region [10]. Biallelic DFNB1 mutations were found in about 30% of the cases, the c.35delG variant being the most frequent (83% of pathogenic alleles), figures that are similar to those observed in other European populations [11]. As regards mutations outside the *GJB2* coding region, Resmerita et al. did find the splice-site variant c.-23+1G>A but not the large deletions that are more frequent in populations of Western Europe. A different DFNB1 landscape is observed in Argentina. Buonfiglio et al. screened a cohort of 600 Argentinean patients with non-syndromic HI by Sanger sequencing of the *GJB2* coding region and flanking sequences, and by PCR-detection of the two more common large deletions in the DFNB1 region [12]. Biallelic pathogenic variants were found in 36% of the familial cases and 15.5% of the sporadic cases. These different figures are a common feature in all tested populations, and illustrate the need to report data for familial and sporadic cases separately to allow for comparison with other studies. The most frequent variant was again c.35delG (52% of pathogenic alleles), and remarkably, the del(*GJB6*-D13S1830) and del(*GJB6*-D13S1854) large deletions accounted for over 8% of the pathogenic alleles. In the third article on DFNB1 in this Special Issue, Zytsar et al. demonstrate common founders and provide estimates of mutation ages for three *GJB2* pathogenic variants in Tuvinians and Altaians, two Turkish-speaking peoples from Southern Siberia [13]. A common founder explains the remarkably high frequency of the c.516G>C variant (up to 63% of pathogenic alleles in Tuvinians). Interestingly, this variant seems to be endemic in these populations, as it has not been reported elsewhere outside this region. Investigating the genetic causes of HI in isolated, less studied populations contributes to broadening our knowledge on the spectra of pathogenic variants and may lead to the identification of novel genes involved in these disorders.

The advent of massively parallel DNA sequencing (MPS) is boosting the studies on genetic epidemiology of HI, as it has solved the long-standing problem of screening a large number of genes in a cost-effective manner. Different screening strategies are being used. Morgan et al. investigated 125 Italian patients through a battery of techniques: Sanger sequencing of *GJB2* and *MTRNR1*, PCR-detection of DFNB1 large deletions, MLPA for deletions and duplications of *STRC* and *OTOA*, and whole-exome sequencing (WES) [14]. *GJB2* pathogenic variants accounted for 20% of the cases. Causative variants were found in an additional 26% of cases, in 24 different genes. In another study, García-García et al. used an MPS panel of 59 genes to investigate a cohort of 118 Spanish patients [15]. Causative variants were found in 40% of cases, in 19 different genes. In both studies, *GJB2* and *STRC* were the most frequently mutated genes among the recessive cases, and *MYO6* among the dominant ones. Finally, in the third broad epidemiological study in this Special Issue, Doll et al. investigated 21 Pakistani consanguineous families with autosomal recessive HI [16]. The cohort included 5 syndromic and 16 non-syndromic cases. The screening strategy combined autozygosity mapping with exome sequencing. Causative pathogenic variants were found in 13 families (62%), in 7 genes. In non-syndromic cases, the most frequently involved gene was *GJB2* (3 families). Pathogenic variants were also found in *MYO7A* (3 families) and *CDH23* (2 families), genes that are involved in non-syndromic HI as well as in Usher syndrome. Indeed, retinitis pigmentosa was present in only two of the *MYO7A* families. The results of these three studies show the diversity of pathogenic variants in different genes among populations. Broad studies on larger cohorts are needed in all populations to reveal the local and global epidemiological landscapes, whose knowledge is essential to orientate the strategies of genetic diagnosis and development of specific therapies.

In contrast to many of the studies in this Special Issue which address monogenic forms of non-syndromic hearing loss, the article by Escalera-Balsera et al. addresses a genetically more complex type of hearing loss, i.e., familial Meniere disease (FMD) (episodic vertigo associated with sensorineural hearing loss) [17]. In a systematic review of the literature, the authors found 20 rare variants in 11 genes to be (potentially) associated with FMD. They classified the variants for their potential deleterious effects and addressed population frequencies. Only a single candidate gene, *OTOG*, was reported to harbor potentially deleterious variants in more than a single family. The authors concluded that associations of genes with FMD need to be replicated in order to determine the causative effect of variants in these candidate genes.

Mice have proven to be excellent models for studying the function and pathophysiology of genes associated with hearing loss in humans, but there are exceptions to this. Tona et al. identified compound heterozygous *TBC1D24* variants in a Pakistani family with intrafamilial phenotypic heterogeneity [18]. Affected family members either suffered from non-syndromic hearing loss or hearing loss and seizures. The authors set out to model *TBC1D24*-associated disease in mice. Although the seizure phenotype was recapitulated in mice with compound heterozygous truncating variants of this gene, none of the models displayed a hearing loss phenotype. This might be explained by differences in the cochlear expression of *TBC1D24/Tbc1d24* in humans and mice. The authors address and discuss additional potential explanations for the phenotypic differences between mice and humans with *Tbc1d24/TBC1D24* defects. For one of the variants, molecular dynamic simulations of peptide structure pointed towards such an explanation.

Perrino et al. employed the mouse to model the potential role of *USH2A* defects in central auditory processing disorder (CAPD), as was indicated in a genome-wide association study (GWAS) [19]. The authors indeed obtained indications for an effect of *Ush2a* defects on the structure of the central auditory system, both in homozygous knockout as well as heterozygous knockout mice. This suggest that cochlear development altered by *USH2A* defects can lead to a secondary effect on the brain regions that function in auditory processing.

Knowledge on the cellular mechanisms that lead to the different types of genetic HI is essential to develop specific therapies. Hayashi et al. reviewed the insights in autophagy in inner ear development and maintenance [20]. These insights are most extensive for hair cells, auditory neurons, and brain stem nuclei. The authors also highlighted the involvement of autophagy in hereditary hearing loss, more specifically for DFNA5 (*GSDME*) and DFNA59 (*PJVK*). Autophagy is essential for cell fate by controlling the balance between cell survival and cell death in conditions of cellular stress. Therefore, the autophagy pathway is an interesting target for therapeutic intervention in hearing loss. One could also hypothesize that variants in genes functioning in autophagy might be modifying factors in dominantly inherited types of hearing loss which display large intrafamilial variability and in which toxic gain of function effects of mutant proteins are often indicated.

The articles and reviews in this Special Issue are representative of the many research lines that are currently active in the field of inherited hearing impairment. These efforts are providing essential data for the comprehension of these highly heterogeneous disorders and for the development of specific new therapies, whose application to humans looks closer than ever.

Acknowledgments: We acknowledge the authors of articles in this Special Issue for their contributions. Research in the laboratories of the authors is being funded by the Heinisius Houbolt Foundation (to H.K.), the VELUX Stiftung (grant 1129 to H.K.), the RNID (grant F111 to H.K.), and by the Instituto de Salud Carlos III (ISCIII), Madrid, Spain, National Plans for Scientific and Technical Research and Innovation 2013–2016, 2017–2020, and 2021–2024, with cofunding from the European Regional Development Fund, "A way to make Europe", grant numbers PI17/00572 and PI20/00619 (to I.d.C).

Conflicts of Interest: The authors declare no conflict of interest.

References

1. Lachgar, M.; Morín, M.; Villamar, M.; del Castillo, I.; Moreno-Pelayo, M.Á. A Novel Truncating Mutation in HOMER2 Causes Nonsyndromic Progressive DFNA68 Hearing Loss in a Spanish Family. *Genes* **2021**, *12*, 411. [CrossRef] [PubMed]
2. Wonkam-Tingang, E.; Schrauwen, I.; Esoh, K.K.; Bharadwaj, T.; Nouel-Saied, L.M.; Acharya, A.; Nasir, A.; Adadey, S.M.; Mowla, S.; Leal, S.M.; et al. Bi-Allelic Novel Variants in CLIC5 Identified in a Cameroonian Multiplex Family with Non-Syndromic Hearing Impairment. *Genes* **2020**, *11*, 1249. [CrossRef] [PubMed]
3. Zazo Seco, C.; Oonk, A.M.; Domínguez-Ruiz, M.; Draaisma, J.M.; Gandía, M.; Oostrik, J.; Neveling, K.; Kunst, H.P.; Hoefsloot, L.H.; del Castillo, I.; et al. Progressive hearing loss and vestibular dysfunction caused by a homozygous nonsense mutation in CLIC5. *Eur. J. Hum. Genet.* **2015**, *23*, 189–194. [CrossRef] [PubMed]

4. Vona, B.; Rad, A.; Reisinger, E. The Many Faces of DFNB9: Relating OTOF Variants to Hearing Impairment. *Genes* **2020**, *11*, 1411. [CrossRef]
5. Domínguez-Ruiz, M.; Rodríguez-Ballesteros, M.; Gandía, M.; Gómez-Rosas, E.; Villamar, M.; Scimemi, P.; Mancini, P.; Rendtorff, N.D.; Moreno-Pelayo, M.A.; Tranebjaerg, L.; et al. Novel Pathogenic Variants in PJVK, the Gene Encoding Pejvakin, in Subjects with Autosomal Recessive Non-Syndromic Hearing Impairment and Auditory Neuropathy Spectrum Disorder. *Genes* **2022**, *13*, 149. [CrossRef] [PubMed]
6. Ramzan, K.; Al-Numair, N.S.; Al-Ageel, S.; Elbaik, L.; Sakati, N.; Al-Hazzaa, S.A.F.; Al-Owain, M.; Imtiaz, F. Identification of Novel CDH23 Variants Causing Moderate to Profound Progressive Nonsyndromic Hearing Loss. *Genes* **2020**, *11*, 1474. [CrossRef]
7. Zafar, S.; Shahzad, M.; Ishaq, R.; Yousaf, A.; Shaikh, R.S.; Akram, J.; Ahmed, Z.M.; Riazuddin, S. Novel Mutations in CLPP, LARS2, CDH23, and COL4A5 Identified in Familial Cases of Prelingual Hearing Loss. *Genes* **2020**, *11*, 978. [CrossRef] [PubMed]
8. Schrauwen, I.; Liaqat, K.; Schatteman, I.; Bharadwaj, T.; Nasir, A.; Acharya, A.; Ahmad, W.; Van Camp, G.; Leal, S.M. Autosomal Dominantly Inherited GREB1L Variants in Individuals with Profound Sensorineural Hearing Impairment. *Genes* **2020**, *11*, 687. [CrossRef] [PubMed]
9. Oziębło, D.; Pazik, J.; Stępniak, I.; Skarżyński, H.; Ołdak, M. Two Novel Pathogenic Variants Confirm RMND1 Causative Role in Perrault Syndrome with Renal Involvement. *Genes* **2020**, *11*, 1060. [CrossRef] [PubMed]
10. Resmerita, I.; Cozma, R.S.; Popescu, R.; Radulescu, L.M.; Panzaru, M.C.; Butnariu, L.I.; Caba, L.; Ilie, O.D.; Gavril, E.C.; Gorduza, E.V.; et al. Genetics of Hearing Impairment in North-Eastern Romania-A Cost-Effective Improved Diagnosis and Literature Review. *Genes* **2020**, *11*, 1506. [CrossRef] [PubMed]
11. del Castillo, I.; Morín, M.; Domínguez-Ruiz, M.; Moreno-Pelayo, M.A. Genetic etiology of non-syndromic hearing loss in Europe. *Hum. Genet.* **2022**, *in press*. [CrossRef] [PubMed]
12. Buonfiglio, P.; Bruque, C.D.; Luce, L.; Giliberto, F.; Lotersztein, V.; Menazzi, S.; Paoli, B.; Elgoyhen, A.B.; Dalamón, V. GJB2 and GJB6 Genetic Variant Curation in an Argentinean Non-Syndromic Hearing-Impaired Cohort. *Genes* **2020**, *11*, 1233. [CrossRef] [PubMed]
13. Zytsar, M.V.; Bady-Khoo, M.S.; Danilchenko, V.Y.; Maslova, E.A.; Barashkov, N.A.; Morozov, I.V.; Bondar, A.A.; Posukh, O.L. High Rates of Three Common GJB2 Mutations c.516G>C, c.-23+1G>A, c.235delC in Deaf Patients from Southern Siberia Are Due to the Founder Effect. *Genes* **2020**, *11*, 833. [CrossRef] [PubMed]
14. Morgan, A.; Lenarduzzi, S.; Spedicati, B.; Cattaruzzi, E.; Murru, F.M.; Pelliccione, G.; Mazzà, D.; Zollino, M.; Graziano, C.; Ambrosetti, U.; et al. Lights and Shadows in the Genetics of Syndromic and Non-Syndromic Hearing Loss in the Italian Population. *Genes* **2020**, *11*, 1237. [CrossRef] [PubMed]
15. García-García, G.; Berzal-Serrano, A.; García-Díaz, P.; Villanova-Aparisi, R.; Juárez-Rodríguez, S.; de Paula-Vernetta, C.; Cavallé-Garrido, L.; Jaijo, T.; Armengot-Carceller, M.; Millán, J.M.; et al. Improving the Management of Patients with Hearing Loss by the Implementation of an NGS Panel in Clinical Practice. *Genes* **2020**, *11*, 1467. [CrossRef] [PubMed]
16. Doll, J.; Vona, B.; Schnapp, L.; Rüschendorf, F.; Khan, I.; Khan, S.; Muhammad, N.; Alam Khan, S.; Nawaz, H.; Khan, A.; et al. Genetic Spectrum of Syndromic and Non-Syndromic Hearing Loss in Pakistani Families. *Genes* **2020**, *11*, 1329. [CrossRef] [PubMed]
17. Escalera-Balsera, A.; Roman-Naranjo, P.; Lopez-Escamez, J.A. Systematic Review of Sequencing Studies and Gene Expression Profiling in Familial Meniere Disease. *Genes* **2020**, *11*, 1414. [CrossRef] [PubMed]
18. Tona, R.; Lopez, I.A.; Fenollar-Ferrer, C.; Faridi, R.; Anselmi, C.; Khan, A.A.; Shahzad, M.; Morell, R.J.; Gu, S.; Hoa, M.; et al. Mouse Models of Human Pathogenic Variants of TBC1D24 Associated with Non-Syndromic Deafness DFNB86 and DFNA65 and Syndromes Involving Deafness. *Genes* **2020**, *11*, 1122. [CrossRef] [PubMed]
19. Perrino, P.A.; Newbury, D.F.; Fitch, R.H. Peripheral Anomalies in USH2A Cause Central Auditory Anomalies in a Mouse Model of Usher Syndrome and CAPD. *Genes* **2021**, *12*, 151. [CrossRef] [PubMed]
20. Hayashi, K.; Suzuki, Y.; Fujimoto, C.; Kanzaki, S. Molecular Mechanisms and Biological Functions of Autophagy for Genetics of Hearing Impairment. *Genes* **2020**, *11*, 1331. [CrossRef] [PubMed]

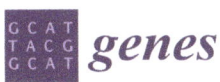

Review

The Many Faces of DFNB9: Relating *OTOF* Variants to Hearing Impairment

Barbara Vona, Aboulfazl Rad and Ellen Reisinger *

Tübingen Hearing Research Centre, Department of Otolaryngology, Head & Neck Surgery, University of Tübingen Medical Center, 72076 Tübingen, Germany; barbara.vona@uni-tuebingen.de (B.V.); Aboulfazl.rad@uni-tuebingen.de (A.R.)
* Correspondence: ellen.reisinger@uni-tuebingen.de; Tel.: +49-7071-29-88184

Received: 3 November 2020; Accepted: 25 November 2020; Published: 26 November 2020

Abstract: The *OTOF* gene encodes otoferlin, a critical protein at the synapse of auditory sensory cells, the inner hair cells (IHCs). In the absence of otoferlin, signal transmission of IHCs fails due to impaired release of synaptic vesicles at the IHC synapse. Biallelic pathogenic and likely pathogenic variants in *OTOF* predominantly cause autosomal recessive profound prelingual deafness, DFNB9. Due to the isolated defect of synaptic transmission and initially preserved otoacoustic emissions (OAEs), the clinical characteristics have been termed "auditory synaptopathy". We review the broad phenotypic spectrum reported in patients with variants in *OTOF* that includes milder hearing loss, as well as progressive and temperature-sensitive hearing loss. We highlight several challenges that must be addressed for rapid clinical and genetic diagnosis. Importantly, we call for changes in newborn hearing screening protocols, since OAE tests fail to diagnose deafness in this case. Continued research appears to be needed to complete otoferlin isoform expression characterization to enhance genetic diagnostics. This timely review is meant to sensitize the field to clinical characteristics of DFNB9 and current limitations in preparation for clinical trials for *OTOF* gene therapies that are projected to start in 2021.

Keywords: DFNB9; otoferlin; sensorineural hearing loss; auditory synaptopathy/neuropathy; temperature-sensitive auditory neuropathy; progressive hearing loss

1. Introduction

Sensorineural hearing loss is one of the most common sensory deficits in humans, affecting one to two per 1000 newborns in developed countries [1]. Over the past 25 years since the discovery of the first deafness gene, more than 120 genes have been causally associated with non-syndromic hearing loss (https://hereditaryhearingloss.org/) and over 6000 disease-causing variants have been identified [2]. As most variants implicated in hearing loss are small insertions/deletions (indels) or single nucleotide variants [2], high-throughput sequencing is a well-suited method to rapidly allow for a deeper understanding of the spectrum of variants involved in deafness and their consequences on the auditory phenotype.

Using a candidate gene approach, the DFNB9 locus (OMIM: 601071) was mapped to chromosome 2p23.1 in 1996 by studying a genetically isolated family from Lebanon [3]. Three years later, the gene *OTOF* (OMIM: 603681), encoding a transmembrane (TM) protein called otoferlin, was mapped to the DFNB9 locus and identified as causing prelingual autosomal recessive, non-syndromic deafness [4]. Biallelic pathogenic variants in *OTOF* cause auditory synaptopathy due to deficient pre-synaptic neurotransmitter release at the ribbon synapse of the inner hair cells (IHCs) [5].

Since its initial identification, about 220 pathogenic and likely pathogenic variants in *OTOF* have been identified. In addition to an expanded understanding of the types of variants in otoferlin that cause deafness, the structure and function of otoferlin have been extensively characterized through functional studies that have greatly informed experimental therapies. This review covers the challenges of clinically diagnosing *OTOF*-associated hearing impairment, the spectrum of phenotypes that have been observed in patients with *OTOF* variants and a current review of genotype-phenotype correlations.

1.1. Mouse Studies Reveal Insights into Otoferlin Function

Otoferlin is distributed throughout the cytoplasm and plasma membrane of IHCs with the exception of the most apical part that forms the cuticular plate and tight junctions with neighboring cells (Figure 1). In addition, type I vestibular hair cells and immature outer hair cells (OHCs) express otoferlin, yet the physiological function for this expression in the mature inner ear is still unclear [6,7]. Although the mRNA of otoferlin can be isolated from several tissues including the brain, clear immunohistochemical proof of otoferlin protein expression outside hair cells is missing. Studies in *Otof*-knock-out mouse models revealed that, in the absence of otoferlin from IHCs, very few neurotransmitter-filled synaptic vesicles fuse with the plasma membrane [5,8]. Thus, acoustic stimuli still generate receptor potentials in the IHCs (and OHCs), but this information is not passed to the auditory pathway. In vitro studies indicating that otoferlin can interact with neuronal SNARE proteins contributed to the hypothesis that otoferlin acts as a synaptotagmin-like Ca^{2+} sensor for exocytosis [5,9]. However, later studies revealed that such neuronal SNAREs are expressed at only very low levels in IHCs and are absent from IHC synapses [10]. Instead, the mechanism of vesicle fusion might rely on a unique molecular mechanism in IHCs [11]. Later studies in a mouse line with the mutation of a presumed Ca^{2+}-binding site revealed a slight delay and slowing down of Ca^{2+}-triggered exocytosis, which would be in line with a Ca^{2+}-dependent acceleration of exocytosis and was interpreted as a Ca^{2+} sensor function for otoferlin in exocytosis and vesicle replenishment [12]. However, the Ca^{2+}-binding capability of the site targeted in this study is still under debate (see Section 5).

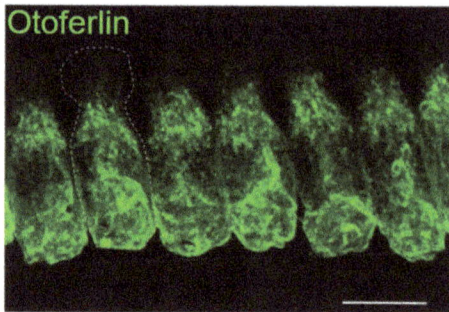

Figure 1. Expression of otoferlin in a row of inner hair cells (IHCs). Maximum projection of optical confocal sections, scale bar: 10 μm (modified from [13]). The dotted white line marks the cell boundary.

Notably, mouse models with reduced levels of otoferlin revealed additional functions for the protein at the synapse: In these models, Ca^{2+}-triggered vesicle fusion still occurred, which allowed for the observation of synaptic processes that are closely linked to exocytosis. In this way, it was uncovered that the rate with which synaptic vesicles are regenerated, supplied to the active zones of the synapses, and rendered competent for Ca^{2+}-triggered fusion depends on the quantity of otoferlin in the basolateral plasma membrane of IHCs [8,13]. A reduction to ~3% of otoferlin protein levels in the plasma membrane in the *pachanga* mouse model still enabled IHCs to release transmitter in response to short (<10 ms) stimuli, but strongly impaired the synaptic transmission for longer stimuli [8,13]. This was attributed to a defect in accomplishing vesicles competent for fusion—also termed "priming" or "vesicle replenishment to the readily releasable pool of vesicles". As a result, in a living organism, such IHC synapses are constantly deficient of fusion-competent synaptic vesicles. Consequently, no auditory brainstem responses (ABRs) can be recorded in these animals [8,14], as this requires the synchronous action potential firing in the auditory pathway for hundreds of stimulus repetitions.

A milder reduction to 35% of wild-type otoferlin levels in the plasma membrane of a mouse model for the human p.Ile515Thr substitution halved the rate of vesicle replenishment compared to normal hearing controls [13]. This only mildly affected the auditory threshold but impaired the ability to detect changes on top of sustained stimuli. In this mouse line, stimulation of exocytosis resulted in enlarged synaptic vesicles. Together with the finding of otoferlin immunoreactivity on endosomal vesicular structures, it was concluded that otoferlin is involved in the reformation of synaptic vesicles from bulk endosomes [13]. This is in agreement with the finding that otoferlin interacts with the clathrin adaptor protein AP2 [15,16]. Presumably, otoferlin is retrieved from the plasma membrane mostly by bulk endocytosis. On the large endosomal structures, clathrin-coated pits appear, supposedly forming novel synaptic vesicles [13,16]. In conclusion, the proper function of the synapse being able to faithfully transmit highly fluctuating acoustic stimuli to the auditory pathway requires a high expression and proper localization of otoferlin. In contrast, low otoferlin levels allow for the transmission of acoustic signals as long as individual synapses are only sparsely activated.

1.2. Otoferlin Isoforms

The structural diversity of *OTOF* has been expanded since its identification to include long and short isoforms that make use of distinctive transcription and translational start sites, as well as alternative splicing of exons 6, 31, and 47. The short and long isoforms range from 28 exons spanning 21 kb [4] to 48 exons across 90 kb [17], respectively. In total, two long and three short isoforms have been identified in humans. Long isoforms are characterized by the presence of six (or seven) C_2 domains and a C-terminal transmembrane (TM) domain, whereas the short isoforms are comprised of only the final three C_2 domains and the TM domain [17]. C_2 domains are globular domains composed of antiparallel β-sheets, which are known for Ca^{2+} and phospholipid binding. In humans, the short isoforms are comprised of isoform b (NP_004793) and d (NP_919304), each with 1230 amino acids and isoform c (NP_919303), with 1307 amino acids, employing an alternate starting exon, compared to the long isoforms a (NP_919224) and e (NP_001274418), which both encode 1997 amino acids.

With respect to a potential functional role of the short isoforms, a review of pathogenic and likely pathogenic variants has shown no indication that variants only affecting the long, but not short, isoforms would cause a milder phenotype. This confirms that the long isoform is critically required for normal hearing function [17].

The two long isoforms of otoferlin can be distinguished by virtue of tissue mRNA expression and subtle differences in exon usage at the 3′ end of the gene. Isoform a was identified from brain cDNA libraries with a termination codon in exon 47 [17]. An alternative splice isoform has been identified in the human cochlea that exclusively uses exon 48 to encode the C-terminus (isoform e, [18]), but lacks exon 47, a finding that was consistent with the mouse [17]. Moreover, pathogenic variants in exon 48, but not exon 47, indicate that the isoform that skips exon 47 and makes use of the termination codon in exon 48 seems to be the predominant isoform in the human cochlea [18–20].

Limitations in obtaining mRNA from human IHCs has presented a major bottleneck in profiling and quantifying the relative fractions of all otoferlin isoforms. According to Yasunaga et al. [17], an alternative splice acceptor site in exon 31 may be employed, eliminating 20 amino acids from the longest variant. This alternative splicing was predicted for the short isoform b and seems to be the predominant variant in mouse inner ear tissue [13]. In the presence of this 20 amino acid "RXR" motif, the p.Ile515Thr substitution caused a retraction of mouse otoferlin from the plasma membrane, which was not the case for the p.Ile515Thr-protein lacking the RXR motif. The authors of this study speculated that the phenotype found in patients with the p.Ile515Thr substitution would be best explained if the human cochlea expresses a mixture of both splice variants [13]. Furthermore, transcript analyses suggest the presence of so far undetected exons (described in Section 3.4 below). Despite these uncertainties, we recommend that human *OTOF* sequence analysis utilizes the reference sequence for variant e,

NM_001287489, encoding the 1997 amino acid protein, NP_001274418. Furthermore, we propose that *OTOF* variants from human molecular genetic diagnostic laboratories that are deposited in clinical variant repositories be adjusted to this reference sequence.

2. Hallmarks of Audiometric Testing in DFNB9 Patients

Since its discovery, *OTOF*-associated hearing loss in humans has presented several challenges, making the selection of clinical diagnostic protocols an essential undertaking for an early diagnosis. Based on the finding that *OTOF* variants disrupt presynaptic function in IHCs rather than neuronal function, a change in terminology from "auditory neuropathy" to "auditory synaptopathy" has been adopted to more precisely describe this. A lesion to the neural pathway that transmits signals from the cochlea to the brain is clinically characterized by an absence of ABRs and the presence of otoacoustic emissions (OAEs). The testing of OAEs indicates proper functioning of cochlear amplification by the OHCs. As OHCs and IHCs employ the same protein machinery for mechanotransduction at their stereocilia bundle, any malfunction of this can be excluded if OAEs are present. Similarly, both hair cell types depend on proper endolymph composition and endocochlear potential as the driving force; a functional deficiency which would be detectable in altered OAE recordings. However, patients with *OTOF* variants lose OHC function, occasionally within the first year, and in about one-third of cases in the second year of life, with only few individuals displaying OAEs in early adulthood [20–22]. Therefore, individuals without OAEs should be considered for genetic testing that includes *OTOF*.

As is true for all forms of auditory neuropathy or synaptopathy, newborn hearing screening that tests for OAEs, e.g., with distortion product otoacoustic emissions (DPOAEs) or transient evoked otoacoustic emissions (TEOAEs), fail to detect a hearing disorder in most cases, as OAEs are initially present. Passing OAE tests despite profound deafness can be misleading and, in the worst-case scenario, prevent parents and pediatricians from pursuing a more complete audiological diagnostic testing. ABRs in patients with synaptopathies are typically absent, even for high sound pressure levels, making them well-suited for the detection of profound deafness. Moreover, even mild forms of hearing loss result in abnormal ABRs in case of DFNB9 (see below). However, as ABR testing is a more time-consuming procedure, this is not routinely applied in newborn hearing screening protocols, delaying the diagnosis of a baby with congenital auditory synaptopathy by months or even years until it is recognized and confirmed. In children with *OTOF* variants, behavioral audiometry, with or without visual reinforcement, can indicate severe to profound hearing loss across all frequencies. While some patients display residual hearing in the low-frequency region (with thresholds of ~75 dB hearing level (HL) for 250 Hz; e.g., [23]), pure tone audiograms may be flat, or bowl-shaped, but in all such cases, average thresholds are above 90 dB HL.

A reliable diagnosis of even mild forms of hearing loss caused by *OTOF* variants is of relevance, especially for young children whose speech acquisition may become strongly impaired. Moreover, a precise diagnosis will also help later in life to specify impairments of speech comprehension, which, for example, may explain why following multiple speakers is much more exhausting for DFNB9 listeners than for normal hearing listeners. Despite pure tone audiograms being only mildly or moderately affected in such cases, ABRs are mostly abnormal, indicating higher thresholds than expected from psychophysical testing. ABR waves I to III are hardly detectable and waves IV and V are delayed [24]. Speech comprehension testing should be performed both in silence and in background noise, the latter of which is typically strongly affected.

A more specific test for this type of synaptopathy would be to quantify the time required for synaptic regeneration. This could be done by gap detection tests, i.e., silent gaps of different length in broadband noise. Intact IHC synapses accurately detect the onset of the white noise after a gap as short as 2–4 ms in humans, at least after some training [25]. This depends on the ability of the IHC synapse to reliably induce a precisely timed postsynaptic action potential at the onset of the white noise after the silent interval, which will require readily releasable synaptic vesicles. Although this has not been systematically tested in patients with mild forms of DFNB9, we expect that silent gaps will need to be substantially longer to be detected by the probands [26]. On average, animal models with the p.Ile515Thr mutation required 17 ms silence (interpolated value, [13]) to detect the gap, whereas normal hearing mice can perceive gaps as short as 1–2 ms [27].

The combination OAE recordings and ABR or pure tone audiometry are, in principle, sufficient to diagnose hearing impairment due to *OTOF* mutations. Other tests do not provide additional information as, for example, even at high sound pressure levels (SPLs), no auditory reflexes can be elicited, which confirms the absence of auditory evoked signal transmission indicated by absent signals in ABRs. In only a few cases, transtympanic electrocochleography (ECochG), with a recording electrode placed at the promontory wall, will be of use for diagnoses. However, since it requires local anesthesia of the tympanic membrane and is rather invasive, it is questionable if this justifies the limited additional information. ECochG is employed to record the summating potential (SP), cochlear microphonics and compound action potentials (CAPs). Cochlear microphonics originate from functional OHCs such that this recording would be redundant to OAE tests, although amplitudes of cochlear microphonics can be highly variable [23,28].

Recording the SP in response to click stimuli may add novel information in particular cases when OAEs are absent, but might be hard to interpret. Since the SP derives from the depolarization of inner and outer hair cells [29], the depolarization of the IHCs may still result in a small but measurable SP even if OHCs are degenerated. This can help to distinguish from forms of hearing loss involving the stereocilia and/or the mechanotransduction channels, since, in this case, no depolarization of hair cells occurs.

CAPs that record the first action potential in the auditory pathway are absent in some DFNB9 patients, while others exhibit a prolonged CAP with reduced amplitude, at least for single click stimuli [23]. Repetitions of click stimuli with short interstimulus intervals of 2.9 ms abolish CAP responses. Findings from a detailed assessment of pre- and postsynaptic function in the *pachanga* mouse model (p.Asp1772Gly) can likely explain this observation: The IHCs in this animal model display intact synaptic signal transmission for short (<10 ms) interspaced stimuli, given that the interstimulus intervals allow for sufficient recovery [8]. Under repetitive stimulation, as in ABR recordings, the strong defect in vesicle replenishment abolishes reliable signal transmission. In single auditory nerve fiber recordings, the first spike was found to be highly variable in timing and was, on average, delayed, which is likely to reflect the prolonged CAP response. The spike rate in *pachanga* mice reached up to 200 spikes/second (compared to >400 spikes/second in wild-type mice), but only when stimuli were presented once every two seconds (0.5 Hz stimulus frequency) [8]. Increasing the stimulus frequency to 10 Hz strongly diminished neural responses (<10 spikes/second) except for the very first trials. Therefore, we infer that the CAP signals for isolated click stimuli in DFNB9 patients indeed originate from an auditory evoked neural response and are prolonged due to the increased first spike latency. Presenting repetitive click stimuli to these patients—a second stimulus after 15 ms and subsequent ones at 33 Hz—strongly reduced or even abolished these CAP responses, which might be the direct equivalent to the diminished neural spiking found in the mouse models. The reason for this is that the replenishment of synaptic vesicles is strongly slowed down when the amount of otoferlin at the IHC plasma membrane is reduced [8,13]. Thus, long silent intervals are required to regenerate the first auditory synapse to enable another cycle of auditory evoked synaptic transmission.

However, why is the CAP response absent in some DFNB9 patients, or prolonged and with a small amplitude in others? This question arose in a study that analyzed CAP responses in patients with various types of variants in the *OTOF* gene. Two frameshift variants were associated with absent CAPs in two patients [23]. Individuals with biallelic premature stop variants exhibited the largest CAP response in this study, while the amplitude of the CAP was intermediate in patients with one frameshift and one premature stop variant. While frameshift variants cause termination of the amino acid chain in all cases, stop codon read-through can occasionally occur with an efficiency of up to 3–4% (reviewed in [30]). As only 3% of the otoferlin protein is localized at the plasma membrane in *pachanga* mice, it is tempting to speculate that an *OTOF* gene with premature stop codons described in this study may have undergone partial natural stop codon read-through, inducing residual synaptic function of an order of magnitude as in *pachanga* mice.

3. Molecular Epidemiology of *OTOF*-Associated Hearing Loss

3.1. Summary of Variants Identified in Otoferlin

By virtue of being one of the first deafness genes identified, *OTOF* has been tested in molecular genetic diagnostic settings for over two decades, allowing an estimate of the global burden of *OTOF*-associated hearing loss. There are presently 219 genetic changes that are classified as pathogenic or likely pathogenic according to the literature or clinical database entries (Leiden Open Variation Database v3.0 (LOVD v3), the Deafness Variation Database (DVD), ClinVar, and the Human Gene Mutation Database (HGMD)) (Table S1). This includes 84 missense, 44 frameshift, 43 nonsense, 36 splice site, 7 in-frame duplications or deletions, 3 copy number variations, as well as 1 stop loss and regulatory variant each (Figures 2 and 3, Table S1).

3.2. Population-Based Diagnostic Rates of Otoferlin

The prevalence of *OTOF*-associated hearing loss varies according to population background. For example, *OTOF* variants account for approximately 5% of genetic diagnoses in the Turkish population [31], and 3.1% of diagnoses in the Pakistani population [32]. A common founder variant (p.Gln829*) was identified in 3% of Spanish cohorts [21,33]. In other populations, *OTOF* has been identified as a cause of hearing impairment in 3.1% of Taiwanese [34], 2.4% (primarily) European-American [35], 2–3% of Pakistani [18,32], 1.9% of French [36] and 1.7% of Japanese [37] patients who were not pre-selected on the basis of auditory neuropathy/synaptopathy. In Iranian patients, a study that included 38 consanguineous patients identified only one family with a homozygous frameshift variant (c.1981dupG, p.Asp661Glyfs*2) and suggested *OTOF* is not a major contributor to hearing loss in the Iranian population [38].

3.3. Diagnostic Rates of Otoferlin in Patients with Auditory Neuropathy/Synaptopathy

Auditory synaptopathy with prelingual onset has been identified in patients with genetic aberrations in a small subset of genes (*PJVK*, *OPA1*, and *DIAPH3* (AUNA1 locus)), and a limited number of suspected cases in a few other genes such as *GJB2* [39–44], although the *GJB2* cases are controversially discussed [45]. The unique phenotypic presentation of DFNB9 makes a targeted selection for *OTOF* screening in patients for genetic testing rather successful. As exemplified by a study that included Japanese patients with auditory neuropathy/synaptopathy, biallelic *OTOF* variants were uncovered in 56% of cases that included the identification of a founder variant (p.Arg1939Gln) [46]. The p.Gln829* founder variant was identified in 87% of patients diagnosed with auditory neuropathy/synaptopathy in the Spanish population [21]. Another founder variant (p.Glu1700Gln) in Taiwanese patients with progressive, moderate-to-profound hearing loss was identified that diagnosed 23% of a selected patient cohort of 22 individuals with auditory neuropathy/synaptopathy [47]. A study that screened the *OTOF* gene in 37 Chinese patients with congenital auditory neuropathy/synaptopathy had a diagnostic yield of 41.2% [48]. On the contrary, a study that involved the screening of 73 Chinese Han patients with auditory neuropathy/synaptopathy resolved only 5.5% of patients and uncovered a temperature-sensitive variant, which was lower than anticipated and demonstrates a high diagnostic variability [49].

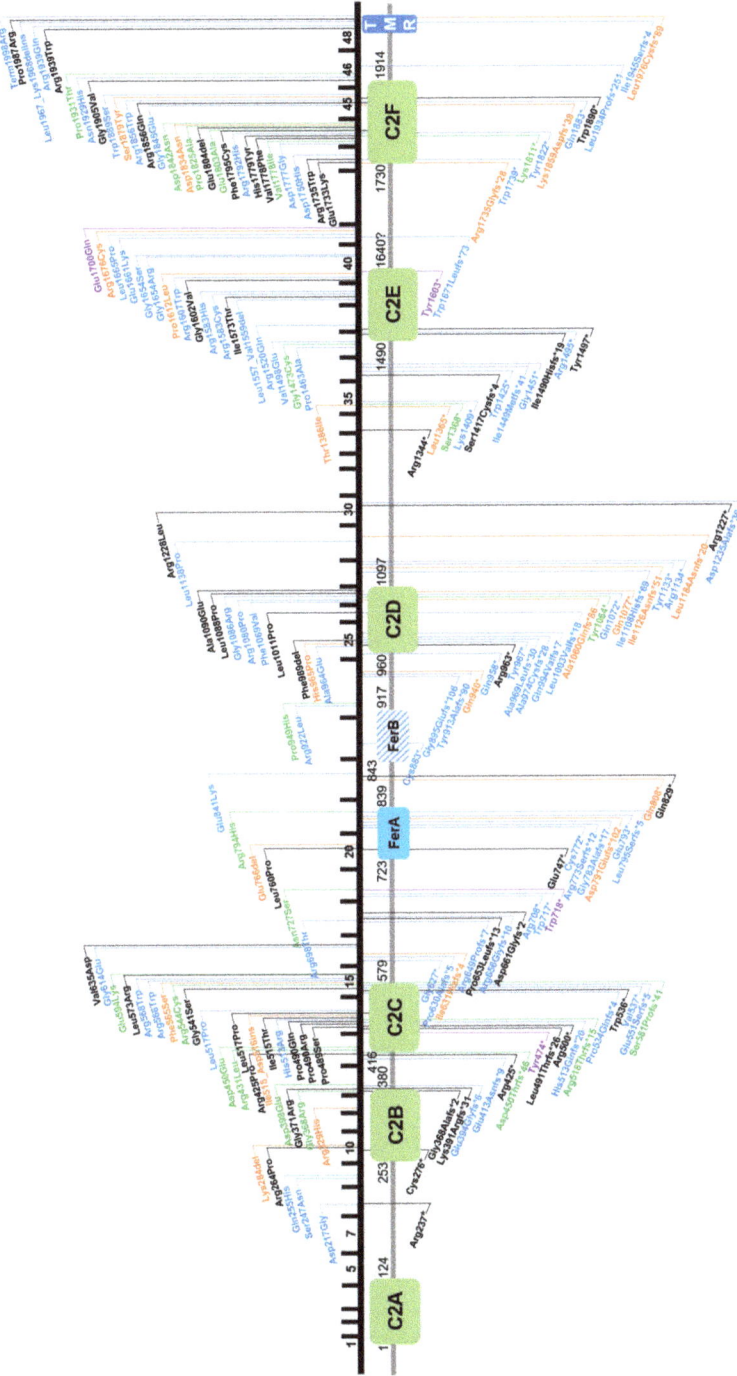

Figure 2. Overview of *OTOF* variants that are classified as pathogenic/likely pathogenic in the databases ClinVar, Leiden Open Variation Database v3.0 (LOVD v3), the Deafness Variation Database (DVD) or Human Gene Mutation Database (HGMD). Variants in the upper part of the figure are non-truncating, variants below are truncating. Black text indicates homozygous variants, blue and green text represents compound heterozygous and heterozygous variants, respectively. Orange text show variants that are reported in databases without a publication reference with undetermined zygosity. Purple text indicates two different variants on the cDNA level that cause the same protein-level change. Variants are annotated according to NM_001287489.1, encoding NP_001274418.1, or isoform e.

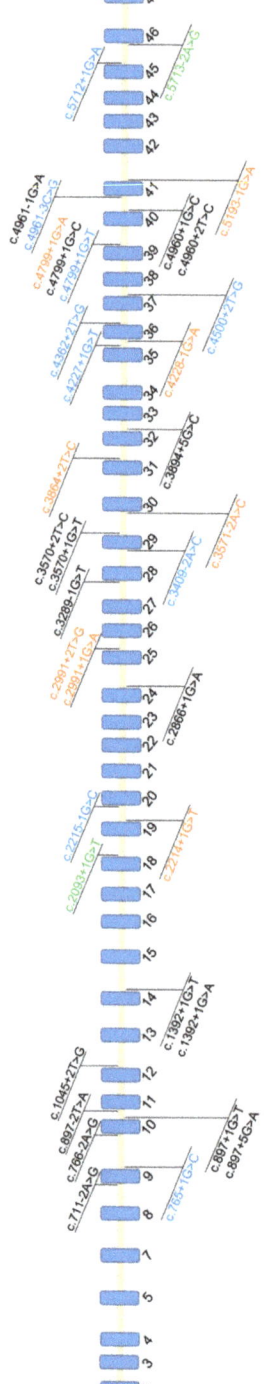

Figure 3. Overview of *OTOF* splice variants according to ClinVar, Leiden Open Variation Database v3.0 (LOVD v3), the Deafness Variation Database (DVD) or the Human Gene Mutation Database (HGMD). Black text indicates homozygous variants, blue and green text represents compound heterozygous and heterozygous variants, respectively. Orange text shows variants that are reported in databases without a publication reference with undetermined zygosity. Variants are annotated according to NM_001287489.1, encoding NP_001274418.1, or isoform e.

3.4. Missing Variants

The diagnostic yield of patients with audiological hallmarks of DFNB9 suggests multifaceted deficits in general isoform and variant knowledge, as well as possible technical limitations. Beyond the possibility of additional genes harboring causally associated variants that evoke the same clinical features, there are several reasons explaining why patients with auditory synaptopathy due to biallelic variants in *OTOF* remain undiagnosed after molecular genetic screening. Such reasons include possible limitations stemming from methodology (e.g., sequencing coverage gaps), missed copy number variations that either fall below the detection resolution of commonly used microarrays in genetic diagnostics or missed due to uneven high-throughput sequencing coverage, especially in the case of exome sequencing, or deep intronic variants that are not captured in targeted enrichment approaches. Furthermore, variant interpretation bottlenecks that could also be due to incorrect transcript usage in variant annotation, current limitations in knowledge about the pathogenicity of rare variants and lack of opportunity for segregation testing in families that can complicate outcomes for definitive statements about variant pathogenicity. Another hypothesis points to variants occurring in currently unannotated exons.

Sequence analysis is primarily focused on exonic regions and relies on the complete understanding of gene isoform structure (i.e., exon annotation). The cochlea is encased in one of the hardest bones of the body, making it one of the least accessible tissues for transcriptome studies. However, many microarray and RNA-seq-based studies using the human and rodent whole cochlea have ensued since the early 2000s [50,51]. Though challenging, single-cell isolation of the inner ear and long read single-cell RNA-seq have recently been performed in mice at several developmental time points [52] to reveal cell-type defining genes and pathways. Long-read sequencing and isoform analysis has identified unappreciated splicing heterogeneity and expression of cell-specific isoforms with unannotated exons [52]. A recent study marked a crucial gap in this understanding in many well-studied genes, such as *Otof*, by mapping a novel non-coding exon 6b and suggesting an in-frame exon 10b (Figure 4). Extending this finding by annotating novel *OTOF* exons in humans could yield significant implications for undiagnosed patients who would otherwise fit the characteristic DFNB9 phenotypic spectrum.

4. Genotype-Phenotype Correlations in DFNB9 Patients

The uniformity of available clinical and genetic information about the current set of identified variants is highly variable. For example, reported variant zygosity (i.e., homozygous versus compound heterozygous) and the extent of audiological characterization and recorded onset in patients are highly heterogeneous. Most variants lack recorded audiological information. Generally, biallelic *OTOF* variants cause congenital or early onset ($n = 114$) hearing impairment. Few variants have been identified with progressive hearing loss ($n = 3$). Seven variants have been linked to temperature-sensitive hearing loss, five of which are located within C_2 domains. While premature stop and frameshift variants typically cause profound prelingual deafness, non-truncating variants can cause a highly variable phenotype. Depending on the localization and the physico-chemical properties of the substituted (or deleted) amino acid residues, variants can severely affect protein stability and contribute to protein degradation. In some cases, the deterioration of protein folding is less severe, leaving some endogenous otoferlin at the plasma membrane that may vary with age and body temperature. This typically results in mildly to moderately elevated thresholds in pure tone audiograms but severely impaired speech comprehension. Notably, patients with point mutations and residual otoferlin expression report perceiving a fading out of a tone burst presented with constant intensity [23,53]. These characteristics of hearing impairment seem to be true for both types of moderate auditory synaptopathy that include the temperature-sensitive and progressive variants.

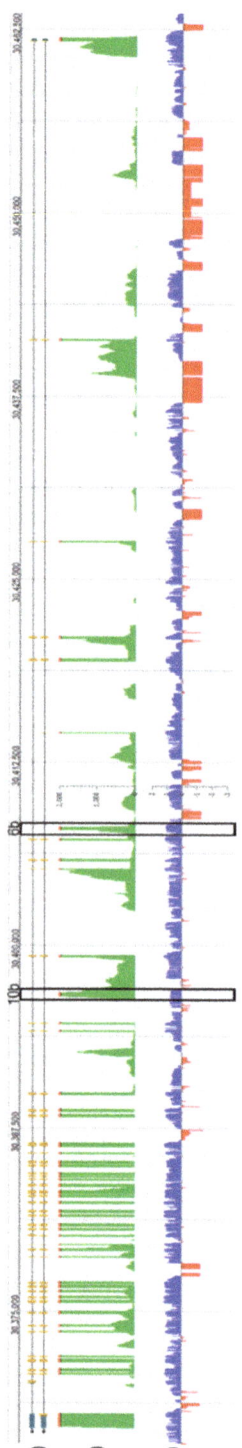

Figure 4. Overview of the *Otof* transcript structure based on single-cell RNA-seq data from mouse IHCs. (**a**) Transcript structure of *Otof*, with exon 1 on the right side of the figure. Exons are depicted as gold bars. Ensembl transcripts *Otof*-201 (upper isoform, encoding 1997 amino acids) and *Otof*-202 (lower isoform, encoding 1992 amino acids) are shown. (**b**) The read depth of each exon is shown in green, with the highest covered regions showing regions in red. Note that maximum read peaks (red) correspond with exons shown in (**a**) if they are expressed in the IHC. (**c**) Mammalian conservation track for *Otof*. Conserved sequences are shown in blue and those not conserved are shown in red. The predicted novel exons 6b and 10b are marked with black boxes. This figure was generated by querying morlscmaseq.org using the "Transcript Structure Browser" tool [52].

4.1. Temperature-Sensitive Auditory Synaptopathy

Temperature-sensitive auditory synaptopathy has been reported by parents observing profound deafness as soon as their children are febrile. Mirroring daytime changes in body temperature, fluctuations in speech comprehension have been described, which was least affected in the early morning and progressed throughout the day to a point where vocal communication is hardly possible [24]. Even a slight increase in body temperature from 36.5 to 36.8 °C in the course of a day seems to attenuate auditory perception. However, in addition to increased body temperature, acoustic exposure is likely higher during the daytime than at night, which may aggravate hearing impairment due to defective synaptic regeneration. Potentially, both body temperature and increased sound stimulation compound to impair speech comprehension during daytime.

When measured in febrile conditions, both an elevation in pure tone thresholds and zero speech comprehension can confirm the diagnosis of temperature-sensitive auditory synaptopathy. The first variant discovered causing temperature-sensitive auditory synaptopathy, p.Ile515Thr [54], has been extensively studied in a mouse model [13]. At normal body temperature, the hearing phenotype of these mice mirrored what is observed in the affected human siblings. When afebrile, they have tremendous difficulties understanding speech in background noise despite having almost normal pure tone audiograms. In the mouse models, ABR thresholds were mildly elevated, 10 dB SPL for click stimuli and ~20 dB SPL across tone burst frequencies at the age of 3–4 weeks. When the same mice were tested again at the age of 8 and 25 weeks, ABR thresholds increased to an average of 80 dB SPL for tone bursts and to 50 (8 weeks) to ~75 dB SPL (25 weeks) for click stimuli. In parallel, ABR wave amplitudes were strongly diminished. In contrast, behavioral tests and auditory nerve fiber recordings revealed only mild threshold shifts in these mice at that age. This correlates well in patients with impaired ABR despite only mild threshold elevations in psychophysical tests. In mice, single auditory nerve fiber recordings were employed to assess the effect of the presynaptic impairment on action potential generation. In agreement with the presynaptic deficiency in replenishing vesicles, the spike rate in the auditory nerve decreased with longer acoustic stimuli or with upscaling of the stimulus frequency, representing a correlate of the auditory fatigue observed in humans. Moreover, the timing of the first spike after sound onset was of greater variability compared to normal hearing controls. In addition, the phase locking to amplitude modulated tones was strongly impaired. If this timely precision of spiking is lower, click sounds or consonants will become blurred. With respect to human hearing, these deficits most likely explain difficulties in speech comprehension and the abolishment of the latter in background noise. At elevated temperature, patch clamp recordings revealed a decrease in exocytosis when cells were heated from near-physiological (35–37 °C) to elevated temperatures (38.5–40 °C). This was especially obvious for wild-type IHCs, indicating that even the wild-type otoferlin protein is very sensitive to elevated temperature and may unfold rather quickly [13]. However, the wild-type protein seemed to be capable of re-folding, as it gained back initial exocytosis when temperature was lowered to <29 °C. In contrast, the IHCs in the p.Ile515Thr model showed impaired recovery, suggesting that the destabilization of the substitution in the C_2C domain reduces the likelihood of proper refolding. This interpretation would be in concordance with the observation that patients regain hearing a few hours after temperature-induced deafening, which would be consistent with the time required for *de novo* synthesis of sufficient quantities of otoferlin.

A similar phenotype to the p.Ile515Thr variant was described in humans with the p.Gly541Ser variant, which also localizes to the C_2C domain of otoferlin [24,46]. In addition, temperature-sensitive auditory neuropathy has been described for the p.Arg1607Trp variant in the C_2E domain [24,49] and for an individual with compound heterozygosity for the p.Gly614Glu and p.Arg1080Pro substitutions, the latter of which resides in the C_2D domain [55]. Remarkably, patients with the p.Arg1607Trp substitution in homozygosity or compound heterozygosity reported hearing loss that ameliorated with increasing age [24]. An in-frame deletion, p.Glu1804del in the C_2F domain, was also attributed to temperature-dependent hearing loss [56]. Notably, no other genes apart from *OTOF* have been associated with temperature-sensitive forms of hearing loss and all cases presenting a similar phenotype in the literature have disclosed pathogenic *OTOF* variants, regardless of population background. All described substitutions seem to cause only slight destabilizations of one C_2 domain. However, since mutations in different otoferlin C_2 domains cause a similar phenotype, we consider it unlikely that each of the substitutions causes heat-sensitivity of the protein. Rather, as shown in Strenzke et al. [13], even the native otoferlin protein is considerably temperature sensitive at 38.5–40 °C. Potentially, any slight destabilization of this highly flexible protein might decrease the chance of re-folding after heat exposure, such that more protein is degraded at a slightly elevated body temperature, thereby exacerbating the hearing disturbance.

4.2. Progressive Hearing Impairment

Progressive forms of *OTOF* hearing impairment have been described for three variants: p.Ile1573Thr, p.Glu1700Gln and p.Ter1998Argext30Ter [46,47,57]. In all cases, the hearing impairment onset was prelingual, but the severity ranged from mild to profound at onset, even for individuals with the same variant.

The homozygous p.Glu1700Gln substitution was identified in several Taiwanese families [47]. In patients from three families, hearing loss was initially mild and became moderate to severe within a few years. In two other families, affected individuals were identified with severe or profound hearing impairment already at the first hearing assessment at the age of two and one years of age, respectively. The reason for hearing loss progression and variability of the onset severity is currently unknown since the linker region between the C_2E and the C_2F domains, in which this substitution lies, has not been studied so far.

A homozygous p.Ile1573Thr substitution was identified in a child with parental consanguinity, in whom hearing deterioration correlated with age [57]. This substitution in the 6th β-strand of the C_2E domain likely reduces the stability of protein folding. The four children of this family were found to have mild (9 years of age), moderate (11 y, 13 y) or severe hearing loss (17 y). All children displayed OAEs. Absence of ABR waves in the 9-year-old child (the only one tested) is in concordance with the severe abnormality described for all DFNB9 patients, even those with only mildly elevated hearing thresholds. A follow-up of the progression of hearing impairment of this family has not been performed so far.

A stop loss variant p.Ter1998Argext30Ter associated with progressive hearing impairment was found in compound heterozygosity with the p.Arg1939Gln substitution [46]. Since the latter causes profound hearing loss in homozygosity, the early onset, moderate hearing loss, with a steeply sloping audiogram in one ear and a gently sloping audiogram in the other, is presumably due to the elongation of the C-terminus. The C-terminal TM domain (amino acids 1964–1984), as well as the 13 amino acids more downstream, are highly sensitive to substitutions (see Section 5.)

In summary, progression of hearing impairment was typically observed over the course of a few months or years, such that affected individuals reached profound deafness in the second decade of life. Presumably due to the residual otoferlin function, OAEs remained preserved in these intermediate forms of hearing impairment; thus, affected individuals may be candidates for gene therapies even in adulthood.

5. Localization and Presumed Effects of Single Amino Acid Substitutions in Otoferlin

Many of the non-truncating variants affect the C_2, FerA and TM domains, meriting a broader discussion about domain functions and deteriorating effects due to substitutions. C_2 domains are globular domains comprised of eight antiparallel β-strands, many of which bind phospholipids and Ca^{2+}. Since the Ca^{2+}-binding site is localized in the structure to five specific aspartate residues in two top loops, the Ca^{2+}-binding ability can be reasonably predicted from the sequence. With respect to the C_2A domain, the structure of the rat protein, which is 91% identical and 96% similar to the human otoferlin C_2A domain, has been solved with X-ray crystallography [58]. Since only one aspartate is present in the two top loops at respective positions, the C_2A domain was predicted not to bind Ca^{2+}, which was confirmed experimentally [58–60].

Different from substitutions in the other otoferlin C_2 domains, neither amino acid replacements in the β-strands nor in the loops of the C_2A domain cause malfunction of the protein. The reasons for this might be first, that the C_2A domain folds much more stably than the other C_2 domains. Crystallization from heterologous expression has been successful for the C_2A domain. However, despite laborious efforts from several research groups, this has not been the case for other C_2 domains so far, presumably because higher protein dynamics prevent the forming of crystals. Notably, the same seems to be true for the myoferlin and dysferlin C_2 domains, of which only the structures of the C_2A domains could be resolved to date [61]. Whether the high flexibility of the ferlin C_2B-C_2F domains is a biological defect or a feature relevant for proper function remains to be determined. The second reason why substitutions may be tolerated well in the C_2A domain is that this domain does not bind Ca^{2+} or phospholipids [58–60] and thus might be not directly involved in the process of Ca^{2+}-triggered vesicle fusion or Ca^{2+}-dependent vesicle replenishment.

Prediction of Ca^{2+}-binding sites or the location of pathogenic substitutions in the other C_2 domains is rather challenging due to the low sequence similarity of the otoferlin C_2B to C_2F domains to C_2 domains with known structure. Automatic domain annotation algorithms such as SMART (EMBL, Heidleberg, Germany) [62] do not predict the extent of these domains reliably. We therefore employed Phyre2 to predict the structures of these domains, which is based on homology modelling and makes use of all structures in the protein data bank (PDB) database [63] (Figure 5). Within the predicted structures, we mapped the substitutions causing profound deafness (shaded in orange), and substitutions causing milder forms of hearing loss (shaded yellow/red; Figure 5). With the exception of the 7th and 8th β-strand of the C_2E domain and the 7th β-strand of the C_2F domain, all β-strands could be localized in the predictions. The first top loop connecting β-strands 1 and 2 and the third top loop between β-strand 5 and 6 comprise five aspartate residues (blue fonts) that coordinate one to three Ca^{2+} ions. Consistent with experimental data revealing that the C_2A domain does not bind Ca^{2+}, its first top loop misses the motif containing the first aspartate, and, in the third top loop, the three aspartate sites are replaced by neutral or positively charged amino acids. Similarly, the C_2B domain comprises only one aspartate residue in the top loops, indicating that this C_2 domain cannot bind Ca^{2+}. Consistent with this prediction, one lab found no Ca^{2+} binding for the C_2B domain using microscale thermophoresis assays [59]; however, other labs did find indications of Ca^{2+} binding with other tests (e.g., [60]).

The same is true for the C_2C domains, for which some labs found Ca^{2+} and phospholipid binding, while one other lab found that this domain binds Ca^{2+} only after including a phosphomimetic mutation in the first top loop (replacing the blue shaded threonine in the first loop by a glutamate, since this threonine is a site for activity-dependent CaMKIIδ phosphorylation [59]). The actual structure prediction reveals a very long top loop 1, even slightly longer than the one on the PKCα C_2 domain, comprising a predicted (otoferlin C_2C) and a confirmed (PKCα) α-helical region. The PKCα C_2 domain does bind phospholipids, but not Ca^{2+}. For the otoferlin C_2C domain, one aspartate resides in the first top loop and two aspartates to a short top loop three, allowing no clear prediction whether this domain can bind Ca^{2+}. We presume that the Ca^{2+} binding of this domain likely depends on posttranslational modifications such as phosphorylation and the direct domain environment, which could be phospholipid membranes, interacting proteins, or both. In a mouse model in which two aspartate residues in the C_2C domain were replaced by alanine residues, exocytosis appeared to be slightly slowed [12]. This finding would be consistent with such a context-dependent Ca^{2+}-binding ability of this domain, but also with interfered phospholipid binding due to altered domain folding.

The C_2D and C_2E domains exhibit the five canonical aspartate residues at respective positions in the top loops, and experimental data confirm that both domains bind Ca^{2+} and phospholipids [60]. Nevertheless, for the C_2E domain, the precise localization of the last two β-strands could not be predicted with the algorithm and the current dataset of structures. Since a growing number of structures is solved and deposited in databases, future structure predictions might result in a reasonable model of the position of the two β-strands. Pathogenic single amino acid substitutions in these domains typically lie within β-strands (Figure 5), likely destabilizing the structure of the domains. The effect is nicely demonstrated in an ENU-mutagenesis induced mouse line, *deaf5Jcs*, with a p.Ile318Asn substitution in the 5th β-strand of the C_2B domain (indicated with green shading in Figure 5). Immunohistochemical analyses of mouse IHCs revealed almost complete absence of the protein, despite mRNA transcripts were present [64], most likely because misfolding of one domain leads to proteasomal degradation of the mutated protein.

```
A    1 --MALLIHLKTVSE-LRGR-----------------GDRIAKVTFRG---QSFYSRVLE--NCEDVADFDETFRWPVASSI
B  251 PMDYQVSITVIEARQLVG---------------LNMDPVVCVEVGD---DKKYTSMKESTNCPYYNEYFVFDFHVSPDVM
C  414 RQWARFYVKIYRAEGLPRMNTSLMANVKKAFIGENKDLVDPYVQVFFAG---QKGKTSVQKSSYEPLWNEQVVFTDLFPP
D  958 QAFQLRAHMYQ-ARSL-------------FAASSGLSDPFARVFFIN---QSQCTEVLNETLCPTWDQMLVFDNLELYGEAHELR
E 1488 DPINVLVRVYVVRATDLH-------------PADINGKADPYIAIRLGK---TDIRDKENYISKQLNPVFGKSFDIEASF
F 1728 KPKKYRLRVIIWNTDEVVL--------EDDDFFTGEKSSDIFVRGWLKGQQEDKQDTDVHYHSLTGEGNFNWRYLFPFDYLAAEEKIVISKKESMFSWDETEY

A   57 DRNEMLEIQVFNYSKVFSNKLIGTFRMVLQKVVEE--------SHVEVTDTLIDDNNAI-----------IKTSLCVEVRYQATDGT---------124
B  313 FDKIIKESVIHSKNLLRSGTLVGSFKMDVGTVYSQ----PEHQFHHKWAILSDPDD--------------ISSGLKGYVKCDVAVVGKGD--------384
C  491 LCK-RMKVQIRDSDKV-NDVAIGTHFEDLRKISNDGDKGFLPTLGPAWVNMYGSTRNYTLLDEHQDLNEGLGEGVSFRARLLLGLAVEIVDTSNP----583
D 1027 DDPPIIVIEIYDQDSMGKADFMGRTFAKPLVKMADEAYCPPRFPPQLEYYQIY--RGNAT-------------AGDLAAPELLQIGPAG---------1101
E 1552 PMESMLTVAVYDWDLVGTDDLLGETKIDLENRFY------SKHRATCGIAQTYSTHGYNIWRDPMKPSQILTRLCKDGKVDGPHFGPPG---------1634
F 1823 KIPARLTLQIWDAEHFSADDFLGAIELDLNRFFPRGAKTAKQCTMEMATGEVDVPLVSIFKQKRVKGWWPLLARNENDEFELTGKVEAELHLLTAEE--1918
```

Figure 5. Alignment of otoferlin C_2 domains A to F with β-strands in brown fonts and α-helices in green fonts. The structure of the C_2A domain was resolved by X-ray crystallography ([58], PDB accession code 3L9B, www.rcsb.org). The structures of the other C_2 domains were modelled by means of Phyre2 [63]. The two last β-strands of the C_2E domain and the 7th β-strand of the C_2F domain could not be reliably predicted due to low sequence homology. In case the modelling of the β-strands is rather uncertain, amino acids are depicted in purple font. The aspartate residues that coordinate Ca^{2+} are depicted in blue fonts, in case several aspartates or glutamates could potentially play a role for Ca^{2+} co-ordination in dark blue fonts. Pathogenic variants leading to profound deafness are shaded in orange. Those causing moderate hearing loss are shaded in yellow, and if the hearing loss appears to be temperature sensitive, in red. Shading in green indicates mutations in deaf mouse models, *deaf5Jcs* in the C_2B domain and *pachanga* in the C_2F domain [14,64]. Threonine or serine residues that were found to be phosphorylated by CaMKIIδ are shaded in blue [59]. Few pathogenic variants affect the CaMKII consensus phosphorylation site, which is RXXS or RXXT.

Structure predictions have hinted to a seventh C_2 domain, termed C_2de, between the C_2D and the C_2E domains that spans amino acids 1143–1220 according to the *Pfam* algorithm. Due to the low sequence similarity and the rather short length of this predicted domain, it is currently unclear if this region folds as a C_2 domain at all. One frameshift and three splice site mutations have been found in this potential domain, but so far no non-truncating pathogenic variant (Table S1).

The C_2F domain seems to be the most unconventional and most susceptible to alterations ultimately leading to protein malfunction. There are presently 18 reported pathogenic/likely pathogenic variants mapping to this domain.

The first top loop comprises eight negatively charged amino acid residues that could potentially contribute to Ca^{2+} co-ordination. Three aspartate residues reside in the canonical positions of the third top loop. Substitution of one of the aspartates in the first top loop (p.Asp1750His) and two in the third top loop (p.Asp1834Asn and p.Asp1842Asn) are each pathogenic. Accordingly, Ca^{2+} co-ordination seems plausible and has experimentally been confirmed [59,60], despite the fact that the precise folding of the first loop is unable to be predicted. Since these Asp>Asn substitutions in the third loop do not change the hydrophobicity, we presume that the Ca^{2+} affinity is strongly reduced by these substitutions, indicating that Ca^{2+} binding to the C_2F domain is essential for proper function.

Different from the other otoferlin C_2 domains, where only two amino acids form the bottom loop between β-strands 2 and 3, the loop in the C_2F domain is predicted to be longer and consists of hydrophobic tryptophane residues flanked by positively charged side chains. This loop comprises the p.Asp1772Gly mutation found in *pachanga* mice which strongly reduced plasma membrane association of otoferlin [8,13,14]. This indicates that this loop structure, also found in other ferlin C_2F

domains [65], seems to be crucial for a partial insertion into phospholipid membranes. Despite homology modelling with alignments with different structures leaving some uncertainty about the beginning of the subsequent β-strand, the consensus prediction of this β-strand includes the position of three consecutive amino acids whose substitutions cause profound hearing loss (p.Asp1777Gly, p.Val1778Ile, p.Val1778Phe, p.His1779Tyr). Moreover, these three amino acids reside just before a CaMKIIδ phosphorylation site, S1782, and might interfere with the binding of the CaMKIIδ and thus phosphorylation [59]. The subsequent bottom loop comprises two glutamate residues. The deletion of one (p.Glu1804del) causes temperature-sensitive auditory neuropathy, presumably because the shortening of this loop destabilizes the domain. Thus, it seems as if the C_2F domain is especially sensitive to point mutations and that Ca^{2+} and phospholipid binding are crucial for proper protein function.

The function of the FerA domain for synaptic transmission is presently less clear. Small-angle X-ray scattering and in vitro experiments indicated that this domain is comprised of four α-helices, which are connected by a dynamic linker region [66]. The FerA domain binds to phospholipid membranes that is enhanced by Ca^{2+}. Four non-truncating substitutions have been identified in the FerA domain so far, but three of those could not be linked to a phenotype (heterozygous, or no reference). The fourth homozygous substitution found in a Taiwanese family alters the second helix (p.Leu760Pro). This suggests that misfolding of the FerA domain is not tolerated, indicating a role for the FerA domain for synaptic transmission that requires further studies.

Substitutions of amino acids in the TM domain cause variable severities of hearing loss. The homozygous p.Pro1987Arg substitution causes early onset, severe to profound hearing impairment, in this specific case, with a bowl-shaped audiogram [19] (Table S1). A three base pair deletion (p.Leu1967_Lys1968delinsGln) at the TM domain caused early onset, mild hearing loss, similar to the p.Ter1998Argext30Ter [46]. This is likely due to the mechanism by which this tail-anchored structure is inserted into the membrane. Once translation of the amino acid chain has been completed, the C-terminal amino acids bind to the chaperone TRC40 and this complex is targeted to the TRC40 receptors WRB and CAML, which insert the C-terminus into the phospholipid membrane [67,68]. These mutations likely interfere with this tail insertion mechanism, thereby reducing the amount of otoferlin at the plasma membrane, leading to a moderate hearing impairment. In contrast, variants truncating the amino acid chain behind the C_2F domain and before the TM domain, such as p.Gln1883Ter or the c.5833delA deletion (p.Ile1945Serfs*4), cause profound deafness, indicating that the TM domain is essential for protein function [48].

6. Current and Future Therapies for DFNB9

The established therapy for individuals with severe to profound hearing loss due to otoferlin deficiency is currently cochlear implantation. Since this prosthetic bridges the first auditory synapse, which is the only part of the auditory pathway involved in DFNB9, patients benefit well from these devices and gain good or even excellent speech understanding. However, the most sensitive period for developing the capability to understand spoken language is within the first two years of life. It is, therefore, critical to implant patients as early as possible. This requires an early diagnosis, but most children with severe to profound hearing loss due to variants in *OTOF* pass newborn hearing testing because, in most countries, the assessment of OAEs is the method of choice for screening. These children are typically diagnosed at a later stage after parents report a severe delay in speech development. Knowing that deafness, either due to biallelic variants in *OTOF* or auditory neuropathies/synaptopathies of other etiologies, cannot be reliably diagnosed with OAE screenings, but could be aided with currently available therapies, requires switching newborn hearing screenings to routine ABR testing. This is not only of importance with respect to cochlear implantation, which will yield much better outcomes if implanted earlier, but also with respect to a gene therapy, which is currently under development.

The currently favored gene therapeutic approach involves replacing the defective gene by transducing IHCs with correct cDNA by means of recombinant adeno-associated viruses (AAVs, reviewed in [69]). These viral vectors have a series of beneficial features: they are non-pathogenic, they evoke the least inflammatory response, they do not integrate into the genome under most conditions, and the choice of their surface protein allows the vector to target different cell types. The main disadvantage is that they can transport only up to 4.9 kb of foreign DNA, which needs to be subcloned between two AAV gene sequences called inverted terminal repeats (ITRs) of 145 bp each. The 6 kb cDNA length encoding otoferlin has successfully been transduced into IHCs by dual-AAV-approaches, where the cDNA is split to two AAV genomes [70,71]. The latter form head-to-tail multimers in the nuclei of target cells, thereby assembling the split cDNA. By means of splice donor and splice acceptor sites, the ITRs are excised, and the otoferlin mRNA transcribed from dual-AAVs has been demonstrated as being correct [70]. Studies in $Otof^{-/-}$ mice have revealed that such dual-AAV strategies successfully and persistently restored hearing [70,71]. At least three companies have prepared for clinical trials with dual-AAV approaches, the first intending to start in 2021 (Akouos, Boston, MA, USA; Decibel Therapeutics, Boston, MA, USA; Sensorion, Montpellier, France). This causal therapy is expected to result in more natural hearing compared to cochlear implants, overcoming limitations such as poor perception of vocal emotions, poor frequency discrimination, or poor speech comprehension in background noise, just to name a few. DFNB9 is predestined for a gene therapy, as all cells develop normally and are in place at birth. However, OHCs degenerate within a few years after birth, as discussed above. For cochlear implantation, the loss of OHCs is not of relevance; however, gene therapy will only yield good outcomes with intact OHC-driven cochlear amplification. Hence, a gene therapy for profoundly deaf DFNB9 patients will need to be applied ideally within the first year of life, both to have OHCs still present and to be within the sensitive time window for language acquisition.

Especially with respect to the envisioned gene therapy, the use of hearing aids for rehabilitation of severe to profound hearing impairment should be critically evaluated. While power hearing aids have successfully induced behavioral responses in DFNB9 children with severe to profound deafness [23], we have to assume that the use of hearing aids is unlikely to assure proper speech comprehension. Studies from animal models indicate that challenging the synapse with a higher rate of acoustic stimuli or more intense stimuli will cause a faster depletion of synaptic transmission. This reduces the capability of the synapse to encode modulations of the input. Moreover, it presumably lowers the timely precision of spiking in the auditory nerve, and thus might blur auditory cues required for speech comprehension.

In addition to being questionable for language acquisition, the use of power hearing aids might accelerate the loss of OHCs, as proposed from observations in retrospective studies [22,72,73]. Whether and potentially why OHCs are more susceptible to noise trauma in DFNB9 patients compared to normal hearing individuals still awaits experimental proof and basic research in animal models. Is the expression of otoferlin in immature OHCs or unknown genetic modifiers related to the loss of DPOAEs (as proposed by [22]) or rather the lack of OHC suppression by efferent inhibition? In intact cochleae, OHCs mechanically amplify the motion of the basilar membrane, which increases the sensitivity of gentle sounds by several orders of magnitude, i.e., they lower hearing thresholds by 50–60 dB SPL. For high SPLs, inhibitory innervation from efferent fibers originating from the medial olivocochlear (MOC) system hyperpolarizes OHCs and thereby suppresses this mechanical amplification. Activation of the MOC efferents occurs through activity in the auditory pathway, which is strongly reduced or missing in absence of otoferlin. Thus, even during exposure to intense sounds, we hypothesize that OHCs do not perceive any inhibitory neurotransmission in DFNB9 patients, as is the case for normal hearing individuals. Chronically high levels of OHC activation, such as, for example, in noise trauma experiments, have been associated with cell death, potentially involving oxidative stress. Thus, power hearing aids should be prescribed and used with caution, potentially only for specialized auditory trainings and not for full day usage.

7. Outlook and Conclusions

A timely clinical and molecular genetic diagnosis of *OTOF* hearing impairment should be made as early as possible. Ideally, a clinical diagnosis should occur within the first few days of life if already apparent at birth, with rapid molecular genetic diagnostic results thereafter. Therefore, changes in newborn hearing screening protocols from OAEs to ABRs, or a combination of the two will support an early diagnosis. This will become increasingly important as promising gene therapies emerge. The structure of otoferlin, particularly of the C_2E and C_2F domains, is provisionally incomplete based on structural modelling. The possibility of an incomplete overall structure is supported by the identification of novel exons in mouse IHC transcriptome data. Therefore, we recommend genetic re-testing of undiagnosed individuals, especially those with auditory neuropathy/synaptopathy to profit from advances in basic knowledge of isoform structure, as well as improvements in sequencing technologies, bioinformatics approaches, and variant interpretation. Diagnostic laboratories critically rely on annotation of variants to the correct transcript in databases such as LOVD, DVD, ClinVar, and HGMD. In many instances in current versions of these databases, the transcript that is used is incorrect. Therefore, careful attention must be exercised by medical geneticists to report variants with the correct transcript until this can be revised.

Supplementary Materials: The following are available online at http://www.mdpi.com/2073-4425/11/12/1411/s1. Table S1: Overview of pathogenic/likely pathogenic *OTOF* variants from literature and database review.

Author Contributions: Conceptualization, E.R.; data curation, B.V., A.R., E.R.; writing, E.R., B.V.; construction of figures, B.V., A.R., E.R. All authors have read and agreed to the published version of the manuscript.

Funding: This research was supported by Intramural Funding (fortüne) at the University of Tübingen (2545-1-0 to B.V.) and the Ministry of Science, Research and Art Baden-Württemberg (to B.V.). The German Research Foundation (DFG) supports E.R. by the Heisenberg-Program (RE 3174/2-1) and a grant (RE 3174/3-1). We acknowledge support by Open Access Publishing Fund of University of Tübingen.

Acknowledgments: We thank Hanan Al-Moyed for the graph in Figure 1, and Youssef Adel for critically reading the manuscript.

Conflicts of Interest: A.R. and B.V. declare no conflict of interest. E.R. is co-inventor on a patent for dual-AAV vectors to restore hearing. The University Medical Center Göttingen has licensed the rights to these parts of the patent exclusively to Akuous Inc. (Boston, MA, USA). The company had no role in the design of the study; in the collection, analyses, or interpretation of data; in the writing of the manuscript, or in the decision to publish the results.

References

1. Morton, C.C.; Nance, W.E. Newborn Hearing Screening—A Silent Revolution. *N. Engl. J. Med.* **2006**, *354*, 2151–2164. [CrossRef] [PubMed]
2. Azaiez, H.; Booth, K.T.; Ephraim, S.S.; Crone, B.; Black-Ziegelbein, E.A.; Marini, R.J.; Shearer, A.E.; Sloan-Heggen, C.M.; Kolbe, D.; Casavant, T.; et al. Genomic Landscape and Mutational Signatures of Deafness-Associated Genes. *Am. J. Hum. Genet.* **2018**, *103*, 484–497. [CrossRef] [PubMed]
3. Chaïb, H.; Place, C.; Salem, N.; Chardenoux, S.; Vincent, C.; Weissenbach, J.; El-Zir, E.; Loiselet, J.; Petit, C. A gene responsible for a sensorineural nonsyndromic recessive deafness maps to chromosome 2p22-23. *Hum. Mol. Genet.* **1996**, *5*, 155–158. [CrossRef]
4. Yasunaga, S.; Grati, M.; Cohen-Salmon, M.; El-Amraoui, A.; Mustapha, M.; Salem, N.; El-Zir, E.; Loiselet, J.; Petit, C. A mutation in OTOF, encoding otoferlin, a FER-1-like protein, causes DFNB9, a nonsyndromic form of deafness. *Nat. Genet.* **1999**, *21*, 363–369. [CrossRef] [PubMed]
5. Roux, I.; Safieddine, S.; Nouvian, R.; Grati, M.; Simmler, M.-C.; Bahloul, A.; Perfettini, I.; Le Gall, M.; Rostaing, P.; Hamard, G.; et al. Otoferlin, defective in a human deafness form, is essential for exocytosis at the auditory ribbon synapse. *Cell* **2006**, *127*, 277–289. [CrossRef] [PubMed]
6. Dulon, D.; Safieddine, S.; Jones, S.M.; Petit, C. Otoferlin Is Critical for a Highly Sensitive and Linear Calcium-Dependent Exocytosis at Vestibular Hair Cell Ribbon Synapses. *J. Neurosci.* **2009**, *29*, 10474–10487. [CrossRef]

7. Beurg, M.; Safieddine, S.; Roux, I.; Bouleau, Y.; Petit, C.; Dulon, D. Calcium- and otoferlin-dependent exocytosis by immature outer hair cells. *J. Neurosci. Off. J. Soc. Neurosci.* **2008**, *28*, 1798–1803. [CrossRef]
8. Pangrsic, T.; Lasarow, L.; Reuter, K.; Takago, H.; Schwander, M.; Riedel, D.; Frank, T.; Tarantino, L.M.; Bailey, J.S.; Strenzke, N.; et al. Hearing requires otoferlin-dependent efficient replenishment of synaptic vesicles in hair cells. *Nat. Neurosci.* **2010**, *13*, 869–876. [CrossRef]
9. Beurg, M.; Michalski, N.; Safieddine, S.; Bouleau, Y.; Schneggenburger, R.; Chapman, E.R.; Petit, C.; Dulon, D. Control of exocytosis by synaptotagmins and otoferlin in auditory hair cells. *J. Neurosci. Off. J. Soc. Neurosci.* **2010**, *30*, 13281–13290. [CrossRef]
10. Nouvian, R.; Neef, J.; Bulankina, A.V.; Reisinger, E.; Pangršič, T.; Frank, T.; Sikorra, S.; Brose, N.; Binz, T.; Moser, T. Exocytosis at the hair cell ribbon synapse apparently operates without neuronal SNARE proteins. *Nat. Neurosci.* **2011**, *14*, 411–413. [CrossRef] [PubMed]
11. Pangršič, T.; Reisinger, E.; Moser, T. Otoferlin: A multi-C2 domain protein essential for hearing. *Trends Neurosci.* **2012**, *35*, 671–680. [CrossRef] [PubMed]
12. Michalski, N.A.; Goutman, J.D.; Auclair, S.M.; De Monvel, J.B.; Tertrais, M.; Emptoz, A.; Parrin, A.; Nouaille, S.; Guillon, M.; Sachse, M.; et al. Otoferlin acts as a Ca^{2+} sensor for vesicle fusion and vesicle pool replenishment at auditory hair cell ribbon synapses. *eLife* **2017**, *6*, e31013. [CrossRef] [PubMed]
13. Strenzke, N.; Chakrabarti, R.; Al-Moyed, H.; Müller, A.; Hoch, G.; Pangrsic, T.; Yamanbaeva, G.; Lenz, C.; Pan, K.-T.; Auge, E.; et al. Hair cell synaptic dysfunction, auditory fatigue and thermal sensitivity in otoferlin Ile515Thr mutants. *EMBO J.* **2016**, *35*, e201694564. [CrossRef] [PubMed]
14. Schwander, M.; Sczaniecka, A.; Grillet, N.; Bailey, J.S.; Avenarius, M.; Najmabadi, H.; Steffy, B.M.; Federe, G.C.; Lagler, E.A.; Banan, R.; et al. A Forward Genetics Screen in Mice Identifies Recessive Deafness Traits and Reveals That Pejvakin Is Essential for Outer Hair Cell Function. *J. Neurosci.* **2007**, *27*, 2163–2175. [CrossRef]
15. Duncker, S.V.; Franz, C.; Kuhn, S.; Schulte, U.; Campanelli, D.; Brandt, N.; Hirt, B.; Fakler, B.; Blin, N.; Ruth, P.; et al. Otoferlin Couples to Clathrin-Mediated Endocytosis in Mature Cochlear Inner Hair Cells. *J. Neurosci.* **2013**, *33*, 9508–9519. [CrossRef]
16. Jung, S.; Maritzen, T.; Wichmann, C.; Jing, Z.; Neef, A.; Revelo, N.H.; Al-Moyed, H.; Meese, S.; Wojcik, S.M.; Panou, I.; et al. Disruption of adaptor protein 2μ (AP-2μ) in cochlear hair cells impairs vesicle reloading of synaptic release sites and hearing. *EMBO J.* **2015**, *34*, 2686–2702. [CrossRef]
17. Yasunaga, S.; Grati, M.; Chardenoux, S.; Smith, T.N.; Friedman, T.B.; Lalwani, A.K.; Wilcox, E.R.; Petit, C. OTOF Encodes Multiple Long and Short Isoforms: Genetic Evidence That the Long Ones Underlie Recessive Deafness DFNB9. *Am. J. Hum. Genet.* **2000**, *67*, 591–600. [CrossRef]
18. Choi, B.Y.; Ahmed, Z.M.; Riazuddin, S.; Bhinder, M.A.; Shahzad, M.; Husnain, T.; Riazuddin, S.; Griffith, A.J.; Friedman, T.B. Identities and frequencies of mutations of the otoferlin gene (OTOF) causing DFNB9 deafness in Pakistan. *Clin. Genet.* **2009**, *75*, 237–243. [CrossRef]
19. Varga, R.; Kelley, P.M.; Keats, B.J.; Starr, A.; Leal, S.M.; Cohn, E.; Kimberling, W.J. Non-syndromic recessive auditory neuropathy is the result of mutations in the otoferlin (OTOF) gene. *J. Med. Genet.* **2003**, *40*, 45–50. [CrossRef]
20. Rodríguez-Ballesteros, M.; del Castillo, F.J.; Martín, Y.; Moreno-Pelayo, M.A.; Morera, C.; Prieto, F.; Marco, J.; Morant, A.; Gallo-Terán, J.; Morales-Angulo, C.; et al. Auditory neuropathy in patients carrying mutations in the otoferlin gene (OTOF). *Hum. Mutat.* **2003**, *22*, 451–456. [CrossRef]
21. Rodríguez-Ballesteros, M.; Reynoso, R.; Olarte, M.; Villamar, M.; Morera, C.; Santarelli, R.; Arslan, E.; Medá, C.; Curet, C.; Völter, C.; et al. A multicenter study on the prevalence and spectrum of mutations in the otoferlin gene (OTOF) in subjects with nonsyndromic hearing impairment and auditory neuropathy. *Hum. Mutat.* **2008**, *29*, 823–831. [CrossRef] [PubMed]
22. Kitao, K.; Mutai, H.; Namba, K.; Morimoto, N.; Nakano, A.; Arimoto, Y.; Sugiuchi, T.; Masuda, S.; Okamoto, Y.; Morita, N.; et al. Deterioration in Distortion Product Otoacoustic Emissions in Auditory Neuropathy Patients With Distinct Clinical and Genetic Backgrounds. *Ear Hear.* **2019**, *40*, 184–191. [CrossRef] [PubMed]
23. Santarelli, R.; Del Castillo, I.; Cama, E.; Scimemi, P.; Starr, A. Audibility, speech perception and processing of temporal cues in ribbon synaptic disorders due to OTOF mutations. *Hear. Res.* **2015**, *330*, 200–212. [CrossRef] [PubMed]
24. Zhang, Q.; Lan, L.; Shi, W.; Yu, L.; Xie, L.-Y.; Xiong, F.; Zhao, C.; Li, N.; Yin, Z.; Zong, L.; et al. Temperature sensitive auditory neuropathy. *Hear. Res.* **2016**, *335*, 53–63. [CrossRef]

25. Mishra, S.K.; Panda, M.R. Rapid auditory learning of temporal gap detection. *J. Acoust. Soc. Am.* **2016**, *140*, EL50. [CrossRef]
26. Michalewski, H.J.; Starr, A.; Nguyen, T.T.; Kong, Y.Y.; Zeng, F.G. Auditory temporal processes in normal-hearing individuals and in patients with auditory neuropathy. *Clin. Neurophysiol.* **2005**, *116*, 669–680. [CrossRef]
27. Radziwon, K.E.; June, K.M.; Stolzberg, D.J.; Xu-Friedman, M.A.; Salvi, R.J.; Dent, M.L. Behaviorally measured audiograms and gap detection thresholds in CBA/CaJ mice. *J. Comp. Physiol. A* **2009**, *195*, 961–969. [CrossRef]
28. Santarelli, R.; Del Castillo, I.; Rodríguez-Ballesteros, M.; Scimemi, P.; Cama, E.; Arslan, E.; Starr, A. Abnormal cochlear potentials from deaf patients with mutations in the otoferlin gene. *J. Assoc. Res. Otolaryngol. JARO* **2009**, *10*, 545–556. [CrossRef]
29. Pappa, A.K.; Hutson, K.A.; Scott, W.C.; Wilson, J.D.; Fox, K.E.; Masood, M.M.; Giardina, C.K.; Pulver, S.H.; Grana, G.D.; Askew, C.; et al. Hair cell and neural contributions to the cochlear summating potential. *J. Neurophysiol.* **2019**, *121*, 2163–2180. [CrossRef]
30. Dabrowski, M.; Bukowy-Bieryllo, Z.; Zietkiewicz, E. Translational readthrough potential of natural termination codons in eucaryotes—The impact of RNA sequence. *RNA Biol.* **2015**, *12*, 950–958. [CrossRef]
31. Duman, D.; Sirmaci, A.; Cengiz, F.B.; Ozdag, H.; Tekin, M. Screening of 38 genes identifies mutations in 62% of families with nonsyndromic deafness in Turkey. *Genet. Test. Mol. Biomark.* **2011**, *15*, 29–33. [CrossRef] [PubMed]
32. Richard, E.M.; Santos-Cortez, R.L.P.; Faridi, R.; Rehman, A.U.; Lee, K.; Shahzad, M.; Acharya, A.; Khan, A.A.; Imtiaz, A.; Chakchouk, I.; et al. Global genetic insight contributed by consanguineous Pakistani families segregating hearing loss. *Hum. Mutat.* **2019**, *40*, 53–72. [CrossRef] [PubMed]
33. Migliosi, V.; Modamio-Hoybjor, S.; Moreno-Pelayo, M.A.; Rodriguez-Ballesteros, M.; Villamar, M.; Telleria, D.; Menendez, I.; Moreno, F.; Del Castillo, I. Q829X, a novel mutation in the gene encoding otoferlin (OTOF), is frequently found in Spanish patients with prelingual non-syndromic hearing loss. *J. Med. Genet.* **2002**, *39*, 502. [CrossRef] [PubMed]
34. Wu, C.-C.; Tsai, C.-Y.; Lin, Y.-H.; Chen, P.-Y.; Lin, P.-H.; Cheng, Y.-F.; Wu, C.-M.; Lin, Y.-H.; Lee, C.-Y.; Erdenechuluun, J.; et al. Genetic Epidemiology and Clinical Features of Hereditary Hearing Impairment in the Taiwanese Population. *Genes* **2019**, *10*, 772. [CrossRef] [PubMed]
35. Sloan-Heggen, C.M.; Bierer, A.O.; Shearer, A.E.; Kolbe, D.L.; Nishimura, C.J.; Frees, K.L.; Ephraim, S.S.; Shibata, S.B.; Booth, K.T.; Campbell, C.A.; et al. Comprehensive genetic testing in the clinical evaluation of 1119 patients with hearing loss. *Hum. Genet.* **2016**, *135*, 441–450. [CrossRef]
36. Baux, D.; Vaché, C.; Blanchet, C.; Willems, M.; Baudoin, C.; Moclyn, M.; Faugère, V.; Touraine, R.; Isidor, B.; Dupin-Deguine, D.; et al. Combined genetic approaches yield a 48% diagnostic rate in a large cohort of French hearing-impaired patients. *Sci. Rep.* **2017**, *7*, 16783. [CrossRef]
37. Iwasa, Y.-I.; Nishio, S.-Y.; Sugaya, A.; Kataoka, Y.; Kanda, Y.; Taniguchi, M.; Nagai, K.; Naito, Y.; Ikezono, T.; Horie, R.; et al. OTOF mutation analysis with massively parallel DNA sequencing in 2,265 Japanese sensorineural hearing loss patients. *PLoS ONE* **2019**, *14*, e0215932. [CrossRef]
38. Mahdieh, N.; Shirkavand, A.; Rabbani, B.; Tekin, M.; Akbari, B.; Akbari, M.T.; Zeinali, S. Screening of OTOF mutations in Iran: A novel mutation and review. *Int. J. Pediatr. Otorhinolaryngol.* **2012**, *76*, 1610–1615. [CrossRef]
39. Delmaghani, S.; del Castillo, F.J.; Michel, V.; Leibovici, M.; Aghaie, A.; Ron, U.; Van Laer, L.; Ben-Tal, N.; Van Camp, G.; Weil, D.; et al. Mutations in the gene encoding pejvakin, a newly identified protein of the afferent auditory pathway, cause DFNB59 auditory neuropathy. *Nat. Genet.* **2006**, *38*, 770–778. [CrossRef]
40. Amati-Bonneau, P.; Guichet, A.; Olichon, A.; Chevrollier, A.; Viala, F.; Miot, S.; Ayuso, C.; Odent, S.; Arrouet, C.; Verny, C.; et al. OPA1 R445H mutation in optic atrophy associated with sensorineural deafness. *Ann. Neurol.* **2005**, *58*, 958–963. [CrossRef]
41. Starr, A.; Isaacson, B.; Michalewski, H.J.; Zeng, F.-G.; Kong, Y.-Y.; Beale, P.; Paulson, G.W.; Keats, B.J.B.; Lesperance, M.M. A Dominantly Inherited Progressive Deafness Affecting Distal Auditory Nerve and Hair Cells. *J. Assoc. Res. Otolaryngol.* **2004**, *5*, 411–426. [CrossRef] [PubMed]
42. Kim, T.B.; Isaacson, B.; Sivakumaran, T.A.; Starr, A.; Keats, B.J.B.; Lesperance, M.M. A gene responsible for autosomal dominant auditory neuropathy (AUNA1) maps to 13q14–21. *J. Med. Genet.* **2004**, *41*, 872. [CrossRef] [PubMed]

43. Cheng, X.; Li, L.; Brashears, S.; Morlet, T.; Ng, S.S.; Berlin, C.; Hood, L.; Keats, B. Connexin 26 variants and auditory neuropathy/dys-synchrony among children in schools for the deaf. *Am. J. Med Genet. Part A* **2005**, *139A*, 13–18. [CrossRef] [PubMed]
44. Santarelli, R.; Cama, E.; Scimemi, P.; Monte, E.D.; Genovese, E.; Arslan, E. Audiological and electrocochleography findings in hearing-impaired children with connexin 26 mutations and otoacoustic emissions. *Eur. Arch. Oto-Rhino-Laryngol.* **2008**, *265*, 43–51. [CrossRef]
45. Del Castillo, F.J.; Del Castillo, I. Genetics of isolated auditory neuropathies. *Front. Biosci.* **2012**, *17*, 1251–1265. [CrossRef]
46. Matsunaga, T.; Mutai, H.; Kunishima, S.; Namba, K.; Morimoto, N.; Shinjo, Y.; Arimoto, Y.; Kataoka, Y.; Shintani, T.; Morita, N.; et al. A prevalent founder mutation and genotype-phenotype correlations of OTOF in Japanese patients with auditory neuropathy. *Clin. Genet.* **2012**, *82*, 425–432. [CrossRef]
47. Chiu, Y.-H.; Wu, C.-C.; Lu, Y.-C.; Chen, P.-J.; Lee, W.-Y.; Liu, A.Y.-Z.; Hsu, C.-J. Mutations in the OTOF gene in Taiwanese patients with auditory neuropathy. *Audiol. Neurootol.* **2010**, *15*, 364–374. [CrossRef]
48. Zhang, Q.-J.; Han, B.; Lan, L.; Zong, L.; Shi, W.; Wang, H.-Y.; Xie, L.-Y.; Wang, H.; Zhao, C.; Zhang, C.; et al. High frequency of OTOF mutations in Chinese infants with congenital auditory neuropathy spectrum disorder. *Clin. Genet.* **2016**, *90*, 238–246. [CrossRef]
49. Wang, D.-Y.; Wang, Y.-C.; Weil, D.; Zhao, Y.-L.; Rao, S.-Q.; Zong, L.; Ji, Y.-B.; Liu, Q.; Li, J.-Q.; Yang, H.-M.; et al. Screening mutations of OTOF gene in Chinese patients with auditory neuropathy, including a familial case of temperature-sensitive auditory neuropathy. *BMC Med. Genet.* **2010**, *11*, 79. [CrossRef]
50. Cho, Y.; Gong, T.-W.L.; Stöver, T.; Lomax, M.I.; Altschuler, R.A. Gene expression profiles of the rat cochlea, cochlear nucleus, and inferior colliculus. *J. Assoc. Res. Otolaryngol. JARO* **2002**, *3*, 54–67. [CrossRef]
51. Cai, T.; Jen, H.-I.; Kang, H.; Klisch, T.J.; Zoghbi, H.Y.; Groves, A.K. Characterization of the transcriptome of nascent hair cells and identification of direct targets of the Atoh1 transcription factor. *J. Neurosci. Off. J. Soc. Neurosci.* **2015**, *35*, 5870–5883. [CrossRef] [PubMed]
52. Ranum, P.T.; Goodwin, A.T.; Yoshimura, H.; Kolbe, D.L.; Walls, W.D.; Koh, J.-Y.; He, D.Z.Z.; Smith, R.J.H. Insights into the Biology of Hearing and Deafness Revealed by Single-Cell RNA Sequencing. *Cell Rep.* **2019**, *26*, 3160–3171.e3. [CrossRef] [PubMed]
53. Wynne, D.P.; Zeng, F.-G.; Bhatt, S.; Michalewski, H.J.; Dimitrijevic, A.; Starr, A. Loudness adaptation accompanying ribbon synapse and auditory nerve disorders. *Brain J. Neurol.* **2013**, *136*, 1626–1638. [CrossRef]
54. Varga, R.; Avenarius, M.R.; Kelley, P.M.; Keats, B.J.; Berlin, C.I.; Hood, L.J.; Morlet, T.G.; Brashears, S.M.; Starr, A.; Cohn, E.S.; et al. OTOF mutations revealed by genetic analysis of hearing loss families including a potential temperature sensitive auditory neuropathy allele. *J. Med. Genet.* **2006**, *43*, 576–581. [CrossRef]
55. Romanos, J.; Kimura, L.; Fávero, M.L.; Izarra, F.A.R.; Auricchio, M.T.B.D.M.; Batissoco, A.C.; Lezirovitz, K.; Abreu-Silva, R.S.; Mingroni-Netto, R.C. Novel OTOF mutations in Brazilian patients with auditory neuropathy. *J. Hum. Genet.* **2009**, *54*, 382–385. [CrossRef] [PubMed]
56. Marlin, S.; Feldmann, D.; Nguyen, Y.; Rouillon, I.; Loundon, N.; Jonard, L.; Bonnet, C.; Couderc, R.; Garabedian, E.N.; Petit, C.; et al. Temperature-sensitive auditory neuropathy associated with an otoferlin mutation: Deafening fever! *Biochem. Biophys. Res. Commun.* **2010**, *394*, 737–742. [CrossRef] [PubMed]
57. Yildirim-Baylan, M.; Bademci, G.; Duman, D.; Ozturkmen-Akay, H.; Tokgoz-Yilmaz, S.; Tekin, M. Evidence for genotype-phenotype correlation for OTOF mutations. *Int. J. Pediatr. Otorhinolaryngol.* **2014**, *78*, 950–953. [CrossRef]
58. Helfmann, S.; Neumann, P.; Tittmann, K.; Moser, T.; Ficner, R.; Reisinger, E. The crystal structure of the C_2A domain of otoferlin reveals an unconventional top loop region. *J. Mol. Biol.* **2011**, *406*, 479–490. [CrossRef]
59. Meese, S.; Cepeda, A.P.; Gahlen, F.; Adams, C.M.; Ficner, R.; Ricci, A.J.; Heller, S.; Reisinger, E.; Herget, M. Activity-Dependent Phosphorylation by CaMKIIδ Alters the Ca2+Affinity of the Multi-C2-Domain Protein Otoferlin. *Front. Synaptic Neurosci.* **2017**, *9*, 13. [CrossRef]
60. Padmanarayana, M.; Hams, N.; Speight, L.C.; Petersson, E.J.; Mehl, R.A.; Johnson, C.P. Characterization of the lipid binding properties of Otoferlin reveals specific interactions between PI(4,5)P2 and the C2C and C2F domains. *Biochemistry* **2014**, *53*, 5023–5033. [CrossRef]
61. Harsini, F.M.; Bui, A.A.; Rice, A.M.; Chebrolu, S.; Fuson, K.L.; Turtoi, A.; Bradberry, M.; Chapman, E.R.; Sutton, R.B. Structural Basis for the Distinct Membrane Binding Activity of the Homologous C2A Domains of Myoferlin and Dysferlin. *J. Mol. Biol.* **2019**, *431*, 2112–2126. [CrossRef] [PubMed]

62. Letunic, I.; Bork, P. 20 years of the SMART protein domain annotation resource. *Nucleic Acids Res.* **2018**, *46*, D493–D496. [CrossRef] [PubMed]
63. Kelley, L.A.; Mezulis, S.; Yates, C.M.; Wass, M.N.; Sternberg, M.J.E. The Phyre2 web portal for protein modeling, prediction and analysis. *Nat. Protoc.* **2015**, *10*, 845–858. [CrossRef] [PubMed]
64. Longo-Guess, C.; Gagnon, L.H.; Bergstrom, D.E.; Johnson, K.R. A missense mutation in the conserved C2B domain of otoferlin causes deafness in a new mouse model of DFNB9. *Hear. Res.* **2007**, *234*, 21–28. [CrossRef] [PubMed]
65. Jiménez, J.L.; Bashir, R. In silico functional and structural characterisation of ferlin proteins by mapping disease-causing mutations and evolutionary information onto three-dimensional models of their C2 domains. *J. Neurol. Sci.* **2007**, *260*, 114–123. [CrossRef]
66. Harsini, F.M.; Chebrolu, S.; Fuson, K.L.; White, M.A.; Rice, A.M.; Sutton, R.B. FerA is a Membrane-Associating Four-Helix Bundle Domain in the Ferlin Family of Membrane-Fusion Proteins. *Sci. Rep.* **2018**, *8*, 10949. [CrossRef]
67. Vilardi, F.; Stephan, M.; Clancy, A.; Janshoff, A.; Schwappach, B. WRB and CAML are necessary and sufficient to mediate tail-anchored protein targeting to the ER membrane. *PLoS ONE* **2014**, *9*, e85033. [CrossRef]
68. Vogl, C.; Panou, I.; Yamanbaeva, G.; Wichmann, C.; Mangosing, S.J.; Vilardi, F.; Indzhykulian, A.A.; Pangršič, T.; Santarelli, R.; Rodriguez-Ballesteros, M.; et al. Tryptophan-rich basic protein (WRB) mediates insertion of the tail-anchored protein otoferlin and is required for hair cell exocytosis and hearing. *EMBO J.* **2016**, *35*, 2536–2552. [CrossRef]
69. Reisinger, E. Dual-AAV delivery of large gene sequences to the inner ear. *Hear. Res.* **2019**, *394*, 107857. [CrossRef]
70. Al-Moyed, H.; Cepeda, A.P.; Jung, S.; Moser, T.; Kügler, S.; Reisinger, E. A dual-AAV approach restores fast exocytosis and partially rescues auditory function in deaf otoferlin knock-out mice. *EMBO Mol. Med.* **2019**, *11*, e9396. [CrossRef]
71. Akil, O.; Dyka, F.; Calvet, C.; Emptoz, A.; Lahlou, G.; Nouaille, S.; De Monvel, J.B.; Hardelin, J.-P.; Hauswirth, W.W.; Avan, P.; et al. Dual AAV-mediated gene therapy restores hearing in a DFNB9 mouse model. *Proc. Natl. Acad. Sci. USA* **2019**, *116*, 4496–4501. [CrossRef] [PubMed]
72. Starr, A.; Picton, T.W.; Sininger, Y.; Hood, L.J.; Berlin, C.I. Auditory neuropathy. *Brain* **1996**, *119*, 741–754. [CrossRef] [PubMed]
73. Rouillon, I.; Marcolla, A.; Roux, I.; Marlin, S.; Feldmann, D.; Couderc, R.; Jonard, L.; Petit, C.; Denoyelle, F.; Garabédian, E.N.; et al. Results of cochlear implantation in two children with mutations in the OTOF gene. *Int. J. Pediatr. Otorhinolaryngol.* **2006**, *70*, 689–696. [CrossRef] [PubMed]

Publisher's Note: MDPI stays neutral with regard to jurisdictional claims in published maps and institutional affiliations.

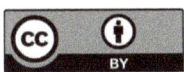

© 2020 by the authors. Licensee MDPI, Basel, Switzerland. This article is an open access article distributed under the terms and conditions of the Creative Commons Attribution (CC BY) license (http://creativecommons.org/licenses/by/4.0/).

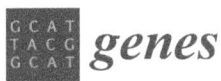

Article

Bi-Allelic Novel Variants in *CLIC5* Identified in a Cameroonian Multiplex Family with Non-Syndromic Hearing Impairment

Edmond Wonkam-Tingang [1], Isabelle Schrauwen [2], Kevin K. Esoh [1], Thashi Bharadwaj [2], Liz M. Nouel-Saied [2], Anushree Acharya [2], Abdul Nasir [3], Samuel M. Adadey [1,4], Shaheen Mowla [5], Suzanne M. Leal [2] and Ambroise Wonkam [1,*]

[1] Division of Human Genetics, Faculty of Health Sciences, University of Cape Town, Cape Town 7925, South Africa; wonkamedmond@yahoo.fr (E.W.-T.); esohkevin4@gmail.com (K.K.E.); smadadey@st.ug.edu.gh (S.M.A.)
[2] Center for Statistical Genetics, Sergievsky Center, Taub Institute for Alzheimer's Disease and the Aging Brain, and the Department of Neurology, Columbia University Medical Centre, New York, NY 10032, USA; is2632@cumc.columbia.edu (I.S.); tb2890@cumc.columbia.edu (T.B.); lmn2152@cumc.columbia.edu (L.M.N.-S.); aa4471@cumc.columbia.edu (A.A.); sml3@cumc.columbia.edu (S.M.L.)
[3] Synthetic Protein Engineering Lab (SPEL), Department of Molecular Science and Technology, Ajou University, Suwon 443-749, Korea; anasirqau@gmail.com
[4] West African Centre for Cell Biology of Infectious Pathogens (WACCBIP), University of Ghana, Accra LG 54, Ghana
[5] Division of Haematology, Department of Pathology, Faculty of Health Sciences, University of Cape Town, Cape Town 7925, South Africa; shaheen.mowla@uct.ac.za
* Correspondence: ambroise.wonkam@uct.ac.za; Tel.: +27-21-4066-307

Received: 28 September 2020; Accepted: 20 October 2020; Published: 23 October 2020

Abstract: DNA samples from five members of a multiplex non-consanguineous Cameroonian family, segregating prelingual and progressive autosomal recessive non-syndromic sensorineural hearing impairment, underwent whole exome sequencing. We identified novel bi-allelic compound heterozygous pathogenic variants in *CLIC5*. The variants identified, i.e., the missense [NM_016929.5:c.224T>C; p.(L75P)] and the splicing (NM_016929.5:c.63+1G>A), were validated using Sanger sequencing in all seven available family members and co-segregated with hearing impairment (HI) in the three hearing impaired family members. The three affected individuals were compound heterozygous for both variants, and all unaffected individuals were heterozygous for one of the two variants. Both variants were absent from the genome aggregation database (gnomAD), the Single Nucleotide Polymorphism Database (dbSNP), and the UK10K and Greater Middle East (GME) databases, as well as from 122 apparently healthy controls from Cameroon. We also did not identify these pathogenic variants in 118 unrelated sporadic cases of non-syndromic hearing impairment (NSHI) from Cameroon. In silico analysis showed that the missense variant *CLIC5*-p.(L75P) substitutes a highly conserved amino acid residue (leucine), and is expected to alter the stability, the structure, and the function of the CLIC5 protein, while the splicing variant *CLIC5*-(c.63+1G>A) is predicted to disrupt a consensus donor splice site and alter the splicing of the pre-mRNA. This study is the second report, worldwide, to describe *CLIC5* involvement in human hearing impairment, and thus confirms *CLIC5* as a novel non-syndromic hearing impairment gene that should be included in targeted diagnostic gene panels.

Keywords: non-syndromic hearing impairment; *CLIC5*; Africa

1. Introduction

Hearing impairment (HI) is the most common sensory disability and is prevalent in about 1 per 1000 live births in high-income countries, with a much higher incidence of up to 6 per 1000 live births in sub-Saharan Africa [1]. When occurring in childhood, HI is associated with impaired language acquisition, learning, and speech development, and affects ~34 million children worldwide (World Health Organisation) [2]. Approximately 30 to 50% of HI cases in Africa have a genetic origin [3,4]. Non-syndromic hearing impairment (NSHI) accounts for about 70% of HI cases of genetic origin and is inherited on an autosomal recessive (AR) mode in approximately 80% of cases [5].

Variants in *GJB2* and *GJB6* genes, which are the major contributors to NSHI in Europeans, Asians, and Arabs, are infrequent in most populations of African descent, with a prevalence close to zero [6–8]. NSHI is highly genetically heterogeneous [3,4]. To date, about 170 loci and 121 genes have been identified as being associated with NSHI (hereditary hearing loss homepage; Appendix A). Targeted sequencing panels that include >100 HI genes have detected a consistently lower rate of pathogenic and likely pathogenic (PLP) variants in sporadic HI cases of African ancestry, e.g., African Americans (26%), and Nigerians and Black South Africans (4%), compared to >70% for Europeans and Asians [9,10]. However, the detection rate was 70% for 10 mutiplex Cameroonian families [11]. Moreover, the prevalence of autosomal recessive non-syndromic hearing impairment (ARNSHI) pathogenic and likely pathogenic (PLP) variants, using data from the genome aggregation database (gnomAD) database [12] were estimated to account for ARNSHI in 5.2 per 100,000 individuals for Africans/African Americans, compared to 96.9 per 100,000 individuals for Ashkenazi Jews based on sequence data [13]. Therefore, there is an urgent need to investigate HI in populations of African ancestry, particularly multiplex families, using next generation sequencing, to improve knowledge a variants and genes which underlie NSHI in African populations.

In this study, we generated whole exome sequence (WES) data for samples obtained from a multiplex non-consanguineous Cameroonian family, segregating progressive ARNSHI, and identified novel bi-allelic PLP variants in *CLIC5* in the locus DFNB103. This gene was previously reported to be associated with HI in a single Turkish family [14]. This gene encodes a member of the chloride intracellular channel (CLIC) family of chloride ion channels. The encoded protein associates with actin-based cytoskeletal structures and may play a role in multiple processes including hair cell stereocilia formation, myoblast proliferation, and glomerular podocyte and endothelial cell maintenance. Alternatively, spliced transcript variants encoding multiple isoforms have been observed for this gene (provided by RefSeq). The corresponding mutant mouse model (jbg mouse), which has an intragenic deletion in *CLIC5* resulting in a truncated protein, presents progressive hearing impairment and vestibular dysfunction [15].

2. Materials and Methods

2.1. Ethics Approval

This study was performed with respect to the Declaration of Helsinki. Ethical approval was granted by the University of Cape Town's Faculty of Health Sciences' Human Research Ethics Committee (HREC 484/2019), the Institutional Research Ethics Committee for Human Health of the Gynaeco-Obstetric and Paediatric Hospital of Yaoundé, Cameroon (No. 723/CIERSH/DM/2018), and the Institutional Review Board of Columbia University (IRB-AAAS2343). Written and signed informed consent was obtained from all participants who were 21 years of age or older, and from parents in the case of minors, with verbal assent from participants.

2.2. Participants' Recruitment

The participants' selection process has been previously reported [16]. The hearing-impaired members of the Cameroonian family (Family 24, Figure 1A) were identified through a community engagement program for the deaf. For all hearing-impaired participants, their detailed personal history and medical records were reviewed by a general practitioner, a medical geneticist, and an ear, nose and throat (ENT) specialist. A general systemic and otological examination was performed, including pure tone audiometry. We followed the recommendation number 02/1 of the Bureau International d'Audiophonologie (BIAP), Belgium.

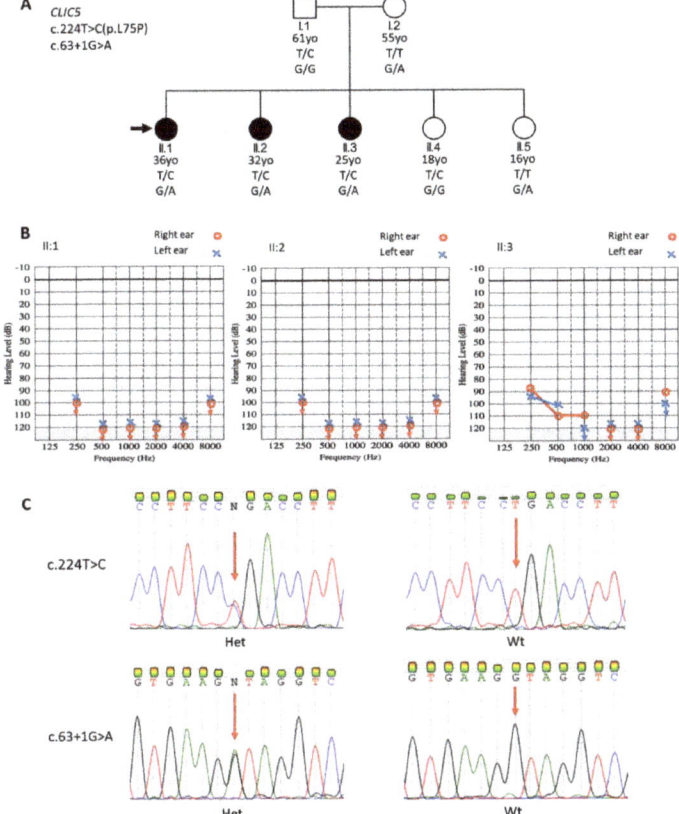

Figure 1. Pedigree of the non-consanguineous family, audiological phenotypes, and electropherogram data of the pathogenic variants in *CLIC5*. (**A**) The pedigree is suggestive of an autosomal recessive mode of inheritance. The missense *CLIC5* variant (NM_016929.5:c.224T>C) and the splicing *CLIC5* variant (NM_016929.5:c.63+1G>A), variants co-segregated with hearing impairment (HI), are compound heterozygous. The black arrow indicates the proband. (**B**) Air conduction of the pure tone audiometry performed for hearing impaired family members. Participants II.1, II.2, and II.3 were presented with a bilateral profound HI. (**C**) Sanger sequencing chromatograms, showing the reference and the alternate alleles of both the missense and the splicing variants. The red arrows indicate the nucleotides affected by the variants. Het, heterozygous for the variant allele; Wt, wild-type (homozygous for the reference allele); yo, years old.

Genomic DNA samples were extracted from peripheral blood, using the chemagic extraction protocol, in the division of Human Genetics, University of Cape Town, South Africa. Additionally, a group of 118 unrelated Cameroonian individuals living with sporadic NSHI of putative genetic origin (Table S1) were recruited, to investigate the frequencies of pathogenic variants that could be found. All hearing impaired family members were previously investigated for variants in *GJB2* (through direct sequencing of the entire coding region of *GJB2*), and *GJB6*-D13S1830 deletion (using a multiplex polymerase chain reaction), and were negative [6].

A total of 122 ethno-linguistically matched Cameroonian controls without personal or familial history of HI were randomly recruited among blood donors at The Central Hospital of Yaoundé, Cameroon.

2.3. Whole Exome Sequencing and Data Analysis

DNA samples from five family members were exome sequenced at Omega Bioservices (Norcross, GA, USA); these samples were obtained from two affected individuals (Figure 1A, II.1, and II.3), their parents (I.1, and I.2), and one unaffected sibling (II.4). Library preparation was performed with an Illumina Nextera Rapid Capture Exome Kit® (Illumina, San Diego, CA, USA) following the manufacturer's instructions, and the resulting libraries were hybridized with a 37 Mb probe pool to enrich exome sequences. Sequencing was performed on an Illumina HiSeq 2500 sequencer using the pair-end 150 bp run format. Sequencing data were processed using the Illumina DRAGEN Germline Pipeline v3.2.8. Briefly, high-quality reads were aligned to the human reference genome GRCh37/hg19 using the DRAGEN software version 05.021.408.3.4.12, and, after sorting and duplicate marking, variants were called, and individual genomic variant call format (gvcf) files were generated. Joint single nucleotide variant (SNV) and Insertion/Deletion (Indel) variant calling was performed using the genome analysis toolkit (GATK) software v4.0.6.0 [17]. The sex of each individual was verified using plinkv1.9 [18]. Familial relationships for all members were verified via Identity-by-Descent sharing (plinkv1.9) and the Kinship-based INference for Gwas (KING) algorithm [18,19].

2.4. Annotation and Filtering Strategy

Variants were annotated and filtered using ANNOVAR [20] and custom scripts. Variants were first prioritized based on the inheritance model, considering both AR and autosomal dominant (AD) modes of inheritance. Subsequently, rare variants with a minor allele frequency (MAF) < 0.005 (for AR) and <0.0005 (for AD) in all populations of the genome aggregation database (gnomAD) were retained. Known pathogenic HI variants listed in ClinVar were also retained, regardless of their frequencies. dbNSFP v3.0 was used to annotate, with 17 bioinformatic tools predicting the deleterious effects of the identified variants [21]. Coding variants were evaluated using Sorting Intolerant from Tolerant (SIFT), polymorphism phenotyping v2 (PolyPhen-2) × 2, MutationAssessor, the likelihood ratio test (LRT), Mendelian clinically applicable pathogenicity (M-CAP) score, Rare Exome Variant Ensemble Learner (REVEL), MutPred, protein variation effect analyzer (PROVEAN), MetaSVM, and MetaLR, while MutationTaster, Eigen, Eigen-PC, functional analysis through Hidden Markov models (FATHMM-MKL), combined annotation dependent depletion (CADD) score, and deleterious annotation of genetic variants using neural networks (DANN) score were used to annotate both coding and non-coding variants [21].

Adaptive boosting (ADA) and random forest (RF) scores derived from dbscSNV v1.1 were used to predict the deleterious effect of variants within splicing consensus regions (−3 to +8 at the 5′ splice site and −12 to +2 at the 3′ splice site) [21,22]. We used phyloP, Genomic Evolutionary Rate Profiling (GERP), SiPhy, and phastCons scores to estimate the evolutionary conservation of the nucleotides and amino acid (aa) residues at which the variants occurred [21,23,24]. The hereditary hearing loss homepage (HHL), online Mendelian inheritance in man (OMIM), human phenotype ontology (HPO), and ClinVar databases were used to determine if there were any existing associations between the identified variants and genes and HI. Candidate variants were considered when: (1) they occurred in known HI genes (and genes expressed in the inner ear); (2) they had a predicted effect on protein function or pre-mRNA splicing (nonsense, missense, start-loss, frameshift, splicing, start-loss, etc.); and (3) they co-segregated with the HI phenotype within the family.

2.5. Sanger Sequencing

Sanger sequencing was performed for all the available family members (I.1, I.2, II.1, II.2, II.3, II.4, and II.5; Figure 1A), 118 unrelated sporadic NSHI cases from Cameroon (Table S1), and 122 apparently healthy controls that were previously recruited as blood donors at The Central Hospital of Yaoundé. Primers to target our variants of interest in exon3 (forward 5′-GAAGGAACATACTGGGGCGA-3′; reverse 5′-AGCGCATTTTTGTTAGGCAGA-3′) and at the exon1-intron1 boundary (forward 5′-CTCTGAGCGAAAGAGAGAAAGAG-3′; reverse 5′-ACTTGTTGCTCCCACGACC-3′) of the *CLIC5* gene were validated using NCBI BLAST. The optimal annealing and extension temperatures for the PCR were 60 °C and 70 °C for 30 s and 1 min, respectively. PCR-amplified DNA products were Sanger sequenced using a BigDye™ Terminator v3.1 Cycle Sequencing Kit and an ABI 3130XL Genetic Analyzer® (Applied Biosystems, Foster City, CA, USA) in the Division of Human Genetics, University of Cape Town, South Africa. Sequencing chromatograms were manually checked using FinchTV v1.4.0, and aligned in UGENE v34.0 to the *CLIC5* reference sequence (ENSG00000112782; retrieved from Ensembl browser).

2.6. Evolutionary Conservation of Amino Acids and Secondary Structure Analysis

We performed a multiple sequence alignment (MSA) of human CLIC5 with non-human similar proteins to provide more evidence on the evolutionary conservation of the amino acid residue at which our candidate missense variant occurred. A PSI-BLAST search against the non-redundant protein database of CLIC5 was performed. Non-redundant, non-synthetic CLIC5 proteins from all the different species in the 500 BLAST hits were manually retrieved as FASTA files. The MSA was performed using CLUSTAL Omega v1.2.4 [25] and the MSA file was visualized using Jalview v2.10.5 [26]. Furthermore, PSIPRED v4.0 [27] and Swiss-Model [28] were used to assess the secondary structural features of both protein forms. Additionally, the InterPro [29] database was queried via the InterProScan web service [30] to identify domains and potential domain changes for both protein forms separately.

2.7. Protein Modelling

Three-dimensional modelling was performed on the longest isoform of the CLIC5 gene as follows: a homology model of the longest isoform (410 amino acids) of wild-type and mutant CLIC5 [NM_001114086.1: c.701T>C:p.(L234P)] was constructed using the program MODELLER based on the available crystal structure of human chloride intracellular channel protein 5 (PDB ID: 6Y2H) as a template [31]. PYMOL viewer was used for structural visualization and image processing.

3. Results

3.1. Participants Phenotypes

A total of seven individuals from "Family 24" were recruited, including three affected individuals (II.1: 36 years old, II.2: 32 years old, and II.3: 25 years old), their parents (I.1: 61 years old, and I.2: 55 years old), and two unaffected siblings (II.4: 18 years old, and II.5: 16 years old) (Figure 1A). The most likely mode of inheritance for the NSHI is AR. From the medical history, no environmental factors were identified as a possible cause of HI, and no HI participant had a history of ophthalmological (blurred or distorted vision, photophobia, eye pain, etc.) or neurological (vertigo, dizziness, etc.) symptoms. Additionally, no vestibular, neurologic, or any other systemic abnormalities were detected by physical examination. A history of prelingual and progressive HI was described for all three affected pedigree members; however, before this study, no formal audiological assessment was performed for any of the family members. Audiological assessment of the three affected individuals revealed bilateral profound sensorineural HI (Figure 1B).

3.2. WES Identification of Candidate Gene and Variants

The average target region coverage was about 225×, with 96.30% of the target region being covered to a depth of 10 X or more. After applying our various filtering criteria described in the methods section, two candidate variants were found to occur in a known HI gene (*CLIC5*; MIM:607293) and to co-segregate with the HI phenotype. These two variants which occurred in a compound heterozygous state are the missense variant NM_016929.5:c.224T>C, and the splice-site variant NM_016929.5:c.63+1G>A. The NM_016929.5:c.224T>C variant leads to the substitution of a leucine by a proline amino acid residue at position 75 [NM_016929.5:p.(L75P)] and was predicted to be damaging by 16 of the 17 bioinformatics tools used (Table S2). The NM_016929.5:c.63+1G>A variant, which occurs in a canonical donor splice site, was predicted damaging by most of the tools that can be used to evaluate non-coding variants, including MutationTaster, FATHMM-MKL, Eigen-PC, CADD, and DANN (Table S2). Both variants were predicted as occurring in conserved positions of the genome and were both absent from the gnomAD, UK10K, Greater Middle East (GME) variome project databases, as well as the Single Nucleotide Polymorphism Database (dbSNP) (Table S2). Based on a human splice finder server (HSF v3.1) and NNSPLICE 0.9, the variant NM_016929.5:c.63+1G>A is predicted to break the consensus 5′ donor site "AAGGTAGGT" (which is altered due to the variation "AAGATAGGT") and probably alter the splicing of the pre-mRNA. The NM_016929.5:c.63+1G>A variant might therefore alter normal protein synthesis and function through various mechanisms. Based on the American College of Medical Genetics' (ACMG) guidelines for the interpretation of sequence variants, both variants were classified as pathogenic (NM_016929.5:c.63+1G>A: PSV1, PP1-S, PM2, and PP3 and NM_016929.5:c.224T>C: PM2, PP3, PM3, PP1, and PP1-S) [32,33]. In addition to *CLIC5*, only the *CEP250* gene shows compound heterozygous synonymous variants that co-segregate with hearing impairment (Table S3), which was unlikely to be the cause of the disease.

3.3. Sanger Sequencing Confirmation of Variants

Sanger sequencing confirms these candidate variants and their co-segregation with the HI phenotype (Figure 1A,C). The three affected individuals (II.1, II.2, and II.3) were compound heterozygous for both variants, the father (I.1) and an unaffected daughter (II.4) were heterozygous for the missense variant, and the mother (I.2) and the other unaffected daughter (II.5) were both heterozygous for the splice-site variant (Figure 1A). Neither of these variants was detected in the 122 controls or 118 sporadic NSHI cases (Table S1) from Cameroon.

3.4. Analysis of the CLIC5—NM_016929.5(CLIC5):p.(L75P) Variant on the Protein

3.4.1. Evolutionary Conservation of Amino Acids

The NCBI PSI-BLAST search of CLIC5 (NP_058625.2) against the non-redundant protein database found the variant position p.(L75P) to be highly conserved across all non-human species retrieved in the top 500 BLAST hits (Figure 2). As expected, there was substantial conservation across an extensive aa block (on which the variant resides) which forms the thioredoxin/Genetic Diversity Statistics (GST)–N-terminal binding domain. This was consistent with the GERP and PhyloP scores for conservation, indicating a strong evolutionary and functional constraint on the region.

3.4.2. Protein Modelling: Secondary Structure Analysis and Domain Search

A significant attenuation of the protein's secondary structural features was predicted for the NM_016929.5(*CLIC5*):p.(L75P) variant using the PSIPRED v4.0 server, whereby; there was an abolishment of the β4 strand (Figure 3 and Figure S1 red box) and multiple changes affecting the lengths of β strands and several helices were inflicted (Figure S1 black boxes). Using Swiss-Model, a similar distortion in the secondary structure of the mutant protein was observed; shortening of the β4 strand, although no β-strand loss was apparent. A domain search with InterProScan (InterPro v80.0) predicted the loss of the N-terminal GST domain due to the variant (Figure S2). This domain loss was also predicted to lead to the abrogation of CLIC5's protein binding function (GO:0005515). Model parameters were refined and showed improvement in model qualities (Table S4).

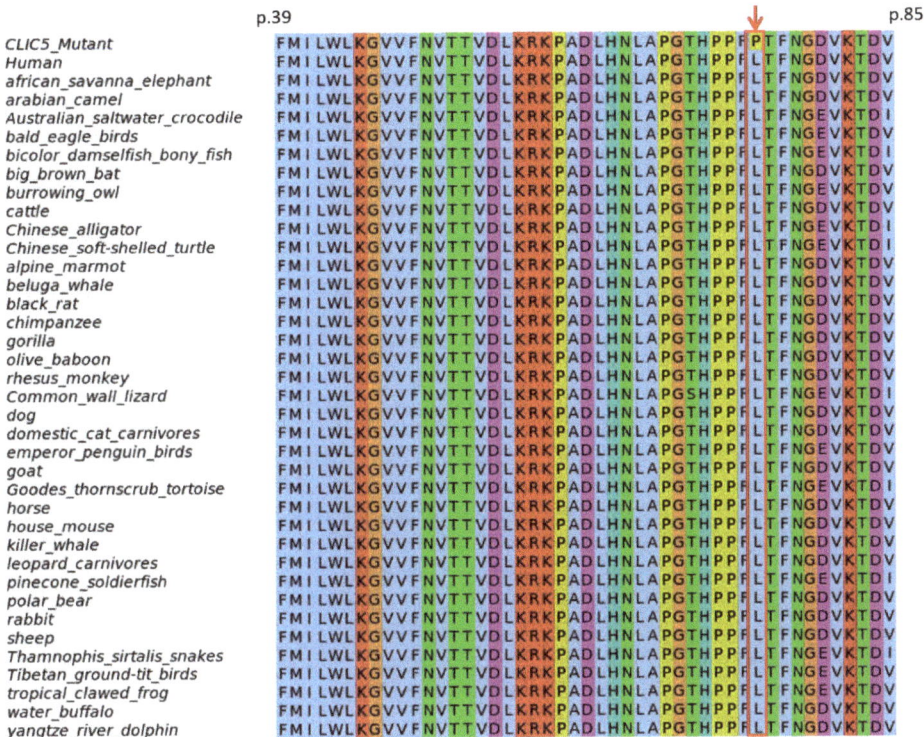

Figure 2. Evolutionary conservation of the *CLIC5*:p.(L75P) variant position (indicated by the red arrow).

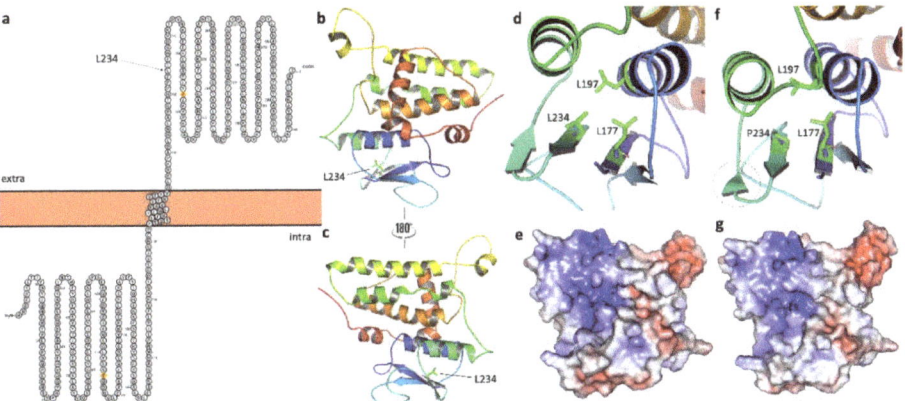

Figure 3. (a) The residue Leu234 of NM_001114086.1:c.701T>C:p.(L234P), representing the long isoform of missense variant NM_016929.5:c.224T>C:p.(L75P) is located in the extracellular domain of the CLIC5 protein. (b,c) The overall structure of CLIC5 and the Leu234 residue (represented by a stick model). (d) Close-up view of the interaction pattern at position 234 of wild-type and mutant protein (f). Due to the mutation, the shortness of the β-strand observed in the mutant protein was highlighted by a dotted-circle. (e) The surface charge distribution of wild and (g) mutant CLIC5. Intra: intracellular; extra: extracellular.

Finally, we performed 3D modelling of the wild-type and mutant long isoform of CLIC5 (Figure 3). The NM_016929.5:c.224T>C missense variant is located in a β-sheet in the extracellular domain of the long isoform of *CLIC5* [NM_001114086.1:c.701T>C:p.(L234P)] (Figure 3c). We found that there was a local perturbation in the hydrophobic interaction of nearby residues at position 234 of the CLIC5 protein (Figure 3d,f). Pro234 affects the shortness of the nearby β-sheet conformation in the mutant protein, as shown in Figure 3f. There was also a difference observed on the surface charge distribution between wild-type and mutant (Figure 3e,g).

4. Discussion

This study is, to our knowledge, the first report highlighting the association of HI with *CLIC5* variants in individuals of African ancestry, and the second to demonstrate this association globally. Thus, the data confirms *CLIC5* as a novel HI gene. Both pathogenic variants reported are novel: (NM_016929.5:c.224T>C) and the splicing variant (NM_016929.5:c.63+1G>A), and were not found in 118 unrelated sporadic cases of NSHI cases, reinforcing the genetic and locus heterogeneity nature of HI, and the importance of investigating diverse populations, particularly the understudied African populations, to help to enhance and refine HI disease-gene curation. The contribution of *CLIC5* to NSHI in humans was first described with the identification of a homozygous nonsense variant [NM_016929.5:c.96T>A; p.(Cys32Ter)] that abrogated the protein function and co-segregated with ARNSHI in a Turkish family [14]. The two affected individuals from the aforementioned Turkish family presented an early onset sensorineural HI, which started mildly and progressed to severe-to-profound HI. This HI phenotype is similar to that described in the present study, as our three affected participants described a history of prelingual HI, and presented profound sensorineural HI at the time of the study [14]. The corresponding mutant mice model (*jbg* mice), which has a deletion in the *CLIC5* mice ortholog gene, resulting in impaired hearing and vestibular dysfunction [15]. *CLIC5* was also studied in 69 unrelated Spanish and 50 predominantly Dutch patients with ARNSHI, and no PLP variants were identified [14]. In the present study, we did not find any clinical evidence of vestibular or renal dysfunctions, unlike what was previously reported in the Turkish family [14], as well as in the corresponding mutant mice model (*jbg* mice) that were also shown to have abnormalities in the foot processes of the kidney podocytes leading to proteinuria [34,35]. Biological exploration of the kidney functions of affected Cameroonian individuals with PLP in *CLIC5* should be performed. In addition to the inner ear and kidney abnormalities, the jbg-mutant mice also exhibited emphysema-like lung pathology, hyperactivity, and gastric haemorrhage [14,36]. Additional studies on more families and populations worldwide are needed to refine the phenotype of *CLIC5*-induced HI in humans.

CLIC5 (mapped on 6p21.1 locus) encodes a protein that belongs to the chloride intracellular ion channel (CLIC) family [37]. The encoded protein (CLIC5) was shown to be highly expressed in the inner ear, and important for sensorineural hearing [15]. CLIC5 protein associates with actin-based cytoskeletal structures and may play a role in multiple processes, including hair cell stereocilia formation [15]. The main function of CLIC5A in the ear is the stabilization of membrane-actin filament linkages at the base of hair cell stereocilia [15]. Therefore, a variant that abrogates CLIC5A or destabilizes its activity would lead to the destabilization of actin-based complexes, fusion, and the elongation of hair cell stereocilia, and consequently, impaired hearing [14,38]. The missense NM_016929.5(*CLIC5*):p.(L75P) variant reported in this study is predicted to lead to the loss of the N-terminal GST domain. This is in turn expected to abrogate CLIC5's protein binding function (GO:0005515), and is therefore likely to affect binding to ERM proteins. Interaction of CLIC5 with the actin-based cytoskeleton is dependent upon its protein–protein interaction with ERM proteins [38].

There are three isoforms of CLIC5 [39]: The canonical isoform CLIC5B (410aa), CLIC5A (251aa) and CLIC5C (205aa). All three isoforms show evidence of expression in the human inner ear, of which CLIC5A shows the highest expression (251aa) [40]. The splice site variant we identified in this study is predicted to affect two of these three isoforms, [NM_016929.5:c.63+1G>A (251 aa; CLIC5A); NM_001256023.1:c.63+1G>A (205 aa; CLIC5C)], including isoform CLIC5A. This splice site variant is located at the 5′ donor canonical splice site of exon 1 of these two isoform transcripts (position +1) and predicted to lead to a loss of the consensus 5′ donor site. The missense variant reported in this study [NM_016929.5: p.(L75P)] is predicted to affect all three isoforms of CLIC5 as a missense change.

Although the identified variants in the present study are predicted to be pathogenic (Table S2), and to also affect the structure and function of the protein (Figure 2, Figures S1 and S2), more studies in other populations will likely inform and strengthen the HI disease gene-pair curation, globally, as illustrated with this case report.

5. Conclusions

We identified bi-allelic novel compound heterozygous pathogenic variants in *CLIC5* (MIM:607293), the missense variant [NM_016929.5:c.224T>C; p.(L75P)] and the splicing variant (NM_016929.5:c.63+1G>A), that co-segregated with non-syndromic autosomal recessive hearing impairment in three affected members of a non-consanguineous family from Cameroon. This study is the second report, worldwide, to describe the *CLIC5*–HI gene-disease pair in humans, and thus confirms *CLIC5* as a novel NSHI that should be included in targeted diagnostic gene panels. Our study emphasizes the urgent need of using WES to investigate hearing impairment in understudied African populations, in order to improve our understanding of hearing pathobiology.

Supplementary Materials: The following are available online at http://www.mdpi.com/2073-4425/11/11/1249/s1, Table S1: Demographic and clinical characteristics of isolated NSHI cases screened for the identified *CLIC5* pathogenic variants. Mean age = 10.92 ± 4.84 (3–31) years, Table S2: Description of pathogenic variants identified in *CLIC5*, Table S3: Synonymous likely benign variants identified in the *CEP250* gene, Table S4: Model parameters before and after refinement showing improvement in protein model qualities, Figure S1: Secondary structure prediction of CLIC5 using the 251 amino acids isoform (NM_016929.5). Boxes indicate positions of difference between the wild-type (CLIC5A:p.75L) and mutant (CLIC5A:p.75P). Red boxes show loss of the fourth strand in the wild-type, while black boxes show changes in the lengths of strands and helices, Figure S2: Domains of CLIC5A:p.75L (wild-type) and CLIC5A:p.75P (mutant) predicted by InterPro, based on the 251 amino acids isoform (NM_016929.5). The GST N-terminal domain is lost in the mutant and its protein-binding activity is abolished.

Author Contributions: Conception of the project: A.W, S.M.L.; recruitment and molecular experiments: E.W.-T.; exclusion of *GJB2* and *GJB6* variants: E.W.-T. and S.M.A.; bioinformatics analysis: I.S., T.B., L.M.N.-S., A.A.; in silico analysis of the pathogenicity of variants: E.W.-T., I.S., K.K.E.; protein modelling: K.K.E., A.N., S.M.; issue of the first draft of the manuscript: E.W.-T.; review and editing: all authors; supervision of the whole project: S.M.L. and A.W. All authors have agreed to the final version of the manuscript.

Funding: This study was possible thanks to funding from the Wellcome Trust, grant number 107755Z/15/Z to GAA and AW (co-applicants); NIH, USA, grant number U01-HG-009716 to AW, the African Academy of Science/Wellcome Trust, grant number H3A/18/001 to AW, and the National Institute of Deafness and other Communication Disorders grants R01 DC01165, DC003594 and DC016593 to S.M.L. The funders were not involved in study design, data collection and analysis, decision to publish, or preparation of the manuscript.

Acknowledgments: We are grateful to patients and their family members for their participation in this research project.

Conflicts of Interest: The authors declare no competing interest.

Appendix A Web Resources

ANNOVAR	https://annovar.openbioinformatics.org/
Bureau international d'audiophonologie (BIAP)	https://www.biap.org/en/recommandations/recommendations/tc-02-classification
ClinVar	https://www.ncbi.nlm.nih.gov/clinvar/
dbNSFP (including dbscSNV)	https://sites.google.com/site/jpopgen/dbNSFP
dbSNP	https://www.ncbi.nlm.nih.gov/snp/
DRAGEN germline pipeline	https://emea.illumina.com/products/by-type/informatics-products/basespace-sequence-hub/apps/edico-genome-inc-dragen-germline-pipeline.html
Ensembl	https://www.ensembl.org/index.html
Gene ontology (GO)	http://geneontology.org/
Genome aggregation database (gnomAD)	https://gnomad.broadinstitute.org/

Genome analysis toolkit (GATK)	https://gatk.broadinstitute.org/hc/en-us
Hereditary hearing loss homepage (HHL)	https://hereditaryhearingloss.org/
Human phenotype ontology (HPO)	https://hpo.jax.org/app/
Human splice finder (HSF)	https://hsf.genomnis.com/home
InterProScan	http://www.ebi.ac.uk/InterProScan/
MODELLER	http://www.salilab.org/modeller
NCBI-BLAST	https://blast.ncbi.nlm.nih.gov/Blast.cgi
Online Mendelian inheritance in man (OMIM)	https://omim.org/
PDB	https://www.wwpdb.org/
PSIPRED	http://bioinf.cs.ucl.ac.uk/psipred/
PYMOL	http://www.pymol.org/
RefSeq	https://www.ncbi.nlm.nih.gov/refseq/
Swiss-Model	https://swissmodel.expasy.org/
Uniprot	https://www.uniprot.org/uniprot/Q9NZA1
UK10K	https://www.uk10k.org/
World Health Organisation	https://www.who.int/news-room/fact-sheets/detail/deafness-and-hearing-loss

References

1. Olusanya, B.O.; Neumann, K.J.; Saunders, J.E. The global burden of disabling hearing impairment: A call to action. *Bull. World Health Organ.* **2014**, *92*, 367–373. [CrossRef] [PubMed]
2. Schrauwen, I.; Liaqat, K.; Schatteman, I.; Bharadwaj, T.; Nasir, A.; Acharya, A.; Ahmad, W.; Van Camp, G.; Leal, S.M. Autosomal dominantly inherited GREB1L variants in individuals with profound sensorineural hearing impairment. *Genes* **2020**, *11*, 687. [CrossRef] [PubMed]
3. Wonkam Tingang, E.; Noubiap, J.J.; Fokouo, J.V.F.; Oluwole, O.G.; Nguefack, S.; Chimusa, E.R.; Wonkam, A. Hearing impairment overview in Africa: The case of Cameroon. *Genes* **2020**, *11*, 233. [CrossRef] [PubMed]
4. Lebeko, K.; Bosch, J.; Noubiap, J.J.N.; Dandara, C.; Wonkam, A. Genetics of hearing loss in Africans: Use of next generation sequencing is the best way forward. *Pan Afr. Med. J.* **2015**, *20*. [CrossRef]
5. Shearer, A.E.; Hildebrand, M.S.; Smith, R.J. Hereditary hearing loss and deafness overview. In *GeneReviews®[Internet]*; University of Washington: Seattle, WA, USA, 2017.
6. Tingang Wonkam, E.; Chimusa, E.; Noubiap, J.J.; Adadey, S.M.; Fokouo, J.V.F.; Wonkam, A. GJB2 and GJB6 mutations in hereditary recessive non-syndromic hearing impairment in Cameroon. *Genes* **2019**, *10*, 844. [CrossRef]
7. Bosch, J.; Noubiap, J.J.N.; Dandara, C.; Makubalo, N.; Wright, G.; Entfellner, J.-B.D.; Tiffin, N.; Wonkam, A. Sequencing of GJB2 in Cameroonians and Black South Africans and comparison to 1000 Genomes project data support need to revise strategy for discovery of nonsyndromic deafness genes in Africans. *OMICS* **2014**, *18*, 705–710. [CrossRef]
8. Bosch, J.; Lebeko, K.; Nziale, J.J.N.; Dandara, C.; Makubalo, N.; Wonkam, A. In search of genetic markers for nonsyndromic deafness in Africa: A study in Cameroonians and Black South Africans with the GJB6 and GJA1 Candidate Genes. *OMICS* **2014**, *18*, 481–485. [CrossRef]
9. Sloan-Heggen, C.M.; Bierer, A.O.; Shearer, A.E.; Kolbe, D.L.; Nishimura, C.J.; Frees, K.L.; Ephraim, S.S.; Shibata, S.B.; Booth, K.T.; Campbell, C.A.; et al. Comprehensive genetic testing in the clinical evaluation of 1119 patients with hearing loss. *Hum. Genet.* **2016**, *135*, 441–450. [CrossRef]
10. Yan, D.; Tekin, D.; Bademci, G.; Foster, J.; Cengiz, F.B.; Kannan-Sundhari, A.; Guo, S.; Mittal, R.; Zou, B.; Grati, M.; et al. Spectrum of DNA variants for nonsyndromic deafness in a large cohort from multiple continents. *Hum. Genet.* **2016**, *135*, 953–961. [CrossRef]
11. Lebeko, K.; Sloan-Heggen, C.M.; Noubiap, J.J.N.; Dandara, C.; Kolbe, D.L.; Ephraim, S.S.; Booth, K.T.; Azaiez, H.; Santos-Cortez, R.L.P.; Leal, S.M.; et al. Targeted genomic enrichment and massively parallel sequencing identifies novel nonsyndromic hearing impairment pathogenic variants in Cameroonian families. *Clin. Genet.* **2016**, *90*, 288–290. [CrossRef]
12. Karczewski, K.J.; Francioli, L.C.; Tiao, G.; Cummings, B.B.; Alföldi, J.; Wang, Q.; Collins, R.L.; Laricchia, K.M.; Ganna, A.; Birnbaum, D.P.; et al. The mutational constraint spectrum quantified from variation in 141,456 humans. *Nature* **2020**, *581*, 434–443. [CrossRef] [PubMed]
13. Chakchouk, I.; Zhang, D.; Zhang, Z.; Francioli, L.C.; Santos-Cortez, R.L.P.; Schrauwen, I.; Leal, S.M. Disparities in discovery of pathogenic variants for autosomal recessive non-syndromic hearing impairment by ancestry. *Eur. J. Hum. Genet.* **2019**, *27*, 1456–1465. [CrossRef] [PubMed]

14. Seco, C.Z.; Oonk, A.M.; Domínguez-Ruiz, M.; Draaisma, J.M.; Gandía, M.; Oostrik, J.; Neveling, K.; Kunst, H.P.; Hoefsloot, L.H.; del Castillo, I.; et al. Progressive hearing loss and vestibular dysfunction caused by a homozygous nonsense mutation in *CLIC5*. *Eur. J. Hum. Genet.* **2015**, *23*, 189–194. [CrossRef] [PubMed]
15. Gagnon, L.H.; Longo-Guess, C.M.; Berryman, M.; Shin, J.-B.; Saylor, K.W.; Yu, H.; Gillespie, P.G.; Johnson, K.R. The chloride intracellular channel protein CLIC5 is expressed at high levels in hair cell stereocilia and is essential for normal inner ear function. *J. Neurosci.* **2006**, *26*, 10188–10198. [CrossRef]
16. Wonkam, A.; Noubiap, J.J.N.; Djomou, F.; Fieggen, K.; Njock, R.; Toure, G.B. Aetiology of childhood hearing loss in Cameroon (sub-Saharan Africa). *Eur. J. Med. Genet.* **2013**, *56*, 20–25. [CrossRef]
17. McKenna, A.; Hanna, M.; Banks, E.; Sivachenko, A.; Cibulskis, K.; Kernytsky, A.; Garimella, K.; Altshuler, D.; Gabriel, S.; Daly, M.; et al. The genome analysis toolkit: A MapReduce framework for analyzing next-generation DNA sequencing data. *Genome Res.* **2010**, *20*, 1297–1303. [CrossRef]
18. Chang, C.C.; Chow, C.C.; Tellier, L.C.; Vattikuti, S.; Purcell, S.M.; Lee, J.J. Second-generation PLINK: Rising to the challenge of larger and richer datasets. *Gigascience* **2015**, *4*. [CrossRef]
19. Manichaikul, A.; Mychaleckyj, J.C.; Rich, S.S.; Daly, K.; Sale, M.; Chen, W.-M. Robust relationship inference in genome-wide association studies. *Bioinformatics* **2010**, *26*, 2867–2873. [CrossRef]
20. Wang, K.; Li, M.; Hakonarson, H. ANNOVAR: Functional annotation of genetic variants from high-throughput sequencing data. *Nucleic Acids Res.* **2010**, *38*, e164. [CrossRef] [PubMed]
21. Liu, X.; Wu, C.; Li, C.; Boerwinkle, E. dbNSFP v3.0: A one-stop database of functional predictions and annotations for human non-synonymous and splice site SNVs. *Hum. Mutat.* **2016**, *37*, 235–241. [CrossRef] [PubMed]
22. Jian, X.; Boerwinkle, E.; Liu, X. In silico prediction of splice-altering single nucleotide variants in the human genome. *Nucleic Acids Res.* **2014**, *42*, 13534–13544. [CrossRef] [PubMed]
23. Cooper, G.M.; Stone, E.A.; Asimenos, G.; Green, E.D.; Batzoglou, S.; Sidow, A. Distribution and intensity of constraint in mammalian genomic sequence. *Genome Res.* **2005**, *15*, 901–913. [CrossRef]
24. Pollard, K.S.; Hubisz, M.J.; Rosenbloom, K.R.; Siepel, A. Detection of nonneutral substitution rates on mammalian phylogenies. *Genome Res.* **2010**, *20*, 110–121. [CrossRef]
25. Sievers, F.; Wilm, A.; Dineen, D.; Gibson, T.J.; Karplus, K.; Li, W.; Lopez, R.; McWilliam, H.; Remmert, M.; Söding, J.; et al. Fast, scalable generation of high-quality protein multiple sequence alignments using Clustal Omega. *Mol. Syst. Biol.* **2011**. [CrossRef]
26. Waterhouse, A.M.; Procter, J.B.; Martin, D.M.A.; Clamp, M.; Barton, G.J. Jalview Version 2—A multiple sequence alignment editor and analysis workbench. *Bioinformatics* **2009**, *25*, 1189–1191. [CrossRef]
27. Buchan, D.W.A.; Jones, D.T. The PSIPRED Protein Analysis Workbench: 20 years on. *Nucleic Acids Res.* **2019**, *47*, W402–W407. [CrossRef]
28. Waterhouse, A.; Bertoni, M.; Bienert, S.; Studer, G.; Tauriello, G.; Gumienny, R.; Heer, F.T.; de Beer, T.A.P.; Rempfer, C.; Bordoli, L.; et al. SWISS-MODEL: Homology modelling of protein structuRes. and complexes. *Nucleic Acids Res.* **2018**, *46*, W296–W303. [CrossRef]
29. Mitchell, A.L.; Attwood, T.K.; Babbitt, P.C.; Blum, M.; Bork, P.; Bridge, A.; Brown, S.D.; Chang, H.-Y.; El-Gebali, S.; Fraser, M.I.; et al. InterPro in 2019: Improving coverage, classification and access to protein sequence annotations. *Nucleic Acids Res.* **2019**, *47*, D351–D360. [CrossRef]
30. Jones, P.; Binns, D.; Chang, H.-Y.; Fraser, M.; Li, W.; McAnulla, C.; McWilliam, H.; Maslen, J.; Mitchell, A.; Nuka, G.; et al. InterProScan 5: Genome-scale protein function classification. *Bioinformatics* **2014**, *30*, 1236–1240. [CrossRef]
31. Mi, W.; Liang, Y.-H.; Li, L.; Su, X.-D. The crystal structure of human chloride intracellular channel protein 2: A disulfide bond with functional implications. *Proteins Struct. Funct. Bioinform.* **2008**, *71*, 509–513. [CrossRef]
32. Richards, S.; Aziz, N.; Bale, S.; Bick, D.; Das, S.; Gastier-Foster, J.; Grody, W.W.; Hegde, M.; Lyon, E.; Spector, E.; et al. Standards and guidelines for the interpretation of sequence variants: A joint consensus recommendation of the American College of Medical Genetics and Genomics and the Association for Molecular Pathology. *Genet. Med.* **2015**, *17*, 405–424. [CrossRef]
33. Oza, A.M.; DiStefano, M.T.; Hemphill, S.E.; Cushman, B.J.; Grant, A.R.; Siegert, R.K.; Shen, J.; Chapin, A.; Boczek, N.J.; Schimmenti, L.A.; et al. Expert specification of the ACMG/AMP variant interpretation guidelines for genetic hearing loss. *Hum. Mutat.* **2018**, *39*, 1593–1613. [CrossRef] [PubMed]
34. Pierchala, B.A.; Muñoz, M.R.; Tsui, C.C. Proteomic analysis of the slit diaphragm complex: CLIC5 is a protein critical for podocyte morphology and function. *Kidney Int.* **2010**, *78*, 868–882. [CrossRef] [PubMed]

35. Wegner, B.; Al-Momany, A.; Kulak, S.C.; Kozlowski, K.; Obeidat, M.; Jahroudi, N.; Paes, J.; Berryman, M.; Ballermann, B.J. CLIC5A, a component of the ezrin-podocalyxin complex in glomeruli, is a determinant of podocyte integrity. *Am. J. Physiol. Ren. Physiol.* **2010**. [CrossRef] [PubMed]
36. Bradford, E.M.; Miller, M.L.; Prasad, V.; Nieman, M.L.; Gawenis, L.R.; Berryman, M.; Lorenz, J.N.; Tso, P.; Shull, G.E. CLIC5 mutant mice are resistant to diet-induced obesity and exhibit gastric hemorrhaging and increased susceptibility to torpor. *Am. J. Physiol. Regul. Integr. Comp. Physiol.* **2010**, *298*, R1531–R1542. [CrossRef]
37. Gururaja Rao, S.; Patel, N.J.; Singh, H. Intracellular chloride channels: Novel biomarkers in diseases. *Front. Physiol.* **2020**, *11*. [CrossRef]
38. Salles, F.T.; Andrade, L.R.; Tanda, S.; Grati, M.; Plona, K.L.; Gagnon, L.H.; Johnson, K.R.; Kachar, B.; Berryman, M.A. CLIC5 stabilizes membrane-actin filament linkages at the base of hair cell stereocilia in a molecular complex with radixin, taperin, and myosin VI. *Cytoskeleton* **2014**, *71*, 61–78. [CrossRef]
39. Breuza, L.; Poux, S.; Estreicher, A.; Famiglietti, M.L.; Magrane, M.; Tognolli, M.; Bridge, A.; Baratin, D.; Redaschi, N. The UniProt Consortium. The UniProtKB guide to the human proteome. *Database* **2016**, *2016*, bav120. [CrossRef]
40. Schrauwen, I.; Hasin-Brumshtein, Y.; Corneveaux, J.J.; Ohmen, J.; White, C.; Allen, A.N.; Lusis, A.J.; Van Camp, G.; Huentelman, M.J.; Friedman, R.A. A comprehensive catalogue of the coding and non-coding transcripts of the human inner ear. *Hear. Res.* **2016**, *333*, 266–274. [CrossRef]

Publisher's Note: MDPI stays neutral with regard to jurisdictional claims in published maps and institutional affiliations.

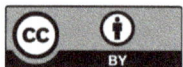

© 2020 by the authors. Licensee MDPI, Basel, Switzerland. This article is an open access article distributed under the terms and conditions of the Creative Commons Attribution (CC BY) license (http://creativecommons.org/licenses/by/4.0/).

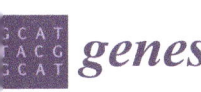

Article

A Novel Truncating Mutation in HOMER2 Causes Nonsyndromic Progressive DFNA68 Hearing Loss in a Spanish Family

María Lachgar [1,2,†], Matías Morín [1,2,†], Manuela Villamar [1,2], Ignacio del Castillo [1,2] and Miguel Ángel Moreno-Pelayo [1,2,*]

1. Servicio de Genética, Hospital Universitario Ramón y Cajal, IRYCIS, Carretera de Colmenar km 9.100, 28034 Madrid, Spain; maria.lachgar95@gmail.com (M.L.); matmorinro@yahoo.es (M.M.); taugen.hrc@salud.madrid.org (M.V.); delcastilloi@hotmail.com (I.d.C.)
2. Centro de Investigación Biomédica en Red de Enfermedades Raras (CIBERER), 28034 Madrid, Spain
* Correspondence: mmorenop@salud.madrid.org
† These authors have contributed equally to this work.

Abstract: Nonsyndromic hereditary hearing loss is a common sensory defect in humans that is clinically and genetically highly heterogeneous. So far, 122 genes have been associated with this disorder and 50 of them have been linked to autosomal dominant (DFNA) forms like DFNA68, a rare subtype of hearing impairment caused by disruption of a stereociliary scaffolding protein (HOMER2) that is essential for normal hearing in humans and mice. In this study, we report a novel HOMER2 variant (c.832_836delCCTCA) identified in a Spanish family by using a custom NGS targeted gene panel (OTO-NGS-v2). This frameshift mutation produces a premature stop codon that may lead in the absence of NMD to a shorter variant (p.Pro278Alafs*10) that truncates HOMER2 at the CDC42 binding domain (CBD) of the coiled-coil structure, a region that is essential for protein multimerization and HOMER2-CDC42 interaction. c.832_836delCCTCA mutation is placed close to the previously identified c.840_840dup mutation found in a Chinese family that truncates the protein (p.Met281Hisfs*9) at the CBD. Functional assessment of the Chinese mutant revealed decreased protein stability, reduced ability to multimerize, and altered distribution pattern in transfected cells when compared with wild-type HOMER2. Interestingly, the Spanish and Chinese frameshift mutations might exert a similar effect at the protein level, leading to truncated mutants with the same Ct aberrant protein tail, thus suggesting that they can share a common mechanism of pathogenesis. Indeed, age-matched patients in both families display quite similar hearing loss phenotypes consisting of early-onset, moderate-to-profound progressive hearing loss. In summary, we have identified the third variant in HOMER2, which is the first one identified in the Spanish population, thus contributing to expanding the mutational spectrum of this gene in other populations, and also to clarifying the genotype–phenotype correlations of DFNA68 hearing loss.

Keywords: hereditary hearing loss; next-generation sequencing; custom panel; HOMER2; CDC42

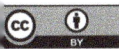

1. Introduction

Hearing loss is the most common sensory deficit in humans, affecting around 1 in 1000 newborns. Its prevalence increases with the age up to 6–8% in the adult population, having a strong impact on the individual's social isolation [1]. Genetic causes account for 50–60% of newborn hearing loss, 30% of which are nonsyndromic forms of deafness [2]. The genetic etiology of hearing impairment is highly heterogeneous. Up to date, 160 nonsyndromic sensorineural hearing loss (NSSNHL) *loci* have been mapped, of which 122 genes have been identified [3]. Sixty-seven of these *loci* and 50 of these genes are associated with autosomal dominant NSSNHL, being, in most cases, rare forms of post-lingual and progressive hereditary hearing impairment.

Autosomal dominant NSSNHL-linked genes encode proteins with a wide variety of functions [4], such as cytoskeleton proteins (*ACTG1*, *DIAPH1*, *PLS1*), adhesion proteins (*GJB2*,

GJB3, *GJB6*, *TJP2*), motor proteins (myosins), scaffolding proteins (*HOMER2*), extracellular matrix proteins (*TECTA*, *COL11A2*), proteins involved in ion homeostasis, such as ionic channels (*KCNQ4*), transcription factors (*EYA4*, *POU4F3*), and even a microRNA (*MIR96*) [5].

The *HOMER2* gene maps to chromosome 15q24.3 [6] within the DFNA68 critical interval and consists of nine exons. Two human transcript variants have been described (NM_004839.4 and NM_199330.3) as encoding the short isoform 1 (NP_004830.2, 343aa) and the long isoform 2 (NP_955362.1, 354aa) of HOMER2, respectively. HOMER2 belongs to a protein family encompassing three members: HOMER1 (MIM604798), HOMER2/CUPIDIN (MIM604799), and HOMER3 (MIM604800). Like HOMER2, members 1 and 3 of the family have long and short isoforms due to alternative splicing [7]. HOMER family members are scaffolding proteins that play a key role in Ca^{2+} signaling [8–10], mostly at the Post-Synaptic-Densities (PSD) [11], where they interact with G-protein coupled metabotropic glutamate receptors (mGluRs) [12] and regulate excitatory signal transduction and receptor plasticity [7]. In their structure, HOMER proteins present a conserved N-terminal domain known as Enabled/vasodilator-stimulated phosphoprotein (Ena/VASP) homology 1 (EVH1) domain [7,13] that binds to proline-rich sequences (i.e. Pro-Pro-x-x-Phe, Pro-x-x-Phe or Leu-Pro-Ser-Ser-Pro, where x represents any amino acid) and a C-terminal domain that consists of a coiled-coil (CC) structure that includes a CDC42 binding domain (CBD) and two Leucine Zipper (LZA and LZB) motifs [7,14]. This C-terminal fragment mediates self-association with other Homer family members [7] and the interaction with the small GTPase CDC42 [15] through its CBD.

In mice, *Homer2* is widespread in the developing and maturing brain [16]. Recently, a study has shown that this gene is also expressed in a wide variety of developing tissues, including tooth, eye, cochlea, salivary glands, olfactory and respiratory mucosae, bone, and taste buds, being highly concentrated at puncta [17]. HOMER2 exhibits overlapping distribution patterns with HOMER1 and HOMER3, although they are distributed at distinct subcellular domains in several cell types [17,18]. Within the inner ear, HOMER2 is expressed in the stria vascularis, the Reissner's membrane, and the inner and outer hair cells of the organ of Corti, especially in the stereocilia but also in perinuclear puncta and the cytoplasm [17,18]. Mild expression is observed in the vascular endothelium of the cochlea and the spiral ganglion [12]. Mice homozygous for the targeted deletion of *Homer2* display early-onset rapidly progressive hearing loss [18].

HOMER2 was firstly associated with hearing loss by Azaiez et al. [18] who identified a heterozygous missense variant (p.Arg196Pro) in a European ascent family. A second mutation in *HOMER2* (c.840_840dup; p.Met281Hisfs*9) was identified by Lu et al. [19] by Whole Exome Sequencing (WES) in a Chinese family segregating with hearing loss. Here, we present a third variant in *HOMER2* (c.832_836delCCTCA, p.Pro278Alafs*10, NM_199330.3). This variant represents the second truncating mutation that affects the CBD and lead, as in the previous two families, to post-lingual and progressive hearing loss. This mutation is the first one identified in the Spanish population, thus increasing the mutational spectrum of this gene associated with DFNA68, a rare form of autosomal dominant nonsyndromic progressive hearing loss.

2. Patients and Methods

2.1. Patients Selection

Patients and healthy relatives of family S1074 (Figure 1A) were recruited from the University Hospital Ramón y Cajal (Madrid-Spain). Clinical history ruled out environmental factors as the cause of the hearing loss in the probands, and physical examination did not reveal any evidence of syndromic features. No other clinically significant manifestations, including balance or visual problems, were reported by any of the affected individuals. The hearing level was evaluated through pure tone audiometry. Air conduction thresholds were determined at frequencies ranging from 250 to 8000 Hz according to standard protocols. This study was designed in compliance with the tenets of the Helsinki Declaration, and patient enrolment was approved by the ethics committee and the human research Institutional Review Boards of Hospital Ramón y Cajal (IRB number: 288-17). All participants of the family approved of the study and signed the Informed Consent.

2.2. Sample Collection

A peripheral blood sample from each subject of the family S1074 enrolled in the study was collected by venipuncture in 5 mM EDTA tubes and genomic DNA was extracted using Chemagen MSM I (Magnetic Separation Module I, PerkinElmer, Massachusetts, MA, USA) according to the manufacturer's instructions. DNA was quantified by the fluorometric method Qubit 3.0 Fluorometer (Thermo Fisher Scientific, Massachusetts, MA, USA).

2.3. Targeted Next-Generation Sequencing

The index case of the family (II:2) was subjected for the genetic screening for causative hearing-loss mutations by using a custom gene panel, OTO-NGS-v2, designed in our laboratory [20]. As the causative mutation was identified following this approach, whole exome sequencing (WES) on the individual II:2 was not further performed. OTO-NGS-v2 is based on IDT probes capture system that included 117 genes associated with NSSNHL. Sequencing of captured enriched-libraries was done on the Illumina MiSeq (Illumina, Inc., San Diego, CA, USA). The sequence data were mapped against the human genome sequence (build GRCh37/hg19), and data analysis was performed using the Sophia Genetics' software that enables the single nucleotide variations (SNVs) and the copy number variation (CNV) analysis of the targeted exonic sequences. Variant prioritization was carried out using a custom filtering strategy [20].

2.4. Sanger Sequencing

The c.832_836delCCTCA mutation in exon 8 of *HOMER2* [NM_199330.3, long transcript] was verified by Sanger sequencing (Figure 1B). Briefly, a forward and a reverse oligonucleotide were designed for amplification of exon 8 (F-oligo 5′-CGTGCACACATTGGTGATTT-3′ and R-oligo 5′-AAGCAGGAAAATGAGTACCATGA-3′) followed by Sanger sequencing using the BigDye™ Terminator v3.1 Cycle Sequencing Kit (Applied Biosystems, Foster City, CA, USA) according to manufacturer's directions in an ABI 3730S sequencer (Perkin Elmer, Waltham, MA, USA). The specificity of the primers designed for the amplification and Sanger sequencing of exon 8 of *HOMER2* was confirmed by BlastN (https://blast.ncbi.nlm.nih.gov/; access date: 9 March 2021). We obtained a unique blast hit for the amplimer at chromosome 15 (NC_000015.10; coordinates 82,851,291 to 82,851,310) within the *HOMER2* genomic region. Segregation analysis was performed by checking the presence of the c.832_836delCCTCA mutation in all the affected and unaffected family members.

3. Results

3.1. Clinical Description of the Family

The clinical history and audiological assessments of the affected members reported a post-lingual bilateral progressive hearing loss consistent with an autosomal dominant inheritance pattern (Figure 1A). Individuals II:2 (8 years old) and II:3 (15 years old) exhibited moderate hearing loss with greater impact on the high frequencies (downsloping profile). Their mother (patient I:2, 39 years old) showed a more severe phenotype, displaying profound hearing loss at frequencies higher than 2000 Hz. The father (I:1, 44 years old) and his healthy son (II:1, 11 years old) showed normal hearing thresholds (Figure 1C) at the time of the study.

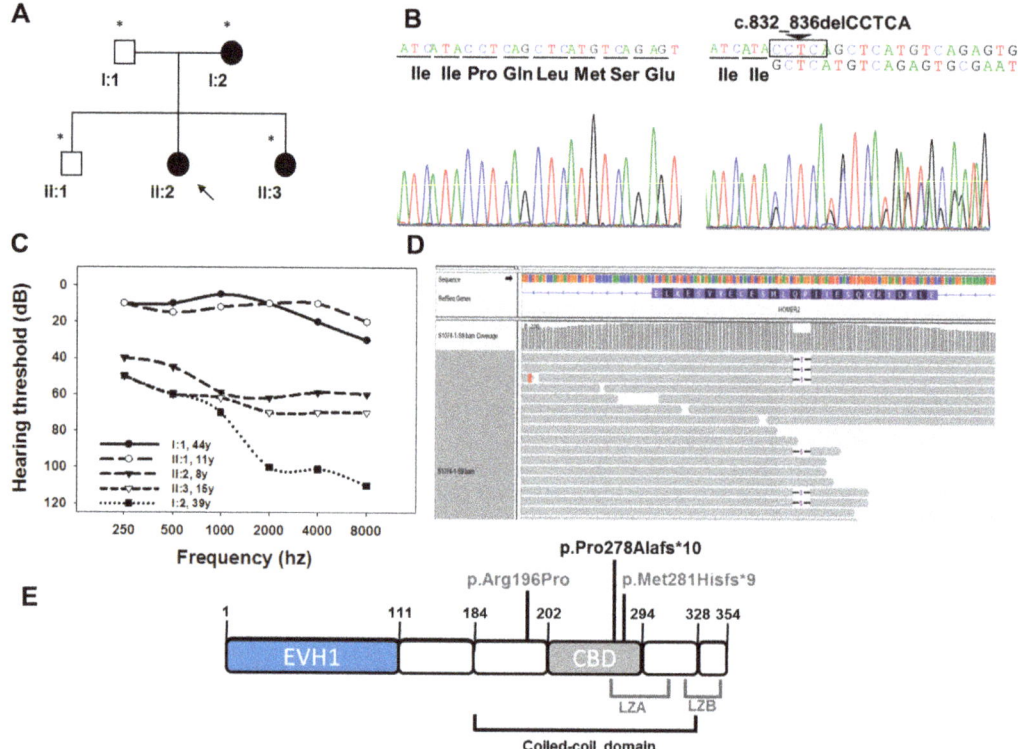

Figure 1. (**A**) Pedigree of the S1074 family indicating the segregation of c.832_836delCCTCA mutation in *HOMER2*. Black symbols indicate affected patients (carrying the mutation in heterozygosis), and white symbols correspond to normal hearing individuals (wild-type for the mutation studied). The subject pointed with an arrow is the index case (studied by OTO-NGS-v2 panel), and the ones marked with an asterisk were analysed by Sanger sequencing for segregation analysis. (**B**) Electropherograms corresponding to the wild-type (left) and mutant (right) sequences of a normal hearing and an affected individual, respectively. (**C**) Audiograms of the S1074 family. The data represented correspond to the average of the audiometric thresholds in both ears. (**D**) Integrative Genomics Viewer (IGV) (Broad Institute) screenshot showing the genomic region corresponding to the c.832_836delCCTCA mutation of *HOMER2* and the translated protein stretch corresponding to exon 8 in the reverse orientation (NP_955362.1, HOMER2 long isoform, amino acid range 292–266), as *HOMER2* is transcribed by using the DNA negative strand. (**E**) Schematic representation of the structure of HOMER2 long isoform (NP_955362.1). The different domains [7,14,21] and the mutations identified so far associated with hearing loss (in grey) are shown. The mutation identified in this work is shown in black. EVH1 (1–111 aa): Enabled/vasodilator-stimulated phosphoprotein (Ena/VASP) homology 1; Coiled-coil domain (184–328 aa); CBD (202–294 aa): CDC42-binding domain. LZA (249–307 aa): Leucine Zipper-A; LZB (322–350 aa): Leucine Zipper-B.

3.2. Genetic Study

By using the OTO-NGS-v2 panel and Sophia DMM software 338 heterozygous genetic variants were retained in the index case (II:2) of the family, 10 of which were classified as potentially pathogenic in *HOMER2*, *MYO7A*, *TMPRSS3*, *COL11A2*, *GPSM2*, *BDP1*, *EPS8*, *EPS8L2*, *OSBPL2*, and *PCDH15* genes, respectively (Table 1). During the tertiary analysis, 9 variants were discarded. Two of them showed high population frequencies in the Genome Aggregation Database (GnomAD) and were classified as benign variants in ClinVar (*MYO7A*, *COL11A2*). The other 6 variants were associated with recessive forms of deafness (*TMPRSS3*, *GPSM2*, *BDP1*, *EPS8*, *EPS8L2*, and *PCDH15*). The variant c.747A>G (rs1309059934) in *OSBPL2* (DFNA67) was classified by Sophia DMM as potentially pathogenic. However, it resulted in a synonymous protein change (p.Arg249Arg) that was classified as likely benign (BP4, BP7, and PM2) according to the American College of Medical Genetics and Genomics (ACMG) guidelines [22,23]. Furthermore, we confirmed by Sanger sequencing that this mutation did not segregate with the hearing loss in the family as it was detected in the normal-hearing subject II:I.

Finally, a novel mutation in *HOMER2* gene, c.832_836delCCTCA, was identified in the *propositus* of the S1074 family (patient II:2). This variant was identified at exon 8 of *HOMER2* and is supposed to alter the two transcript variants with known reported expression (NM_004839.4, short transcript, and NM_199330.3, long transcript). The variant leads to a frameshift generating a premature stop codon that in the absence of nonsense-mediated decay (NMD) may produce a truncated HOMER2 protein (p.Pro278Alafs*10). This mutation was classified as pathogenic (PVS1, PM2 and PP3) according to the ACMG guidelines [22,23]. The variant was not present in the GnomAD [24], in the Collaborative Spanish Variant Server-CSVS database [25] nor in the Deafness Variation Database (DVD, http://deafnessvariationdatabase.org/; access date: 9 March 2021;) [26,27]. Additionally, we confirmed by Sanger sequencing (Figure 1B) it segregated with the hearing loss in the family. The novel *HOMER2* variant c.832_836delCCTCA has been deposited in ClinVar (accession# SCV001499845). Comparison of the genetic and clinical data of the S1074 family with previously reported cases is made in Table 2.

4. Discussion

Hearing loss caused by *HOMER2* mutations is an extremely rare disorder. In this study, we have used OTO-NGS-v2, a custom targeted NGS panel, for the identification of a novel mutation (c.832_836delCCTCA; p.Pro278Alafs*10) in this gene linked to DFNA68 hearing loss. To date, only two different mutations in *HOMER2* have been documented to cause hearing loss. The first mutation was a missense substitution (c.587G>C; p.Arg196Pro; NM_199330.3) that affects a highly conserved residue in the coiled-coil (CC) structure, a region that is required for homo/hetero-multimerization to form tetrameric hubs (in which the CC domains align in a parallel fashion) and for interaction through the CBD with Rho family GTPase proteins like CDC42, a GTPase that mediates actin-turnover [28] and is responsible for planar polarity establishment in hair cells [29,30]. Functional assessment of the p.Arg196Pro in zebrafish strongly suggests that this mutation exerts its effect through a dominant-negative mechanism on wild-type protein by either inhibiting multimerization or competing for partner proteins [18]. The second mutation, c.840_840dup, p.Met281Hisfs*9 (NM_199330.3) was identified in a Chinese family with symmetric ADSNHL [19]. This frameshift variant at the CDC42-binding domain leads to the generation of a premature stop codon supposed to produce a truncated HOMER2 protein of 288 amino acids, with an aberrant protein tail of 8 amino acids from position 281 onwards.

In this work, we have identified a novel frameshift mutation, c.832_836delCCTCA, p.Pro278Alafs*10 in *HOMER2* that represents the second truncating mutation identified in the CDC42-binding domain. The Spanish mutation also creates a premature stop codon that may lead to generate a truncated shorter protein of 286 amino acids with an aberrant tail of 9 amino acids from position 278, thus lacking the canonical C-terminal end. Interestingly, the alignment of both truncated proteins revealed an identical sequence of the last 8 amino acids of the aberrant tails (Figure 2).

Table 1. Genetic variants with potential pathogenicity identified by SOPHIA DDM software in the index case (II:2) of family S1074.

Gene Transcript	Exon	cDNA and Protein Alteration	Variant Fraction Coverage (Ref/Alt)	Coding Consequence	Pathogenicity Prediction by SOPHIA DDM	ACMG	ClinVar Rating	GnomAD	Locus
HOMER2 NM_199330	8	c.832_836delCCTCA p.Pro278Alafs*10	34.98% (145/78)	frameshift	Highly Pathogenic	Pathogenic (PVS1, PM2, PP3)	-	0	DFNA68
MYO7A NM_001127179	27	c.3515_3536del p.Gly1172*1179del	49.0% (582/306)	No-stop	Highly Pathogenic	Benign (PVS1, BA1, BS2, BP6)	Benign rs111033223	0.391	DFNA11 DFNB2
TMPRSS3 NM_001256317	8	c.617-3_617-2dupTA p.?	46.73% (421/372)	Splice acceptor	Highly Pathogenic	(PVS1, PP3, BA1, BP6)	Benign rs34966432	0.118	DFNB8 DFNB10
COL11A2 NM_080679	32	c.2307+3G>A p.?	50.43% (402/409)	splice_donor_+3	Potentially Pathogenic	Benign (BA1, BS2)	Benign rs970901	0.601	DFNA13 DFNB53
GPSM2 NM_013296	13	c.1572_1574delTTC p.Ser525del	48.55% (278/267)	inframe_3	Potentially Pathogenic	Benign(PP3, BA1, BP3, BP6)	Benign rs35029887	0.291	DFNB82
BDP1 NM_018429	23	c.5068G>C p.Gly1690Arg	44.54% (335/269)	missense	Potentially Pathogenic	Likely Benign (PM2, BP1, BP4)	rs193135814	7.48×10^{-5}	DFNB112
EPS8 NM_004447	20	c.2230G>A p.Val744Ile	44.34% (359/286)	missense	Potentially Pathogenic	Benign (BS1, BS2, BP1, BP6)	Likely Benign rs77967764	2.06×10^{-3}	DFNB102
EPS8L2 NM_022772	9	c.710C>T p.Arg237Leu	50.22% (560/565)	missense	Potentially Pathogenic	VUS (PM2, BP4)	-	7.1×10^{-6}	DFNB106
OSBPL2 NM_014835	9	c.747A>G p.Arg249Arg	51.09% (157/164)	synonymous	Potentially Pathogenic	Likely Benign (BP4, BP7, PM2)	Benign rs1309059934	0	DFNA67
PCDH15 NM_001142771	21	c.2596G>A p.Val866Met	49.09% (446/430)	missense	Potentially Pathogenic	VUS (PM1, PM2)	Uncertain Significance rs142512524	6.37×10^{-4}	DFNB23

Table 2. Clinical data and classification of the different variants described in *HOMER2* causing hearing loss.

DNA Change	Protein Change	Exon	Origin	Phenotype	Detection Decade	Degree	Audiogram Profile	ACMG Classification	Number of Scores Supporting Pathogenicity	Pathogenicity	DVD	CSVS Allele Freq	GnomAD Allele Freq.	References
c.587G>C	p.Arg196Pro	6	European descent	SNHL	1st	Mild-profound	Down-sloping	Uncertain significance (PM2, PP3, PP5, BP1)	20/22	Pathogenic	N.A	0	0	Azaiez et al. 2015
c.840_840dup	p.(Met281Hisfs*9)	8	Chinese	SNHL	1st	Moderate-profound	Down-sloping	Pathogenic (PVS1, PM2, PP3, PP5)	N.A	N.A	N.A	0	0	Lu et al. 2018
c.832_836delCCTCA	p.(Pro278Alafs*10)	8	Spanish	SNHL	1st	Moderate-profound	Down-sloping	Pathogenic (PVS1, PM2, PP3)	N.A	N.A	N.A	0	0	This work

All the variants are named according to NM_199330.3 long transcript and the nomenclature was checked using Mutalyzer 2.0.32. ACMG criteria [22,23]: PVS1 (Pathogenic Very Strong): null variant (nonsense, frameshift, canonical ±1 or 2 splice sites, initiation codon, single or multiexon deletion) in a gene where LOF is a known mechanism of disease. PM2 (Pathogenic Moderate 2): absent from controls (or at extremely low frequency if recessive) in Exome Sequencing Project, 1000 Genomes Project, or Exome Aggregation Consortium. PP3 (Pathogenic Supporting 3): multiple lines of computational evidence support a deleterious effect on the gene or gene product (conservation, evolutionary, splicing impact, etc.). PP5 (Pathogenic Supporting 5): reputable source recently reports variant as pathogenic, but the evidence is not available to the laboratory to perform an independent evaluation. BP1 (Benign Supporting 1): missense variant in a gene for which primarily truncating variants are known to cause disease. The databases GnomAD [24], CSVS [25], and Deafness Variation Database (DVD) [26] were searched on the 20th December 2020. SNHL: sensorineural hearing loss, NA: not available.

```
Wt human HOMER2      266  ELKDLRKQSEIIPQLMSECEYVSEKLE  292
                          |||||||||||||||........
p.Met281Hisfs*9      266  ELKDLRKQSEIIPQLHVRVRICL      288
                          |||||||||||| .|||||||||
p.Pro278Alafs*10     266  ELKDLRKQSEII--AHVRVRICL      286
```

Figure 2. Alignment of the wild-type protein fragment encoded by exon 8 of *HOMER2* long isoform (NP_955362.1) and the truncating mutations in the CDC42-binding domain (CBD) identified in the Chinese (p.Met281Hisfs*9) and Spanish (p.Pro278Alafs*10) families. The amino acid sequence shared between both aberrant protein tails is shown in bold face.

Based on the similar effect that the two different frameshift mutations may cause at the protein level, both supposed to truncate the protein at the CDB and resulting in the same aberrant tail, it might be reasonable to suggest that the Chinese and Spanish mutations may share a similar mechanism of pathogenesis. Lu et al. demonstrated that the p.Met281Hisfs*9 mutant protein was less stable than the wild-type protein and it showed an altered subcellular localization in HEK293T and HEI-OC1 cells. Whereas the wild-type proteins were mainly aggregated near the nucleus, the p.Met281Hisfs*9 mutants were more widely distributed throughout the cytoplasm. Furthermore, these authors demonstrated that p.Met281Hisfs*9 showed a decreased ability to oligomerize [19]. It has also been postulated that HOMER2 could play an important role in maintaining stereocilia through its interaction with CDC42 [19], therefore the truncation of HOMER2 in the CBD could eventually prevent its interaction with other HOMER protein family members and with other proteins like CDC42. Indeed, targeted deletion of Cdc42 in murine hair cells causes a progressive hearing loss phenotype that is comparable to the hearing loss phenotype in the Spanish and Chinese families [19]. Another possibility is that the *HOMER2* mutation identified in this study may cause nonsense-mediated decay (NMD), a mechanism that affects the processing of the transcripts at different extent depending on the type of mutation and gene involved as previously reported in other pathologies like Neurofibromatosis I [31]. In this regard, and in contrast to mouse mutants homozygous for the targeted deletion of *Homer2* that display early-onset rapidly progressive hearing loss, mice heterozygous for the targeted deletion of exon 3 in *Homer2* (*Homer*$^{-/+}$) displayed normal hearing levels [18]. It may indicate that a moderate or even low extent NMD might be associated with *HOMER2* frameshift mutations thus suggesting that the pathophysiology of the DFNA68 hearing loss in the Spanish and Chinese families would not be mediated by haploinsufficiency, but by a gain-of-function of the Ct aberrant tail or by a dominant-negative mechanism as it has been postulated for the p.Arg196Pro missense mutation [18]. However, more experiments to detect *HOMER2* mutant transcripts levels by using a gene-editing tool to mimic actual mutation in cell lines or the generation of knock-in murine models are necessary to fully understand the underlying mechanism of pathogenesis linked to DFNA68 frameshift mutations.

Regarding the clinical phenotype, the hearing loss observed in *HOMER2* patients caused by the missense (p.Arg196Pro) and two truncating mutations seems to be quite similar in the three studied families. Affected individuals show progressive hearing loss affecting mainly the high frequencies (downsloping profile) with a typical onset in the first decade of life (7–9 years old), although a more severe phenotype was detected in patients bearing the truncating mutations when age-matched hearing-impaired subjects of the three families were compared. For individuals in a similar age-range, those carrying the missense p.Arg196Pro mutation [18] displayed minor affectation on the entire range of frequencies (i.e., subject IV:2, 8y.o, IV:10, 15y.o, and III:4, 34y.o, European ascent family) than patients carrying the p.Met281Hisfs*9 (subject IV:7, 7y.o; III:10, 34y.o, and III:8, 39y.o in the Chinese family) or the p.Pro278Alafs*10 variant (subject II:2, 8y.o; II:3, 15y.o, and I:2, 39y.o in the Spanish family). The presence of tinnitus or cranial tinnitus, however, has only been displayed by some affected members of the Chinese family and this phenotype was not present in any of the other two families. The identification of other *HOMER2* cases is, therefore, necessary to further establish more accurate genotype–phenotype correlations.

In summary, we have identified a third variant in *HOMER2*; the first one reported in the Spanish population, thus contributing to expanding the mutational spectrum of this gene in other populations. Our study also highlights the importance of using NGS-based diagnostic methods to identify mutations in low-prevalence deafness genes like *HOMER2*, thus helping to improve our knowledge about the pathophysiology of DFNA68 and to define more accurate genotype–phenotype correlations in this disorder.

Author Contributions: Conceptualization, M.M. and M.Á.M.-P.; Data curation, M.L., M.V. and I.d.C.; Formal analysis, M.L. and M.M.; Funding acquisition, M.Á.M.-P.; Methodology, M.M.; Supervision, M.Á.M.-P.; Writing—original draft, M.L., M.M. and M.Á.M.-P. All authors have read and agreed to the published version of the manuscript.

Funding: This research was supported by grants from the Spanish Institute of Health Carlos III (ISCIII) cofunded with the European Regional Development Fund (ERDF) within the "Plan Estatal de Investigación Científica y Técnica y de Innovación 2017–2020" (PI14-948, PI17-1659 and PI20/0429 to MAMP), the Spanish Center for Biomedical Network Research on Rare Diseases (CIBERER, 06/07/0036 grant, to MAMP) and by the Regional Government of Madrid (CAM, B2017/ BMD3721 grant to MAMP).

Institutional Review Board Statement: The study was conducted according to the guidelines of the Declaration of Helsinki, and approved by the Institutional Review Board (or Ethics Committee) of Hospital Ramón y Cajal (protocol code 288-17; 29 January 2018).

Informed Consent Statement: Informed consent was obtained from all subjects involved in the study.

Data Availability Statement: The data presented in this study are openly available in ClinVar (accession# SCV001499845).

Acknowledgments: The authors sincerely thank the family for their participation in this study.

Conflicts of Interest: The authors declare no conflict of interest. The funders had no role in the design of the study; in the collection, analyses, or interpretation of data; in the writing of the manuscript, or in the decision to publish the results.

References

1. Petit, C.; Levilliers, J.; Hardelin, J.P. Molecular genetics of hearing loss. *Annu. Rev. Genet.* **2001**, *35*, 589–646. [CrossRef]
2. Morton, C.C.; Nance, W.E. Newborn hearing screening-a silent revolution. *N. Engl. J. Med.* **2006**, *354*, 2151–2164. [CrossRef]
3. Van Camp, G.; Smith, R.J. Hereditary Hearing Loss Homepage. Available online: https://hereditaryhearingloss.org (accessed on 20 December 2020).
4. Hilgert, N.; Smith, R.J.; Van Camp, G. Function and expression pattern of nonsyndromic deafness genes. *Curr. Mol. Med.* **2009**, *9*, 546–564. [CrossRef]
5. Mencía, A.; Modamio-Høybjør, S.; Redshaw, N.; Morín, M.; Mayo-Merino, F.; Olavarrieta, L.; Aguirre, L.A.; del Castillo, I.; Steel, K.P.; Dalmay, T.; et al. Mutations in the seed region of human miR-96 are responsible for nonsyndromic progressive hearing loss. *Nat. Genet.* **2009**, *41*, 609–613. [CrossRef] [PubMed]
6. Norton, N.; Williams, H.J.; Williams, N.M.; Spurlock, G.; Zammit, S.; Jones, G.; Jones, S.; Owen, R.; O'Donovan, M.C.; Owen, M.J. Mutation screening of the Homer gene family and association analysis in schizophrenia. *Am. J. Med. Genet. B Neuropsychiatr. Genet.* **2003**, *120*, 18–21. [CrossRef]
7. Shiraishi-Yamaguchi, Y.; Furuichi, T. The Homer family proteins. *Genome Biol.* **2007**, *8*, 206. [CrossRef]
8. Worley, P.F.; Worley, P.F.; Zeng, W.; Huang, G.; Kim, J.Y.; Shin, D.M.; Kim, M.S.; Yuan, J.P.; Kiselyov, K.; Muallem, S. Homer proteins in Ca^{2+} signaling by excitable and non-excitable cells. *Cell Calcium* **2007**, *42*, 363–371. [CrossRef] [PubMed]
9. Yang, Y.M.; Lee, J.; Jo, H.; Park, S.; Chang, I.; Muallem, S.; Shin, D.S. Homer2 protein regulates plasma membrane Ca^{2+}-ATPase-mediated Ca^{2+} signaling in mouse parotid gland acinar cells. *J. Biol. Chem.* **2014**, *289*, 24971–24979. [CrossRef] [PubMed]
10. Jardin, I.; López, J.J.; Berna-Erro, A.; Salido, G.M.; Rosado, J.A. Homer proteins in Ca^{2+} entry. *IUBMB Life* **2013**, *65*, 497–504. [CrossRef] [PubMed]
11. Tao-Cheng, J.H.; Thein, S.; Yang, Y.; Reese, T.S.; Gallant, P.E. Homer is concentrated at the postsynaptic density and does not redistribute after acute synaptic stimulation. *Neuroscience* **2014**, *266*, 80–90. [CrossRef]
12. Kato, A.; Ozawa, F.; Saitoh, Y.; Fukazawa, Y.; Sugiyama, H.; Inokuchi, K. Novel members of the Vesl/Homer family of PDZ proteins that bind metabotropic glutamate receptors. *J. Biol. Chem.* **1998**, *273*, 23969–23975. [CrossRef] [PubMed]

3. Barzik, M.; Carl, U.D.; Schubert, W.D.; Frank, R.; Wehland, J.; Heinz, D.W. The N-terminal domain of Homer/Vesl is a new class II EVH1 domain. *J. Mol. Biol.* **2001**, *309*, 155–169. [CrossRef] [PubMed]
4. Sun, J.; Tadokoro, S.; Imanaka, T.; Murakami, S.D.; Nakamura, M.; Kashiwada, K.; Ko, J.; Nishida, W.; Sobue, K. Isolation of PSD-Zip45, a novel Homer/vesl family protein containing leucine zipper motifs, from rat brain. *FEBS Lett.* **1998**, *437*, 304–308. [CrossRef]
5. Shiraishi, Y.; Mizutani, A.; Bito, H.; Fujisawa, K.; Narumiya, S.; Mikoshiba, K.; Furuichi, T. Cupidin, an isoform of Homer/Vesl, interacts with the actin cytoskeleton and activated rho family small GTPases and is expressed in developing mouse cerebellar granule cells. *J. Neurosci.* **1999**, *19*, 8389–8400. [CrossRef] [PubMed]
6. Shiraishi, Y.; Mizutani, A.; Yuasa, S.; Mikoshiba, K.; Furuichi, T. Differential expression of Homer family proteins in the developing mouse brain. *J. Comp. Neurol.* **2004**, *473*, 582–599. [CrossRef] [PubMed]
7. Reibring, C.G.; Hallberg, K.; Linde, A.; Gritli-Linde, A.G. Distinct and Overlapping Expression Patterns of the Homer Family of Scaffolding Proteins and Their Encoding Genes in Developing Murine Cephalic Tissues. *Int. J. Mol. Sci.* **2020**, *21*, 1264. [CrossRef]
8. Azaiez, H.; Decker, A.R.; Booth, K.T.; Simpson, A.C.; Shearer, A.E.; Huygen, P.L.M.; Bu, F.; Hildebrand, M.S.; Ranum, P.T.; Shibata, S.B.; et al. HOMER2, a stereociliary scaffolding protein, is essential for normal hearing in humans and mice. *PLoS Genet.* **2015**, *11*, e1005137. [CrossRef] [PubMed]
9. Lu, X.; Wang, Q.; Gu, H.; Zhang, X.; Qi, Y.; Liu, Y. Whole exome sequencing identified a second pathogenic variant in HOMER2 for autosomal dominant nonsyndromic deafness. *Clin. Genet.* **2018**, *94*, 419–428. [CrossRef]
10. Morín, M.; Borreguero, L.; Booth, K.T.; Lachgar, M.; Huygen, P.; Villamar, M.; Mayo, F.; Barrio, L.C.; Santos Serrão de Castro, L.; Morales, M.; et al. Insights into the pathophysiology of DFNA10 hearing loss associated with novel EYA4 variants. *Sci. Rep.* **2020**, *10*, 6213. [CrossRef]
11. Shiraishi, Y.; Sato, Y.; Sakai, R.; Mizutani, A.; Knöpfel, T.; Mori, N.; Mikoshiba, K.; Furuichi, T. Interaction of Cupidin/Homer2 with two actin cytoskeletal regulators, Cdc42 small GTPase and Drebrin, in dendritic spines. *BMC Neurosci.* **2009**, *10*, 25.
12. Richards, S.; Aziz, N.; Bale, S.; Bick, D.; Das, S.; Gastier-Foster, J.; Grody, W.W.; Hegde, M.; Lyon, E.; Spector, E.; et al. Standards and guidelines for the interpretation of sequence variants: A joint consensus recommendation of the American College of Medical Genetics and Genomics and the Association for Molecular Pathology. *Genet. Med.* **2015**, *17*, 405–424. [CrossRef] [PubMed]
13. Kopanos, C.; Tsiolkas, V.; Kouris, A.; Chapple, C.E.; Albarca Aguilera, M.; Meyer, R.; Massouras, A. VarSome: The human genomic variant search engine. *Bioinformatics* **2019**, *35*, 1978–1980. [CrossRef]
14. Karczewski, K.J.; Francioli, L.C.; Tiao, G.; Cummings, B.B.; Alföldi, J.; Wang, Q.; Collins, R.L.; Laricchia, K.M.; Ganna, A.; Birnbaum, D.P.; et al. The mutational constraint spectrum quantified from variation in 141,456 humans. *Nature* **2020**, *581*, 434–443. [CrossRef]
15. Peña-Chilet, M.; Roldán, G.; Perez-Florido, J.; Ortuño, J.M.; Carmona, R.; Aquino, V.; Lopez-Lopez, D.; Loucera, C.; Fernandez-Rueda, J.L.; Gallego, A.; et al. CSVS, a crowdsourcing database of the Spanish population genetic variability. *Nucleic Acid Res.* **2020**, *49*, D1130–D1137. [CrossRef] [PubMed]
16. Azaiez, H.; Booth, K.T.; Ephraim, S.S.; Crone, B.; Black-Ziegelbein, E.A.; Marini, R.J.; Shearer, A.E.; Sloan-Heggen, C.M.; Kolbe, D.; Casavant, T.; et al. Genomic Landscape and Mutational Signatures of Deafness-Associated Genes. *Am. J. Hum. Genet.* **2018**, *103*, 484–497. [CrossRef]
17. Deafness Variation Database. Available online: http://deafnessvariationdatabase.org/ (accessed on 20 December 2020).
18. Ueyama, T.; Sakaguchi, H.; Nakamura, T.; Goto, A.; Morioka, S.; Shimizu, A.; Nakao, K.; Hishikawa, Y.; Ninoyu, Y.; Kassai, H.; et al. Maintenance of stereocilia and apical junctional complexes by Cdc42 in cochlear hair cells. *J. Cell. Sci.* **2014**, *127*, 2040–2052. [CrossRef] [PubMed]
19. Kirjavainen, A.; Laos, M.; Anttonen, T.; Pirvola, U. The Rho GTPase Cdc42 regulates hair cell planar polarity and cellular patterning in the developing cochlea. *Biol. Open* **2015**, *4*, 516–526. [CrossRef]
20. Wildeman, M.; Ophuizen, E.V.; den Dunnen, J.T.; Taschner, P.E.M. Improving sequence variant descriptions in mutation databases and literature using the Mutalyzer sequence variation nomenclature checker. *Hum. Mutat.* **2008**, *29*, 6–13. [CrossRef] [PubMed]
21. Pros, E.; Larriba, S.; López, E.; Ravella, A.; Gili, M.L.; Kruyer, H.; Valls, J.; Serra, E.; Lázaro, C. NF1 mutation rather than individual genetic variability is the main determinant of the NF1-transcriptional profile of mutations affecting splicing. *Hum. Mutat.* **2006**, *27*, 1104–1114. [CrossRef]

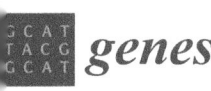

Article

Novel Pathogenic Variants in *PJVK*, the Gene Encoding Pejvakin, in Subjects with Autosomal Recessive Non-Syndromic Hearing Impairment and Auditory Neuropathy Spectrum Disorder

María Domínguez-Ruiz [1,2,†], Montserrat Rodríguez-Ballesteros [1,2,†], Marta Gandía [1,2], Elena Gómez-Rosas [1,2], Manuela Villamar [1,2], Pietro Scimemi [3,4], Patrizia Mancini [5], Nanna D. Rendtorff [6], Miguel A. Moreno-Pelayo [1,2], Lisbeth Tranebjaerg [6,7], Carme Medà [8], Rosamaria Santarelli [3,4] and Ignacio del Castillo [1,2,*]

1. Servicio de Genética, Hospital Universitario Ramón y Cajal, IRYCIS, 28034 Madrid, Spain; mdominguezr@salud.madrid.org (M.D.-R.); montserodrig@yahoo.es (M.R.-B.); martagandia04@gmail.com (M.G.); elenagomez_tel@yahoo.es (E.G.-R.); taugen.hrc@salud.madrid.org (M.V.); mmorenop@salud.madrid.org (M.A.M.-P.)
2. Centro de Investigación Biomédica en Red de Enfermedades Raras (CIBERER), 28034 Madrid, Spain
3. Department of Neurosciences, University of Padua, 35121 Padua, Italy; pietro.scimemi@unipd.it (P.S.); rosamaria.santarelli@unipd.it (R.S.)
4. Audiology Service, Santi Giovanni e Paolo Hospital, 30122 Venice, Italy
5. Department of Sense Organs, University La Sapienza, 00162 Rome, Italy; p.mancini@uniroma1.it
6. Department of Clinical Genetics, University Hospital, Copenhagen/The Kennedy Centre, DK-2600 Glostrup, Denmark; nanna.dahl.rendtorff@regionh.dk (N.D.R.); tranebjaerg@sund.ku.dk (L.T.)
7. Department of Clinical Medicine, University of Copenhagen, DK-2100 Copenhagen, Denmark
8. Unidad de Prevención de Enfermedades del Oído, Conselleria de Salut, Illes Balears, 07120 Palma de Mallorca, Spain; cmeda@dgsanita.caib.es
* Correspondence: ignacio.castillo@salud.madrid.org
† These authors have contributed equally to this work.

Abstract: Pathogenic variants in the *PJVK* gene cause the DFNB59 type of autosomal recessive non-syndromic hearing impairment (AR-NSHI). Phenotypes are not homogeneous, as a few subjects show auditory neuropathy spectrum disorder (ANSD), while others show cochlear hearing loss. The numbers of reported cases and pathogenic variants are still small to establish accurate genotype-phenotype correlations. We investigated a cohort of 77 Spanish familial cases of AR-NSHI, in whom DFNB1 had been excluded, and a cohort of 84 simplex cases with isolated ANSD in whom *OTOF* variants had been excluded. All seven exons and exon-intron boundaries of the *PJVK* gene were sequenced. We report three novel DFNB59 cases, one from the AR-NSHI cohort and two from the ANSD cohort, with stable, severe to profound NSHI. Two of the subjects received unilateral cochlear implantation, with apparent good outcomes. Our study expands the spectrum of *PJVK* mutations, as we report four novel pathogenic variants: p.Leu224Arg, p.His294Ilefs*43, p.His294Asp and p.Phe317Serfs*20. We review the reported cases of DFNB59, summarize the clinical features of this rare subtype of AR-NSHI and discuss the involvement of *PJVK* in ANSD.

Keywords: non-syndromic hearing impairment; auditory neuropathy spectrum disorder; DFNB59; *PJVK*; pejvakin; genetic epidemiology

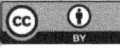

1. Introduction

Inherited hearing impairment is clinically and genetically very heterogeneous. Hearing loss can be an isolated condition (non-syndromic hearing impairment, NSHI) or it can be part of the clinical signs that are characteristic of specific genetic syndromes [1]. Over 120 genes are currently known to be involved in NSHI, and it is estimated that many more remain to be identified [2]. For most of the known genes, few affected subjects have been reported to carry causative variants, and this poor knowledge of the mutational spectra is hindering the investigation of genotype-phenotype correlations in the different genetic types of NSHI [3].

The DFNB59 type of autosomal recessive (AR) NSHI (MIM #610220) is caused by pathogenic variants in the *PJVK* gene (MIM #610219) [4], which is located on 2q31.2, spanning 9950 bp of genomic sequence. It contains seven exons and codes for pejvakin, a 352-residue protein that belongs to the gasdermin family. Six different gasdermins are known in humans (gasdermins A to E, and pejvakin) [5]. The five canonical members of the family (gasdermins A-E) contain an N-terminal membrane-permeabilizing domain, a short linker region, and a C-terminal autoinhibitory domain. Proinflammatory signals result in the separation of the two domains through caspase-mediated cleavage at the linker region, so that the N-terminal domain is released and can form pores in the plasma membrane. Depending on which gasdermin is activated, this mechanism triggers different types of programmed cell death (pyroptosis, secondary necrosis or NETosis) [6]. In contrast, pejvakin is a non-canonical gasdermin, as it lacks the cleavable linker and the C-terminal autoinhibitory domain, which is substituted by a zinc-finger domain whose function is unknown. Pejvakin has been reported to localize to the stereociliary rootlets of the inner ear hair cells, where it would be needed for stereocilia maintenance [7]. In other studies, pejvakin has been reported to be associated with peroxisomes, where it would mediate their autophagic degradation (pexophagy) as a protective mechanism against the oxidative stress that is caused by noise overexposure [8,9].

Up to 19 different variants in *PJVK* have been reported as causative of AR-NSHI in families from diverse geographic origins [4,10–26]. In a study performed on four Iranian families, three of them carrying the same homozygous variant (c.547C>T, p.Arg183Trp), the hearing impairment showed features of auditory neuropathy spectrum disorder (ANSD), i.e., abnormal or absent auditory brainstem responses but normal otoacoustic emissions [4]. This clinical feature is in accordance with the phenotype observed in a knock-in mouse model for the p.Arg183Trp variant [4]. However, ANSD was not observed in any of the few other reported DFNB59 cases in whom this condition was tested, nor in the *sirtaki* mouse, which was obtained by ENU mutagenesis and carries a nonsense variant in *Pjvk* [13]. Clarification of this controversial issue needs a better knowledge of the *PJVK* variant spectrum and the resulting phenotypes, through the investigation of large cohorts of hearing-impaired subjects, with or without ANSD.

In this study, we have screened a cohort of 77 familial cases of non-DFNB1 AR-NSHI, and a cohort of 84 subjects with isolated ANSD. We report the first European cases of DFNB59 NSHI. Five *PJVK* pathogenic variants, four of them novel, were found in three unrelated cases whose clinical characterization further illustrates the phenotypic variability of the *PJVK* type of hearing impairment.

2. Materials and Methods
2.1. Human Subjects

Two cohorts of subjects were enrolled in this study. The first cohort consisted of 140 Spanish familial cases of autosomal recessive NSHI (AR-NSHI), with at least two affected siblings and unaffected parents. Prior to this work, they were investigated by Sanger sequencing of the coding region and splice sites of the *GJB2* gene and by testing for the common del(*GJB6*-D13S1830) and del(*GJB6*-D13S1854) deletions, which revealed causative variants in 63 families. The remaining 77 families were investigated for variants in the *PJVK* gene. The second cohort consisted of 84 simplex cases (40 from Spain, 23 from Italy, 21 from Denmark) with isolated AN in whom pathogenic variants in the *OTOF* gene, encoding otoferlin, had been excluded previously. After approval by the Ethical Committee of Hospital Universitario Ramón y Cajal (in accordance with the 1964 Declaration of Helsinki), written informed consent was obtained from all participating subjects.

2.2. Clinical Tests

Hearing was evaluated by pure-tone audiometry, testing for air conduction (frequencies 250–8000 Hz) and bone conduction (frequencies 250–4000 Hz). The degree of hearing impairment was defined by the pure tone average (PTA) threshold levels at 0.5, 1, 2 and 4 kHz, and was classified as mild (21–40 dB HL), moderate (41–70 dB HL), severe (71–95 dB HL) and profound (>95 dB HL). ANSD was diagnosed on the basis of absent or grossly abnormal auditory-evoked brainstem responses (ABR) and preserved otoacoustic emissions (OAE) [27]. Speech perception tests were performed on Italian subject E1471 II:1 in the auditory-only listening condition using live-voice presentation. The speech material consisted of disyllabic words obtained from an Italian adaptation [28] of the word lists in the Northwestern University-Children's Perception of Speech (NU-CHIPs) tool [29].

2.3. DNA Purification, Genotyping and Sequencing

DNA was extracted from peripheral blood samples by using the Chemagic MSM I automated system (Chemagen, Baesweiler, Germany). Microsatellite markers D2S148, D2S2173, D2S324 and D2S2310 were amplified using fluorescently-labeled primers and PCR conditions as previously reported [30]. Amplified alleles were resolved by capillary electrophoresis in an ABI Prism 3100 Avant Genetic Analyzer (Applied Biosystems, Waltham, MA, USA). Primers and conditions for PCR amplification of all seven exons of the *PJVK* gene are shown in Table 1. Sanger DNA sequencing was performed in an ABI Prism 3100 Avant Genetic Analyzer (Applied Biosystems, Waltham, MA, USA).

Table 1. Primers and conditions for PCR amplification of all exons of *PJVK*.

Exon	Primer Sequences (5′-3′)	[MgCl$_2$]
1	F: CTAGGCCGCAGTTCTTTGTCCTTAG R: TCCCAGGCAAACGCCATTACA	2.5 mM
2	F: GCAGAGGCAGGGAATTATACAGT R: ACAAACTTTTGGCATTGTTAATCTT	2.0 mM
3	F: TGGTGAGTCATGTTGCCTTTCT R: CAACCTCAATGTTTTAAGCATTCTT	1.5 mM
4	F: CTGACTATTAGGATTGCCTTGATTT R: CAGCTCTTTCATCAGAACATTTCA	1.5 mM
5	F: TTGTTTTTGGTAGGATTATAGGAAA R: GAGAGCACATGCCCTAATGAAT	2.5 mM
6	F: TCATCACCCCATCAAACAATAA R: GAATAGAAAACCTCATGTGTTAAGC	1.5 mM
7	F: GCTGTTTGCATTATGTATTTTCA R: TGTGGCACAACTGCACCTAA	2.0 mM

F, forward; R, reverse; annealing temperature of 60 °C for all amplicons.

2.4. Assessment of Pathogenicity of DNA Variants

Pathogenicity of DNA variants was assessed according to the guidelines from the American College of Medical Genetics and Genomics and the Association for Molecular Pathology (ACMG/AMP) [31], as implemented by Varsome [32], using GRCh38 as human reference genome. Scores were subsequently modified manually to delete criterion PP2 and to take into consideration criterion PM3, as recommended in the disease-specific ACMG/AMP guidelines for hearing loss [33].

3. Results
3.1. Genetic Study

We investigated a cohort of 77 Spanish familial cases of autosomal recessive nonsyndromic hearing loss, with at least two affected siblings, in whom DFNB1 pathogenic variants had been previously excluded. Firstly, all siblings in the family and their parents were genotyped for microsatellite markers D2S148, D2S2173, D2S324 and D2S2310, closely linked to *PJVK*. In 23 families in which haplotype analysis could not exclude genetic linkage, we sequenced all exons and exon/intron boundaries of *PJVK* from one affected sibling. We found likely causative variants in Spanish family S269. The two affected brothers were compound heterozygous for the novel variants c.671T>G (p.Leu224Arg) and c.880del (p.His294Ilefs*43), whereas the father carried c.671T>G, and the mother carried c.880del (Figure 1). The family had no siblings with normal hearing.

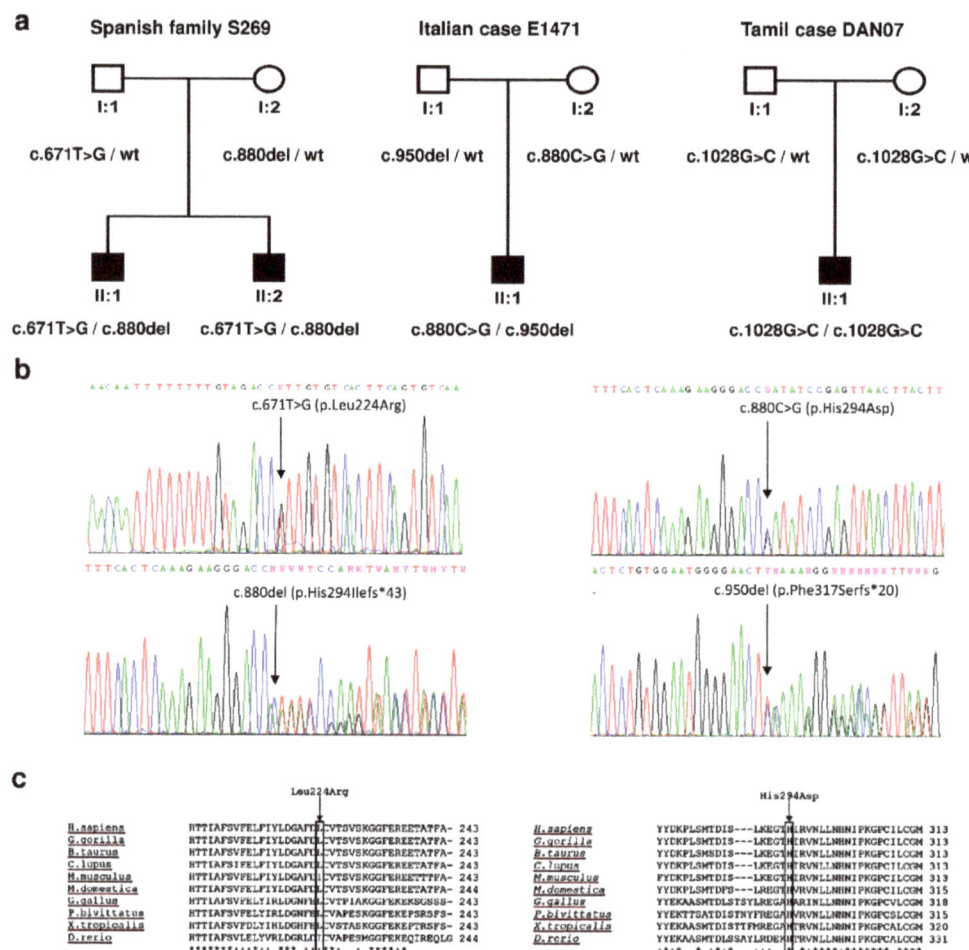

Figure 1. Novel pathogenic variants that were found in this study. (**a**) Pedigrees showing the segregation of variants. (**b**) Electropherograms from subject S269 II:1 (left panel) and from subject E1471 II:1 (right panel). (**c**) Alignment of pejvakin orthologous sequences from human and nine other vertebrates. Asterisks indicate identical residues across all sequences; colons, conserved positions (residues of strongly similar properties); periods, semi-conserved positions (residues of weakly similar properties). Sequence accesion numbers: *Homo sapiens* (NP_001036167.1); *Gorilla gorilla* (XP_004032916.1); *Bos taurus* (NP_001180112.1); *Canis lupus* (XP_535979.2); *Mus musculus* (NP_001074180.1); *Monodelphis domestica* (XP_001368857.1); *Gallus gallus* (XP_426573.2); *Python bivittatus* (XP_007337246.1); *Xenopus tropicalis* (XP_012826511.1); *Danio rerio* (XP_009300492.1).

We also screened a cohort of 84 simplex cases (40 from Spain, 23 from Italy, 21 from Denmark) with isolated ANSD in whom pathogenic variants in the *OTOF* gene, encoding otoferlin, had been excluded previously. All exons and exon/intron boundaries of the *PJVK* gene were sequenced in every case. We found likely causative variants in two unrelated subjects, who had no siblings with normal hearing. Italian subject E1471-1 was compound heterozygous for the novel variants c.880C>G (p.His294Asp) and c.950del (p.Phe317Serfs*20). His father carried c.950del, and his mother c.880C>G. Subject DAN7-1, from the cohort recruited in Denmark but of Tamil ethnic origin, was homozygous for the previously reported c.1028G>C (p.Cys343Ser) variant. His parents were heterozygous carriers for this variant. Cys-343 has been shown to play a crucial role in the interaction between pejvakin and LC3B, an autophagosomal marker in the pexophagy pathway [9].

Two of the novel variants are single-base deletions that result in frame shifts, leading to truncated polypeptides or mRNA degradation by nonsense-mediated decay. The two other novel variants are missense, which affect evolutionarily conserved residues in the pejvakin polypeptide (Figure 1C). They were classified as deleterious/probably damaging according to the scores provided by SIFT and Polyphen-2 (Table 2). They segregate with the disease as expected from an autosomal recessive pattern, and each variant is in trans with a truncating variant in affected subjects (Figure 1A). They were found at very low frequencies in the Genome Aggregation Database [34]. Both variants were classified as "likely pathogenic" according to the ACMG/AMP guidelines [31,33] (Table 2). Therefore, the reported novel genotypes in cases S269 and E1471 are considered to be causative of the hearing impairment of the affected subjects.

Table 2. Assessment of pathogenicity of the novel missense variants in *PJVK*.

Variant		SIFT Score	Polyphen-2 Score	Minor Allele Frequency (MAF) [31]	ACMG Criteria	Classification
DNA	Protein					
c.671T->G	p.Leu224Arg	0.01 (deleterious)	0.959 (Probably damaging)	2×10^{-5} (global) 4×10^{-5} (Non-Finnish Europeans)	PM2 (strong), PM3 (strong), PP1 (supporting)	Likely pathogenic
c.880C>G	p.His294Asp	0.00 (deleterious)	0.981 (Probably damaging)	4×10^{-6} (global) 8×10^{-6} (Non-Finnish Europeans)	PM2 (strong), PM3 (moderate)	Likely pathogenic

3.2. Clinical Study

In Spanish family S269, the two affected brothers had not been subjected to newborn hearing screening. Subject II:1 was diagnosed with non-syndromic hearing impairment by age four years. Because of this familial history, his brother (II:2) received a similar diagnosis earlier, at age two years. Both presented with a severe hearing loss, which seems to be stable, as shown by serial pure-tone audiograms along 10 years of evolution (Figure 2a–d). Their parents had normal hearing. The two brothers were tested for otoacoustic emissions at ages six and three years, respectively, with no response bilaterally. ABR recordings were performed at these same ages, and the results were consistent with a severe hearing impairment. Computed Tomography (CT) scan of subject II:1 did not reveal any abnormal findings.

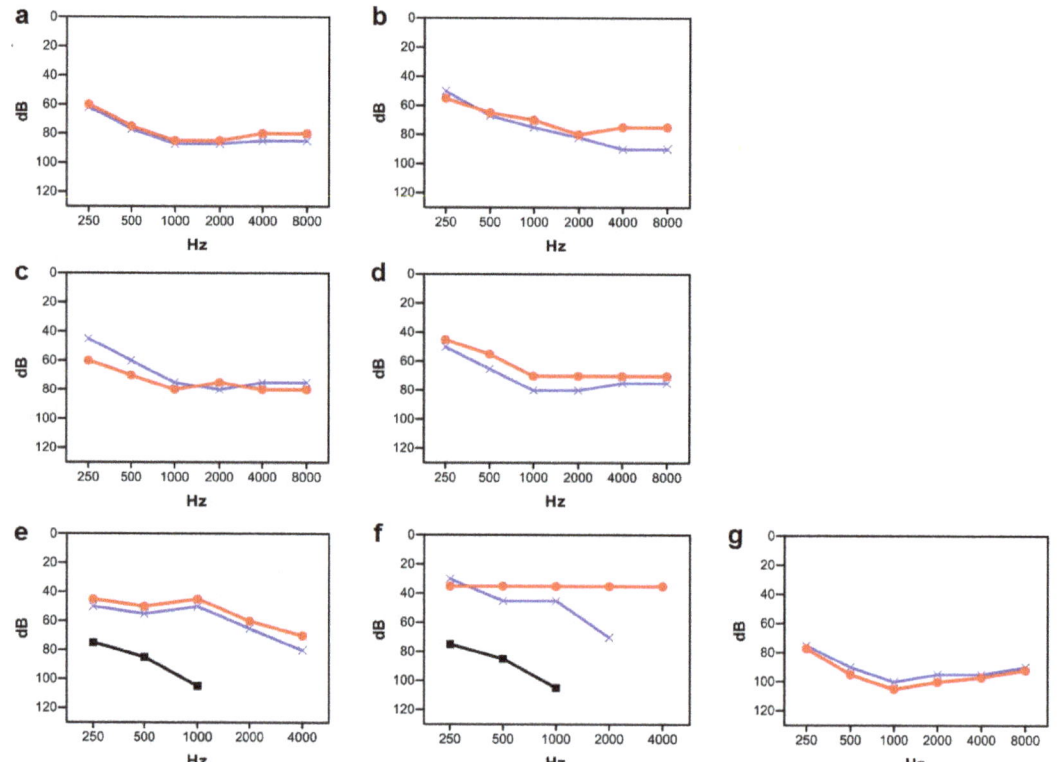

Figure 2. Audiograms from subjects with *PJVK* variants causing sensorineural hearing loss. Only results for air conduction are shown. Red line, right ear. Blue line, left ear. (**a**,**b**) Subject S269 II:1 at ages 7 yr and 14 yr, respectively. (**c**,**d**) Subject S269 II:2 at ages 5 yr and 11 yr, respectively. (**e**) Subject E1471 II:1, while using hearing aids in both ears (red and blue lines); black line, unaided hearing. (**f**) Subject E1471 II:1, while using the cochlear implant in the right ear (red line) and a hearing aid in the left ear (blue line); black line, unaided hearing. (**g**) Subject DAN07 II:1 at age 12 yr, before unilateral cochlear implantation.

In Italian case E1471, subject II:1 had normal growth and motor development, and he showed no risk factors for hearing loss. He had not been subjected to newborn hearing screening and was referred for assessment because of parental concern regarding his hearing at the age of two years. ABR recordings showed no response at the maximum stimulation intensity (90 dB nHL) while OAE were detected in both ears and disappeared thereafter. Behavioral reinforced audiometry, performed at the age of four years, indicated profound hearing loss. Pure tone average (PTA) threshold at 0.5, 1, 2 and 4 kHz measured in the free field was higher than 110 dB HL. The child was first fitted with power hearing aids, which resulted in a considerable improvement in pure tone sensitivity (Figure 2e); however, the aided thresholds were above the range of conversational speech and there was a considerable delay in development of language skills. Both CT and magnetic resonance imaging (MRI) head and ear (including internal acoustic canal) scans were normal.

At age five years, the child received a cochlear implant (MED-EL Synchrony, MED-EL, Innsbruck, Austria) in the right ear. Electrically-evoked auditory nerve responses (electrically-evoked compound action potentials, e-CAPs) were recorded through the cochlear implant. The aided thresholds, measured in the free field with the child wearing the cochlear implant (Figure 2f), fell within the estimated range of estimated conversational speech [35]. Disyllable recognition scores improved from the pre-implant value of 20% to 90% within one year of cochlear implant use.

At age nine years, the child was using the cochlear implant in the right ear and a hearing aid in the other ear. Scores of the speech perception tests were as follows: recognition of disyllabic words, in bimodal configuration and quiet environment: 85%; recognition of sentences, in bimodal configuration and quiet environment: 90%; recognition of disyllabic words, with cochlear implant only, in quiet environment: 70%. Overall, speech perception is satisfactory. In contrast, language is poorly developed for the chronological age. Indeed, scores on lexical comprehension and production would be adequate only for the age of five years (standardized tests in Italian language: Peabody, Rustioni).

Case DAN07 was recruited in Denmark, but the family is of Tamil origin. Subject II:1 was diagnosed with hearing impairment at age six months. Both CT and MRI scans were normal. ABR recordings and pure-tone audiometry revealed a profound hearing loss (Figure 2g). Electrocochleography records were abnormal and compatible with auditory neuropathy. He was initially treated with hearing aids. At age 12 years, he received a cochlear implant in the right ear, with apparent good outcomes in aided hearing thresholds, but a careful follow-up is needed to confirm this conclusion.

4. Discussion

Here we report the first European cases of DFNB59 hearing impairment, including four novel pathogenic variants that expand the mutational spectrum of *PJVK*. Both the Spanish and Italian cases had only Spanish and Italian ancestors, respectively, beyond at least three generations, which supports their European origins. Taking into account the four novel variants, 23 pathogenic variants have hitherto been reported in this gene (Table 3), all of them in cases of AR-NSHI. The list includes 15 truncating variants, seven missense variants and one in-frame deletion of a single codon. Most of the variants have been reported in the homozygous state in cases from Iran, Pakistan and Turkey (Table 4). In European populations, pathogenic *PJVK* variants seem to be a rare cause of, as observed in our study (1 case out of 140 families with AR-NSHI, i.e., 0.7%) and in previous works, which did not find any DFNB59 case in a series of cohorts from different European countries (reviewed in [36]).

Although clinical data in the literature are far from being complete (Table 4), it is possible to start delineating some clinical features of the DFNB59 AR-NSHI. Onset is prelingual in a great majority of cases, and subjects with the onset reported in early childhood are likely to reflect a delay in diagnosis because they were not subjected to newborn hearing screening (e.g., cases S269 and E1471 of this study). The evolution of the hearing impairment has been reported to be stable or progressive in equal proportions (Table 4). In most cases, the hearing loss ranges from severe to profound (Table 4). In one of the two cases in whom it is moderate, it progressed to profound over the years [13]. None of these features is associated to any specific combination of truncating or non-truncating variants.

ANSD was postulated to be a clinical feature of DFNB59 on the basis of the study of four Iranian families, in the first report of *PJVK* variants as a cause of AR-NSHI [4]. In three of the families, affected subjects were homozygous for p.Arg183Trp, and in the other one, they were homozygous for p.Thr54Ile. In 11 of 12 affected subjects (four with p.Arg183Trp, and eight with p.Thr54Ile), normal synchronized spontaneous OAE (SSOAE) were recorded (ages of subjects at testing, 12–23 years). In contrast, ABR were absent or showed thresholds higher than 80 dB in all subjects. Unfortunately, ANSD was not specifically investigated in most of the DFNB59 cases that were reported subsequently (Table 4). However, in 10 of the 12 remaining cases who were tested (one of them, case S269 in this study), normal OAE could not be recorded. In case E1471 (this work), OAE were recorded at an early age and they disappeared thereafter. Of note, all cases with a diagnosis of ANSD share the feature of carrying at least one allele with a missense variant [4], this work. This would suggest that ANSD could be associated with specific non-truncating variants. However, cases without

ANSD have been reported with the same genotypes (p.Arg183Trp or p.Cys343Ser in the homozygous state) as cases with ANSD.

Table 3. Pathogenic variants reported to date in *PJVK* (NM_001042702.3).

Exon	DNA Level	Protein Level	Reference
2	c.113dup	p.Lys41Glufs*8	[11,26]
2	c.122del	p.Lys41Serfs*18	[13,16]
2	c.147T>A	p.Tyr49*	[23]
2	c.158C>G	p.Ser53*	[24]
2	c.161C>T	p.Thr54Ile	[4]
2	c.162_172del	p.Pro55fs*23	[24]
intron 2	c.211+1G>T		[18]
3	c.274C>T	p.Arg92*	[16,18]
3	c.406C>T	p.Arg136*	[14,15,24,26]
4	c.485G>A	p.Ser162Asn	[25]
4	c.499C>T	p.Arg167*	[12,18,20]
4	c.547C>T	p.Arg183Trp	[4,12,21,22]
6	c.671T>G	p.Leu224Arg	This work
6	c.726del	p.Phe242Leufs*7	[10]
6	deletion of whole exon		[18]
7	c.880del	p.His294Ilefs*43	This work
7	c.880C>G	p.His294Asp	This work
7	c.908_910del	p.Asn303del	[24]
7	c.930_931del	p.Cys312Trpfs*19	[19]
7	c.950del	p.Phe317Serfs*20	This work
7	c.970G>T	p.Gly324Trp	[18]
7	c.988del	p.Val330Leufs*7	[10]
7	c.1028G>C	p.Cys343Ser	[17], This work

Murine models do not shed light on this issue, as they reproduce the situation that has been observed in humans. A knock-in mouse model for the p.Arg183Trp variant in *PJVK* shows ANSD [4]. However, OAE records were abnormal in the *sirtaki* mouse, which carries a nonsense variant in *Pjvk* [13], and in *Pjvk*-null mice carrying a deletion of whole exon 2 [8]. Moreover, the expression and function of pejvakin in the inner ear and auditory pathway still need clarification. Expression of pejvakin was reported in the hair cells of the organ of Corti, in the spiral ganglion neurons, and in the first three relays of the afferent auditory pathway (cell bodies of neurons from the cochlear nuclei, superior olivary complex and inferior colliculus) [4,13]. However, selective ablation of murine *Pjvk* in spiral ganglion neurons did not result in hearing impairment [7]. As regards pejvakin function, two different roles have been postulated. Pejvakin would be needed for stereocilia maintenance in hair cells, by interacting with proteins of the stereociliary rootlets [7]. Pejvakin has also been reported to mediate pexophagy, the autophagic degradation of peroxisomes, as a protective mechanism against the oxidative stress that is caused by noise overexposure [8,9]. Accordingly, the lack of this protective mechanism may explain the progressive hearing impairment that is observed in some DFNB59 patients. If the primary lesion in DFNB59 patients occurred in the hair cells, it could be hypothesized that inner hair cells would be affected earlier than outer hair cells in some subjects [7]. Consequently, ABR would be abnormal whereas OAE could be recorded during a short period of time, as in case E1471. If tested later, those DFNB59 patients would not be diagnosed with ANSD.

Table 4. Genotypes and phenotypes observed in subjects with the DFNB59 type of autosomal recessive hearing impairment.

Genotype	Families	Features of the Hearing Loss				Reference
		Onset	Severity	Evolution	AN	
p.[Lys41Glufs*8];[Lys41Glufs*8]	1 (Moroccan)	Prelingual	S-P	Progressive	No	[11]
	1 (Moroccan)	Prelingual	P	NR	NT	[26]
p.[Lys41Serfs*18];[Lys41Serfs*18]	1 (Iranian)	NR	M-P	Progressive	NT	[13]
	1 (Iranian)	Prelingual	P	Progressive	NT	[16]
p.[Tyr49*];[Tyr49*]	1 (Pakistani)	Prelingual	NR	NR	NT	[23]
p.[Ser53*];[Ser53*]	1 (Pakistani)	NR	NR	NR	NT	[24]
p.[Thr54Ile];[Thr54Ile]	1 (Iranian)	Prelingual	S	NR	Yes	[4]
p.[Pro55fs*23];[Pro55fs*23]	1 (Pakistani)	NR	NR	NR	NT	[24]
c.[211 + 1G > T];[211 + 1G > T]	1 (Iranian)	Prelingual	NR	NR	NT	[18]
p.[Arg92*];[Arg92*]	1 (Iranian)	Prelingual	S-P	Stable	NT	[16]
	1 (Iranian)	Prelingual	S	NR	NT	[18]
p.[Arg136*];[Arg136*]	1 (Palestinian)	Prelingual	P	NR	No	[14]
	3 (Israeli Arab)	Prelingual	M-S	Stable	No	[15]
	1 (Pakistani)	NR	NR	NR	NT	[24]
	1 (Moroccan)	Prelingual	P	NR	NT	[26]
p.[Ser162Asn];[p.Ser162Asn]	1 (Pakistani)	Prelingual	P	NR	NT	[25]
p.[Arg167*];[Arg167*]	1 (Turkish)	NR	S-P	NR	No	[12]
	1 (Iranian)	Prelingual	P	NR	NT	[18]
	1 (Turkish)	Prelingual	NR	NR	NT	[20]
p.[Arg183Trp];[Arg183Trp]	3 (Iranian)	Prelingual	P	NR	Yes	[4]
	1 (Turkish)	Prelingual	S-P	NR	No	[12]
	1 (Iranian)	Prelingual	NR	NR	NT	[21]
	1 (Iranian)	NR	NR	NR	NT	[22]
p.[Leu224Arg];[His294Ilefs*43]	1 (Spanish)	Early childhood	S	Stable	No	This work
p.[Phe242Leufs*7];[Phe242Leufs*7]	1 (Iranian)	NR	P	NR	NT	[10]
Homozygous deletion of exon 6	1 (Iranian)	Prelingual	NR	NR	NT	[18]
p.[His294Asp];[Phe317Serfs*20]	1 (Italian)	Early childhood	P	Stable	Yes	This work
p.[Asn303del];[Asn303del]	1 (Pakistani)	NR	NR	NR	NT	[24]
p.[Cys312Trpfs*19];[Cys312Trpfs*19]	1 (Chinese)	Prelingual	S-P	Progressive	No	[19]
p.[Gly324Trp];[Gly324Trp]	1 (Iranian)	Prelingual	S-P	NR	NT	[18]
p.[Val330Leufs*7];[Val330Leufs*7]	1 (Iranian)	NR	P	NR	No	[10]
p.[Cys343Ser];[Cys343Ser]	1 (Pakistani)	Early childhood	S-P	Progressive	NT	[17]
	1 (Tamil)	Prelingual	P	Stable	Yes	This work

AN, auditory neuropathy; M, moderate; S, severe; P, profound; NR, not reported; NT, not tested.

On the basis of the expression of pejvakin in the auditory pathway, it was hypothesized that the outcomes of cochlear implants in DFNB59 patients may not be good. Here we report case E1471, with an early diagnosis of ANSD, who received a cochlear implant in the right ear at the age of five years. Four years later, speech perception tests show good results, but language development is delayed. Although this delay could be related to the relatively late age of implantation, careful follow-up is needed for a correct evaluation of this case. Data on the outcome of cochlear implants in many other DFNB59 patients should be collected before any recommendation may be issued to orientate the choice of therapy in subjects with this subtype of AR-NSHI.

Author Contributions: Conceptualization, L.T., R.S. and I.d.C.; methodology, M.D.-R. and M.R.-B.; investigation, M.D.-R., M.R.-B., M.G., E.G.-R., P.S., P.M., N.D.R. and C.M.; resources, P.M., M.A.M.-P., L.T., C.M. and R.S.; data curation, M.D.-R., M.V., L.T., R.S. and I.d.C.; writing—original draft preparation, I.d.C., M.D.-R. and M.R.-B.; writing—review and editing, all authors; supervision, L.T., R.S. and I.d.C.; funding acquisition, I.d.C., M.A.M.-P. and R.S. All authors have read and agreed to the published version of the manuscript.

Funding: This research was funded by the Instituto de Salud Carlos III (ISCIII), Madrid, Spain, National Plan for Scientific and Technical Research and Innovation 2013–2016, with cofounding from the European Regional Development Fund, "A way to make Europe") (to I.d.C.), grant number PI17/00572; by the Regional Government of Madrid (to M.A.M-P.), grant number S2017/ BMD3721; and by the 'Department of Excellence 2018–2022' initiative of the Italian Ministry of Education (MIUR) awarded to the Department of Neurosciences, University of Padua.

Institutional Review Board Statement: The study was conducted according to the guidelines of the Declaration of Helsinki and approved by the Ethics Committee of Hospital Universitario Ramón y Cajal (protocol code 337-18, 28 February 2018).

Informed Consent Statement: Written informed consent was obtained from all subjects involved in the study.

Data Availability Statement: Data on the novel pathogenic variants that are reported in this study are available in ClinVar (accession numbers SCV002043792 to SCV002043795).

Acknowledgments: We kindly thank the patients and their relatives who participated in this study.

Conflicts of Interest: The authors declare no conflict of interest. The funders had no role in the design of the study; in the collection, analyses, or interpretation of data; in the writing of the manuscript, or in the decision to publish the results.

References

1. Dror, A.A.; Avraham, K.B. Hearing impairment: A panoply of genes and functions. *Neuron* **2010**, *68*, 293–308. [CrossRef]
2. Van Camp, G.; Smith, R.J. Hereditary Hearing Loss Homepage. Available online: https://hereditaryhearingloss.org (accessed on 15 December 2021).
3. Hoefsloot, L.H.; Feenstra, I.; Kunst, H.P.; Kremer, H. Genotype phenotype correlations for hearing impairment: Approaches to management. *Clin. Genet.* **2014**, *85*, 514–523. [CrossRef] [PubMed]
4. Delmaghani, S.; del Castillo, F.J.; Michel, V.; Leibovici, M.; Aghaie, A.; Ron, U.; Van Laer, L.; Ben-Tal, N.; Van Camp, G.; Weil, D.; et al. Mutations in the gene encoding pejvakin, a newly identified protein of the afferent auditory pathway, cause DFNB59 auditory neuropathy. *Nat. Genet.* **2006**, *38*, 770–778. [CrossRef] [PubMed]
5. De Schutter, E.; Roelandt, R.; Riquet, F.B.; Van Camp, G.; Wullaert, A.; Vandenabeele, P. Punching Holes in Cellular Membranes: Biology and Evolution of Gasdermins. *Trends Cell Biol.* **2021**, *31*, 500–513. [CrossRef]
6. Rogers, C.; Alnemri, E.S. Gasdermins in apoptosis: New players in an old game. *Yale J. Biol. Med.* **2019**, *92*, 603–617. [PubMed]
7. Kazmierczak, M.; Kazmierczak, P.; Peng, A.W.; Harris, S.L.; Shah, P.; Puel, J.L.; Lenoir, M.; Franco, S.J.; Schwander, M. Pejvakin, a Candidate Stereociliary Rootlet Protein, Regulates Hair Cell Function in a Cell-Autonomous Manner. *J. Neurosci.* **2017**, *37*, 3447–3464. [CrossRef] [PubMed]
8. Delmaghani, S.; Defourny, J.; Aghaie, A.; Beurg, M.; Dulon, D.; Thelen, N.; Perfettini, I.; Zelles, T.; Aller, M.; Meyer, A.; et al. Hypervulnerability to Sound Exposure through Impaired Adaptive Proliferation of Peroxisomes. *Cell* **2015**, *163*, 894–906. [CrossRef]
9. Defourny, J.; Aghaie, A.; Perfettini, I.; Avan, P.; Delmaghani, S.; Petit, C. Pejvakin-mediated pexophagy protects auditory hair cells against noise-induced damage. *Proc. Natl. Acad. Sci. USA* **2019**, *116*, 8010–8017. [CrossRef]
10. Chaleshtori, M.H.; Simpson, M.A.; Farrokhi, E.; Dolati, M.; Hoghooghi-Rad, L.; Amani Geshnigani, S.; Crosby, A.H. Novel mutations in the pejvakin gene are associated with autosomal recessive non-syndromic hearing loss in Iranian families. *Clin. Genet.* **2007**, *72*, 261–263. [CrossRef]

1. Ebermann, I.; Walger, M.; Scholl, H.P.; Charbel Issa, P.; Lüke, C.; Nürnberg, G.; Lang-Roth, R.; Becker, C.; Nürnberg, P.; Bolz, H.J. Truncating mutation of the DFNB59 gene causes cochlear hearing impairment and central vestibular dysfunction. *Hum. Mutat.* **2007**, *28*, 571–577. [CrossRef]
2. Collin, R.W.; Kalay, E.; Oostrik, J.; Caylan, R.; Wollnik, B.; Arslan, S.; den Hollander, A.I.; Birinci, Y.; Lichtner, P.; Strom, T.M.; et al. Involvement of DFNB59 mutations in autosomal recessive nonsyndromic hearing impairment. *Hum. Mutat.* **2007**, *28*, 718–723. [CrossRef] [PubMed]
3. Schwander, M.; Sczaniecka, A.; Grillet, N.; Bailey, J.S.; Avenarius, M.; Najmabadi, H.; Steffy, B.M.; Federe, G.C.; Lagler, E.A.; Banan, R.; et al. A forward genetics screen in mice identifies recessive deafness traits and reveals that pejvakin is essential for outer hair cell function. *J. Neurosci.* **2007**, *27*, 2163–2175. [CrossRef]
4. Shahin, H.; Walsh, T.; Rayyan, A.A.; Lee, M.K.; Higgins, J.; Dickel, D.; Lewis, K.; Thompson, J.; Baker, C.; Nord, A.S.; et al. Five novel loci for inherited hearing loss mapped by SNP-based homozygosity profiles in Palestinian families. *Eur. J. Hum. Genet.* **2010**, *18*, 407–413. [CrossRef]
5. Borck, G.; Rainshtein, L.; Hellman-Aharony, S.; Volk, A.E.; Friedrich, K.; Taub, E.; Magal, N.; Kanaan, M.; Kubisch, C.; Shohat, M.; et al. High frequency of autosomal-recessive DFNB59 hearing loss in an isolated Arab population in Israel. *Clin. Genet.* **2012**, *82*, 271–276. [CrossRef] [PubMed]
6. Babanejad, M.; Fattahi, Z.; Bazazzadegan, N.; Nishimura, C.; Meyer, N.; Nikzat, N.; Sohrabi, E.; Najmabadi, A.; Jamali, P.; Habibi, F.; et al. A comprehensive study to determine heterogeneity of autosomal recessive nonsyndromic hearing loss in Iran. *Am. J. Med. Genet.* **2012**, *158A*, 2485–2492. [CrossRef] [PubMed]
7. Mujtaba, G.; Bukhari, I.; Fatima, A.; Naz, S. A p.C343S missense mutation in *PJVK* causes progressive hearing loss. *Gene* **2012**, *504*, 98–101. [CrossRef]
8. Sloan-Heggen, C.M.; Babanejad, M.; Beheshtian, M.; Simpson, A.C.; Booth, K.T.; Ardalani, F.; Frees, K.L.; Mohseni, M.; Mozafari, R.; Mehrjoo, Z.; et al. Characterising the spectrum of autosomal recessive hereditary hearing loss in Iran. *J. Med. Genet.* **2015**, *52*, 823–829. [CrossRef] [PubMed]
9. Zhang, Q.J.; Lan, L.; Li, N.; Qi, Y.; Zong, L.; Shi, W.; Yu, L.; Wang, H.; Yang, J.; Xie, L.Y.; et al. Identification of a novel mutation of PJVK in the Chinese non-syndromic hearing loss population with low prevalence of the PJVK mutations. *Acta Otolaryngol.* **2015**, *135*, 211–216. [CrossRef]
10. Bademci, G.; Foster, J.; Mahdieh, N.; Bonyadi, M.; Duman, D.; Cengiz, F.B.; Menendez, I.; Diaz-Horta, O.; Shirkavand, A.; Zeinali, S.; et al. Comprehensive analysis via exome sequencing uncovers genetic etiology in autosomal recessive nonsyndromic deafness in a large multiethnic cohort. *Genet. Med.* **2016**, *18*, 364–371. [CrossRef]
11. Yan, D.; Tekin, D.; Bademci, G.; Foster, J.; Cengiz, F.B.; Kannan-Sundhari, A.; Guo, S.; Mittal, R.; Zou, B.; Grati, M.; et al. Spectrum of DNA variants for non-syndromic deafness in a large cohort from multiple continents. *Hum. Genet.* **2016**, *135*, 953–961. [CrossRef]
12. Alimardani, M.; Hosseini, S.M.; Khaniani, M.S.; Haghi, M.R.; Eslahi, A.; Farjami, M.; Chezgi, J.; Derakhshan, S.M.; Mojarrad, M. Targeted Mutation Analysis of the SLC26A4, MYO6, PJVK and CDH23 Genes in Iranian Patients with AR Nonsyndromic Hearing Loss. *Fetal Pediatr. Pathol.* **2019**, *38*, 93–102. [CrossRef]
13. Khan, A.; Han, S.; Wang, R.; Ansar, M.; Ahmad, W.; Zhang, X. Sequence variants in genes causing nonsyndromic hearing loss in a Pakistani cohort. *Mol. Genet. Genomic Med.* **2019**, *7*, e917. [CrossRef] [PubMed]
14. Richard, E.M.; Santos-Cortez, R.L.P.; Faridi, R.; Rehman, A.U.; Lee, K.; Shahzad, M.; Acharya, A.; Khan, A.A.; Imtiaz, A.; Chakchouk, I.; et al. Global genetic insight contributed by consanguineous Pakistani families segregating hearing loss. *Hum. Mutat.* **2019**, *40*, 53–72. [CrossRef]
15. Zhou, Y.; Tariq, M.; He, S.; Abdullah, U.; Zhang, J.; Baig, S.M. Whole exome sequencing identified mutations causing hearing loss in five consanguineous Pakistani families. *BMC Med. Genet.* **2020**, *21*, 151. [CrossRef] [PubMed]
16. Salime, S.; Charif, M.; Bousfiha, A.; Elrharchi, S.; Bakhchane, A.; Charoute, H.; Kabine, M.; Snoussi, K.; Lenaers, G.; Barakat, A. Homozygous mutations in PJVK and MYO15A genes associated with non-syndromic hearing loss in Moroccan families. *Int. J. Pediatr. Otorhinolaryngol.* **2017**, *101*, 25–29. [CrossRef]
17. Starr, A.; Picton, T.W.; Sininger, Y.; Hood, L.J.; Berlin, C.I. Auditory neuropathy. *Brain* **1996**, *119*, 741–753. [CrossRef]
18. Arslan, E.; Genovese, E.; Orzan, E.; Turrini, M. *Valutazione della Percezione Verbale nel Bambino Ipoacusico*; Ecumenica: Roma, Italy, 1997; pp. 1–79.
19. Elliott, L.L.; Katz, D. *Development of a New Children's Test of Speech Discrimination (Technical Manual)*; Auditec: St. Louis, MO, USA, 1980.
20. Dib, C.; Fauré, S.; Fizames, C.; Samson, D.; Drouot, N.; Vignal, A.; Millasseau, P.; Marc, S.; Hazan, J.; Seboun, E.; et al. A comprehensive genetic map of the human genome based on 5,264 microsatellites. *Nature* **1996**, *380*, 152–154. [CrossRef] [PubMed]
21. Richards, S.; Aziz, N.; Bale, S.; Bick, D.; Das, S.; Gastier-Foster, J.; Grody, W.W.; Hegde, M.; Lyon, E.; Spector, E.; et al. ACMG Laboratory Quality Assurance Committee. Standards and guidelines for the interpretation of sequence variants: A joint consensus recommendation of the American College of Medical Genetics and Genomics and the Association for Molecular Pathology. *Genet. Med.* **2015**, *17*, 405–424. [CrossRef]
22. VarSome: The Human Genomic Variant Search Engine. Available online: https://varsome.com/ (accessed on 15 December 2021).

33. Oza, A.M.; DiStefano, M.T.; Hemphill, S.E.; Cushman, B.J.; Grant, A.R.; Siegert, R.K.; Shen, J.; Chapin, A.; Boczek, N.J.; Schimmenti, L.A.; et al. ClinGen Hearing Loss Clinical Domain Working Group. Expert specification of the ACMG/AMP variant interpretation guidelines for genetic hearing loss. *Hum. Mutat.* **2018**, *39*, 1593–1613. [CrossRef] [PubMed]
34. Genome Aggregation Database (gnomAD). Available online: https://gnomad.broadinstitute.org/ (accessed on 15 December 2021).
35. Boothroyd, A. The acoustic speech signal. In *Pediatric audiology: Diagnosis, technology, and management*; Madell, J.R., Flexer, C., Eds.; Thieme: New York, NY, USA, 2008; pp. 159–167.
36. Del Castillo, I.; Morín, M.; Domínguez-Ruiz, M.; Moreno-Pelayo, M.A. Genetic Etiology of Non-Syndromic Hearing Loss in Europe. *Hum. Genet.* 2022; *in press*.

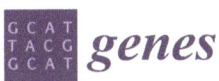

Article

Identification of Novel *CDH23* Variants Causing Moderate to Profound Progressive Nonsyndromic Hearing Loss

Khushnooda Ramzan [1,*], Nouf S. Al-Numair [1], Sarah Al-Ageel [2], Lina Elbaik [1], Nadia Sakati [3], Selwa A. F. Al-Hazzaa [4], Mohammed Al-Owain [3,4] and Faiqa Imtiaz [1]

1. Department of Genetics, King Faisal Specialist Hospital and Research Centre, P.O. Box 3354, Riyadh 11211, Saudi Arabia; alnumair@kfshrc.edu.sa (N.S.A.-N.); lelbaik@kfshrc.edu.sa (L.E.); fahmad@kfshrc.edu.sa (F.I.)
2. Department of Otolaryngology Head and Neck Surgery, King Faisal Specialist Hospital and Research Centre, P.O. Box 3354, Riyadh 11211, Saudi Arabia; salageel97@kfshrc.edu.sa
3. Department of Medical Genetics, King Faisal Specialist Hospital and Research Centre, P.O. Box 3354, Riyadh 11211, Saudi Arabia; nsakati@kfshrc.edu.sa (N.S.); alowain@kfshrc.edu.sa (M.A.-O.)
4. College of Medicine, Alfaisal University, Riyadh 11533, Saudi Arabia; salhazzaa@alfaisal.edu
* Correspondence: kramzan@kfshrc.edu.sa; Tel.: +966-11-4647272 (ext. 36484)

Received: 1 November 2020; Accepted: 26 November 2020; Published: 9 December 2020

Abstract: Mutant alleles of *CDH23*, a gene that encodes a putative calcium-dependent cell-adhesion glycoprotein with multiple cadherin-like domains, are responsible for both recessive *DFNB12* nonsyndromic hearing loss (NSHL) and Usher syndrome 1D (*USH1D*). The encoded protein cadherin 23 (CDH23) plays a vital role in maintaining normal cochlear and retinal function. The present study's objective was to elucidate the role of *DFNB12* allelic variants of *CDH23* in Saudi Arabian patients. Four affected offspring of a consanguineous family with autosomal recessive moderate to profound NSHL without any vestibular or retinal dysfunction were investigated for molecular exploration of genes implicated in hearing impairment. Parallel to this study, we illustrate some possible pitfalls that resulted from unexpected allelic heterogeneity during homozygosity mapping due to identifying a shared homozygous region unrelated to the disease locus. Compound heterozygous missense variants (p.(Asp918Asn); p.(Val1670Asp)) in *CDH23* were identified in affected patients by exome sequencing. Both the identified missense variants resulted in a substitution of the conserved residues and evaluation by multiple in silico tools predicted their pathogenicity and variable disruption of CDH23 domains. Three-dimensional structure analysis of human CDH23 confirmed that the residue Asp918 is located at a highly conserved DXD peptide motif and is directly involved in "Ca^{2+}" ion contact. In conclusion, our study identifies pathogenic *CDH23* variants responsible for isolated moderate to profound NSHL in Saudi patients and further highlights the associated phenotypic variability with a genotypic hierarchy of *CDH23* mutations. The current investigation also supports the application of molecular testing in the clinical diagnosis and genetic counseling of hearing loss.

Keywords: nonsyndromic hearing loss; *DFNB12*; *CDH23*; whole exome sequencing; missense variants; phenotypic variability; Saudi Arabia

1. Introduction

Hearing loss (HL), an etiologically heterogeneous trait, is the most frequent sensory impairment affecting 1–3 out of every 1000 children at birth or during early childhood [1,2]. HL can be caused by genetic or environmental factors, due to an association between these factors, and has major clinical, social, and quality of life implications. Approximately more than 50% of all congenital cases are hereditary, with nonsyndromic hearing loss (NSHL) being the most common, accounting for 75% of all the cases [2,3]. NSHL is often sensorineural and can be transmitted as autosomal recessive (*DFNB*, 80%), autosomal dominant (*DFNA*, 15–20%), and X-linked trait (*DFN*, 1%), or by a mitochondrial pattern of inheritance (<1%) [4,5]. To date, a total of 170 loci and 115 genes responsible for NSHL have been identified (Hereditary Hearing Loss Homepage; Appendix A).

Recessive mutations of the *CDH23* gene (MIM#605516) are responsible for both nonsyndromic deafness 12 (*DFNB12*, MIM#601386) and Usher syndrome type 1D (*USH1D*, MIM#601067) [6–8]. *DFNB12* is characterized by prelingual-onset sensorineural NSHL, without the impairment of visual or vestibular functions. Conversely, individuals with *USH1D* are associated with severe manifestations, including congenital severe to profound deafness, variable vestibular areflexia, and progressive adolescent-onset vision loss due to retinitis pigmentosa (RP) [9–11].

The significance of *CDH23* as a deafness gene and the associated phenotypic spectrum of *CDH23* mutations has been widely studied among different ethnic populations, and an interesting genotype-phenotype correlation is suggested based on the pathogenic potential of the variants (The Human Gene Mutation Database, HGMD). Missense *CDH23* variants usually underlie a milder phenotype of NSHL, known as *DFNB12*. In contrast, protein-truncating *CDH23* mutations due to frameshift, splice site, or nonsense pathogenic variants are causative of the severe phenotype of Usher syndrome [8,9,12]. The encoded protein, cadherin 23 (CDH23), belongs to the cadherin superfamily, which constitutes a family of transmembrane proteins that mediate calcium-dependent cell-cell adhesion. CDH23 has essential roles in establishing and maintaining the proper organization of the stereocilia bundle of hair cells in the cochlea and vestibule during late embryonic and early postnatal development. It is a part of the functional network formed by CDH23, MYO7A, USH1C, and USH1G, which regulates hair bundle morphogenesis and is essential for proper mechanotransduction in hair bundles of the inner-ear neurosensory cells [13].

We describe a consanguineous Saudi family in which four siblings had moderate to severe high-frequency progressive NSHL, without any vestibular or ocular involvement. Detailed clinical and molecular genetic analyses were performed. Autozygosity mapping followed by whole-genome SNP genotyping, failed to identify any possible block of homozygosity encompassing a known NSHL gene. Whole exome sequencing (WES) was further used to identify compound heterozygous *CDH23* variants as the probable genetic cause of the *DFNB12* phenotype in this family. Moreover, the effects of the identified variants on protein structure were assessed, and we discuss the pathogenic potential and clinical fate of the identified *CDH23* variants.

2. Materials and Methods

2.1. Study Subjects and Ethical Considerations

A Saudi family (NSHD4; Figure 1A) was referred to the Department of Medical Genetics at King Faisal Specialist Hospital and Research Centre (KFSH&RC), Riyadh, Saudi Arabia, for molecular exploration of genes implicated in HL. The family consists of four siblings presenting with HL (IV-3, IV-4, IV-5, IV-6), two unaffected siblings (IV-1, IV-2), and healthy first cousin parents (III-1, III-2). Family information to draw the pedigree was obtained by interviewing the parents (Figure 1A). The study was approved by the institutional review board (RAC#2100001). Written informed consent was obtained from all the participating individuals. The experimental procedures were carried out in the First Arabian Hereditary Deafness (FAHD) Unit of KFSH&RC following the Declaration of Helsinki.

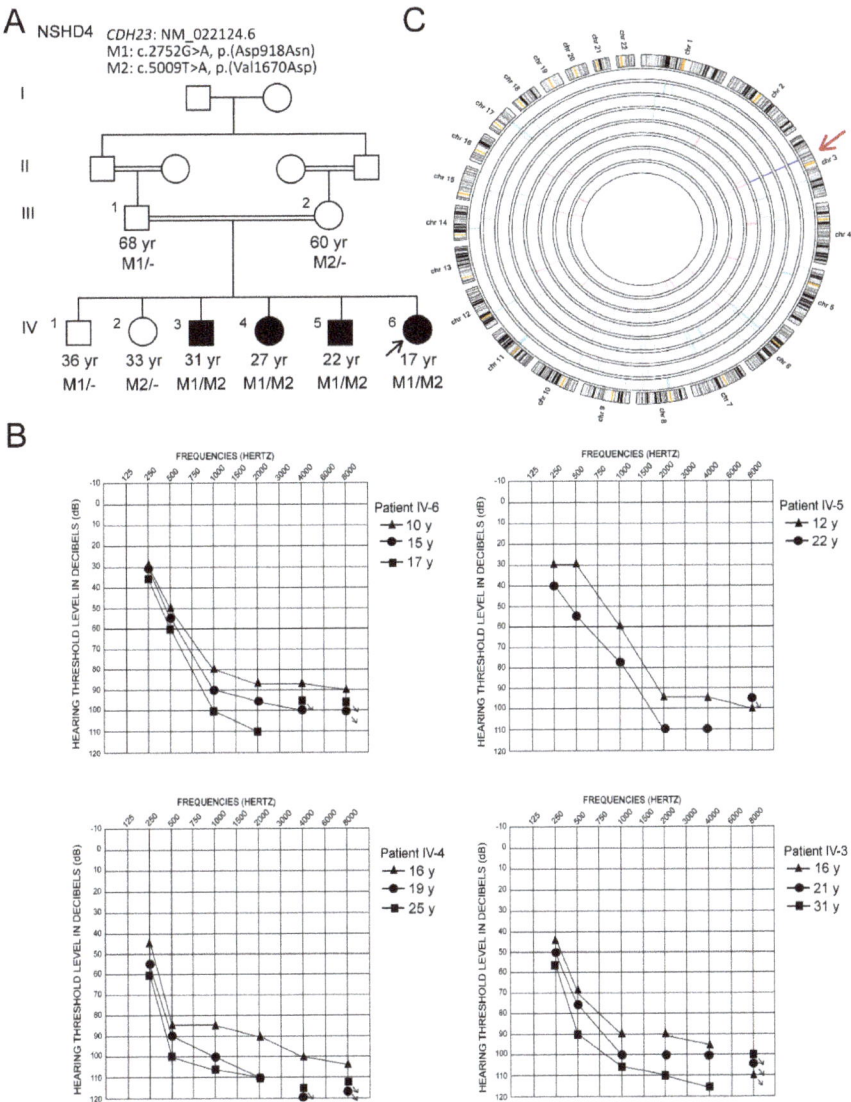

Figure 1. (**A**) Pedigree of the study family (NSHD4), segregating nonsyndromic hearing loss. Circles and squares denote females and males, respectively (solid symbols indicate affected individuals). Genotypes for the two identified mutations in *CDH23* are shown below the symbols of each tested family member. *CDH23*: M1/- or M2/- indicate heterozygous carriers of the c.2752G>A, p.(Asp918Asn) and c.5009T>A, p.(Val1670Asp), respectively. *CDH23*: M1/M2 indicates compound heterozygous individuals. (**B**) Representative pure-tone audiometric results in the best ear of the patients. Hearing-impaired family members illustrate mild sloping to profound hearing loss for the younger siblings (IV-5 and IV-6) and moderate sloping to profound hearing loss for older siblings (IV-3 and IV-4). The affected patients showed progressive nature of HL, as confirmed by audiograms obtained at different ages. (**C**) AgileMultiIdeogram output of autozygosity analysis showing a single common region of homozygosity (ROH) between the four affected members of the family (IV-3, IV-4, IV-5, IV-6, dark blue) on chromosome 3, which is not shared with any of the unaffected individuals (III-1, III-2, IV-1, IV-2, pink). The shared ROH is indicated by a red arrow.

2.2. Clinical Evaluation of Subjects

The affected siblings were thoroughly examined in the Department of Otolaryngology at KFSH&RC. Detailed medical histories and physical examinations were carried out to exclude any possible environmental causes or syndromic forms of HL. Pure-tone audiometry on affected individuals was performed at frequencies between 250 and 8000 Hz in a sound-treated room, following current clinical standards. The severity of hearing loss was defined as mild (26–40 dB), moderate (41–60 dB), severe (61–80 dB), or profound (>81 dB). A computerized tomography (CT) scan of the temporal bone was obtained to look for inner ear anomalies. The vestibular function was evaluated via tandem gait and Romberg testing. The ophthalmological evaluation included the eye fundus and visual field examination.

2.3. DNA Extraction and Whole-Genome SNP Genotyping Using Axiom^{TM} 6.0 Array

Blood samples were obtained from the four affected individuals and their family members. The genomic DNA was extracted using Gentra Puregene Blood kit (Qiagen, Germantown, MD, USA). The integrity and quantity of the extracted DNA samples were assessed through NanoDrop spectrophotometer (Thermo Scientific, Wilmington, DE, USA). DNA of both the affected and unaffected individuals was subjected to genome-wide single nucleotide polymorphism (SNP) genotyping, using Axiom^{TM} CEU Human Array 6.0 and Gene Titan MC Instrument (Affymetrix Inc., Santa Clara, CA, USA), which provide high genetic coverage of 587,352 SNPs across the whole genome. Analyses for annotated regions of the absence of heterozygosity (AOH) for each sample and shared runs of homozygosity (ROH) in the affected cases were performed using AgileMultiIdeogram.

2.4. Whole Exome Sequencing (WES), Data Processing, and Variant Analysis

DNA samples from two affected individuals (IV-5 and IV-6; Figure 1A) underwent exome sequencing. The exonic library preparation was performed using the Agilent SureSelectXT human all exon platform, which provides high end-to-end coverage of the complete coding regions of the genome. In short, after initial sample quality control, 50 ng of DNA was fragmented using QXT enzymatic protocol followed by adaptor tagging (Agilent Technologies, Santa Clara, CA, USA). Paired-end sequencing was performed on a HiSeq2000 instrument (Illumina Inc., San Diego, CA, USA) according to the manufacture's protocol. The raw data were evaluated for read quality with FastQC software (Babraham Bioinformatics). After removing low-quality reads, Burrows–Wheeler Aligner [14] and SAMTOOLS [15] were used to align sequences, copy number variants (CNVs), and small indels, to the UCSC Human Genome Database (UCSC, GRCh37/hg19). Variants were called using the Genome Analysis Toolkit (GATK; The Broad Institute, Cambridge, MA, USA) [16], and the variant annotation and filtering were performed using ANNOVAR [17]. A web-based tool, VCF2CNA, was used to detect CNVs in the Variant Call Format (VCF) files. Minor allele frequency (MAF) of the variants was determined using publicly available variant databases: dbSNP147, 1000Genomes (NCBI browser), ExAC and gnomAD (The Broad Institute). Furthermore, the variants that are frequent in our in-house Saudi Human Genome Program (SHGP) database, which is based on >3000 Saudi individuals, were also filtered out.

2.5. Sanger Validation and Segregation Analysis

Bidirectional sequencing was carried out to verify the variants of interest identified by WES. Primers flanking candidate variants were designed using Primer3 software. The amplified PCR products were sequenced using the BigDye Terminator v3.1 Cycle Sequencing kit and an ABI3130xl sequencer (Applied Biosystems, Foster City, CA, USA). Sequencing data were examined with the SeqManII module of Lasergene (DNA Star Inc., Madison, WI, USA) software. All family members were screened for the filtered candidate variants to establish their segregation with the disease phenotype.

2.6. Pathogenicity Computation and In Silico Modeling

Possible pathogenic effects of the missense single-nucleotide variants (SNVs) on CDH23 protein function were evaluated using multiple pathogenicity-computation tools, including PolyPhen-2, SIFT, DANN, MutationTaster, FATHMM-MKL, MetaSVM, MetaLR, MutationAssessor, and CADD. Clustal Omega and the Genomic Evolutionary Rate Profiling (GERP++) algorithm were used to estimate the conservation of mutated residues (Asp918 and Val1670).

To predict the impact of both the identified missense variants, located in the protein domains cadherin 9 and cadherin 16, CDH23 sequences were obtained from the Uniprot database (Q9H251). Homology models for both the domains affected by the SNVs were predicted by performing template search with BLASTp [18] and HHBlits [19] against the SWISS-MODEL template library (SMTL version 2019-10-02) utilizing the solved molecular models in the Protein Data Bank (PDB). The best structure templates matching the target sequences were selected for each domain: cadherin 9 (3q2w.1.A) and cadherin 16 (5wjm.1.A). ProMod3 was used to build models based on the target–template alignment [20]. The conserved coordinates between the template and the target were copied to the model. Global and per-residue model qualities were estimated using the QMEAN scoring function [21]. The molecular graphics program PyMOL was used to visualize the model, examine the consequences of introducing the mutations, p.(Asp918Asn) and p.(Val1670Asp), and produce figures. Mutagenesis tool within PyMOL was used to mutate the native residue and the native side chain was then substituted by the "best" rotamer of the mutant amino acid, which totalizes the lowest score based on the lowest energy (least collisions and most favorable hydrogen bonds).

3. Results

3.1. Clinical Description and Hearing Characteristics

A consanguineous Saudi family (NSHD4) presented with hearing loss in four of their children (Figure 1A). The ages for the patients were 17 to 31 years at the time of the study. A thorough clinical examination of the patients showed a mild sloping to profound sensorineural HL for the younger two siblings (IV-5 and IV-6) and a moderate sloping to profound sensorineural HL for the two older siblings (IV-3 and IV-4). The affected patients showed a progressive nature of HL, as confirmed by audiograms obtained at different ages (Figure 1B). All four patients are using binaural hearing aids with significant benefits. They were able to identify words in a close-set with no visual cues at normal conversation levels. However, they rely on lip-reading for communication. Their aided scores with current hearing aids were in the range of mild to moderate HL (thresholds between 30 and 55 dB HL), suggesting significant functional gain with amplification. CT of the temporal bone revealed that both mastoids were normally pneumatized. The inner ear structures, including the left and right cochlear, vestibules, semicircular canals, and middle ear structures, were normal. No gross vestibular dysfunction was reported by any of the patients, and there was no delay in the motor milestones. The patients did not display RP or any other ophthalmological manifestations. There were no extended family members with congenital or progressive HL. There was no history of head trauma, exposure to ototoxic noise levels, aminoglycoside antibiotics, or systemic or otic infections that might underlie the HL in the four affected siblings. These findings suggested the possibility of genetic involvement underlying NSHL in the main family, and the DNA samples from all available family individuals were used for genetic analysis.

3.2. Genetic Analysis

3.2.1. Autozygome Analysis

SNP genotypes were analyzed using AgileMultiIdeogram to determine regions of AOH and common ROHs in affected four siblings (V-3, V-4, V-5, and V-6; Figure 1A). A single shared region of homozygosity at chromosome 3q13.2–11q23.2 (chr3: 65,010,372–68,988,334 bp; UCSC hg19) was identified (Figure 1C). This region corresponded to a 3.97-Mb region on the human Genome Data Viewer (annotation release 109), which contained seven labeled genes. The affected individuals were products of a consanguineous union, and as presumed from the pedigree, the possibility of homozygous mutation was more likely, but this region did not contain any known or potential HL gene; therefore, we next proceeded with exome sequencing.

3.2.2. Identification of Mutations by Whole Exome Sequencing

Exome data of two affected individuals (IV-5 and IV-6; Figure 1A) were obtained from the HiSeq 2000 platform (Illumina Inc., San Diego, CA, USA), with an average sequence depth of on-target regions of 97× for affected individual IV-5 and 106× for IV-6. The average percentage of bases in the target region was 97.8% and 93.2%, with a 10× and 20× coverage, respectively. Variants with a quality score (QUAL) of ≤30 (Q30) were selected only. For CNV detection, a VCF file containing paired patient and normal control individual data was uploaded and analyzed by the VCF2CNA algorithm using the standard parameters. A CNV profile of the patient IV-5 was obtained containing 453 CNVs, overlapping at least one coding exon. These CNVs were also present in the normal control individuals from the same ethnic population; therefore, they were not considered further.

The VCF files of the two affected individuals were annotated and filtered using Illumina Variant Studio software to ascertain potentially damaging variants underlying the HL phenotype. A workflow for variant filtering scheme of exome data used for variants prioritization and following the genetic analysis is illustrated in Figure 2. In short, the variants' genomic positions were taken into account, and the variants located in intergenic, intronic, and untranslated regions (UTRs) were excluded. For individual IV-5, a total of 109,306 variants (41,389 homozygous and 67,917 heterozygous) and for individual IV-6, 107,264 variants (41,770 homozygous and 65,494 heterozygous) were identified. Based on family history and pedigree, an autosomal recessive mode of inheritance was considered, and homozygous or compound heterozygous variants were anticipated. The variants from WES were filtered such that: coding/splicing variants, novel or variants with MAF below 0.01% in 1000Genomes, ExAC and gnomAD, variants not frequently observed in our in-house Saudi exomes database, variants that are predicted to be likely pathogenic/pathogenic, and shared among the two affected siblings, were considered as likely causal variants. A list of last filtered variants shared among the exome data of two affected siblings is in Table S1. The indels detected in the exome data were filtered out in the variant filtration strategy and were not prioritized further. MultiIdeogram analysis for regions of AOH for each affected sample and the few shared ROHs among the siblings' pair (Figure 1C) could explain a shortlist of shared homozygous variants in the exome data of the affected siblings IV-5 and IV-6. The in-house exome database has also led us to more filtration power and made this list even shorter.

In short, the variants identified in any gene associated with HL phenotype were carefully prioritized by allele frequency and predicted molecular phenotypic effect. According to the clinical phenotypes and autosomal recessive inheritance patterns combined with the database analysis, two variants of the *CDH23* gene (NM_022124.6); c.2752G>A, p.(Asp918Asn) in exon 24, and c.5009T>A, p.(Val1670Asp) in exon 38, were considered as likely pathogenic compound heterozygous variants causing the disease presentation (Figure 3A). The identified genetic variants were validated by Sanger sequencing (Figure 3B). Genotyping in the parents confirmed that these mutations co-segregated with deafness within the family; the variant c.2752G>A was inherited from the father (III-1), while c.5009T>A was inherited from the mother (III-2) (Figure 3B). The unaffected siblings (IV-1 and IV-2) were also carriers (Figure 1A).

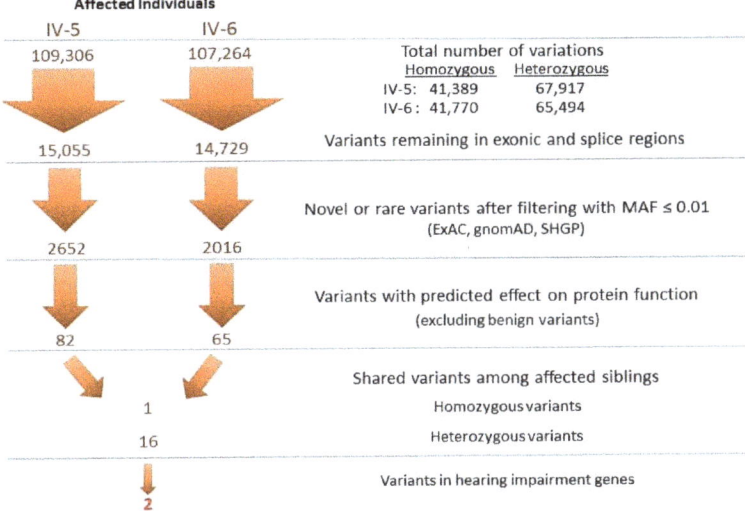

Figure 2. Whole exome sequencing and variant filtering strategy adapted to narrow down the most promising causative mutations in Family NSHD4. The exome was interrogated for variants present in genes shared by two affected individuals under an autosomal recessive model.

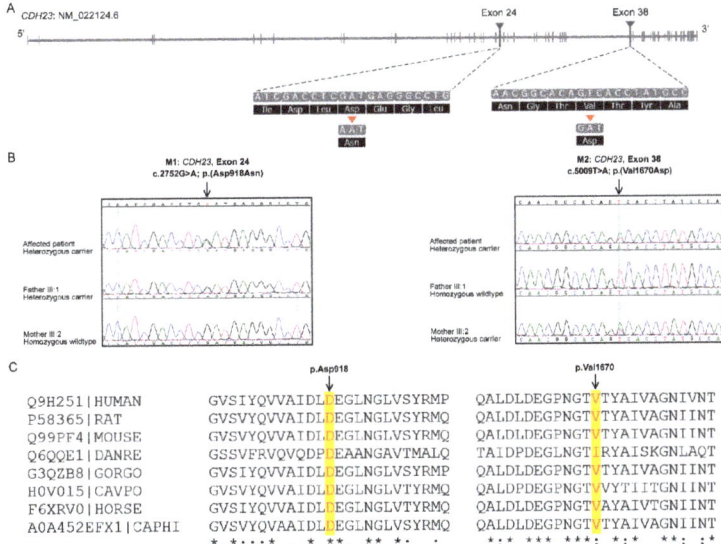

Figure 3. Identification of *CDH23* (NM_022124.6) mutations by whole exome sequencing. (**A**) The schematic of the *CDH23* gene that is 290 kb in length. The triangles locate the positions of the two heterozygous mutations identified in exons 24 and 38 by exome sequencing. (**B**) Electropherogram profiles of the index patient and unaffected parents showing the inheritance of the missense mutations, (c.2752G>A, p.(Asp918Asn) and c.5009T>A, p.(Val1670Asp)). (**C**) Conservation of Asp918 and Val1670 amino acids is observed across species (highlighted in yellow). Asterisk (*) indicates positions which have a single, fully conserved residue. Colon (:) indicates conservation between groups of strongly similar properties-scoring > 0.5.

3.2.3. Prediction of the Pathogenic Significance of the Mutations

The pathogenicity scores of CDH23 SNVs by multiple in silico bioinformatics tools predicted the variants to be damaging for the protein function (Table 1). The p.(Asp918Asn) and p.(Val1670Asp) variants have a CADD score of 28.3 and 24.5, respectively. Upon sequence comparison across various species, a high degree of evolutionary conservation was observed for both the amino acid residues at the mutation sites (Figure 3C). The GERP++ score of 5.4 and 5.76 was obtained for Asp918 and Val1670, respectively (Table 1). The p.(Asp918Asn) has already been reported as a causative *CDH23* mutation in HL patient (HGMD: CM140352 [22]), while the p.(Val1670Asp) is a novel variant.

Table 1. *CDH23* variants associated with nonsyndromic hearing loss identified in family NSHD4.

		CDH23 (10q22.1)	
		Variant 1	Variant 2
Genomic Coordinates and nomenclature	Genomic Position (hg19/GRCh37)	chr10:73464686	chr10:73537600
	dbSNP ID	rs769870573	rs397517333
	HGVS RefSeq:NM_022124.6	exon 24 of 70 c.2752G>A, p.(Asp918Asn)	exon 38 of 70 c.5009T>A, p.(Val1670Asp)
Global minor allele frequency (MAF)	GnomAD_exomes	A = 0.000008 (2/246770)	A = 0.000068 (17/249302)
	ExAC	A = 0.000017 (2/117490)	A = 0.000058 (7/120554)
	SHGP	0	0
In silico pathogenicity prediction tool	CADD Score [a]	Pathogenic (28.3)	Pathogenic (24.5)
	PolyPhen-2	Probably damaging (0.999)	Possibly damaging (0.735)
	SIFT	Deleterious (0)	Deleterious (0)
	MutationTaster	Disease causing (1)	Disease causing (0.9954)
	Mutation assessor	High (3.985)	High (3.82)
	DANN	Pathogenic (0.9991)	Pathogenic (0.9807)
	FATHMM-MKL	Damaging (0.9939)	Damaging (0.9695)
	MetaSVM	Damaging (0.3538)	Damaging (0.5357)
	MetaLR	Damaging (0.5892)	Damaging (0.6209)
	Conservation GERP++ [b]	Conserved (5.4)	Conserved (5.76)
	ACMG variant classification [c]	PM1, PM2, PP1, PP2, PP3	PM2, PP1, PP2, PP3
		"Pathogenic"	"Likely Pathogenic"

[a] CADD scores are derived from several different functional annotation tools. A score of 20 indicates that a variant is amongst the top 1% of deleterious variants in the human genome. The higher the score, the more likely that variant is predicted to be damaging to the protein. [b] Genomic Evolutionary Rate Profiling (GERP) is a conservation score calculated by quantifying substitution deficits across multiple alignments of orthologues using the genomes of 35 mammals. It ranges from −12.3 to 6.17, with 6.17 being the most conserved. [c] Classified based on the American College of Medical Genetics (ACMG) guidelines.

3.2.4. Impact of p.(Asp918Asn) and p.(Val1670Asp) Mutations on the CDH23 3D Structure

The identified variant p.(Asp918Asn) is located in the Cadherin 9 domain of the CDH23 protein. Analysis of the homology model of the crystal structure of human CDH23 showed that Asp918 is directly involved in a metal "Ca^{2+}" ion contact, H-bond with aspartic acid at position 5, and a salt bridge with lysine 64. The mutant residue "Asn" is neutral compared to negatively charged wild-type residue "Asp". In the p.(Asp918Asn) mutant structure, the difference in charge disturbs the ionic interactions made by the wild-type residue. Notably, loss of negative charge (oxygen atoms of the Asp "−COO−") results in the loss of binding with the Ca^{2+}, thus disturbing the domain (Figure 4A). The second variant p.(Val1670Asp) is located within the Cadherin 16 domain on the protein's surface; replacement of the native amino acid with a negatively charged mutant residue results in loss of hydrophobic interactions with other molecules or other parts of the protein. The bigger-sized mutant residue may also cause a clash and repulsion with the neighboring residues, affecting the domain's stability (Figure 4B). CDH23 homology models confirm the variable disruption of both structurally and functionally critical CDH23 domains, which may impact the normal development of hearing.

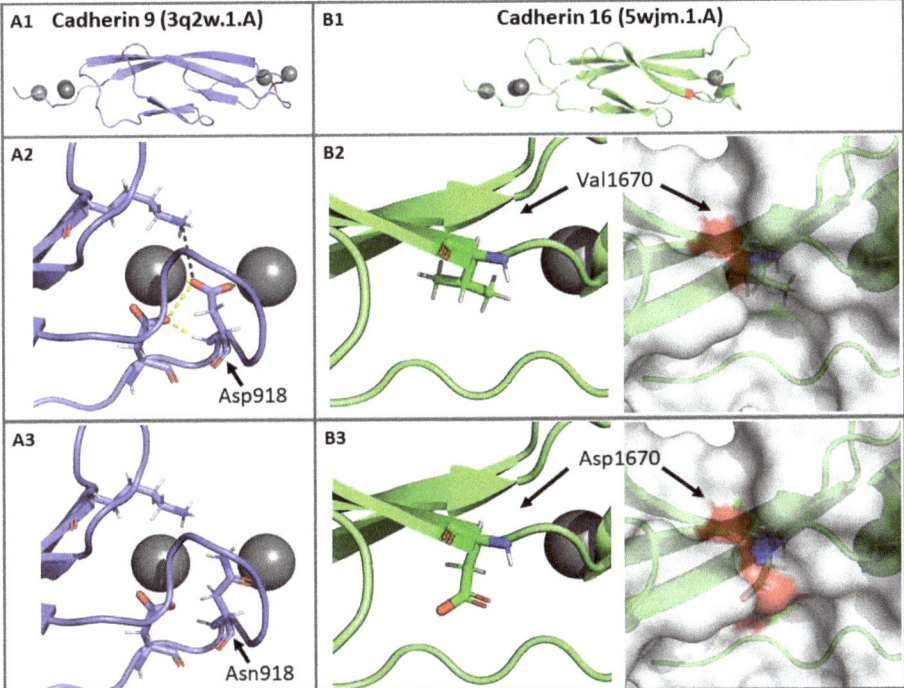

Figure 4. The generated 3D homology model of the CDH23 protein. The Asp918 and Val1670 mutation sites are located at extracellular cadherin domains EC9 and EC16, respectively. CDH23 sequences were obtained from the Uniprot database (Q9H251), and the best structure templates matching the target sequences were selected for each domain (**A1**) cadherin 9 (3q2w.1.A) and (**B1**) cadherin 16 (5wjm.1.A). (**A2**) A close-up view of the wild-type residue p.Asp918 at the mutation site, with the hydrogen bond interaction shown as a yellow dashed line. Asp918 amino acid is part of a highly conserved peptide motif DXD and is directly involved in "Ca^{2+}" ion contact required for the interdomain rigidification of the cadherin repeat domains. (**A3**) The introduction of Asn residue at position 918 would abrogate the "Ca^{2+}" ion contact and other bonds, thereby disrupting the structure of the Cadherin 9 domain. (**B2**) A close-up view of the wild-type residue p.Val1670 at the mutation site. (**B3**) The bigger negatively charged mutant residue Asp at position 1670 results in loss of hydrophobic interactions causing a clash or repulsion with the neighboring residues, thus affecting the stability of the domain. Homology models confirm the variable disruption of structurally and functionally critical CDH23 domains.

4. Discussion

Autosomal recessive NSHL (arNSHL), one of the most frequent genetic disorders in humans, is subjected to extensive genetic heterogeneity, therefore rendering molecular diagnosis difficult. Homozygosity mapping in consanguineous families provides a means to detect genes causing recessive Mendelian disorders by identifying chromosomal regions with shared ROH among the affected family members [23–26]. Although it is much more probable for a related spouse to carry the same recessive mutation than a different mutation, compound heterozygosity can still occur in the setting of consanguinity [27,28]. In the study family (NSHD4) with four affected siblings with arNSHL, initial autozygosity analysis suggested a novel locus, but none of the genes within the autozygome explained the HL phenotype. The potential pitfalls that arose during the course of homozygosity mapping of the family's NSHL gene resulted from unexpected allelic heterogeneity and identification of a shared ROH region unrelated to the disease locus. Consistent with the recessive inheritance of this family, we later identified compound heterozygous *CDH23* mutations by successfully and efficiently applying WES for the molecular diagnosis of arNSHL in all four siblings. With the more recent availability of next-generation sequencing (NGS) technologies, pathogenic variant identification, especially in highly heterogeneous disorders including hearing impairment phenotype, has been significantly improved by obviating the prerequisite to prioritize genes for sequencing within candidate autozygous loci.

The *CDH23*, located on chromosome 10q21-q22, encompasses more than 290 kb and consists of 70 exons. The gene encodes a 3354 amino acid protein with 27 extracellular cadherin (EC) repeat domains (exons 2–64), a single transmembrane domain (exon 65), and a short cytoplasmic domain (exons 66–70). The encoded protein, cadherin 23 (CDH23), is among the 113 human cadherin superfamily members, which constitutes a family of integral transmembrane proteins that mediate Ca^{2+}-dependent cell-cell adhesion. CDH23 is involved in the establishment of cell-cell contacts and the organization of the EC matrix. The EC domains interact with other cadherin molecules in cis and trans to form homo-dimeric interactions, which are essential to mechanically hold the opposing cell surfaces together. This stability is achieved by binding of Ca^{2+} ions to highly conserved cadherin-specific amino acids motifs such as LDRE, DXD, and DXNDN located in each EC domain. These conserved peptide sequences are required for Ca^{2+} binding, linearization, rigidification, and dimerization of the cadherin molecules [29,30]. Protein structure analyses suggest that mutations in such domains perturb CDH23 dimerization and might impair the interactions, change the local surface structure, and destabilize CDH23 protein structure affecting the function of the protein [31]. Both p.(Asp918Asn) and p.(Val1670Asp) mutations identified in our patients involved conserved CDH23 amino acids (Figure 3C) and were predicted to have severe detrimental effects by multiple in silico tools (Table 1). The altered protein conformations indicated that both the wild-type residues are indispensable for the protein function of CDH23 (Figure 4). The mutation p.(Asp918Asn) disrupts the highly conserved peptide motif DXD at cadherin domain 9, where Asp918 is directly involved in binding to the Ca^{2+} ions for the interdomain rigidification of the cadherin repeat domains. Biallelic pathogenic mutations at position 918 have been previously associated with arNSHL; c.2752G>A, p.(Asp918Asn) mutation was identified in an Indian family [22] and c.2752G>C, p.(Asp918His) in Chinese Hans [32]. Based on the American College of Medical Genetics (ACMG) guidelines for variant classification [33], variant p.(Asp918Asn) was classified as pathogenic (PM1, PM2, PP1, PP2, PP3), and p.(Val1670Asp) as a likely pathogenic variant (PM2, PP1, PP2, PP3). The novel *CDH23* variant p.(Val1670Asp) is deposited in the Leiden Open Variation Database (LOVD#00314956) and ClinVar (accession#SUB8608268). The variants are also registered as mutations in the Saudi Human Genome Program database.

The allelic disorders *DFNB12* and *USH1D* were first mapped to the long arm of chromosome 10 [34,35], and the causative mutations in *CDH23* were subsequently identified [7,8]. The mutation spectrum of *CDH23* phenotypes is diverse, and a total of 400 different mutations in this gene have been described to date with an interesting genotype-phenotype correlation [9,12,36]. *CDH23* mutations can cause distinct disease outcomes. The patients with recessive *CDH23* variants display a wide range of hearing and vision loss phenotypes differing in severity, age at onset, and presence or absence of vestibular areflexia. The majority of *CDH23* mutations have been associated with congenital or prelingual-onset, severe-to-profound sensorineural HL either as nonsyndromic *DFNB12* or syndromic *USH1D* [6,37,38]. Individuals with NSHL usually carry *CDH23* missense mutations, which are assumed to be hypomorphic alleles with sufficient residual activity for retinal and vestibular function, but not sufficient for the auditory cochlear function, thereby causing hearing loss *DFNB12* phenotype. On the contrary, *CDH23* null alleles (due to frameshift, splice-site, or nonsense variants), and some missense *CDH23* mutations cause deafness/blindness syndrome, *USH1D* [6,8]. It was further hypothesized that *USH1D* occurs only in the presence of two *USH1D* alleles in trans, while a *DFNB12* allele in trans with a *USH1D* allele results in *DFNB12* phenotype, suggesting the phenotypically dominant nature of a *DFNB12* allele, which can preserve the normal retinal and vestibular function even in the presence of a *USH1D* allele [38].

HL progression is also reported as an essential clinical feature caused by *CDH23* mutations. The contribution of *CDH23* to adult-onset postlingual progressive sensorineural HL in Caucasians, Japanese and Korean adults has been documented [38–40]. Four affected siblings with progressive hearing impairment in our study carried a known pathogenic missense *CDH23* variant, previously known as the prelingual *DFNB12* variant, in a trans configuration with another rare novel *CDH23* missense variant. Taken together, both the detected variants were missense mutations, thereby corroborating the previous reports regarding the *DFNB12* phenotype, as the affected individuals in our family had isolated sensorineural NSHL with no extra-audiological features.

CDH23 is expressed in various structures within the inner ear: the utricular–saccular foramen, ductus reuniens, Reissner's membrane, and particularly in sensory inner and outer hair cells, where it is a component of the tip-links in the hair cell stereocilia [41–43]. CDH23 is supposed to be critical for the crosslinking of the stereocilia. CDH23 co-localizes with protocadherin-15 (PCDH15) and both are localized in the upper and lower parts of the tip-link complex, respectively. CDH23 homodimers interact in trans with PCDH15 homodimers to form tip-link filaments, and they play a crucial role in mechanoelectrical transduction channels in the hair bundles of cochlear hair cells [42,44]. Mutations in *CDH23* or *PCDH15* that affect their interaction severely disrupt hair-bundle morphology, causing sensory impairment [45]. The murine ortholog, which carries a *Cdh23* null allele, gives rise to waltzer phenotype and leads to disorganized, splayed stereocilia, and mimic *USH1D* exhibiting deafness and vestibular dysfunction [46,47]. While in contrast, the salsa mice suffer from progressive HL due to a *Cdh23* missense mutation that is predicted to disturb Ca^{2+} binding by the EC CDH23 domain, modeling the *DFNB12* phenotype. Unlike the mice with *Cdh23* null alleles, hair cell development in salsa mice with a *Cdh23* missense mutation is unaffected. Instead, tip-links were found to be progressively lost, resulting in hair cell death, suggesting that similar mutations in *DFNB12* patients lead to HL by affecting the tip links [48]. Moreover, $Cdh23^{ahl}$ mutant alleles in mice have been linked to age-related progressive HL with varying degrees of progression, as explained by allelism and modifier genes [49,50]. A strain-specific *Cdh23* is also implicated in noise-induced HL susceptibility [47,51,52]. The *CDH23* variants in human subjects have been associated with age-related and noise-induced HL; however, its relative contribution has not been adequately investigated [39,40,53]. The underlying mechanisms responsible for different phenotypes of *CDH23* mutations have not yet been thoroughly elucidated.

5. Conclusions

In conclusion, our analyses identified compound heterozygous mutations in the *CDH23* gene associated with congenital high-frequency recessively inherited hearing loss phenotype. Our findings add to the mutation spectrum of the *CDH23*, explain the phenotypic variability associated with *CDH23* mutant alleles, and further provide a basis for the genotypic hierarchy of *CDH23* mutations, depending on the pathogenic potential of the variants. Moreover, we support the application of NGS in the early diagnosis of HL, effective rehabilitation, and its implications for informed genetic counseling.

Supplementary Materials: The following are available online at http://www.mdpi.com/2073-4425/11/12/1474/s1, Table S1: contains list of shared variants among the two affected siblings (IV-5 and IV-6, Figure 1A) after strategic filtration as depicted in Figure 2, with the *CDH23* pathogenic variants highlighted.

Author Contributions: Conceptualization, experiment design: K.R. and F.I.; WES Data interpretation, Bioinformatics analysis and Sanger validation: K.R., N.S.A.-N. and L.E.; patient recruitment and audiological assessment: N.S., M.A.-O., S.A.-A. and S.A.F.A.-H.; manuscript preparation: K.R., N.S.A.-N. and F.I. All authors have read and agreed to the published version of the manuscript.

Funding: This research was funded by KFSH&RC (RAC#2100001), the King Salman Centre for Disability Research (KSCDR#85722), and the King Abdulaziz City for Science and Technology (KACST/NSTIP#14-MED2979-20).

Acknowledgments: We are thankful to the patients and their families for their participation and contribution to this study. We would like to acknowledge the support of the genotyping and sequencing core facility at KFSH&RC, Riyadh and the Saudi Human Genome Program (SHGP) at KACST and KFSH&RC.

Conflicts of Interest: The authors declare no conflict of interest.

Appendix A. Web Resources

1000Genome	http://browser.1000genomes.org/
ANNOVAR	http://annovar.openbioinformatics.org/
Burrows-Wheeler Aligner (BWA) aligner	(http://bio-bwa.sourceforge.net/)
ClustalW2 for Multiple Sequence Alignment	http://www.ebi.ac.uk/Tools/msa/clustalw2/
Combined Annotation Dependent Depletion (CADD)	https://cadd.gs.washington.edu/
dbSNP	http://www.ncbi.nlm.nih.gov/snp/
ExAC	http://exac.broadinstitute.org/
FATHMM-MKL	http://fathmm.biocompute.org.uk/fathmmMKL.htm
Genome Aggregation Database (gnomAD)	http://gnomad.broadinstitute.org/
Genomic evolutionary rate profiling (GERP)	http://mendel.stanford.edu/SidowLab/downloads/gerp/
Hereditary hearing loss homepage	http://hereditaryhearingloss.org/
Human gene mutation database	http://www.hgmd.cf.ac.uk/ac/
Human genome data viewer	https://www.ncbi.nlm.nih.gov/genome/gdv/
Leiden open variation database (LOVD)	http://databases.lovd.nl/shared/genes/CDH23
MutationAssessor	http://mutationassessor.org/r3/
MutationTaster	http://www.mutationtaster.org/
National Center for Biotechnology Information (NCBI)	http://www.ncbi.nlm.nih.gov/
Online Mendelian inheritance of man (OMIM)	https://www.omim.org/
Polyphen-2 (Polymorphism Phenotyping)	http://genetics.bwh.harvard.edu/pph2/
Primer3web (v4.1.0)	https://primer3.ut.ee/
Protein Data Bank (PDB)	http://www.wwpdb.org/
PyMOL Molecular Graphics System, Schrodinger, LLC	https://pymol.org/
SAMTOOLS	http://samtools.sourceforge.net/
Saudi Human Genome Program (SHGP)	https://shgp.sa/
SIFT (Sorting Intolerant from Tolerant)	http://sift.jcvi.org/
UCSC Human Genome Database	http://www.genome.ucsc.edu/
VCF2CNA	http://vcf2cna.stjude.org/

References

1. Marazita, M.L.; Ploughman, L.M.; Rawlings, B.; Remington, E.; Arnos, K.S.; Nance, W.E. Genetic epidemiological studies of early-onset deafness in the U.S. school-age population. *Am. J. Med Genet.* **1993**, *46*, 486–491. [CrossRef] [PubMed]
2. Morton, N.E. Genetic Epidemiology of Hearing Impairment. *Ann. N. Y. Acad. Sci.* **1991**, *630*, 16–31. [CrossRef] [PubMed]
3. Smith, R.J.; Bale, J.F., Jr.; White, K.R. Sensorineural hearing loss in children. *Lancet* **2005**, *365*, 879–890. [CrossRef]
4. Alford, R.L.; Arnos, K.S.; Fox, M.; Lin, J.W.; Palmer, C.G.; Pandya, A.; Rehm, H.L.; Robin, N.H.; Scott, D.A.; Yoshinaga-Itano, C. American College of Medical Genetics and Genomics guideline for the clinical evaluation and etiologic diagnosis of hearing loss. *Genet. Med. Off. J. Am. Coll. Med Genet.* **2014**, *16*, 347–355.
5. Toriello, H.V.S.S. *Hereditary Hearing Loss and Its Syndromes*, 3rd ed.; Oxford University Press: New York, NY, USA, 2013.
6. Astuto, L.M.; Bork, J.M.; Weston, M.D.; Askew, J.W.; Fields, R.R.; Orten, D.J.; Ohliger, S.J.; Riazuddin, S.; Morell, R.J.; Khan, S.; et al. CDH23 mutation and phenotype heterogeneity: A profile of 107 diverse families with Usher syndrome and nonsyndromic deafness. *Am. J. Hum. Genet.* **2002**, *71*, 262–275. [CrossRef]
7. Bolz, H.; Von Brederlow, B.; Ramírez, A.; Bryda, E.C.; Kutsche, K.; Nothwang, H.G.; Seeliger, M.; Cabrera, M.D.C.-S.; Vila, M.C.; Molina, O.P.; et al. Mutation of CDH23, encoding a new member of the cadherin gene family, causes Usher syndrome type 1D. *Nat. Genet.* **2001**, *27*, 108–112. [CrossRef]

8. Bork, J.M.; Peters, L.M.; Riazuddin, S.; Bernstein, S.L.; Ahmed, Z.M.; Ness, S.L.; Polomeno, R.; Ramesh, A.; Schloss, M.; Srisailpathy, C.R.S.; et al. Usher Syndrome 1D and Nonsyndromic Autosomal Recessive Deafness DFNB12 Are Caused by Allelic Mutations of the Novel Cadherin-Like Gene CDH. *Am. J. Hum. Genet.* **2001**, *68*, 26–37. [CrossRef]
9. Bork, J.M.; Morell, R.J.; Khan, S.; Riazuddin, S.; Wilcox, E.R.; Friedman, T.B.; Griffith, A.J. Clinical presentation of DFNB12 and Usher syndrome type 1D. *Adv. Oto-Rhino-Laryngol.* **2002**, *61*, 145–152.
10. Friedman, T.B.; Schultz, J.M.; Ahmed, Z.M.; Tsilou, E.T.; Brewer, C. Usher Syndrome: Hearing Loss with Vision Loss. *Gene Ther. Cochlear Deaf.* **2011**, *70*, 56–65. [CrossRef]
11. Oshima, A.; Jaijo, T.; Aller, E.; Millan, J.; Carney, C.; Usami, S.; Moller, C.; Kimberling, W. Mutation profile of theCDH23 gene in 56 probands with Usher syndrome type I. *Hum. Mutat.* **2008**, *29*, E37–E46. [CrossRef]
12. Bolz, H.J.; Roux, A.F. Clinical utility gene card for: Usher syndrome. *Eur. J. Hum. Genet. EJHG* **2011**, *19*, 4. [CrossRef] [PubMed]
13. Frolenkov, G.I.; Belyantseva, I.A.; Friedman, T.B.; Griffith, A.J. Genetic insights into the morphogenesis of inner ear hair cells. *Nat. Rev. Genet.* **2004**, *5*, 489–498. [CrossRef] [PubMed]
14. Li, H.; Durbin, R. Fast and accurate short read alignment with Burrows-Wheeler transform. *Bioinformatics* **2009**, *25*, 1754–1760. [CrossRef]
15. Li, H.; Handsaker, B.; Wysoker, A.; Fennell, T.; Ruan, J.; Homer, N.; Marth, G.; Abecasis, G.; Durbin, R. 1000 Genome Project Data Processing Subgroup. The Sequence Alignment/Map format and SAMtools. *Bioinformatics* **2009**, *25*, 2078–2079. [CrossRef]
16. McKenna, A.; Hanna, M.; Banks, E.; Sivachenko, A.; Cibulskis, K.; Kernytsky, A.; Garimella, K.; Altshuler, D.; Gabriel, S.B.; Daly, M.J.; et al. The Genome Analysis Toolkit: A MapReduce framework for analyzing next-generation DNA sequencing data. *Genome Res.* **2010**, *20*, 1297–1303. [CrossRef] [PubMed]
17. Yang, H.; Wang, K. Genomic variant annotation and prioritization with ANNOVAR and wANNOVAR. *Nat. Protoc.* **2015**, *10*, 1556–1566. [CrossRef]
18. Camacho, C.; Coulouris, G.; Avagyan, V.; Ma, N.; Papadopoulos, J.S.; Bealer, K.; Madden, T.L. BLAST+: Architecture and applications. *BMC Bioinform.* **2009**, *10*, 421. [CrossRef] [PubMed]
19. Remmert, M.; Biegert, A.; Hauser, A.; Söding, J. HHblits: Lightning-fast iterative protein sequence searching by HMM-HMM alignment. *Nat. Methods* **2012**, *9*, 173–175. [CrossRef] [PubMed]
20. Biasini, M.; Schmidt, T.; Bienert, S.; Mariani, V.; Studer, G.; Haas, J.; Johner, N.; Schenk, A.D.; Philippsen, A.; Schwede, T. OpenStructure: An integrated software framework for computational structural biology. *Acta Crystallogr. Sect. D Biol. Crystallogr.* **2013**, *69*, 701–709. [CrossRef]
21. Benkert, P.; Biasini, M.; Schwede, T. Toward the estimation of the absolute quality of individual protein structure models. *Bioinformatics* **2011**, *27*, 343–350. [CrossRef]
22. Ganapathy, A.; Pandey, N.; Srisailapathy, C.R.S.; Jalvi, R.; Malhotra, V.; Venkatappa, M.; Chatterjee, A.; Sharma, M.; Santhanam, R.; Chadha, S.; et al. Non-Syndromic Hearing Impairment in India: High Allelic Heterogeneity among Mutations in TMPRSS3, TMC1, USHIC, CDH23 and TMIE. *PLoS ONE* **2014**, *9*, e84773. [CrossRef] [PubMed]
23. Botstein, D.; Risch, N. Discovering genotypes underlying human phenotypes: Past successes for mendelian disease, future approaches for complex disease. *Nat. Genet.* **2003**, *33*, 228–237. [CrossRef] [PubMed]
24. Alkuraya, F.S. Discovery of rare homozygous mutations from studies of consanguineous pedigrees. *Curr. Protoc. Hum. Genet.* **2012**, *6*, 6–12. [CrossRef] [PubMed]
25. Ramzan, K.; Taibah, K.; Tahir, A.I.; Al Tassan, N.; Berhan, A.; Khater, A.M.; Al-Hazzaa, S.A.; Al-Owain, M.; Imtiaz, F. ILDR1: Novel mutation and a rare cause of congenital deafness in the Saudi Arabian population. *Eur. J. Med. Genet.* **2014**, *57*, 253–258. [CrossRef] [PubMed]
26. Ramzan, K.; Al-Owain, M.; Al-Numair, N.S.; Afzal, S.; Al-Ageel, S.; Al-Amer, S.; Al-Baik, L.; Al-Otaibi, G.F.; Hashem, A.; Al-Mashharawi, E.; et al. Identification of TMC1 as a relatively common cause for nonsyndromic hearing loss in the Saudi population. *Am. J. Med. Genet. Part B Neuropsychiatr. Genet.* **2019**, *183*, 172–180. [CrossRef] [PubMed]
27. Miano, M.G.; Jacobson, S.G.; Carothers, A.; Hanson, I.; Teague, P.; Lovell, J.; Cideciyan, A.V.; Haider, N.; Stone, E.M.; Sheffield, V.C.; et al. Pitfalls in homozygosity mapping. *Am. J. Hum. Genet.* **2000**, *67*, 1348–1351. [CrossRef]

28. Ramzan, K.; Al-Owain, M.; Huma, R.; Al-Hazzaa, S.A.; Al-Ageel, S.; Imtiaz, F.; Al-Sayed, M. Utility of whole exome sequencing in the diagnosis of Usher syndrome: Report of novel compound heterozygous MYO7A mutations. *Int. J. Pediatr. Otorhinolaryngol.* **2018**, *108*, 17–21. [CrossRef]
29. Angst, B.D.; Marcozzi, C.; I Magee, A. The cadherin superfamily: Diversity in form and function. *J. Cell Sci.* **2001**, *114*, 629–641.
30. Rowlands, T.M.; Symonds, J.M.; Farookhi, R.; Blaschuk, O.W. Cadherins: Crucial regulators of structure and function in reproductive tissues. *Rev. Reprod.* **2000**, *5*, 53–61. [CrossRef]
31. Nollet, F.; Kools, P.F.J.; Van Roy, F. Phylogenetic analysis of the cadherin superfamily allows identification of six major subfamilies besides several solitary members 1 1Edited by M. Yaniv. *J. Mol. Biol.* **2000**, *299*, 551–572. [CrossRef]
32. Yang, T.; Wei, X.; Chai, Y.; Li, L.; Wu, H. Genetic etiology study of the non-syndromic deafness in Chinese Hans by targeted next-generation sequencing. *Orphanet J. Rare Dis.* **2013**, *8*, 85. [CrossRef] [PubMed]
33. Richards, S.; Aziz, N.; Bale, S.; Bick, D.; Das, S.; Gastier-Foster, J.; Grody, W.W.; Hegde, M.; Lyon, E.; Spector, E.; et al. Standards and guidelines for the interpretation of sequence variants: A joint consensus recommendation of the American College of Medical Genetics and Genomics and the Association for Molecular Pathology. *Genet. Med.* **2015**, *17*, 405–423. [CrossRef] [PubMed]
34. Chaib, H.; Place, C.; Salem, N.; Dodé, C.; Chardenoux, S.; Weissenbach, J.; El Zir, E.; Loiselet, J.; Petit, C. Mapping of DFNB12, a gene for a non-syndromal autosomal recessive deafness, to chromosome 10q21-22. *Hum. Mol. Genet.* **1996**, *5*, 1061–1064. [CrossRef]
35. Wayne, S.; Der Kaloustian, V.M.; Schloss, M.; Polomeno, R.; Scott, D.A.; Hejtmancik, J.F.; Sheffield, V.C.; Smith, R.J.H. Localization of the Usher syndrome type ID gene (Ush1D) to chromosome 10. *Hum. Mol. Genet.* **1996**, *5*, 1689–1692. [CrossRef]
36. Mizutari, K.; Mutai, H.; Namba, K.; Miyanaga, Y.; Nakano, A.; Arimoto, Y.; Masuda, S.; Morimoto, N.; Sakamoto, H.; Kaga, K.; et al. High prevalence of CDH23 mutations in patients with congenital high-frequency sporadic or recessively inherited hearing loss. *Orphanet J. Rare Dis.* **2015**, *10*, 1–9. [CrossRef] [PubMed]
37. Pennings, R.; Topsakal, V.; Astuto, L.; De Brouwer, A.P.M.; Wagenaar, M.; Huygen, P.L.M.; Kimberling, W.J.; Deutman, A.F.; Kremer, H.; Cremers, C.W.R.J. Variable Clinical Features in Patients with CDH23 Mutations (USH1D-DFNB12). *Otol. Neurotol.* **2004**, *25*, 699–706. [CrossRef]
38. Schultz, J.M.; Bhatti, R.; Madeo, A.C.; Turriff, A.; A Muskett, J.; Zalewski, C.K.; A King, K.; Ahmed, Z.M.; Riazuddin, S.; Ahmad, N.; et al. Allelic hierarchy of CDH23 mutations causing non-syndromic deafness DFNB12 or Usher syndrome USH1D in compound heterozygotes. *J. Med. Genet.* **2011**, *48*, 767–775. [CrossRef]
39. Kim, B.J.; Kim, A.R.; Lee, C.; Kim, S.Y.; Kim, N.K.D.; Chang, M.Y.; Rhee, J.; Park, M.-H.; Koo, S.K.; Kim, M.Y.; et al. Discovery of CDH23 as a Significant Contributor to Progressive Postlingual Sensorineural Hearing Loss in Koreans. *PLoS ONE* **2016**, *11*, e0165680. [CrossRef]
40. Miyagawa, M.; Nishio, S.Y.; Usami, S. Prevalence and clinical features of hearing loss patients with CDH23 mutations: A large cohort study. *PLoS ONE* **2012**, *7*, e40366. [CrossRef]
41. Müller, U. Cadherins and mechanotransduction by hair cells. *Curr. Opin. Cell Biol.* **2008**, *20*, 557–566. [CrossRef]
42. Siemens, J.; Lillo, C.; Dumont, R.A.; Reynolds, A.; Williams, D.S.; Gillespie, P.G.; Müller, U. Cadherin 23 is a component of the tip link in hair-cell stereocilia. *Nature* **2004**, *428*, 950–955. [CrossRef] [PubMed]
43. Wilson, S.M.; Householder, D.B.; Coppola, V.; Tessarollo, L.; Fritzsch, B.; Lee, E.-C.; Goss, D.; Carlson, G.A.; Copeland, N.G.; Jenkins, N.A. Mutations in Cdh23 Cause Nonsyndromic Hearing Loss in waltzer Mice. *Genomics* **2001**, *74*, 228–233. [CrossRef] [PubMed]
44. Kazmierczak, P.; Sakaguchi, H.; Tokita, J.; Wilson-Kubalek, E.M.; Milligan, R.A.; Müller, U.; Kachar, B. Cadherin 23 and protocadherin 15 interact to form tip-link filaments in sensory hair cells. *Nat. Cell Biol.* **2007**, *449*, 87–91. [CrossRef] [PubMed]
45. Alagramam, K.N.; Goodyear, R.J.; Geng, R.; Furness, D.N.; Van Aken, A.F.J.; Marcotti, W.; Kros, C.J.; Richardson, G.P. Mutations in Protocadherin 15 and Cadherin 23 Affect Tip Links and Mechanotransduction in Mammalian Sensory Hair Cells. *PLoS ONE* **2011**, *6*, e19183. [CrossRef]
46. Di Palma, F.; Holme, R.H.; Bryda, E.C.; Belyantseva, I.A.; Pellegrino, R.; Kachar, B.; Steel, K.P.; Noben-Trauth, K. Mutations in Cdh23, encoding a new type of cadherin, cause stereocilia disorganization in waltzer, the mouse model for Usher syndrome type 1D. *Nat. Genet.* **2001**, *27*, 103–107. [CrossRef]

47. Holme, R.H.; Steel, K.P. Stereocilia defects in waltzer (Cdh23), shaker1 (Myo7a) and double waltzer/shaker1 mutant mice. *Hear. Res.* **2002**, *169*, 13–23. [CrossRef]
48. Schwander, M.; Xiong, W.; Tokita, J.; Lelli, A.; Elledge, H.M.; Kazmierczak, P.; Sczaniecka, A.; Kolatkar, A.; Wiltshire, T.; Kuhn, P.; et al. A mouse model for nonsyndromic deafness (DFNB12) links hearing loss to defects in tip links of mechanosensory hair cells. *Proc. Natl. Acad. Sci. USA* **2009**, *106*, 5252–5257. [CrossRef]
49. Kane, K.L.; Longo-Guess, C.M.; Gagnon, L.H.; Ding, D.; Salvi, R.J.; Johnson, K.R. Genetic background effects on age-related hearing loss associated with Cdh23 variants in mice. *Hear. Res.* **2012**, *283*, 80–88. [CrossRef]
50. McHugh, R.K.; Friedman, R.A. Genetics of hearing loss: Allelism and modifier genes produce a phenotypic continuum. *Anat. Rec. Part A Discov. Mol. Cell. Evol. Biol.* **2006**, *288*, 370–381. [CrossRef]
51. Davis, R.R.; Newlander, J.; Ling, X.-B.; Cortopassi, G.A.; Krieg, E.F.; Erway, L.C. Genetic basis for susceptibility to noise-induced hearing loss in mice. *Hear. Res.* **2001**, *155*, 82–90. [CrossRef]
52. Noben-Trauth, K.; Zheng, Q.Y.; Johnson, K.R. Association of cadherin 23 with polygenic inheritance and genetic modification of sensorineural hearing loss. *Nat. Genet.* **2003**, *35*, 21–23. [CrossRef] [PubMed]
53. Kowalski, T.J.; Pawelczyk, M.; Rajkowska, E.; Dudarewicz, A.; Sliwinska-Kowalska, M. Genetic variants of CDH23 associated with noise-induced hearing loss. *Otol. Neurotol.* **2014**, *35*, 358–365. [CrossRef] [PubMed]

Publisher's Note: MDPI stays neutral with regard to jurisdictional claims in published maps and institutional affiliations.

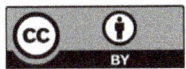

© 2020 by the authors. Licensee MDPI, Basel, Switzerland. This article is an open access article distributed under the terms and conditions of the Creative Commons Attribution (CC BY) license (http://creativecommons.org/licenses/by/4.0/).

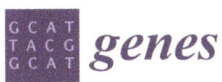 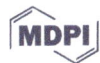

Brief Report

Novel Mutations in *CLPP*, *LARS2*, *CDH23*, and *COL4A5* Identified in Familial Cases of Prelingual Hearing Loss

Saba Zafar [1], Mohsin Shahzad [2], Rafaqat Ishaq [3,4], Ayesha Yousaf [1], Rehan S. Shaikh [1], Javed Akram [5], Zubair M. Ahmed [2] and Saima Riazuddin [2,*]

1. Institute of Molecular Biology & Biotechnology, Bahauddin Zakariya University, Multan 60800, Pakistan; saba.zafar28@yahoo.com (S.Z.); ayesha_yousaf2007@yahoo.com (A.Y.); rehansadiq80@bzu.edu.pk (R.S.S.)
2. Department of Molecular Biology, Shaheed Zulfiqar Ali Bhutto Medical University, Islamabad 44000, Pakistan; mohsinzoologist@gmail.com (M.S.); zmahmed@som.umaryland.edu (Z.M.A.)
3. Department of Otorhinolaryngology Head and Neck Surgery, University of Maryland School of Medicine, Baltimore, MD 21201, USA; rafaqatishaq@gmail.com
4. University Institute of Biochemistry & Biotechnology, PMAS-Arid Agriculture University, Rawalpindi 46000, Pakistan
5. University of Health Sciences, Lahore 54600, Pakistan; vc@uhs.edu.pk
* Correspondence: sriazuddin@som.umaryland.edu

Received: 30 July 2020; Accepted: 18 August 2020; Published: 22 August 2020

Abstract: We report the underlying genetic causes of prelingual hearing loss (HL) segregating in eight large consanguineous families, ascertained from the Punjab province of Pakistan. Exome sequencing followed by segregation analysis revealed seven potentially pathogenic variants, including four novel alleles c.257G>A, c.6083A>C, c.89A>G, and c.1249A>G of *CLPP*, *CDH23*, *COL4A5*, and *LARS2*, respectively. We also identified three previously reported HL-causing variants (c.4528C>T, c.35delG, and c.1219T>C) of *MYO15A*, *GJB2*, and *TMPRSS3* segregating in four families. All identified variants were either absent or had very low frequencies in the control databases. Our in silico analyses and 3-dimensional (3D) molecular modeling support the deleterious impact of these variants on the encoded proteins. Variants identified in *MYO15A*, *GJB2*, *TMPRSS3*, and *CDH23* were classified as "pathogenic" or "likely pathogenic", while the variants in *CLPP* and *LARS2* fall in the category of "uncertain significance" based on the American College of Medical Genetics and Genomics/Association for Molecular Pathology (ACMG/AMP) variant pathogenicity guidelines. This paper highlights the genetic diversity of hearing disorders in the Pakistani population and reports the identification of four novel mutations in four HL families.

Keywords: prelingual hearing loss; genetic heterogeneity; whole-exome sequencing; genetic testing; Pakistan

1. Introduction

Hearing loss (HL) is an etiologically heterogeneous trait that can present itself at any age and degree of severity. This condition affects 1 in 500 newborns and >360 million people worldwide [1,2]. Unlike genetic disorders caused by single-gene pathogenic variants (e.g., cystic fibrosis), over 120 distinct autosomal genetic loci are already linked to just the nonsyndromic form of recessively inherited HL [3]. It is estimated that up to 1% of human genes are essential for hearing function [4], and at least 1000 genes are associated with inherited HL, based upon studies on HL-associated diseases, unique inner-ear transcripts [5–9], and model organisms [10–15]. Intriguingly, of the 72 known nonsyndromic HL genes, 34 were initially identified in Pakistani families [3], and eventually, the variants in these genes were identified in populations around the world [16–21]. The Pakistani population is ideal for genetic studies because of its rich anthropogeneological background, via successive waves of invasions due to its pivotal location at crossroads of South Asia, the Middle East, and Central Asia, as well as its high consanguinity. Parental consanguinity accounts for a 0.25–20% higher chance of recessive genetic disorders [22]. Specific clans and high consanguinity in Pakistan provide a unique genetic resource (62.7% of marriages are consanguineous, of which ~80% are between first cousins) [23].

In the present study, we performed exome sequencing on the DNA samples of eight large consanguineous Pakistani families segregating prelingual HL. Four novel and three previously reported variants in seven known HL genes were identified, including five missense, one nonsense, and one frameshifting truncation allele. The results of this study further support the utility of exome sequencing and genetic screening of HL families to catalog the novel disease-causing variants of known genes, which will certainly aid in improving the clinical genetic diagnostic rate, as well as in establishing the frequency of previously reported alleles in the Pakistani population.

2. Materials and Methods

2.1. Subjects and Clinical Evaluation

All procedures in this study were approved by the Institutional Review Board (IRB) Committees (HP-00061036) of the University of Maryland School of Medicine, Baltimore, MD, USA; the Institute of Molecular Biology & Biotechnology, Bahauddin Zakariya University, Multan, Pakistan; and the Shaheed Zulfiqar Ali Bhutto Medical University, Islamabad, Pakistan. The tenets of the Declaration of Helsinki for human subjects were followed and informed written consent from adults and assent from minors was obtained from all the participating individuals prior to inclusion in the study. Family histories were taken from multiple members to establish family structure, comorbidities, the onset of disease, and treatment. Clinical phenotyping was performed through a detailed review of medical history, physical examination, pure tone audiometry, a tandem gait test, a Romberg test, and an ophthalmic examination. Genomic DNA was extracted from blood samples of participating individuals via an inorganic method [24].

2.2. Exome Sequencing and Bioinformatic Analyses

Exome sequencing was performed on probands of all families. Exome-enriched genomic libraries were prepared using the Agilent SureSelect Human Expanded All Exon V5 kit and sequenced on an Illumina HiSeq4000 with an average of 100× coverage. Data alignment, variant calling, and filtration were performed as described previously [25,26]. The Primer3 web resource (http://bioinfo.ut.ee/primer3-0.4.0/) was used to design primers for Sanger sequencing of the selected variants.

Clustal Omega (https://www.ebi.ac.uk/Tools/msa/clustalo/) multiple sequence alignment was used to appraise the evolutionary conservation of the identified variants. Mutation Taster (http://www.mutationtaster.org/), Polyphen-2 (http://genetics.bwh.harvard.edu/pph2/), Mutation Assessor (http://mutationassessor.org/r3/), SIFT (https://sift.bii.a-star.edu.sg/), and Combined Annotation Dependent Depletion score (https://cadd.gs.washington.edu/score) were used to evaluate the impact of the identified variants on the encoded proteins. Finally, the Varsome (https://varsome.com) online tool was used for the classification of HL-associated variants according to the American College of Medical Genetics and Genomics (ACMG) guidelines.

2.3. Structural Modeling

To further evaluate the impact of variants on secondary structure, 3D protein models were generated through the Phyre2 server (http://www.sbg.bio.ic.ac.uk/phyre2/html/page.cgi?id=index) and analyzed through the HOPE protein prediction tool (https://www3.cmbi.umcn.nl/hope/). The University of California, San Francisco (UCSF) CHIMERA online tool (https://www.cgl.ucsf.edu/chimera/) was used to visualize the impact of amino acid change on protein folding and ionic interactions.

3. Results

After IRB approval and informed consent, eight large consanguineous families (Figure 1A) were enrolled from the Punjab province of Pakistan (Figure 1A). According to family medical histories, all affected individuals had prelingual hearing loss (HL). Pure tone audiometric analysis revealed a bilateral mild to profound sensorineural hearing loss in all the tested individuals (Figure 1B). Consequently, to determine the genetic causes of HL segregating in these eight families, exome sequencing was performed for the proband of each family. Autosomal recessive inheritance, both homozygous and compound heterozygous, was assumed during the exome data filtering stages. We detected four novel variants, c.257G>A (p.(Cys86Tyr)), c.6083A>C (p.(Asp2028Ala)), c.89A>G (p.(Tyr30Cys)), and c.1249A>G (p.(Met417Val)), in *CLPP, CDH23, COL4A5,* and *LARS2,* and three previously reported variants, c.4528C>T (p.(Gln1510*)), c.35delG (p.(Gly12Valfs*2)), and c.1219T>C (p.(Cys407Arg)), in *MYO15A, GJB2,* and *TMPRSS3,* respectively (Figure 2A, Table 1). Except for the *COL4A5* allele, variants identified in this study were present in the evolutionarily conserved regions (Figure 2B) of the encoded proteins and were absent or had very low frequencies in the ExAC database (Table 1).

Next, to assess the predicted impact of identified HL-associated variants on the secondary structures of the encoded proteins, we performed 3D molecular modeling with Phyre2 and HOPE online programs. These models were generated using available structural information of the closely related proteins available in the NCBI protein database (https://www.ncbi.nlm.nih). The p.(Gln1510*) nonsense variant of myosin 15A and the p.(Gly12Val*2) frameshift variant of connexin 26 (encoded by *GJB2*), segregating with HL in three families, are likely to yield complete loss of function of both proteins, as the mRNAs harboring these alleles will likely be degraded through the nonsense-mediated decay (NMD) machinery [27]. In the unlikely event that *MYO15A* mRNA escapes NMD, the insertion of a nonsense codon at amino acid position 1510 is predicted to remove the carboxy tail, which will severely hamper the cargo function of the encoded protein [28,29].

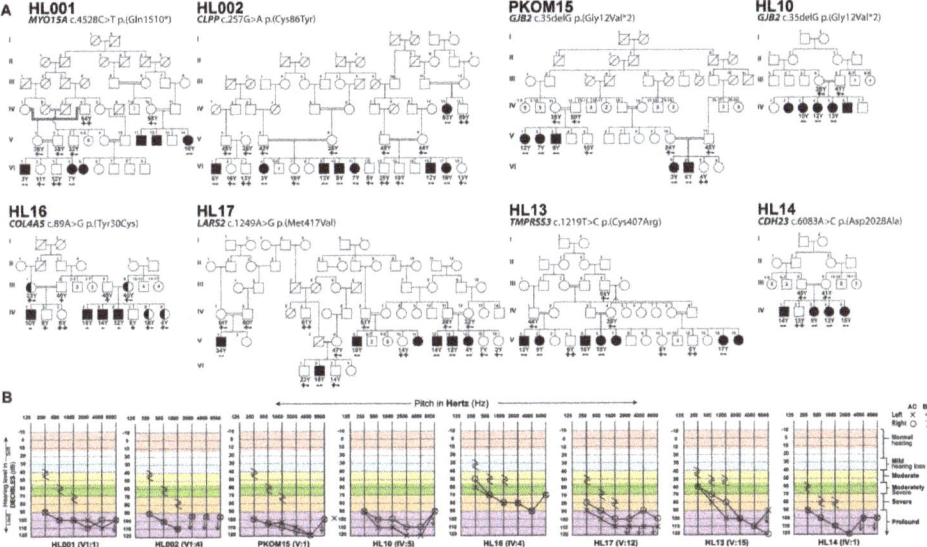

Figure 1. Hearing loss (HL) family pedigrees and causative variants. (**A**) Segregation of disease-causing alleles in eight Pakistani families. Filled and empty symbols represent affected and unaffected individuals, respectively, while half-filled symbols in family HL16 indicate carriers of identified X-linked variants.

Double lines indicate consanguineous marriages. The genotypes (wild type, heterozygous, homozygous, or hemizygous) of the identified mutant alleles are also shown for each of the participating family members. All families had autosomal recessive mode of inheritance for HL, except for the family that had sex-linked (X-chromosome) inheritance. (**B**) Representative audiometric air (AC) and bone (BC) conduction thresholds from the affected individuals of eight Pakistani families revealed bilateral sensorineural hearing loss.

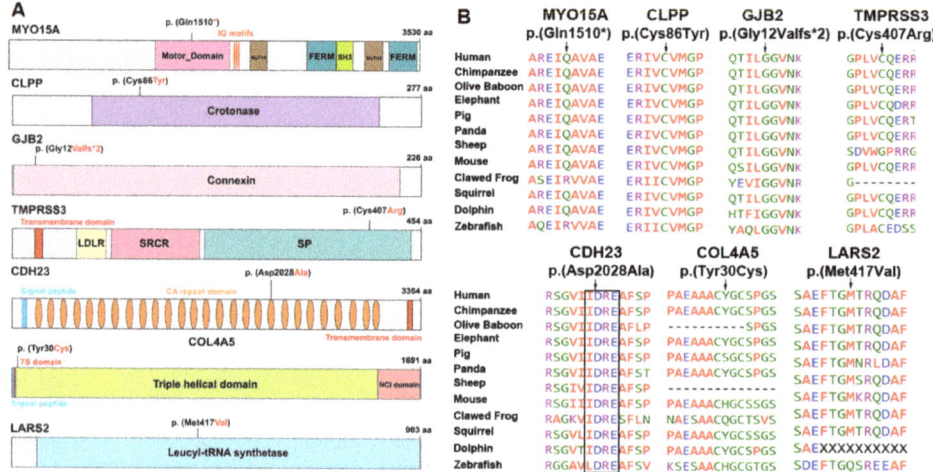

Figure 2. Protein structures and amino acid sequence alignments of orthologs. (**A**) Schematic representation of MYO15A, CLPP, GJB2, CDH23, COL4A5, and LARS2 proteins along with HL-associated variants identified in Pakistani families. (**B**) Clustal-W multiple amino acid sequence alignments of orthologous proteins showed evolutionarily conserved mutated residues across different species, except for the p.(Tyr30Cys) variant of COL4A5. However, none of the evaluated species had cysteine at position 30 in COL4A5 orthologs.

The nonconservative p.(Cys86Tyr) variant of CLPP is predicted to change the torsion angle (Figure 3) since wild-type cystine is a sulfur-containing residue. This residue generally serves two essential biological roles: the site of redox reactions and participation in mechanical linkage for 3D folding of protein secondary structure. Replacement with tyrosine, which has a larger molecular size and different stereotypic properties, would likely impact protein folding and function (Figure 3). The p.Cys407 residue was located in the peptidase S1 enzymatic domain of TMPRSS3 and the p.(Cys407Arg) missense variant, found in family HL13, is predicted to cause loss of hydrophobic interactions in the core of the protein (Figure 3), leading to distortion of protein folding and thus abolishing the related function. The p.(Asp2028Ala) variant identified in family HL14 is predicted to alter the classical calcium-binding motif (LDRE; Figure 2B) within the cadherin repeat of CDH23, and is thus predicted to impair the calcium-binding ability (Figure 3). In contrast, the p.(Met417Val) variant, found in family HL17, was located in the transfer RNA (tRNA) synthetase domain of encoded leucyl-tRNA synthetase 2 (LARS2) protein. Replacement of methionine at position 417 with valine is predicted to alter the ionic interactions (hydrogen bonding) and folding of the secondary structure (Figure 3). Finally, the p.(Tyr30Cys) hemizygous variant of COL4A5, found in family HL16, could not be modeled due to lack of reasonable similarity to protein structures in the NCBI database. However, evaluation through the HOPE algorithm indicated that incorporation of a more-hydrophobic residue at position 30 could result in loss of hydrogen bonds and/or disturb the normal folding properties of COL4A5.

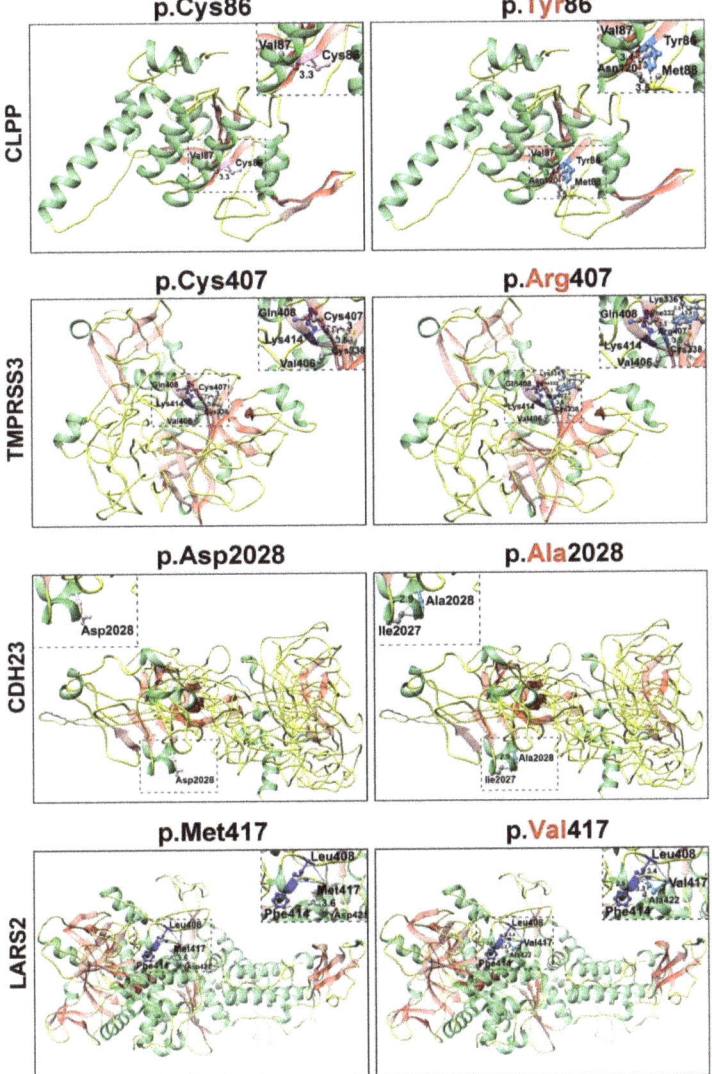

Figure 3. Protein 3D secondary structures generated by Phyre2 are shown in the respective colors: helix, green; strand, reddish pink; and coils, yellow. Pink and Dodger blue colors are used to show wild-type and mutant amino acids, respectively. Hydrogen bonding is shown by solid blue lines and concerned amino acids in dark blue color. Dotted lines represent the distance of the amino acids of interest with nearby residues in Angstroms respect. However, nearby residues are shown in color by element. The differences in size, charge, and hydrophobic properties of cysteine versus tyrosine at position 86 of CLPP might impact the interactions with other molecules on the surface of the protein. Similarly, the p.(Cys407Arg) missense substitution in TMPRSS3 is predicted to impact the core of the protein due to the larger size and different hydrophobic properties. The p.(Asp2028Ala) change mutates the calcium-binding motif (LDRE) of the cadherin repeat in CDH23, and causes a loss of interaction with the p.(Glu2030) residue. Finally, the p.(Met417Val) missense variant of LARS2 is predicted to induce aberrant ionic interactions with p.(Leu408).

Table 1. Genes, identified variants, and their ACMG classification.

Family	Gene	cDNA Change	Protein Change	CADD	ExAC	Mutation Taster	Mutation Assessor	Polyphen 2	SIFT	ACMG Classification (Criteria Used)	Reference
HL001	MYO15A	c.4528C>T	p.(Gln1510*)	42	8×10^{-6}	Disease causing	N/A	N/A	N/A	Pathogenic (PVS1, PM1, PM2, PP3, PP5)	[30]
HL002	CLPP	c.257G>A	p.(Cys86Tyr)	33	0	Disease causing	Low	Probably damaging	Damaging	Uncertain significance (PM2, PP3)	This study
HL10	GJB2	c.35delG	p.(Gly12Valfs*2)	N/A	0.006	Disease causing	Medium	Probably damaging	Damaging	Pathogenic (PVS1, PS3, PM1, PP3, BS2)	[31]
PKOM15	GJB2	c.35delG	p.(Gly12Valfs*2)	N/A	0.006	Disease causing	Medium	Probably damaging	Damaging	Pathogenic (PVS1, PS3, PM1, PP3, BS2)	[31]
HL13	TMPRSS3	c.1219T>C	p.(Cys407Arg)	27.5	0.00005	Disease causing	Medium	Possibly damaging	Tolerated	Pathogenic (PS1, PM1, PM2, PP2, PP3, PP5)	[32]
HL14	CDH23	c.6083A>C	p.(Asp2028Ala)	21.9	0.00001	Disease causing	High	Possibly damaging	Damaging	Likely pathogenic (PM1, PM2, PP3, PP5, BP1)	This study
HL16	COL4A5	c.89A>G	p.(Tyr30Cys)	22.8	0.0003	Benign	Neutral	Possibly damaging	Tolerated	Benign (PM1, PP2, BS1, BS2, BP4)	This study
HL17	LARS2	c.1249A>G	p.(Met417Val)	16.83	0.00002	Disease causing	Medium	Benign	Tolerated	Uncertain significance (PM2, PP2, BP4)	This study

N/A: Not applicable. CADD: Combined Annotation Dependent Depletion, https://cadd.gs.washington.edu/. ExAC: Exome Aggregation Consortium, http://exac.broadinstitute.org/. PVS1: pathogenic very strong (null variant (nonsense, frameshift, canonical ±1 or 2 splice sites, initiation codon, single or multiexon deletion) in a gene where loss of function is a known mechanism of disease)). PM1: pathogenic moderate 1 (located in a mutational hot spot and/or critical and well-established functional domain (e.g., active site of an enzyme) without benign variation). PM2: pathogenic moderate 2 (absent from controls (or at extremely low frequency if recessive) in Exome Sequencing Project, 1000 Genomes Project, or Exome Aggregation Consortium). PP3: pathogenic supporting 3 (multiple lines of computational evidence support a deleterious effect on the gene or gene product (conservation, evolutionary, splicing impact, etc.)). PP5: pathogenic supporting 5 (reputable source recently reports variant as pathogenic, but the evidence is not available to the laboratory to perform an independent evaluation). BP1: benign supporting 1 (missense variant in a gene for which primarily truncating variants are known to cause disease). BP4: benign supporting 4 (benign computational verdict because one benign prediction from GERP vs. no pathogenic predictions). BS1: benign supporting 1 (allele frequency is greater than expected for disorder). BS2: benign supporting 2 (observed in a healthy adult individual for a recessive (homozygous), dominant (heterozygous), or X-linked (hemizygous) disorder, with full penetrance expected at an early age).

4. Discussion

Advancements in molecular genetics screening and bioinformatics tools have been tremendously helpful in deciphering the causal variants for Mendelian disorders, including HL. Combinatorial approaches to identify individuals with actionable variants in highly penetrant genetic forms of common diseases like HL are essential if genomic medicine is to have its promised impact. With the advent of improved gene manipulation and delivery strategies to mitigate inherited HL [33–36], within the perceivable future, genetic testing will not only be useful for genetic diagnosis but also for personalized medicine. Here, we report the identification of seven HL-associated variants in eight multiplexed Pakistani families, including four novel alleles of *CLPP*, *LARS2*, *CDH23*, and *COL4A5* (Table 1). In addition, we also identified three previously reported variants of *MYO15A*, *GJB2*, and *TMPRSS3* in four large families (Figure 1A). All of these genes are highly expressed in the inner and outer hair cells of the cochlea [8,9], and their encoded protein products are required for the development, organization, maintenance, or ionic homeostasis of organ of Corti mechanosensory epithelia (e.g., [28,29]).

Affected individuals of families HL002 and HL17 were homozygous for the presumptive missense variants p.(Cys86Tyr) and p.(Met417Val) in CLPP and LARS2, respectively (Figure 1A). Biallelic variants in *CLPP* and *LARS2* are known to cause Perrault syndrome, a rare autosomal recessive disorder characterized by sensorineural HL in both sexes and primary ovarian failure in females [37,38]. In family HL002, four affected males and four affected females were found to have profound prelingual sensorineural HL. Affected female IV:11 (age 53 years) is currently at the menopausal stage; however, she and affected female IV:17 (age 19 years) were reported to have a history of normal menstrual cycles, although formal evaluation of hormonal profiles was not possible. Similarly, in family HL17, five affected males and two affected females were present. The only affected female that is still alive (V:14) has not reached puberty (age 4 years). Identification of a variant in *LARS2* that segregates in family HL17 is highly clinically relevant, considering that, without this genetic screening, the diagnosis of Perrault syndrome would not be considered in disease clinical management, prognosis, and counseling.

In family HL14, all the affected individuals were homozygous for a missense variant (p.(Asp2028Ala)) of CDH23 (Figure 1A). Biallelic variants in *CDH23* are a frequent cause of both nonsyndromic HL (DFNB12) as well as Usher syndrome type 1, an autosomal recessive disorder characterized by prelingual HL, vestibular areflexia, and progressive retinitis pigmentosa [39]. CDH23 encodes a large protein with 27 extracellular calcium-binding cadherin motifs and a single transmembrane domain [39]. The p.(Asp2028Ala) variant identified in family HL14 is predicted to alter the classical calcium-binding motif (LDRE; Figure 2B) of the cadherin repeat. Mutations in the calcium-binding motifs often cause nonsyndromic HL with preserved retinal and balance functions [40,41]. Similarly, the affected individuals of family HL14 did not report any vision problems and appeared to have normal gait sophisticated function (evaluated through Romberg and Tandem gait tests). However, we cannot rule out the possibility that night vision problems, retinal degeneration, or balance areflexia might develop as these children age.Finally, in family HL16 with an X-linked HL inheritance pattern, we found a novel hemizygous missense variant p.(Tyr30Cys) of COL4A5 (Figure 1). As of March 2020, around 865 variants of *COL4A5* have been documented in the literature. They are known to cause Alport syndrome, a hereditary progressive kidney disease accompanied by ocular lesions and progressive or high tone sensorineural hearing loss [42]. However, currently, the affected individuals have no visual or renal problems. Parents of HL children with *COL4A5* variants should be made aware that alleles of this gene are associated with Alport syndrome. Subsequently, the parents should be offered genetic counseling to explain this potential outcome, and the children should undergo regular nephrological and ophthalmologic screening for kidney and ocular problems. In summary, for families living in remote areas of Pakistan with limited economic resources and sparse health facilities, genetic screening might further help in forming a complete diagnosis, enhancing family counseling, and advancing disease management.

Author Contributions: S.Z., Z.M.A., and S.R., conceived and designed the experiments; S.Z., M.S., R.I., and A.Y., enrolled the families, performed the experiments, and/or performed clinical evaluation; R.S.S., J.A., Z.M.A., and S.R., contributed reagents/materials/analysis tools; and S.Z., R.I., Z.M.A., and S.R. wrote the manuscript. All authors have read and agreed to the published version of the manuscript.

Funding: This study has been supported by grants from the National Institutes of Health (NIH)–National Institute on Deafness and Other Communication Disorders (NIDCD) R56DC011803 (to S.R.), R01DC016295 (to Z.M.A.), and Pakistan Science Foundation project Med450 (to M.S.).

Acknowledgments: We would like to thank the participating patients, their families, and the health care professionals involved in their care.

Conflicts of Interest: The authors declare no conflict of interest.

References

1. Morton, C.C.; Nance, W.E. Newborn hearing screening—A silent revolution. *N. Engl. J. Med.* **2006**, *354*, 2151–2164. [CrossRef] [PubMed]
2. Morton, N.E. Genetic epidemiology of hearing impairment. *Ann. N. Y. Acad. Sci.* **1991**, *630*, 16–31. [CrossRef] [PubMed]
3. Van Camp, G.; Smith, R.J.H. Hereditary Hearing Loss Homepage. 2019. Available online: https://hereditaryhearingloss.org (accessed on 6 July 2020).
4. Friedman, T.B.; Griffith, A.J. Human nonsyndromic sensorineural deafness. *Annu. Rev. Genom. Hum. Genet.* **2003**, *4*, 341–402. [CrossRef] [PubMed]
5. Burns, J.C.; Kelly, M.C.; Hoa, M.; Morell, R.J.; Kelley, M.W. Single-cell RNA-Seq resolves cellular complexity in sensory organs from the neonatal inner ear. *Nat. Commun.* **2015**, *6*, 8557. [CrossRef]
6. Elkon, R.; Milon, B.; Morrison, L.; Shah, M.; Vijayakumar, S.; Racherla, M.; Leitch, C.C.; Silipino, L.; Hadi, S.; Weiss-Gayet, M.; et al. RFX transcription factors are essential for hearing in mice. *Nat. Commun.* **2015**, *6*, 8549. [CrossRef]
7. Hertzano, R.; Elkon, R. High throughput gene expression analysis of the inner ear. *Hear. Res.* **2012**, *288*, 77–88. [CrossRef]
8. Liu, H.; Pecka, J.L.; Zhang, Q.; Soukup, G.A.; Beisel, K.W.; He, D.Z.Z. Characterization of Transcriptomes of Cochlear Inner and Outer Hair Cells. *J. Neurosci.* **2014**, *34*, 11085–11095. [CrossRef]
9. Scheffer, D.I.; Shen, J.; Corey, D.P.; Chen, Z.Y. Gene Expression by Mouse Inner Ear Hair Cells during Development. *J. Neurosci.* **2015**, *35*, 6366–6380. [CrossRef]
10. Ayadi, A.; Birling, M.C.; Bottomley, J.; Bussell, J.; Fuchs, H.; Fray, M.; Gailus-Durner, V.; Greenaway, S.; Houghton, R.; Karp, N.; et al. Mouse large-scale phenotyping initiatives: Overview of the European Mouse Disease Clinic (EUMODIC) and of the Wellcome Trust Sanger Institute Mouse Genetics Project. *Mamm. Genome* **2012**, *23*, 600–610. [CrossRef]
11. Brown, S.D.; Hardisty-Hughes, R.E.; Mburu, P. Quiet as a mouse: Dissecting the molecular and genetic basis of hearing. *Nat. Rev. Genet.* **2008**, *9*, 277–290. [CrossRef]
12. Hrabe de Angelis, M.; Nicholson, G.; Selloum, M.; White, J.; Morgan, H.; Ramirez-Solis, R.; Sorg, T.; Wells, S.; Fuchs, H.; Fray, M.; et al. Analysis of mammalian gene function through broad-based phenotypic screens across a consortium of mouse clinics. *Nat. Genet.* **2015**, *47*, 969–978. [CrossRef] [PubMed]
13. Potter, P.K.; Bowl, M.R.; Jeyarajan, P.; Wisby, L.; Blease, A.; Goldsworthy, M.E.; Simon, M.M.; Greenaway, S.; Michel, V.; Barnard, A.; et al. Novel gene function revealed by mouse mutagenesis screens for models of age-related disease. *Nat. Commun.* **2016**, *7*, 12444. [CrossRef] [PubMed]
14. Schwander, M.; Sczaniecka, A.; Grillet, N.; Bailey, J.S.; Avenarius, M.; Najmabadi, H.; Steffy, B.M.; Federe, G.C.; Lagler, E.A.; Banan, R.; et al. A forward genetics screen in mice identifies recessive deafness traits and reveals that pejvakin is essential for outer hair cell function. *J. Neurosci.* **2007**, *27*, 2163–2175. [CrossRef] [PubMed]
15. Stottmann, R.W.; Moran, J.L.; Turbe-Doan, A.; Driver, E.; Kelley, M.; Beier, D.R. Focusing forward genetics: A tripartite ENU screen for neurodevelopmental mutations in the mouse. *Genetics* **2011**, *188*, 615–624. [CrossRef] [PubMed]
16. Ammar-Khodja, F.; Bonnet, C.; Dahmani, M.; Ouhab, S.; Lefevre, G.M.; Ibrahim, H.; Hardelin, J.P.; Weil, D.; Louha, M.; Petit, C. Diversity of the causal genes in hearing impaired Algerian individuals identified by whole exome sequencing. *Mol. Genet. Genom. Med.* **2015**, *3*, 189–196. [CrossRef] [PubMed]

17. Bademci, G.; Foster, J.; Mahdieh, N.; Bonyadi, M.; Duman, D.; Cengiz, F.B.; Menendez, I.; Diaz-Horta, O.; Shirkavand, A.; Zeinali, S.; et al. Comprehensive analysis via exome sequencing uncovers genetic etiology in autosomal recessive nonsyndromic deafness in a large multiethnic cohort. *Genet. Med.* **2016**, *18*, 364–371. [CrossRef] [PubMed]
18. Masindova, I.; Soltysova, A.; Varga, L.; Matyas, P.; Ficek, A.; Huckova, M.; Surova, M.; Safka-Brozkova, D.; Anwar, S.; Bene, J.; et al. MARVELD2 (DFNB49) mutations in the hearing impaired Central European Roma population—Prevalence, clinical impact and the common origin. *PLoS ONE* **2015**, *10*, e0124232. [CrossRef]
19. Meyer, C.G.; Gasmelseed, N.M.; Mergani, A.; Maqzoub, M.M.A.; Muntau, B.; Thye, T.; Horstmann, R.D. Novel TMC1 structural and splice variants associated with congenital nonsyndromic deafness in a Sudanese pedigree. *Hum. Mutat.* **2005**, *25*, 100. [CrossRef]
20. Riahi, Z.; Bonnet, C.; Zainine, R.; Louha, M.; Bouyacoub, Y.; Laroussi, N.; Chargui, M.; Kefi, R.; Jonard, L.; Dorboz, I.; et al. Whole exome sequencing identifies new causative mutations in Tunisian families with non-syndromic deafness. *PLoS ONE* **2014**, *9*, e99797. [CrossRef]
21. Vozzi, D.; Morgan, A.; Vuckovic, D.; Eustacchio, A.D.; Abdulhadi, K.; Rubinato, E.; Badii, R.; Gasparini, P.; Girotto, G. Hereditary hearing loss: A 96 gene targeted sequencing protocol reveals novel alleles in a series of Italian and Qatari patients. *Gene* **2014**, *542*, 209–216. [CrossRef]
22. Bittles, A. Consanguinity and its relevance to clinical genetics. *Clin. Genet.* **2001**, *60*, 89–98. [CrossRef] [PubMed]
23. Hussain, R.; Bittles, A.H. The prevalence and demographic characteristics of consanguineous marriages in Pakistan. *J. Biosoc. Sci.* **1998**, *30*, 261–275. [CrossRef] [PubMed]
24. Grimberg, J.; Nawoschik, S.; Belluscio, L.; McKee, R.; Turck, A.; Eisenberg, A. A simple and efficient non-organic procedure for the isolation of genomic DNA from blood. *Nucleic Acids Res.* **1989**, *17*, 8390. [CrossRef] [PubMed]
25. Noman, M.; Ishaq, R.; Bukhari, S.A.; Ahmed, Z.M.; Riazuddin, S. Delineation of Homozygous Variants Associated with Prelingual Sensorineural Hearing Loss in Pakistani Families. *Genes (Basel)* **2019**, *10*, 1031. [CrossRef] [PubMed]
26. Riazuddin, S.; Hussain, M.; Razzaq, A.; Iqbal, Z.; Shahzad, M.; Polla, D.L.; Song, Y.; Beusekom, E.V.; Khan, A.A.; Roca, L.T.; et al. Exome sequencing of Pakistani consanguineous families identifies 30 novel candidate genes for recessive intellectual disability. *Mol. Psychiatry* **2017**, *22*, 1604–1614. [CrossRef]
27. Maquat, L.E. Nonsense-mediated mRNA decay: Splicing, translation and mRNP dynamics. *Nat. Rev. Mol. Cell Biol.* **2004**, *5*, 89–99. [CrossRef]
28. Belyantseva, I.A.; Boger, E.T.; Naz, S.; Frolenkov, G.I.; Sellers, J.R.; Ahmed, Z.M.; Griffith, A.J.; Friedman, T.B. Myosin-XVa is required for tip localization of whirlin and differential elongation of hair-cell stereocilia. *Nat. Cell Biol.* **2005**, *7*, 148–156. [CrossRef]
29. Delprat, B.; Michel, V.; Goodyear, R.; Yamasaki, Y.; Michalski, N.; Amraoui, A.; Perfettini, I.; Legrain, P.; Richardson, G.; Hardelin, J.P.; et al. Myosin XVa and whirlin, two deafness gene products required for hair bundle growth, are located at the stereocilia tips and interact directly. *Hum. Mol. Genet.* **2005**, *14*, 401–410. [CrossRef]
30. Rehman, A.; Bird, J.E.; Faridi, R.; Shahzad, M.; Shah, S.; Lee, K.; Khan, S.N.; Imtiaz, A.; Ahmed, Z.M.; Riazuddin, S.; et al. Mutational Spectrum of MYO15A and the Molecular Mechanisms of DFNB3 Human Deafness. *Hum. Mutat.* **2016**, *37*, 991–1003. [CrossRef]
31. Kelsell, D.P.; Dunlop, J.; Stevens, H.P.; Lench, N.J.; Liang, J.N.; Parry, G.; Mueller, R.F.; Leigh, I.M. Connexin 26 mutations in hereditary non-syndromic sensorineural deafness. *Nature* **1997**, *387*, 80–83. [CrossRef]
32. Yosef, T.B.; Wattenhofer, M.; Riazuddin, S.; Ahmed, Z.M.; Scott, H.S.; Kudoh, J.; Shibuya, K.; Antonarakis, S.E.; Tamir, B.B.; Radhakrishna, U.; et al. Novel mutations of TMPRSS3 in four DFNB8/B10 families segregating congenital autosomal recessive deafness. *J. Med. Genet.* **2001**, *38*, 396–400. [CrossRef] [PubMed]
33. Akil, O.; Seal, R.P.; Burke, K.; Wang, C.; Alemi, A.; During, M.; Edwards, R.H.; Lustig, L.R. Restoration of hearing in the VGLUT3 knockout mouse using virally mediated gene therapy. *Neuron* **2012**, *75*, 283–293. [CrossRef] [PubMed]
34. Alagramam, K.N.; Gopal, S.R.; Geng, R.; Chen, D.; Nemet, I.; Lee, R.; Tian, G.; Miyagi, G.; Malagu, K.F.; Lock, C.J.; et al. A small molecule mitigates hearing loss in a mouse model of Usher syndrome III. *Nat. Chem. Biol.* **2016**, *12*, 444–451. [CrossRef] [PubMed]

35. Askew, C.; Rochat, C.; Pan, B.; Asai, Y.; Ahmed, H.; Child, E.; Schneider, B.L.; Aebischer, P.; Holt, J.R. Tmc gene therapy restores auditory function in deaf mice. *Sci. Transl. Med.* **2015**, *7*, 295ra108. [CrossRef] [PubMed]
36. Lentz, J.J.; Jodelka, F.M.; Hinrich, H.L.; McCaffrey, K.E.; Farris, H.E.; Spalitta, M.J.; Bazan, N.G.; Duelli, D.M.; Rigo, F.; Hastings, M.L. Rescue of hearing and vestibular function by antisense oligonucleotides in a mouse model of human deafness. *Nat. Med.* **2013**, *19*, 345–350. [CrossRef]
37. Emma M Jenkinson, E.M.; Rehman, A.; Walsh, T.; Smith, J.; Lee, K.; Morell, R.J.; Drummond, M.C.; Khan, S.N.; Naeem, M.A.; Rauf, B.; et al. Perrault syndrome is caused by recessive mutations in CLPP, encoding a mitochondrial ATP-dependent chambered protease. *Am. J. Hum. Genet.* **2013**, *92*, 605–613. [CrossRef]
38. Pierce, S.B.; Gersak, J.; Cohen, R.M.; Walsh, T.; Lee, M.K.; Malach, D.; Klevit, R.E.; King, M.; Lahad, E. Mutations in LARS2, encoding mitochondrial leucyl-tRNA synthetase, lead to premature ovarian failure and hearing loss in Perrault syndrome. *Am. J. Hum. Genet.* **2013**, *92*, 614–620. [CrossRef]
39. Bork, J.M.; Peters, L.M.; Riazuddin, S.; Bernstein, S.L.; Ahmed, Z.M.; Ness, S.L.; Polomeno, R.; Ramesh, A.; Schloss, M.; Srisailpathy, C.R.; et al. Usher syndrome 1D and nonsyndromic autosomal recessive deafness DFNB12 are caused by allelic mutations of the novel cadherin-like gene CDH23. *Am. J. Hum. Genet.* **2001**, *68*, 26–37. [CrossRef]
40. Brouwer, A.P.M.; Pennings, R.J.E.; Roeters, M.; Hauwe, P.V.; Astuto, L.M.; Hoefsloot, L.H.; Huygen, P.L.M.; Helm, B.; Deutman, A.F.; Bork, J.M.; et al. Mutations in the calcium-binding motifs of CDH23 and the 35delG mutation in GJB2 cause hearing loss in one family. *Hum. Genet.* **2003**, *112*, 156–163. [CrossRef]
41. Astuto, L.M.; Bork, J.M.; Weston, M.D.; Askew, J.W.; Fields, R.R.; Orten, D.J.; Ohliger, S.J.; Riazuddin, S.; Morell, R.J.; Khan, S.N.; et al. CDH23 mutation and phenotype heterogeneity: A profile of 107 diverse families with Usher syndrome and nonsyndromic deafness. *Am. J. Hum. Genet.* **2002**, *71*, 262–275. [CrossRef]
42. Barker, D.F.; Hostikka, S.L.; Zhou, J.; Chow, L.T.; Oliphant, A.R.; Gerken, S.C.; Gregory, M.C.; Skolnick, M.H.; Atkin, C.L.; Tryggvason, K.; et al. Identification of mutations in the COL4A5 collagen gene in Alport syndrome. *Science* **1990**, *248*, 1224–1227. [CrossRef] [PubMed]

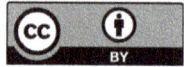

© 2020 by the authors. Licensee MDPI, Basel, Switzerland. This article is an open access article distributed under the terms and conditions of the Creative Commons Attribution (CC BY) license (http://creativecommons.org/licenses/by/4.0/).

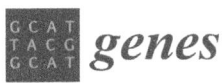

Article

Autosomal Dominantly Inherited GREB1L Variants in Individuals with Profound Sensorineural Hearing Impairment

Isabelle Schrauwen [1,*], Khurram Liaqat [2], Isabelle Schatteman [3], Thashi Bharadwaj [1], Abdul Nasir [4], Anushree Acharya [1], Wasim Ahmad [5], Guy Van Camp [6] and Suzanne M. Leal [1]

1. Center for Statistical Genetics, Sergievsky Center, Taub Institute for Alzheimer's Disease and the Aging Brain, and the Department of Neurology, Columbia University Medical Center, New York, NY 10032, USA; tb2890@cumc.columbia.edu (T.B.); aa4471@cumc.columbia.edu (A.A.); sml3@cumc.columbia.edu (S.M.L.)
2. Department of Biotechnology, Faculty of Biological Sciences, Quaid-i-Azam University, Islamabad 45320, Pakistan; khurramliaqat89@gmail.com
3. Department of ENT, St-Augustinus Hospital Antwerp, 2610 Antwerp, Belgium; Isabelle.Schatteman@gza.be
4. Synthetic Protein Engineering Lab (SPEL), Department of Molecular Science and Technology, Ajou University, Suwon 443-749, Korea; anasirqau@gmail.com
5. Department of Biochemistry, Faculty of Biological Sciences, Quaid-i-Azam University, Islamabad 45320, Pakistan; wahmad@qau.edu.pk
6. Center of Medical Genetics, University of Antwerp & Antwerp University Hospital, 2650 Antwerp, Belgium; guy.vancamp@uantwerpen.be
* Correspondence: is2632@cumc.columbia.edu; Tel.: +1-(212)-304-5272

Received: 1 June 2020; Accepted: 20 June 2020; Published: 23 June 2020

Abstract: Congenital hearing impairment is a sensory disorder that is genetically highly heterogeneous. By performing exome sequencing in two families with congenital nonsyndromic profound sensorineural hearing loss (SNHL), we identified autosomal dominantly inherited missense variants [p.(Asn283Ser); p.(Thr116Ile)] in *GREB1L*, a neural crest regulatory molecule. The p.(Thr116Ile) variant was also associated with bilateral cochlear aplasia and cochlear nerve aplasia upon temporal bone imaging, an ultra-rare phenotype previously seen in patients with de novo *GREB1L* variants. An important role of GREB1L in normal ear development has also been demonstrated by $greb1l^{-/-}$ zebrafish, which show an abnormal sensory epithelia innervation. Last, we performed a review of all disease-associated variation described in *GREB1L*, as it has also been implicated in renal, bladder and genital malformations. We show that the spectrum of features associated with *GREB1L* is broad, variable and with a high level of reduced penetrance, which is typically characteristic of neurocristopathies. So far, seven *GREB1L* variants (14%) have been associated with ear-related abnormalities. In conclusion, these results show that autosomal dominantly inherited variants in *GREB1L* cause profound SNHL. Furthermore, we provide an overview of the phenotypic spectrum associated with *GREB1L* variants and strengthen the evidence of the involvement of *GREB1L* in human hearing.

Keywords: autosomal dominant inheritance; exome sequencing; *GREB1L*; profound nonsyndromic hearing impairment; cochlear aplasia; cochlear nerve aplasia; neural crest; neurocristopathy

1. Introduction

Childhood hearing impairment (HI) is associated with impaired language acquisition, learning, speech development and affects 34 million children worldwide (World Health Organization). Approximately 1/1000 children are born with hearing loss, of which approximately 80% is genetic [1]. HI can be part of a syndrome with the presence of other medical anomalies, or it can be nonsyndromic.

Currently, 120 nonsyndromic HI genes have been identified, with 59% having an autosomal recessive (AR), 37% an autosomal dominant (AD), and 5% an X-linked mode of inheritance (Hereditary hearing loss homepage). However, many genes remain to be identified due to the complexity of the hearing system and due to the understudy of some ancestries [2].

Nonsyndromic HI has no association with additional features or abnormalities. However, it can be associated with abnormalities of the middle ear and/or inner ear [1]. A large number of these abnormalities are mild, but bilateral cochlear aplasia, i.e., bilateral absence of the cochlea, is an ultra-rare and severe developmental abnormality of the inner ear. Approximately 0.3% of children with congenital sensorineural HI are estimated to have bilateral cochlear aplasia [3]. However, this estimate is predominantly based on children who were candidates for a cochlear implant, and they usually present with severe-to-profound HI [3–5].

We previously identified de novo loss-of-function variants in *GREB1L* in two individuals with profound nonsyndromic HI with inner ear and cochleovestibular nerve (or 8th cranial) malformations (Table 1) [5,6]. Affected individuals had either absent cochleae bilaterally [p.(Glu1410fs)] or an absent cochlea on the right and incomplete partition type I on the left [p.(Arg328*)]. Both individuals also displayed abnormalities of their vestibules and absent 8th cranial nerves [6]. In addition, $greb1l^{-/-}$ zebrafish exhibit a loss of and/or abnormal sensory epithelia innervation, including a loss of the anterior cristae nerve and an abnormal innervation pathway from the occipital lateral line neuromast. These findings in humans and model organisms confirm the importance of *GREB1L* in sensory innervation [6]. Furthermore, Greb1l is widely expressed during craniofacial development, including the otic vesicle [6,7], and $Greb1l^{-/-}$ mice are embryological lethal and demonstrate severe abnormalities, including craniofacial and renal abnormalities [8]. $Greb1l^{+/-}$ mice show an abnormal embryo size, growth retardation [9] and mild abnormalities to their kidneys and ureters [8].

Table 1. Variants identified in *GREB1L* associated with nonsyndromic hearing impairment.

Family Type	Variant Segregation	Inheritance Model	Predicted Variant Effect	cDNA Change [1]	AA Change	gnomAD	CADD Score (v1.3)	GERP++RS	Splicing Effect Prediction [2]	Phenotype	ACMG [3]	Study
Trio	de novo	AD	splicing	c.4368G>T	p.(Glu1410fs)	absent	26	5.17	splice site loss	profound bilateral SNHI; UCA (right); UIP-I (left); BVES + SCC; BCNA	P	[6]
Trio	de novo	AD	nonsense	c.982C>T	p.(Arg328*)	absent	38	4.52	NA	profound bilateral SNHI; BCA; BVES + SCC; BCNA	P	[6]
Family	inherited	AD	missense/ splicing	c.848A>G	p.(Asn283Ser)	absent	10	3.44	ESE site loss	profound bilateral SNHI [4]	LP	This study (Family 1)
Trio	inherited [5]	AD	missense	c.347C>T	p.(Thr116Ile)	absent	30	5.25	NA	profound bilateral SNHI; BCA; BVES + SCC; BCNA	VUS	This study (Family 2)

[1] Based on NM_001142966.2; [2] Based on Human splicing finder (v.3.1), ESEfinder (v2.0) [10,11]; [3] Classified based on the American College of Medical Genetics (ACMG) guidelines: P, Pathogenic; LP, likely pathogenic; VUS, variant of unknown significance [12]. [4] Inner ear not evaluated via imaging. [5] Maternal reduced penetrance; AD, Autosomal Dominant; BCA, bilateral cochlear aplasia; BCNA, bilateral cochlear nerve aplasia; BVES + SCC: bilateral dysplastic vestibule and semicircular canals; ESE, exonic splicing enhancer; NA, Not applicable; SNHI, sensorineural hearing impairment; UCA, unilateral cochlear aplasia; UIP-I, unilateral incomplete partition type I.

In addition, de novo or autosomal dominantly inherited variants (often with reduced penetrance) have previously been implicated in individuals with renal, bladder and genital malformations [8,13,14]. Renal hypoplasia/aplasia 3 (RHDA3) is a severe developmental disorder characterized by abnormal kidney development and is caused by heterozygous *GREB1L* variants. Although the phenotype can be highly variable, the disorder falls within the most severe end of the spectrum of congenital anomalies of the kidney and urinary tract. In many of these cases, children were aborted or stillborn due to the severity of the malformations, such as bilateral renal aplasia [8,13,14].

In this article, we have, for the first time, identified a family with congenital profound HI that segregates a missense variant in *GREB1L* with an AD mode of inheritance and also report on an additional case with bilateral cochlear and cochlear nerve aplasia with a *GREB1L* variant.

2. Materials and Methods

2.1. Patient Recruitment and Clinical Assessment

The study was approved by the ethics committee of the Quaid-i-Azam University (IRB-QAU-153), University of Antwerp (B3002020000073) and the Institutional review board of Columbia University (IRB-AAAS2343). Informed consent and peripheral blood samples were obtained from all individuals of a non-consanguineous Pakistani family with deafness (Family 1 [4697]; Figure 1A) and a non-consanguineous Egyptian family with deafness (Family 2 [BAIE1]; Figure 1B). DNA was extracted using a phenol-chloroform procedure for the Pakistani family [15] and using magnetic beads with the chemagic™ blood DNA kit on a chemagic™ Prime™ instrument (PerkinElmer, Waltham, MA, USA) for the Egyptian family. The patient evaluation included a clinical history, physical, audiological and vestibular examination. Computed tomography (CT) and magnetic resonance imaging (MRI) of the temporal bone were performed in the Egyptian patient to identify the presence of cochleovestibular malformations (Family 2). Unfortunately, we were unable to perform CT or MRI on the Pakistani family (Family 1) due to the remote location of these individuals in the Khyber Pakhtunkhwa province, Pakistan.

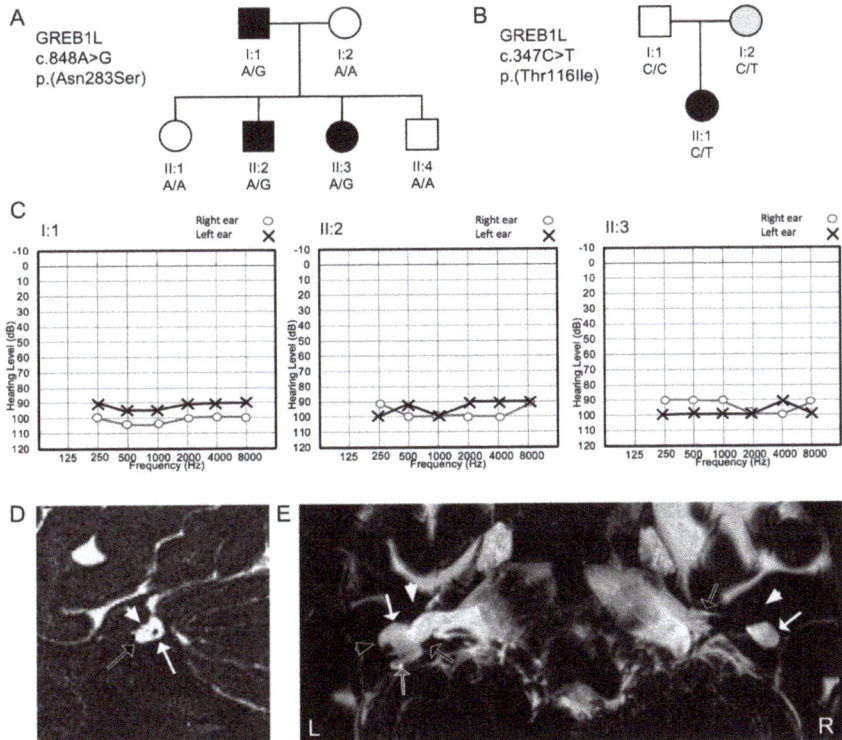

Figure 1. Segregation of the *GREB1L* missense variants in both families, audiological and imaging data. **A/B.** Segregation of the p.(Asn283Ser) *GREB1L* variant in family 1 (4697) (**A**) and p.(Thr116Ile) variant in family 2 (BAIE1) (**B**). Solid black symbols represent affected individuals and clear symbols unaffected family members. Grey symbols represent unaffected individuals that are also heterozygous for the variant (reduced penetrance). Females are represented by circles and males by squares. (**C**) Pure-tone audiograms of hearing-impaired family members of family 1 illustrate that each one presents with bilateral profound HI. (**D**) Oblique sagittal T2 sequence across the right internal auditory canal (IAC) of patient II:1 of family 2. The white arrow indicates the vestibular nerve (black dot). The arrowhead indicates a hypoplastic facial nerve (small grey dot). The black arrow indicates the area in the IAC where the cochlear nerve is expected but not observed. (**E**) Maximum intensity projection of a heavily T2 weighted sequence to the inner ear of the affected individual (II:1) of family 2. Bilateral cochlear aplasia and dysplasia of the vestibular system is visualized. The white arrowhead indicates the area where the cochlea is expected but not seen (bilaterally). The white arrow indicates a dysplastic cystic dilated vestibule on each side. The black arrow indicates a left narrow IAC and the right broad IAC with wide communication between the fundus of the IAC and the vestibule. The black arrowhead indicates a right dilated lateral semicircular canal. The grey arrow indicates a right rudimentary posterior semicircular canal. L, Left; R, right.

2.2. Exome Sequencing

For family 1, Sanger sequencing was performed to exclude coding variants in the HI gene *GJB2* prior to exome sequencing. Additional variants were also excluded by Sanger sequencing that are common causes of HI in the Pakistani population: i.e., p.(Phe91Ser) and p.(Cys99Trp) within *CIB2*, two intronic variants in *HGF* (c.482+1986_1988delTGA and c.482+1991_2000delGATGATGAAA) and p.(Gln446Arg) and p.(Val239Asp) in *SLC26A4* [16–18]. Next, a DNA sample from the affected member (II:2, family 1) underwent exome sequencing. From family 2, the affected patient (II:2) and both normal hearing parents (I:1; I:II) underwent exome sequencing. In short, exomic library preparation was performed using the SureSelect human all exon V6 kit (60.46 Mb target region) for family 1 and SeqCap EZ Exome Probes v3 (64 Mb target region) for family 2. Paired-end sequencing was performed on a HiSeq2500/4000 instrument (Illumina Inc, San Diego, CA, USA), with an average sequencing depth of on target regions of 61× for family 1 (II:2) and 119× (II:1), 97× (I:1), 106× (I:2) for family 2 and the fraction of targets covered >10× was 98.95% for family 1 and 96.80% for family 2. After removing low-quality reads, the filtered reads were aligned to the human reference genome (GRCh37/Hg19) using Burrows–Wheeler Aligner-MEM (BWAv0.7.15) [19]. Duplicate reads were marked using Picard-tools (v2.5.0). An insertions/deletion (Indel)-realignment and base quality score recalibration were performed with Genome Analysis Toolkit (GATK) (v3.7), and single nucleotide variants (SNVs) and InDels were called by the GATK HaplotypeCaller [20]. Variant annotation and filtering were performed using ANNOVAR [21]. In short for the analysis, (1) exonic and splice region variants +/− 12 bp from intron-exon boundary were retained; (2) An AD mode (including de novo for family 2) and AR mode of inheritance was considered for both families; (3) Variants with a predicted effect on protein function or pre-mRNA splicing (missense, nonsense, frameshift, start-loss, splice region, etc.) with a population-specific minor allele frequency (MAF) of <0.005 (for AR) and <0.0005 (for AD) in all populations of the Genome Aggregation Database (gnomAD) [22] and the Greater Middle East Variome Project (GME) [23] were retained to test for segregation; and (4) Bioinformatic prediction scores were annotated from dbnsfp35a and dbscSNV1.1 to evaluate missense and splice site variants respectively [24,25], including Combined Annotation Dependent Depletion (CADD) and Genomic Evolutionary Rate Profiling (GERP++) scores [26,27]. Genes previously involved in human/animal HI or genes expressed in the inner ear were prioritized [28,29]. Candidate variants obtained from filtering were visualized with the Integrative Genomics Viewer (IGV2.4.3). Sanger sequencing performed using an ABI3130XL Genetic Analyzer was used to validate the variants in both families and check the segregation of variants in additional family 1 members for which DNA was available.

Copy number variants (CNVs) were called in exome data from both families using CONiFER (v0.2.2) [30]. Gene annotation was done using the BioMart Database [31] and variant frequency was assessed using the Database of Genomic Variants [32] and gnomAD [22] using the same frequency cut-offs as above for SNV/InDels.

3. Results

3.1. Clinical Findings

In the Pakistani family (Family 1), hearing impairment was prelingual for the three affected family members, and pure-tone audiometry revealed bilateral profound sensorineural HI (Figure 1). No gross vestibular dysfunction was observed via a tandem gait test, and Romberg test in affected individuals I:1, II:2, and II:3. Clinical histories were obtained, and the patients underwent a physical exam at the ages of 45 years of age (y) (I:2), 15y (II:2), and 17y (II:3) with no other health problems reported, including no kidney or bladder issues, however asymptomatic kidney disease could not be excluded. History of head trauma, severe infections or ototoxic treatment was not present. None of the other family members displayed HI or any other clinical features, and the parents have no reported consanguinity.

In the Egyptian patient (Family 2), auditory brainstem responses and cochlear microphonic potentials were bilaterally absent. Vestibular testing showed bilateral aberrant head impulse test, minimal nystagmi on the rotational chair test, and no nystagmus response on the caloric test (with water 44 °C), suggesting a reduced canalar function. C-Vemp (cervical-vestibular evoked myogenic potentials) were bilaterally present at 130 dBSPL, implying a functioning vestibule. MRI and CT imaging showed bilateral cochlear aplasia, aplasia of the cochlear nerve and dysplasia of the vestibule and semicircular canals (Figure 1). The vestibular nerve was present on both sides. On the left side, a hypoplastic narrow internal auditory canal (IAC) was found. On the right side, the IAC was wide with deficient fundus and wide communication between the IAC and vestibule. The facial nerve had a hypoplastic aspect bilaterally. The patient did not have any other known health issues, however, mild kidney disease could not be excluded. The parents have normal hearing, reported no health issues and are non-consanguineous. There is no family history of congenital or progressive HI.

3.2. Exome Sequencing

In family 1, exome sequencing and variant filtering identified variants in *MYO15A*, *POLE* and *GREB1L* as candidates and were validated and tested for segregation (Table S1). Only a missense [(NM_001142966.2:c.848A>G:p.(Asn283Ser)] variant in *GREB1L*, a gene previously associated with HI, segregated with HI in pedigree 4697 with an AD mode of inheritance (Table 1, Figures 1 and S1) [6]. The variant is absent from gnomAD and GME. It is located at a conserved position amongst species (GERP++ RS: 3.44; phastCons20way_mammalian: 1.00). The variant has a CADD score = 10 and is predicted damaging by fathmm-MKL. Based on ESEfinder (v2.0) [10], the variant is located in an exonic splicing enhancer motif (ACAGTAG; score 2.74; threshold >2.67) predicted responsive to Pre-MRNA-Splicing Factor SRp40, which is lost due to the variant (GCAGTAG; score 1.28; threshold >2.67). Therefore, the variant might impact normal protein functioning through various mechanisms, however, we do not know its exact effect in vivo as we were unable to obtain RNA from the patients. *GREB1L* is intolerant to loss-of-function (LoF) variants and is likely under selection against them (pLI = 1; o/e = 0.02 [0.01–0.07]) [22], with only 2% of the expected LoF variants observed. In addition, only 52% of the expected missense variants are observed in *GREB1L* (z score = 5.37; o/e = 0.52 [0.49–0.56]) [22]. The p.(Asn283Ser) missense variant is located in a position and region with a gene-specific missense tolerance ratio (MTR) percentile of <25 [33], which signifies that this region of the protein is also less likely to tolerate missense variants. Pathogenic missense variants are enriched within the 25th percentile of the intolerant region of the gene's MTR distribution [33].

In family 2, all family members were sequenced via exome sequencing. We also identified a variant in *GREB1L* [(NM_001142966.2:c.347C>T:p.(Thr116Ile)], which was verified with Sanger sequencing (Figure S1). None of the other identified variants were likely to be related to HI (Table S1). The p.(Thr116Ile) variant in *GREB1L* was inherited from the unaffected mother, and the variant is absent from gnomAD and GME. It is located at a conserved position amongst species (GERP++ RS: 5.25; phastCons20way_mammalian: 0.935), has a CADD score = 30, and is predicted damaging by fathmm-MKL. The temporal bone imaging phenotype of the patient in this family is remarkably similar to patients previously described with *de novo GREB1L* variants (Table 1), a phenotype that is ultra-rare [6].

Based on the ACMG guidelines for variant classification, p.(Asn283Ser) was classified as likely pathogenic (PM2, PP1-M [Bayes Factor = 16 [34]], PP2 and PP3) and p.(Thr116Ile) was classified as a variant of unknown significance (PM2, PP2, PP3 and PP4) [12]. Finally, no CNVs were identified in either family that were likely to be involved in disease etiology.

3.3. Phenotypic Spectrum of GREB1L Variation

We performed a detailed literature search of all disease-associated variation (N = 49) reported in *GREB1L*, which are listed in Table 2 and displayed in Figure 2. This illustrates that variants are present over the entire length of the gene, with some clustered in or near the TAGT domain. Although previous studies were mostly focused on renal malformations, this table shows that a variety of malformations can be present in affected individuals, including renal, bladder, uterus, ear and other issues such as skeletal abnormalities. Reduced penetrance was observed in 50% of the reported variants in which parents or unaffected siblings were also assessed. In addition, variants were inherited maternally in a large majority of cases (71%). Three patients previously studied for renal malformations also showed ear-related issues. Therefore, of the total of 49 variants that have been reported, 7 variants (14%) have been associated with a hearing or an ear abnormality.

Table 2. All variants reported in *GREB1L* and their associated phenotypic features.

cDNA Variant [1]	Amino Acid Variant	Urinary Phenotype	Genital Phenotype	Ear Phenotype [2]	Other Phenotypes	Inheritance	Reduced Penetrance	Reference
c.37C>T	p.(Arg13*)	unilateral MCD, congenital megaureter	-	-	-	NA	NA	[14]
c.293C>G	p.(Ser98*)	BKA	-	-	-	de novo	no	[13]
c.347C>T	p.(Thr116Ile)			profound bilateral SNHI, BCA; BVES+SCC; BCNA		mat	yes (mat)	This study
c.371G>T	p.(Gly124Val)	BKA, UKA, bladder hypoplasia	-	-	Potter sequence	suspected pat [4]	NA	[35]
c.383G>A	p.(Arg128His)	UKA	unicornate uterus, agenesis of left ovary	-	-	NA	NA	[14]
c.575G>T	p.(Arg192Leu)	BKA, UKA	unique fallopian trump and ovary	-	insulin-dependent diabetes	mat	no	[8]
c.705G>T	p.(Trp235Cys)	BKA, UKA, renal cysts, clear cell renal carcinoma	MRKH, arcuate uterus	-	-	AD family (2 mat, 2 pat)	yes (2 mat, 1 unaffected female sib)	[36]
c.818G>T	p.(Gly273Val)	UKA	-	-	-	NA	NA	[14]
c.848A>G	p.(Asn283Ser) + splicing	-	-	profound bilateral SNHI [3]	-	AD family (1 pat)	no	This study
c.982C>T	p.(Arg328*)	-	-	profound bilateral SNHI, BCA; BVES+SCC; BCNA	-	de novo	no	[6]
c.983G>A	p.(Arg328Gln)	pelvic kidney, MCD, VUR	-	-	-	mat	no	[8]

Table 2. Cont.

cDNA Variant [1]	Amino Acid Variant	Urinary Phenotype	Genital Phenotype	Ear Phenotype [2]	Other Phenotypes	Inheritance	Reduced Penetrance	Reference
c.1490C>G	p.(Ala497Gly)	UKA	-	-	-	NA	NA	[14]
c.1582delC	p.(Gln528Argfs*12)	BKA, UKA	UA, unicornuated uterus	-	clinodactyly	mat	yes (mat)	[8]
c.1780G>T	p.(Glu594*)	BKA, UKA, VUR	UA, fallopian trumps absence, ovarian hernia, uterine left artery absent	-	-	mat	no	[8]
c.1813A>C	p.(Ser605Arg)	UKA, multilocular cyst	blind ending hemi-vagina and bicornuated uterus	-	-	pat	yes (pat)	[8]
c.1852G>A	p.(Asp618Asn)	Ectopic kidney, VUR, duplicated ureter	MRKH type 2	-	unilateral polydactyly, facial asymmetry	NA	NA	[37]
c.2148G>T	p.(Leu716Phe)	VUR	-	-	iris anomaly	NA	NA	[8]
c.2227del	p.(Gln743Argfs*10)	UKA, MCD	MRKH type 2, UA	-	scoliosis	AD family (1 mat)	yes (mat)	[37]
c.2251C>T	p.(Arg751Cys)	BKA, unilateral hypoplasia	unicornuated uterus	-	-	mat	no	[8]
c.2252G>A	p.(Arg751His)	UKA, MCD, megaurethra	-	-	hepatic portal fibrosis	mat [5]	NA	[8]
c.2281G>C	p.(Glu761Gln)	UKA, duplication of the ureter, unilateral MCD, congenital megaureter	-	-	-	pat	yes (pat)	[14]

Table 2. Cont.

cDNA Variant [1]	Amino Acid Variant	Urinary Phenotype	Genital Phenotype	Ear Phenotype [2]	Other Phenotypes	Inheritance	Reduced Penetrance	Reference
c.2312C>T	p.(Pro771Leu)	UKA, MCD	UA, streak ovaries, rudimentary follopian tubes	–	Right unique umbilical artery, 11 pairs of ribs, 6 cervical hemivertebrae with 1 hemivertebrae	NA	NA	[37]
c.2787_2788dep.(Asp930Profs*12)		BKA, UKA, MCD	UA	–	–	AD family (1 mat; 1pat)	yes (mat)	[37]
c.2903C>T	p.(Ala968Val)	BKA, with agenesis of ureters, bladder hypoplasia	–	–	–	de novo	no	[13]
c.2926C>T	p.(Gln976*)	BKA, UKA	–	–	–	mat	no	[8]
c.3197G>C	p.(Arg1066Pro)	UKA	–	–	–	NA	NA	[14]
c.3295C>T	p.(Gln1099*)	unilateral MCD	–	–	–	mat	no	[14]
c.3970-20A>G	splicing	BKA, ureter and bladder aplasia	UA	–	Unilateral hexadactyly	pat	yes (pat)	[37]
c.3983G>A	p.(Gly1328Asp)	UKA	MRKH type 2	–	–	NA	NA	[37]
c.3998_3999insC(Leu1334Profs*18)		UKA	–	–	–	mat	no	[14]
c.4368G>T	splicing	–	–	profound bilateral SNHL, UCA (right); UIP-I (left); BVES+SCC; BCNA	–	de novo	no	[37]
c.4369−1G>C	splicing	BKA	UA	–	thickened left ventricular wall, 10 pairs of ribs	mat	yes (mat)	[8]

Table 2. Cont.

cDNA Variant [1]	Amino Acid Variant	Urinary Phenotype	Genital Phenotype	Ear Phenotype [2]	Other Phenotypes	Inheritance	Reduced Penetrance	Reference
c.4505T>C	p.(Met1502Thr)	BKA	–	–	retro-esophageal subclavian artery, adrenal gland hypoplasia, enlarged thymus, one pair of cervical ribs	mat [5]	NA	[8]
c.4526A>T	p.(Asp1509Val)	BKA	–	–	adrenal cytomegaly	NA	NA	[8]
c.4607A>G	p.(His1536Arg)	BKA, UKA, MCD, horseshoe kidney	UA	–	11 pairs of ribs	mat	no	[8]
c.4646T>C	p.(Val1549Ala)	UKA	UA	–	Henoch Schönlein Purpura	NA	NA	[14]
c.4672C>A	p.(Arg1558Ser)	BKA	–	–	–	mat	yes (mat)	[8]
c.4680C>A	p.(Tyr1560*)	BKA, bladder agenesis, VUR	uterus anomaly	–	Potter sequence	AD family (1 mat)	no	[14]
c.4700T>C	p.(Leu1567Pro)	UKA	–	–	–	de novo	no	[14]
c.4727C>T	p.(Ala1576Val)	BKA	–	auricular tag	hypertrophic left ventricle, aortic stenosis	NA	NA	[8]
c.4843G>A	p.(Val1615Ile)	BRHD, congenital hydronephrosis	–	–	–	mat	yes (mat)	[14]

Table 2. Cont.

cDNA Variant [1]	Amino Acid Variant	Urinary Phenotype	Genital Phenotype	Ear Phenotype [2]	Other Phenotypes	Inheritance	Reduced Penetrance	Reference
c.4964T>C	p.(Ile1655Thr)	UKA	–	unilateral SNHI	genu valgum, flat feet	pat	yes (pat)	[14]
c.4991A>C	p.(Tyr1664Cys)	UKA	–	–	–	NA	NA	[14]
c.5068G>A	p.(Val1690Met)	UKA, VUR	–	–	–	pat [5]	NA	[14]
c.5198A>G	p.(Asn1733Ser)	BKA, UKA, ureter and bladder aplasia	UA, hemi-uterus, streak ovaries	–	–	AD family (1 mat, 1 pat)	yes (mat; unaffected female sib)	[37]
c.5323G>A	p.(Asp1775Asn)	BKA	–	preauricular tag, lop ear	–	NA	NA	[8]
c.5378T>G	p.(Leu1793Arg)	BKA, RKA, hypertrophy of the kidney	–	–	–	AD family (2 mat)	yes (1 mat)	[38]
c.5608+1delG	splicing	BKA, UKA, bladder agenesis	undifferentiated external female genitalia	–	Potter sequence	de novo, mat	yes (2 male siblings)	[35,38]
c.5651G>A	p.(Arg1884His)	URHD	–	–	–	NA	NA	[14]

[1] Based on NM_001142966.2. [2] Many of the children with renal malformations listed here were aborted/stillborn, in which hearing could not have been assessed. [3] Inner ear not evaluated via imaging. [4] No genetic evaluation. [5] Parent not evaluated via renal ultrasound. AD, Autosomal Dominant; AD family, family with multiple affected (>2) showing autosomal dominant inheritance; BCA, bilateral cochlear aplasia; BCNA, bilateral cochlear nerve aplasia; BKA, bilateral kidney agenesis; BVES + SCC, bilateral dysplastic vestibule and semicircular canals; ESE, exonic splicing enhancer; mat, maternal inheritance; MCD, multi-cystic dysplasia; MRKH, Mayer-Rokitansky-Küster-Hauser syndrome; NA, Not assessed; pat, paternal inheritance; SNHI, sensorineural hearing impairment; UCA, unilateral cochlear aplasia; UIP-I, unilateral incomplete partition type I; UKA, unilateral kidney agenesis; UA, uterovaginal aplasia or uterus aplasia; VUR, vesicoureteral reflux.

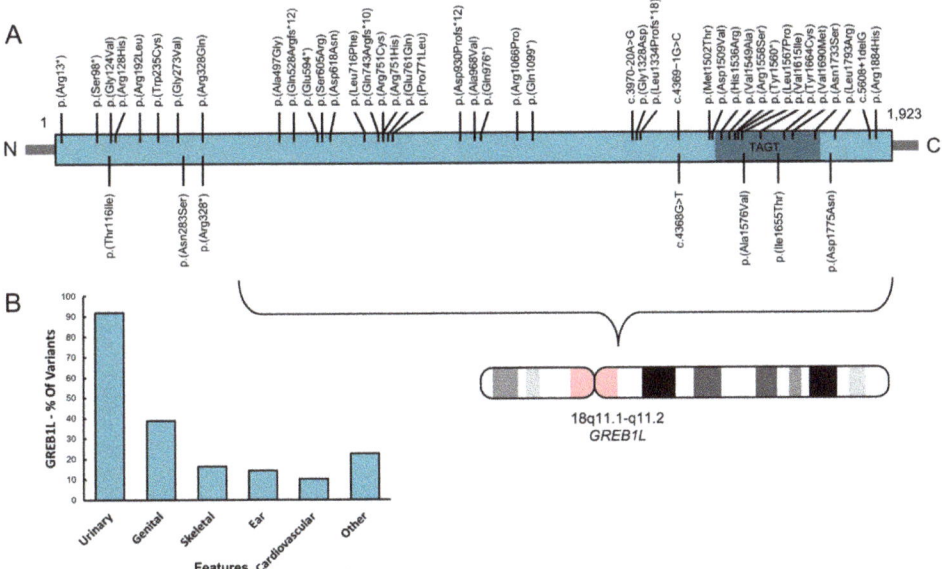

Figure 2. All variants reported in GREB1L and their associated phenotypic features. **A.** GREB1L protein structure with all variants indicated. The seven bottom variants are associated with ear-related abnormalities. Dark green, TAGT or Ten-eleven translocation/J binding protein (TET/JBP)-associated glycosyltrasferase domain [39]. **B.** The percentage (%) of variants associated with the most prevalent phenotypic features seen in affected individuals.

4. Discussion

HI in children is both genetically and phenotypically heterogeneous. Identification of novel genes implicated in congenital HI is important to understand normal hearing and ear development, for patient management and intervention and for the development of novel therapeutic strategies.

We identified two families with congenital profound nonsyndromic sensorineural HI that segregate missense variants [p.(Asn283Ser) and p.(Thr116Ile)] in *GREB1L* (Figure 1). GREB1L is a premigratory neural crest (NC) regulatory molecule implicated in the embryonic development of many tissues [40]. The cranial NC is important in the development of the peripheral nervous system and non-neural tissues, including craniofacial connective and skeletal tissues [41]. In addition, it also gives rise to the stria vascularis of the inner ear and the glia cells of the cochleovestibular nerve and inner ear ganglion [42]. *greb1l* has also been implicated in Hoxb1 and Shh$_a$ signaling in zebrafish [14], important pathways in the inner ear and cranial nerve development [43–45].

Previous reports on disease-related *GREB1L* variants showed that a variable phenotype is present, including within families segregating the same variant (e.g., left vs. right ear) [36,37]. In addition, a high level of reduced penetrance has been reported, including in family 2 of this study. There is no evidence that variants cluster within specific domains of the protein (Table 2; Figure 2). This finding is similar to what was observed for *EYA1*, an NC regulatory molecule which is involved branchio-oto-renal (BOR)/branchio-otic (BO) syndrome etiology [46]. *EYA1* is also characterized by a high level of phenotypic variation between patients, even within the same family, and the severity of the phenotype does not correlate with the type of variant nor with the domain involved. In BOR patients with *EYA1* variants, which presents with both ear and renal abnormalities, normal kidneys were often observed in family members with BOR while other family members had renal abnormalities [46]. Many neurocristopathies typically show this variable phenotypic profile amongst patients, even within families or within the same individual (left vs. right) [47], and multiple hypotheses have been suggested to explain this phenomenon, such as environmental factors and genetic modifiers [6,46,48]. However, as the NC is a transient and migratory cell population during development, there are also complex micro-regulations that could disturb NC migration during development. Because of this, the path of NC migration that ends up affected due to *GREB1L* dysfunction could perhaps be attributed to chance. An example of this can be found in knockout (Wv/Wv) mice. These mice have a defect in c-kit, a NC migration regulatory molecule involved in the migration and proliferation of melanocytes in the inner ear. Wv/Wv mice show uni- or bilateral inner ear issues with variable hearing levels, and this variability in inner-ear phenotype was found to be reflected by the number of melanocytes present and how far they migrated along each cochlea during development [49].

The particular link between renal and ear abnormalities has previously been demonstrated [47], including in neurocristopathies. Several neural crest regulatory molecules are known to cause ear/kidney syndromes with variable expression of both ear and kidney phenotypes (e.g., *EYA1*, *SIX1*, *SIX5*, *CHD7*, *MASP1*, *TBX1*), involved in BOR/BO syndrome, CHARGE syndrome, 3MC syndrome and DiGeorge syndrome [5,47]. In addition to these, there are also several other disorders with a specific renal/ear link, such as Alport syndrome and Bartter syndrome [50,51]. Interestingly, when reviewing all variants reported in *GREB1L* to date, we also demonstrate that 14% of *GREB1L* variants (N = 7) have been associated with ear-related issues. It is to be noted however, that many of the previous reports (focused on renal malformations) included aborted/stillborn fetuses, in which hearing could not have been assessed. In addition, inner ear and cochlear nerve malformations cannot be assessed via prenatal ultrasound and if an autopsy was performed and would usually not be detected on routine autopsy. Therefore, the number of ear malformations associated with *GREB1L* variants is likely under-reported. Last, this renal/ear link is also seen in Mayer-Rokitansky-Kuster-Hauser (MRKH) syndrome, characterized by abnormal development of the internal reproductive system in females, and is also caused by *GREB1L* variants (Table 2). Interestingly, HI is reported in 10–25% of individuals with MRKH syndrome [37].

We also detected a maternal bias in the inheritance of *GREB1L* variants (Table 2). This maternal bias has previously observed and two mechanisms have been suggested: (1) imprinting [8,36] (2) or *GREB1L* variants could affect male fertility resulting in a low rate of paternal inheritance [8]. Genital issues, including uterus aplasia, are common and have been reported in many females (Table 2), but the presence in males may be underestimated as the defect might not be a gross morphological abnormality that causes infertility.

De novo *GREB1L* variants have been previously implicated in a phenotype which consists of profound HI and inner ear and cochleovestibular nerve malformations [6]. The inner ear malformation seen in family 2 is remarkably similar to the patients previously reported with *de novo GREB1L* variants (Table 1) [6], and includes cochlear aplasia, cochlear nerve aplasia and bilateral dysplastic vestibules and semicircular canals (Figure 1), an ultra-rare phenotype. The finding of multiple independent cases with *GREB1L* variants and this exact ultra-rare phenotype is significant [6]. In addition, $greb1l^{-/-}$ zebrafish (p.Gln408Ter) exhibit a loss of or abnormal sensory epithelia innervation [6], supporting the importance of *GREB1L* in the inner ear and nerve development.

Unfortunately, we were unable to perform temporal bone imaging in the affected members of family 1 since they are located in a remote village in Pakistan. The profound bilateral congenital HI phenotype observed for affected members of this family suggests that it may also be due to inner ear/cochleovestibular nerve malformations. Since sample collection for DNA extraction and genetic screening is easier to implement in areas with limited access to modern healthcare systems than temporal bone imaging, we believe including *GREB1L* in diagnostic screening for nonsyndromic HI is valuable.

In conclusion, we demonstrate that autosomal dominantly inherited variants in *GREB1L* are involved in profound sensorineural HI etiology and show that *GREB1L* behaves with a similar phenotypic variance compared to other neurocristopathies. In addition, we recommend including *GREB1L* in diagnostic screening panels for nonsyndromic HI.

Supplementary Materials: The following are available online at http://www.mdpi.com/2073-4425/11/6/687/s1, Table S1: Candidate variants identified in both families, genotypes and annotations. Figure S1: Sanger traces of the *GREB1L* variants in both families.

Author Contributions: Conceptualization, methodology, I.S. (Isabelle Schrauwen), W.A., G.V.C. and S.M.L.; formal analysis, I.S. (Isabelle Schrauwen) T.B., and A.N.; investigation: K.L., I.S. (Isabelle Schatteman) and A.A.; data curation, K.L. and I.S. (Isabelle Schatteman); writing—original draft preparation, I.S. (Isabelle Schrauwen); writing—review and editing, all authors. All authors have read and agreed to the published version of the manuscript.

Funding: This study was supported by the American Hearing Research Foundation to I.S., the Higher Education Commission of Pakistan (to W.A.) and the National Institute of Deafness and other Communication Disorders grants R01 DC011651 and DC003594 to S.M.L.

Acknowledgments: We would like to thank the families for their participation in this study.

Conflicts of Interest: The authors have no conflicts of interest related to the work in this manuscript.

Web Resources:

ANNOVAR	http://annovar.openbioinformatics.org/
Burrows-Wheeler aligner	http://bio-bwa.sourceforge.net/
ClinVar	https://www.ncbi.nlm.nih.gov/clinvar/
combined annotation dependent depletion (CADD)	http://cadd.gs.washington.edu/
dbSNFP	https://sites.google.com/site/jpopgen/dbNSFP
dbSNP	https://www.ncbi.nlm.nih.gov/projects/SNP/
gEAR	https://umgear.org/
genome aggregation database (gnomAD)	http://gnomad.broadinstitute.org/
genome analysis toolkit (GATK)	https://software.broadinstitute.org/gatk/
genomic evolutionary rate profiling (GERP)	http://mendel.stanford.edu/SidowLab/downloads/gerp/
Greater Middle East (GME) variome project	http://igm.ucsd.edu/gme
Hereditary hearing loss homepage	https://hereditaryhearingloss.org
Online Mendelian inheritance of man (OMIM)	https://www.omim.org/
PhastCons and PhyloP	http://compgen.cshl.edu/phast/
Picard	http://broadinstitute.github.io/picard/
SHIELD	https://shield.hms.harvard.edu/
World Health Organization	https://www.who.int/news-room/fact-sheets/detail/deafness-and-hearing-loss

References

1. Shearer, A.E.; Hildebrand, M.S.; Smith, R.J. Hereditary hearing loss and deafness overview. In *GeneReviews®*; Adam, M.P., Ardinger, H.H., Pagon, R.A., Wallace, S.E., Bean, L.J., Stephens, K., Amemiya, A., Eds.; University of Washington: Seattle, WA, USA, 1993.
2. Chakchouk, I.; Zhang, D.; Zhang, Z.; Francioli, L.C.; Santos-Cortez, R.L.P.; Schrauwen, I.; Leal, S.M. Disparities in discovery of pathogenic variants for autosomal recessive non-syndromic hearing impairment by ancestry. *Eur. J. Hum. Genet.* **2019**, *27*, 1456–1465. [CrossRef] [PubMed]
3. Kaplan, A.B.; Kozin, E.D.; Puram, S.V.; Owoc, M.S.; Shah, P.V.; Hight, A.E.; Sethi, R.K.V.; Remenschneider, A.K.; Lee, D.J. Auditory brainstem implant candidacy in the United States in children 0–17 years old. *Int. J. Pediatr. Otorhinolaryngol.* **2015**, *79*, 310–315. [CrossRef] [PubMed]
4. Sennaroglu, L.; Saatci, I. A new classification for cochleovestibular malformations. *Laryngoscope* **2002**, *112*, 2230–2241. [CrossRef] [PubMed]
5. Kari, E.; Llaci, L.; Go, J.L.; Naymik, M.; Knowles, J.A.; Leal, S.M.; Rangasamy, S.; Huentelman, M.J.; Liang, W.; Friedman, R.A.; et al. Genes Implicated in Rare Congenital Inner Ear and Cochleovestibular Nerve Malformations. *Ear Hear.* **2020**. [CrossRef]
6. Schrauwen, I.; Kari, E.; Mattox, J.; Llaci, L.; Smeeton, J.; Naymik, M.; Raible, D.W.; Knowles, J.A.; Crump, J.G.; Huentelman, M.J.; et al. De novo variants in GREB1L are associated with non-syndromic inner ear malformations and deafness. *Hum. Genet.* **2018**, *137*, 459–470. [CrossRef]
7. Brunskill, E.W.; Potter, A.S.; Distasio, A.; Dexheimer, P.; Plassard, A.; Aronow, B.J.; Potter, S.S. A gene expression atlas of early craniofacial development. *Dev. Biol.* **2014**, *391*, 133–146. [CrossRef]

8. De Tomasi, L.; David, P.; Humbert, C.; Silbermann, F.; Arrondel, C.; Tores, F.; Fouquet, S.; Desgrange, A.; Niel, O.; Bole-Feysot, C.; et al. Mutations in GREB1L cause bilateral kidney agenesis in humans and mice. *Am. J. Hum. Genet.* **2017**, *101*, 803–814. [CrossRef]
9. Cacheiro, P.; Haendel, M.A.; Smedley, D. International Mouse Phenotyping Consortium and the Monarch Initiative New models for human disease from the International Mouse Phenotyping Consortium. *Mamm. Genome* **2019**, *30*, 143–150. [CrossRef]
10. Cartegni, L.; Wang, J.; Zhu, Z.; Zhang, M.Q.; Krainer, A.R. ESEfinder: A web resource to identify exonic splicing enhancers. *Nucleic Acids Res.* **2003**, *31*, 3568–3571. [CrossRef]
11. Desmet, F.-O.; Hamroun, D.; Lalande, M.; Collod-Béroud, G.; Claustres, M.; Béroud, C. Human splicing finder: An online bioinformatics tool to predict splicing signals. *Nucleic Acids Res.* **2009**, *37*, e67. [CrossRef]
12. Richards, S.; Aziz, N.; Bale, S.; Bick, D.; Das, S.; Gastier-Foster, J.; Grody, W.W.; Hegde, M.; Lyon, E.; Spector, E.; et al. Standards and guidelines for the interpretation of sequence variants: A joint consensus recommendation of the American College of Medical Genetics and Genomics and the Association for Molecular Pathology. *Genet. Med.* **2015**, *17*, 405–424. [CrossRef] [PubMed]
13. Boissel, S.; Fallet-Bianco, C.; Chitayat, D.; Kremer, V.; Nassif, C.; Rypens, F.; Delrue, M.-A.; Soglio, D.D.; Oligny, L.L.; Patey, N.; et al. Genomic study of severe fetal anomalies and discovery of GREB1L mutations in renal agenesis. *Genet. Med.* **2018**, *20*, 745–753. [CrossRef] [PubMed]
14. Sanna-Cherchi, S.; Khan, K.; Westland, R.; Krithivasan, P.; Fievet, L.; Rasouly, H.M.; Ionita-Laza, I.; Capone, V.P.; Fasel, D.A.; Kiryluk, K.; et al. Exome-wide Association Study Identifies GREB1L Mutations in Congenital Kidney Malformations. *Am. J. Hum. Genet.* **2017**, *101*, 789–802. [CrossRef]
15. Sambrook, J.; Russell, D.W. Purification of nucleic acids by extraction with phenol: Chloroform. *CSH Protoc.* **2006**, *2006*. [CrossRef] [PubMed]
16. Schultz, J.M.; Khan, S.N.; Ahmed, Z.M.; Riazuddin, S.; Waryah, A.M.; Chhatre, D.; Starost, M.F.; Ploplis, B.; Buckley, S.; Velásquez, D.; et al. Noncoding mutations of HGF are associated with nonsyndromic hearing loss, DFNB39. *Am. J. Hum. Genet.* **2009**, *85*, 25–39. [CrossRef] [PubMed]
17. Riazuddin, S.; Belyantseva, I.A.; Giese, A.P.J.; Lee, K.; Indzhykulian, A.A.; Nandamuri, S.P.; Yousaf, R.; Sinha, G.P.; Lee, S.; Terrell, D.; et al. Alterations of the CIB2 calcium- and integrin-binding protein cause Usher syndrome type 1J and nonsyndromic deafness DFNB48. *Nat. Genet.* **2012**, *44*, 1265–1271. [CrossRef]
18. Shahzad, M.; Sivakumaran, T.A.; Qaiser, T.A.; Schultz, J.M.; Hussain, Z.; Flanagan, M.; Bhinder, M.A.; Kissell, D.; Greinwald, J.H.; Khan, S.N.; et al. Genetic Analysis through OtoSeq of Pakistani Families Segregating Prelingual Hearing Loss. *Otolaryngol. -Head Neck Surg.* **2013**, *149*, 478–487. [CrossRef]
19. Li, H.; Durbin, R. Fast and accurate short read alignment with Burrows-Wheeler transform. *Bioinformatics* **2009**, *25*, 1754–1760. [CrossRef]
20. McKenna, A.; Hanna, M.; Banks, E.; Sivachenko, A.; Cibulskis, K.; Kernytsky, A.; Garimella, K.; Altshuler, D.; Gabriel, S.; Daly, M.; et al. The genome analysis toolkit: A MapReduce framework for analyzing next-generation DNA sequencing data. *Genome Res.* **2010**, *20*, 1297–1303. [CrossRef]
21. Yang, H.; Wang, K. Genomic variant annotation and prioritization with ANNOVAR and wANNOVAR. *Nat. Protoc.* **2015**, *10*, 1556–1566. [CrossRef]
22. Lek, M.; Karczewski, K.J.; Minikel, E.V.; Samocha, K.E.; Banks, E.; Fennell, T.; O'Donnell-Luria, A.H.; Ware, J.S.; Hill, A.J.; Cummings, B.B.; et al. Analysis of protein-coding genetic variation in 60,706 humans. *Nature* **2016**, *536*, 285–291. [CrossRef] [PubMed]
23. Scott, E.M.; Halees, A.; Itan, Y.; Spencer, E.G.; He, Y.; Azab, M.A.; Gabriel, S.B.; Belkadi, A.; Boisson, B.; Abel, L.; et al. Characterization of Greater Middle Eastern genetic variation for enhanced disease gene discovery. *Nat. Genet.* **2016**, *48*, 1071–1076. [CrossRef] [PubMed]
24. Liu, X.; Wu, C.; Li, C.; Boerwinkle, E. dbNSFP v3.0: A one-stop database of functional predictions and annotations for human Nonsynonymous and splice-site SNVs. *Hum. Mutat.* **2016**, *37*, 235–241. [CrossRef] [PubMed]
25. Jian, X.; Boerwinkle, E.; Liu, X. In silico prediction of splice-altering single nucleotide variants in the human genome. *Nucleic Acids Res.* **2014**, *42*, 13534–13544. [CrossRef]
26. Davydov, E.V.; Goode, D.L.; Sirota, M.; Cooper, G.M.; Sidow, A.; Batzoglou, S. Identifying a High Fraction of the Human Genome to be under Selective Constraint Using GERP++. *PLoS Comput. Biol.* **2010**, *6*, e1001025. [CrossRef] [PubMed]

27. Rentzsch, P.; Witten, D.; Cooper, G.M.; Shendure, J.; Kircher, M. CADD: Predicting the deleteriousness of variants throughout the human genome. *Nucleic Acids Res.* **2019**, *47*, D886–D894. [CrossRef] [PubMed]
28. Shen, J.; Scheffer, D.I.; Kwan, K.Y.; Corey, D.P. SHIELD: An integrative gene expression database for inner ear research. *Database (Oxford)* **2015**, *2015*. [CrossRef]
29. Schrauwen, I.; Hasin-Brumshtein, Y.; Corneveaux, J.J.; Ohmen, J.; White, C.; Allen, A.N.; Lusis, A.J.; Van Camp, G.; Huentelman, M.J.; Friedman, R.A. A comprehensive catalogue of the coding and non-coding transcripts of the human inner ear. *Hear. Res.* **2016**, *333*, 266–274. [CrossRef]
30. Krumm, N.; Sudmant, P.H.; Ko, A.; O'Roak, B.J.; Malig, M.; Coe, B.P.; Quinlan, A.R.; Nickerson, D.A.; Eichler, E.E. Copy number variation detection and genotyping from exome sequence data. *Genome Res.* **2012**, *22*, 1525–1532. [CrossRef]
31. Zhang, J.; Haider, S.; Baran, J.; Cros, A.; Guberman, J.M.; Hsu, J.; Liang, Y.; Yao, L.; Kasprzyk, A. BioMart: A data federation framework for large collaborative projects. *Database (Oxford)* **2011**, *2011*. [CrossRef]
32. MacDonald, J.R.; Ziman, R.; Yuen, R.K.C.; Feuk, L.; Scherer, S.W. The Database of Genomic Variants: A curated collection of structural variation in the human genome. *Nucleic Acids Res.* **2014**, *42*, D986–D992. [CrossRef] [PubMed]
33. Optimizing Genomic Medicine in Epilepsy Through a Gene-Customized Approach to Missense Variant Interpretation. Available online: https://genome.cshlp.org/content/27/10/1715/F1.expansion.html (accessed on 6 March 2020).
34. Jarvik, G.P.; Browning, B.L. Consideration of Cosegregation in the Pathogenicity Classification of Genomic Variants. *Am. J. Hum. Genet.* **2016**, *98*, 1077–1081. [CrossRef]
35. Rasmussen, M.; Sunde, L.; Nielsen, M.L.; Ramsing, M.; Petersen, A.; Hjortshøj, T.D.; Olsen, T.E.; Tabor, A.; Hertz, J.M.; Johnsen, I.; et al. Targeted gene sequencing and whole-exome sequencing in autopsied fetuses with prenatally diagnosed kidney anomalies. *Clin. Genet.* **2018**, *93*, 860–869. [CrossRef] [PubMed]
36. Herlin, M.K.; Le, V.Q.; Højland, A.T.; Ernst, A.; Okkels, H.; Petersen, A.C.; Petersen, M.B.; Pedersen, I.S. Whole-exome sequencing identifies a GREB1L variant in a three-generation family with Müllerian and renal agenesis: A novel candidate gene in Mayer-Rokitansky-Küster-Hauser (MRKH) syndrome. A case report. *Hum. Reprod.* **2019**, *34*, 1838–1846. [CrossRef]
37. Adeline, J.; Bouchra, B.; Corinne, F.; Jerôme, T.; Claire, J.; Aimé, L.; Elise, B.-B.; Christèle, D.; Véronique, D.; Laurent, P.; et al. GREB1L variants in familial and sporadic hereditary urogenital adysplasia and Mayer-Rokitansky-Kuster-Hauser syndrome. *Clin. Genet.* **2020**. [CrossRef]
38. Brophy, P.D.; Rasmussen, M.; Parida, M.; Bonde, G.; Darbro, B.W.; Hong, X.; Clarke, J.C.; Peterson, K.A.; Denegre, J.; Schneider, M.; et al. A Gene Implicated in Activation of Retinoic Acid Receptor Targets Is a Novel Renal Agenesis Gene in Humans. *Genetics* **2017**, *207*, 215–228. [CrossRef] [PubMed]
39. Iyer, L.M.; Zhang, D.; Burroughs, A.M.; Aravind, L. Computational identification of novel biochemical systems involved in oxidation, glycosylation and other complex modifications of bases in DNA. *Nucleic Acids Res.* **2013**, *41*, 7635–7655. [CrossRef] [PubMed]
40. Plouhinec, J.-L.; Roche, D.D.; Pegoraro, C.; Figueiredo, A.-L.; Maczkowiak, F.; Brunet, L.J.; Milet, C.; Vert, J.-P.; Pollet, N.; Harland, R.M.; et al. Pax3 and Zic1 trigger the early neural crest gene regulatory network by the direct activation of multiple key neural crest specifiers. *Dev. Biol.* **2014**, *386*, 461–472. [CrossRef]
41. Shakhova, O.; Sommer, L. Neural crest-derived stem cells. In *StemBook*; Harvard Stem Cell Institute: Cambridge, MA, USA, 2008.
42. Whitfield, T.T. Development of the inner ear. *Curr. Opin. Genet. Dev.* **2015**, *32*, 112–118. [CrossRef]
43. Webb, B.D.; Shaaban, S.; Gaspar, H.; Cunha, L.F.; Schubert, C.R.; Hao, K.; Robson, C.D.; Chan, W.-M.; Andrews, C.; MacKinnon, S.; et al. HOXB1 founder mutation in humans recapitulates the phenotype of Hoxb1-/- mice. *Am. J. Hum. Genet.* **2012**, *91*, 171–179. [CrossRef]
44. Vogel, M.; Velleuer, E.; Schmidt-Jiménez, L.F.; Mayatepek, E.; Borkhardt, A.; Alawi, M.; Kutsche, K.; Kortüm, F. Homozygous HOXB1 loss-of-function mutation in a large family with hereditary congenital facial paresis. *Am. J. Med. Genet. A* **2016**, *170*, 1813–1819. [CrossRef] [PubMed]
45. Brown, A.S.; Epstein, D.J. Otic ablation of smoothened reveals direct and indirect requirements for Hedgehog signaling in inner ear development. *Development* **2011**, *138*, 3967–3976. [CrossRef] [PubMed]
46. Orten, D.J.; Fischer, S.M.; Sorensen, J.L.; Radhakrishna, U.; Cremers, C.W.R.J.; Marres, H.A.M.; Van Camp, G.; Welch, K.O.; Smith, R.J.H.; Kimberling, W.J. Branchio-oto-renal syndrome (BOR): Novel mutations in the

EYA1 gene, and a review of the mutational genetics of BOR. *Hum. Mutat.* **2008**, *29*, 537–544. [CrossRef] [PubMed]
47. Vega-Lopez, G.A.; Cerrizuela, S.; Tribulo, C.; Aybar, M.J. Neurocristopathies: New insights 150 years after the neural crest discovery. *Dev. Biol.* **2018**, *444* (Suppl 1), S110–S143. [CrossRef] [PubMed]
48. Marques, A.H.; O'Connor, T.G.; Roth, C.; Susser, E.; Bjørke-Monsen, A.-L. The influence of maternal prenatal and early childhood nutrition and maternal prenatal stress on offspring immune system development and neurodevelopmental disorders. *Front. Neurosci.* **2013**, *7*, 120. [CrossRef]
49. Cable, J.; Barkway, C.; Steel, K.P. Characteristics of stria vascularis melanocytes of viable dominant spotting (Wv/Wv) mouse mutants. *Hear. Res.* **1992**, *64*, 6–20. [CrossRef]
50. Mochizuki, T.; Lemmink, H.H.; Mariyama, M.; Antignac, C.; Gubler, M.C.; Pirson, Y.; Verellen-Dumoulin, C.; Chan, B.; Schröder, C.H.; Smeets, H.J. Identification of mutations in the alpha 3(IV) and alpha 4(IV) collagen genes in autosomal recessive Alport syndrome. *Nat. Genet.* **1994**, *8*, 77–81. [CrossRef]
51. Birkenhäger, R.; Otto, E.; Schürmann, M.J.; Vollmer, M.; Ruf, E.M.; Maier-Lutz, I.; Beekmann, F.; Fekete, A.; Omran, H.; Feldmann, D.; et al. Mutation of BSND causes Bartter syndrome with sensorineural deafness and kidney failure. *Nat. Genet.* **2001**, *29*, 310–314. [CrossRef]

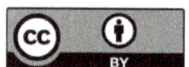

© 2020 by the authors. Licensee MDPI, Basel, Switzerland. This article is an open access article distributed under the terms and conditions of the Creative Commons Attribution (CC BY) license (http://creativecommons.org/licenses/by/4.0/).

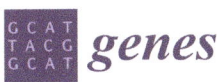

Article

Two Novel Pathogenic Variants Confirm *RMND1* Causative Role in Perrault Syndrome with Renal Involvement

Dominika Oziębło [1,2], Joanna Pazik [3], Iwona Stępniak [1], Henryk Skarżyński [4] and Monika Ołdak [1,*]

1. Department of Genetics, Institute of Physiology and Pathology of Hearing, 02-042 Warsaw, Poland; d.ozieblo@ifps.org.pl (D.O.); neurogenetyka@protonmail.com (I.S.)
2. Postgraduate School of Molecular Medicine, Medical University of Warsaw, 02-091 Warsaw, Poland
3. Department of Transplantation Medicine, Nephrology and Internal Diseases, Medical University of Warsaw, 02-091 Warsaw, Poland; jt.pazik@gmail.com
4. Oto-Rhino-Laryngology Surgery Clinic, Institute of Physiology and Pathology of Hearing, 02-042 Warsaw, Poland; h.skarzynski@ifps.org.pl
* Correspondence: m.oldak@ifps.org.pl; Tel.: +48-22-356-03-66

Received: 21 July 2020; Accepted: 3 September 2020; Published: 8 September 2020

Abstract: *RMND1* (required for meiotic nuclear division 1 homolog) pathogenic variants are known to cause combined oxidative phosphorylation deficiency (COXPD11), a severe multisystem disorder. In one patient, a homozygous *RMND1* pathogenic variant, with an established role in COXPD11, was associated with a Perrault-like syndrome. We performed a thorough clinical investigation and applied a targeted multigene hearing loss panel to reveal the cause of hearing loss, ovarian dysfunction (two cardinal features of Perrault syndrome) and chronic kidney disease in two adult female siblings. Two compound heterozygous missense variants, c.583G>A (p.Gly195Arg) and c.818A>C (p.Tyr273Ser), not previously associated with disease, were identified in *RMND1* in both patients, and their segregation with disease was confirmed in family members. The patients have no neurological or intellectual impairment, and nephrological evaluation predicts a benign course of kidney disease. Our study presents the mildest, so far reported, *RMND1*-related phenotype and delivers the first independent confirmation that *RMND1* is causally involved in the development of Perrault syndrome with renal involvement. This highlights the importance of including *RMND1* to the list of Perrault syndrome causative factors and provides new insight into the clinical manifestation of *RMND1* deficiency.

Keywords: *RMND1* (required for meiotic nuclear division 1 homolog); Perrault syndrome; renal disease; hearing loss; ovarian dysfunction; COXPD11 (combined oxidative phosphorylation deficiency); mitochondria

1. Introduction

RMND1 (required for meiotic nuclear division 1 homolog) is a nuclear gene that encodes a protein needed for proper functioning of mitochondria. Although the data on its exact role are still limited, it has been shown that the RMND1 protein belongs to a large mitochondrial inner membrane complex that supports translation of the mtDNA-encoded polypeptides [1,2], all of which represent essential structural components of the oxidative phosphorylation (OXPHOS) complexes. It has been proposed that RMND1 tethers mitochondrial ribosomes close to the sites where the primary mRNAs are matured, spatially coupling mitochondrial transcription with translation [3]. In line with this, *RMND1* pathogenic variants cause a generalized mitochondrial translation defect and are detected in patients with combined oxidative phosphorylation deficiency (COXPD11; MIM #614922), a severe recessive condition characterized by the presence of lactic acidosis, deafness, renal and liver dysfunction, central nervous system and muscle involvement with an onset at birth or early infancy [4,5].

In 2018, a different clinical presentation consistent with a diagnosis of Perrault syndrome (PRLTS) was associated with a known *RMND1* (c.713A>G; p.Asn238Ser) homozygous variant. The individual reported by Demain et al. suffered from sensorineural hearing loss (HL) and primary ovarian insufficiency (POI), defining clinical features of PRLTS, in addition to renal dysfunction and short stature. The phenotype was delineated based on exome sequencing data from a single patient [6]. Considering the absence of another reported disease-causing variant, a doubt may arise as to whether *RMND1* is related to PRLTS development. Here, we present novel data delivering the first independent confirmation that *RMND1* is causally involved in the development of PRLTS with chronic kidney disease.

2. Materials and Methods

2.1. Study Subjects

Two affected sisters from a nonconsanguineous Polish family, together with their parents and two other unaffected sisters, participated in the study (Figure 1A). The proband was born at term after an uneventful pregnancy, and her development in the first years of life was considered normal until the age of four, when bilateral HL was diagnosed. She received hearing aids at the age of six; the degree of HL progressed gradually and was accompanied by tinnitus and vertigo from the age of 31. No ear malformations were observed on temporal bone CT scans. Cochlear implantation was performed for the right ear at the age of 34 and for the left ear at the age of 36 with a good outcome. From the age of 17, she was under gynecological care due to irregular and scanty menstruation (menarche at age 14). Hypergonadotropic hypogonadism and small ovaries and uterus were recognized. Infertility was diagnosed, and hormone replacement therapy was introduced at the age of 28. Hypertension was diagnosed at the age of 31. At the age of 33, her left adrenal gland was removed because of lymphangioma, and chronic kidney disease (CKD) was diagnosed.

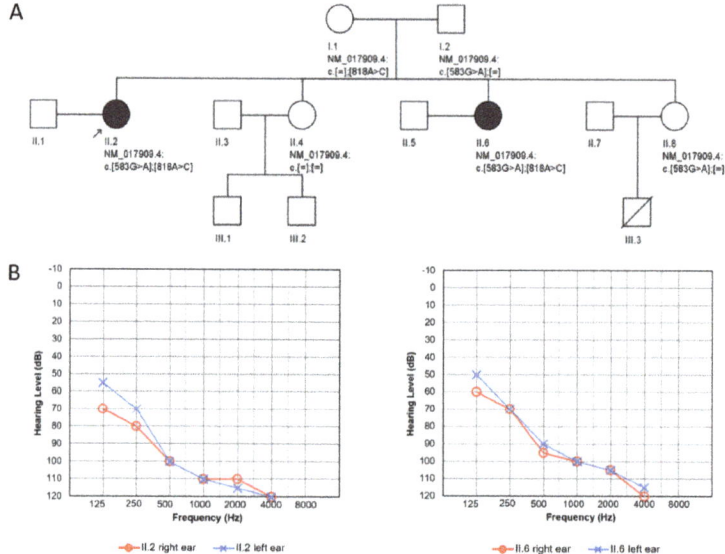

Figure 1. Pedigree and audiological data of the investigated family. (**A**) Pedigree showing affected family members (proband II.2, proband's sister II.6) and the identified *RMND1* variants. (**B**) Pure tone audiometry results of the proband (left panel) and her sister (right panel) at the age of 32.

The proband's younger sister was also born at term without any complications, and her development was normal. Bilateral HL was diagnosed at the age of 3. She does not have tinnitus or vertigo, and her HL is stable. She is using hearing aids sporadically and prefers to communicate with sign language. Evaluation for primary amenorrhea and delayed pubertal development at the age of 18 revealed gonadal dysgenesis with a normal female karyotype 46,XX. Vitamin B12 deficiency anemia and osteoporosis were diagnosed at the age of 26. At the age of 32, hypertension and CKD were recognized. Due to hypertension, enarenal and indapamide were implemented in the proband and amlodipine and torasemide in her sister. Both receive oestradiol and dydrogesterone supplementation to reduce the complications of POI.

Written informed consent was obtained from all participants. The study was approved by the ethics committee at the Institute of Physiology and Pathology of Hearing (KB.IFPS.25/2017) and performed according to the Declaration of Helsinki.

2.2. Nephrological and Neurological Examinations

The proband and her sister underwent thorough nephrological evaluation including whole blood count, electrolytes, venous blood gases, serum creatinine, calcium/phosphate balance, uric acid, lipid profile, urinalysis as well as urine albumin to creatinine ratio (UACR), urinary tract ultrasound with kidney size, and cortical thickness evaluation. To estimate glomerular filtration rate (eGFR), CKD-EPI (CKD Epidemiology Collaboration) creatinine equation was used [7]. A detailed neurological examination was performed. To assess the occurrence of neurological signs, the scale for assessment rating of ataxia—5th version (SARA) and Inventory of Non-Ataxia symptoms—6th version (INAS) were used [8,9].

2.3. Targeted HL Gene Panel, Data Analysis and Interpretation

Genomic DNA was extracted using a standard salting out procedure. Libraries were prepared with a custom HL 237-gene panel (SeqCap EZ Choice, Roche, Switzerland), containing genes related to PRLTS, i.e., *HSD17B4, HARS2, LARS2, TWNK, ERAL1, CLPP,* and *RMND1* and sequenced on a MiSeq Illumina platform. The quality control of raw FASTQ reads was performed, followed by adapter trimming and low quality reads removal with Trimmomatic [10]. Burrows–Wheeler Aligner [11] was used to map reads on hg38, followed by sorting and duplication removal using Samblaster [12]. Variant identification was done using multiple algorithms: HaplotypeCaller from GATK (Genome Analysis Toolkit) [13], Freebayes [14], DeepVariant [15], and MuTect2 [16]. Identified variants were annotated using Ensembl VEP [17] as well as multiple databases, including dbSNP [18], dbNSFP [18], GnomAD [19], ClinVar [20], and HGMD [21]. Inhouse databases of previously identified variants were used for annotation, to identify sequencing artifacts as well as variants common in the Polish population. The pathogenicity of identified variants was predicted based on the biochemical properties of the codon change and degree of evolutionary conservation using PolyPhen-2 [22], SIFT [23], Mutation Taster [24], LRT [25], and CADD [26]. Pathogenicity of the identified single nucleotide (SNV) and INDEL variants was evaluated by analyzing allele frequency, in silico predictions, annotations from public variant databases, matches in the inhouse variants database, and related medical literature. Evolutionary conservation was evaluated using GERP++ score [27]. Multiple protein sequence alignment was performed using COBALT [28], and variant localization across evolutionary diverse species was visualized with Jalview v2.11.1.0 software [29]. Detected variants were assigned according to standards and guidelines for the interpretation of sequence variants [30,31]. Selected probably causative variants were confirmed using direct Sanger sequencing and reported based on the *RMND1* NM_017909.4 and NP_060379.2 reference sequences.

3. Results

3.1. Clinical Presentation

The major clinical features of the proband, a 44-year old female, and her sister, a 36-year old female, were severe-to-profound bilateral sensorineural HL (Figure 1B) and ovarian dysfunction accompanied by CKD that developed in the fourth decade of life. Both had a normal stature. Laboratory findings on renal involvement, blood lactate concentration and core parameters of venous acid-base balance are given in Table 1, as shown by eGFR and UACR both patients were in stage G3, A1 of CKD [32]. The proband's calculated one-year eGFR decline was −0.45 mL/min and in her sister −0.66 mL/min. On repeated ultrasound evaluations, the size and cortex thickness of the kidneys was slightly diminished, but generally, the kidneys' dimensions did not change within a twelve-year follow up. The proband's sister had a more complex nephrological profile. Although on ultrasound, both kidneys and their cortex were of normal size, on scintigraphy at the age of 32, substantial asymmetry of ERPL (effective renal plasma flow; 64% left, 36% right kidney) with uneven radiotracer accumulation in the right organ was found. It was interpreted as post-inflammatory scars even though the patient denied urinary tract infections.

Neurological assessment did not reveal any features of cerebellar, pyramidal or extrapyramidal syndromes either in the proband or her affected sister. They presented normal muscle tone and strength as well as reflexes in the upper and lower limbs. Both have completed higher education.

3.2. Identification of Pathogenic Variants

After performing next-generation sequencing (NGS), two heterozygous variants, c.583G>A and c.818A>C in *RMND1*, corresponding to missense changes p.Gly195Arg and p.Tyr273Ser, respectively, were identified in the proband (Figure 2A). The vast majority of computational algorithms predicted a probably pathogenic character of detected variants, and they were identified only in heterozygous, individual cases in the gnomAD population database (Table 2). Conservation analyses showed 100% identity of the analyzed regions among all tested species (Figure 2B), with GERP++ scores of 4.57 and 5.95. Based on the applicable standards and guidelines, we have classified the identified *RMND1* variants as likely pathogenic. No other pathogenic variants related to isolated or syndromic hereditary HL, in particular to PRLTS, were found. The same *RMND1* variant constellation was identified in her affected younger sister. Both parents and another healthy sister were heterozygous carriers of one of the *RMND1* variants. In the third sister, none of the *RMND1* variants was identified (Figure 1A).

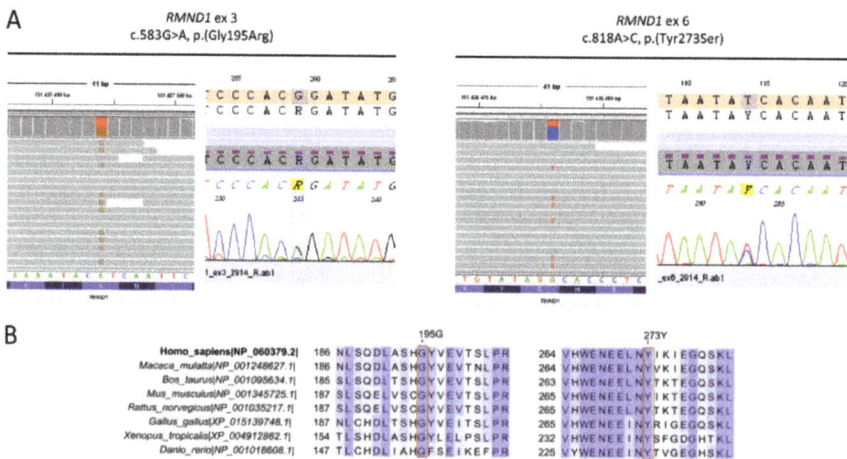

Figure 2. Genetic data of the investigated family. (**A**) Results of next-generation sequencing (NGS) and Sanger sequencing showing c.583G>A transition (p.Gly195Arg) and c.818A>C transversion (p.Tyr273Ser) in the *RMND1* gene. (**B**) Multiple protein sequence alignment of selected RMND1 regions among different species.

Table 1. Laboratory results of the proband and her sister.

	RBC (T/L)	Hb (g/dL)	Creatinine (mg/dL)	eGFR CKD EPI (mL/min)	Acid Base Venous Balance	Blood Lipids (mg/dL)	Calcium (mg/dL)	Phosphates (mg/dL)	PTH (pg/mL)	UACR (mg/g)
proband	4.49 (4.2–6.3)	13.3 (12–16)	**1.53** (0.6–1.3)	**41** (>90)	pH **7.31** (7.35–7.45) HCO$_3^-$ **20.7** (22–26 mmol/L) BE **−1.7** (−2 to +2mmol/l) Anion gap 12 (12 ± 4 mEq/L) Cl$^-$ 105 (98–106 mmol/L) Lactic acid 1.2 (0.5–1.6 mmol/L) K$^+$ **5.4** (3.4–4.5 mEq/L) Na$^+$ 137 (136–146 mEq/L)	T chol 159 (<190) HDL 71 (35–65) LDL 72 (<115) TG 76 (<150)	9.2 (8.5–10.1)	3.6 (2.5–4.9)	**72.6** (12–68.3)	2.9 (<30)
proband's sister	4.08 (4.2–6.3)	12.4 (12–16)	**1.38** (0.6–1.3)	**49** (>90)	pH **7.35** (7.35–7.45) HCO$_3^-$ **22** (22–26 mmol/L) BE **−0.6** (−2 to +2mmol/L) Anion gap 8.9 (12 ± 4 mEq/L) Cl$^-$ 105 (98–106 mmol/L) Lactic acid **1.7** (0.5–1.6 mmol/L) K$^+$ **5.2** (3.4–4.5 mEq/L) Na$^+$ 138 (136–146 mEq/L)	T chol **213** (<190) HDL 68 (35–65) LDL **145** (<115) TG 57 (<150)	9.4 (8.5–10.1)	3.6 (2.5–4.9)	**148.8** (12–68.3)	6.5 (<30)

Abnormal values are given in bold; reference values are in parentheses.

Table 2. Characteristics of *RMND1* variants detected in this study.

Variant cDNA Level	Variant Protein Level	Reference SNP ID	Population Frequencies			Pathogenicity Predictions					ACMG Classification *
			gnomAD	1000 Genomes	ESP 6500	SIFT	PolyPhen-2	Mutation Taster	LRT	CADD	
c.583G>A	p.(Gly195Arg)	rs776083030	0.00002388 (6/251308)	0	0	D (0.011)	PD (0.997)	D (1)	D (0)	D (29.7)	LP (PM2, PP1_M, PP3, PP4)
c.818A>C	p.(Tyr273Ser)	rs766739125	0.00000399 (1/250612)	0	0	D (0)	PD (1)	D (0.99)	N (0.001742)	D (26.4)	LP (PM2, PP1_M, PP3, PP4)

Abbreviations: D, damaging; PD, probably damaging; N, neutral; * ACMG classification criteria legend: LP, likely pathogenic; PM, moderate pathogenicity evidence; PP, supporting pathogenicity evidence; _M, moderate.

4. Discussion

Our clinical and genetic investigation shows that a combination of HL, ovarian dysfunction, and CKD constitutes a milder end of the *RMND1*-related phenotypic spectrum. Presence of the three clinical features can be defined as Perrault-like syndrome [6], PRLTS with renal involvement or just PRLTS with a respective consecutive number, according to the nomenclature used by OMIM (Online Mendelian Inheritance in Man, https://omim.org/), where subsequent numbers are assigned to a syndrome in order to distinguish the causative gene. PRLTS is characterized by the presence of sensorineural HL in both males and females and ovarian dysfunction ranging from gonadal dysgenesis to POI in females. These are the two PRLTS cardinal features; however, in some individuals additional, usually neurological conditions (e.g., developmental delay, cognitive impairment, ataxia or sensory axonal neuropathy) have been also reported (Table 3) [33]. Taking into account the heterogeneity of PRLTS phenotypic manifestations, in our opinion, it seems justified to recognize *RMND1* as the seventh PRLTS gene, where renal involvement represents an additional characteristic finding and no neurological signs or symptoms are found (neither in the patient reported by Demain [6] nor in our patients).

Kidney function is frequently affected in patients with RMND1 deficiency. Analyzing a large group of patients with COXPD11 due to *RMND1* pathogenic variants, Ng et al. found that renal involvement was present in more than two thirds of patients [4]. It was manifested by cystic dysplasia, renal tubular acidosis (persistent hyponatremia and hyperkalemia), end stage renal failure with subsequent kidney transplantation, anemia, proteinuria or CKD at different stages. The single, so far described, patient with PRLTS and *RMND1* homozygous pathogenic variant [6] had distal renal tubular acidosis with hyperchloremic metabolic acidosis, a normal anion gap, mildly elevated uric acid, low urine citrate levels, normal calcium levels, and a normal renal ultrasound. CKD was mentioned, but exact kidney function has not been given. In our patients, we found CKD of mild to moderate severity. The proband was affected by metabolic acidosis with normal fasting lactic acid concentration, hyperkalemia, normal chloride, and a normal anion gap. In her sister, we did not find metabolic acidosis, although the fasting lactic acid concentration was slightly above normal values. Both sisters presented with hypertension that may be secondary to CKD, and applied antihypertensive medications might have had an influence on electrolyte abnormalities. The calculated yearly filtration losses that we assessed in the patients were similar to the value of eGFR slope (−0.48 mL/min) found in women aged 35 to 49 years and renal stage IIIa (45–59 mL/min) [34]. This, together with a low-grade UACR of our patients, predicts a benign kidney disease course and makes reaching kidney failure and a requirement of renal replacement therapy less likely [32].

Ovarian dysfunction (ovarian atrophy and hypergonadotropic hypogonadism) as a consequence of *RMND1* pathogenic variants has been previously reported only once in a patient described by Demain et al. [6] and in none of the approximately 40 patients with OXPHOS deficiency. This could be explained by the early, prepubertal age at which the majority of children were investigated [4,5,35,36]. In only two patients examined at the age of 14 and 17, no reference was made to their sexual development [36]. Thus, at the moment, it is not clear how frequently ovaries are affected in patients with RMND1 deficiency.

RMND1 is a nuclear-encoded protein involved in mitochondrial translation. Disruption of this process is a well-known mechanism leading to PRLTS development (Table 3). In this study, we have identified two likely pathogenic *RMND1* variants not previously associated with disease. Presence of the detected *RMND1* variants in a trans configuration is consistent with the autosomal recessive mode of inheritance. Our study provides an independent confirmation on the causative role of *RMND1* in Perrault syndrome with renal involvement. Hearing loss and renal dysfunction are typical for of *RMND1*-related disorders. These two clinical features accompanied by ovarian dysfunction were present in our patients and they are consistent with the phenotype reported in the original study by Demain et al. [6]. The identification of two ultra-rare *RMND1* variants that are in a *trans* configuration, co-occur in two affected family members (having an almost identical phenotype) and do not co-occur in two other healthy siblings, strongly supports their pathogenic potential.

One of the identified variants (p.Gly195Arg) localizes close to the DUF155 domain at the protein N-terminus and the second one (p.Tyr273Ser) within the DUF155 domain (Figure 3). Considering that *RMND1* has three protein-encoding transcripts all of which contain the DUF155 domain [1], one may assume that all three proteins arising from the p.(Tyr273Ser)-carrying allele will be dysfunctional. It is not applicable for the second *RMND1* variant, that will affect two out of three alternative transcripts, leaving some functional RMND1 protein in the cells. Although the tissue-specific ratio of *RMND1* transcripts remains unknown, this observation may provide a possible explanation for the milder phenotype in our patients. It could also be owed to some other yet unidentified modifying factors. It is still a conundrum why the single patient with a homozygous p.(Asn238Ser) variant, localizing within the DUF155 domain, presented a relatively mild phenotype resembling PRLTS [6], in contrast to the, currently, four other patients with the same causative variant and a more severe infantile-onset multisystem disorder [4,5,37].

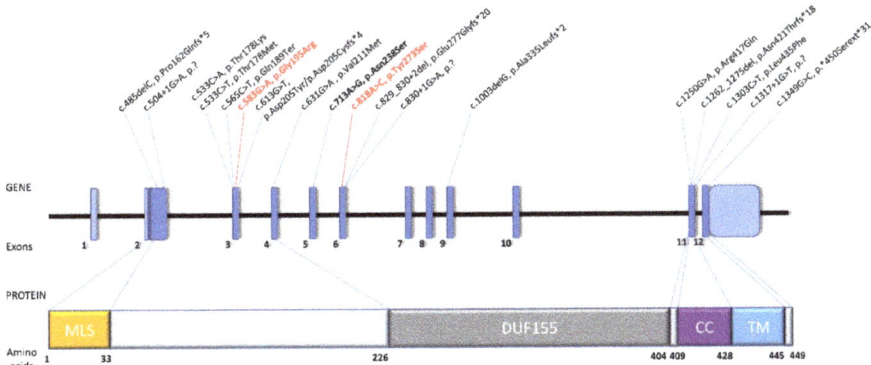

Figure 3. Schematic representation of *RMND1* gene and protein organization. Gene and protein structure is depicted based on the canonical transcript NM_017909.4 and reference protein sequence NP_060379.2. Previously reported *RMND1* pathogenic variants involved in development of combined oxidative phosphorylation deficiency (COXPD11) are written in black. Variants identified in this study are shown in red. Bolded are variants involved in the development of Perrault syndrome (PRLTS) with renal involvement. Abbreviations: MLS, mitochondrial localization sequence; DUF155, domain of unknown function; CC, coiled-coil; TM, transmembrane.

Table 3. Genes causally involved in the development of PRLTS and PRLTS-like features.

Gene (Locus)	Protein	Subcellular Localization	Function	Additional Clinical Features *	Inheritance Mode	Ref.
CLPP (19p13.3)	caseinolytic mitochondrial matrix peptidase proteolytic subunit	mitochondrial	mitochondrial protein degradation (component of a proteolytic complex)	• neurologic (e.g., ataxia, polyneuropathy, epilepsy, learning and developmental delay, spastic diplegia) • microcephaly • growth retardation	AR	[33,38–43]
ERAL1 (17q11.2)	Era like 12S mitochondrial rRNA chaperone 1	mitochondrial	mitochondrial protein translation (assembly of mitochondrial ribosomal subunit)	• not reported	AR	[44]
GGPS1 (1q42.3)	geranylgeranyl diphosphate synthase 1	cytoplasmic	acts on peroxisomal products, part of mevalonate pathway	• neurologic (muscular dystrophy, myopathy)	AR	[33,45]
HARS2 (5q31.3)	histidyl-tRNA synthetase 2	mitochondrial	mitochondrial protein translation (synthesis of histidyl-transfer RNA)	• not reported	AR	[39,46,47]
HSD17B4 (17q12.1)	hydroxysteroid 17-β dehydrogenase 4	peroxisomal	β-oxidation pathway for fatty acids in peroxisomes	• neurologic (e.g., ataxia, polyneuropathy, cerebellar atrophy, spastic diplegia, hypertonia, dysarthria, nystagmus, oculomotor apraxia, tremor, delayed motor development, cognitive impairment) • growth retardation • skeletal (e.g., pes cavus, pes equinovarus, scoliosis)	AR	[39,41,48–51]
LARS2 (3p21.31)	leucyl-tRNA synthetase	mitochondrial	mitochondrial protein translation (synthesis of leucyl-transfer RNA)	• neurologic (e.g., ataxia, cerebellar syndrome, epilepsy, developmental delay, intellectual impairment, behavior disorder, leukodystrophy) • macrocephaly	AR	[33,39,41,52–60]
PEX6 (6p21.1)	peroxisomal biogenesis factor 6	peroxisomal	peroxisomal protein import (ATPase activity)	• not reported	AR	[33]
RMND1 (6q25.1)	required for meiotic nuclear division 1 homolog	mitochondrial	mitochondrial protein translation	• kidney disease • short stature	AR	[6] Present study
TFAM (10q21.1)	transcription factor A, mitochondrial	mitochondrial	key mitochondrial transcription factor	• intellectual impairment	AR	[33]
TWNK (10q24.31)	twinkle mtDNA helicase	mitochondrial	mitochondrial DNA replication and transcription (unwinds double-stranded DNA)	• neurologic (e.g., ataxia, polyneuropathy, limb paresis, muscle atrophy, muscle weakness, atrophy of cerebellum, diminished cervical enlargement, epilepsy, impaired eye movements, nystagmus, dysarthria)	AR	[39,41,61–65]

* Clinical features additional to hearing loss (HL) and ovarian dysfunction observed in some patients. AR, autosomal recessive.

5. Conclusions

In summary, we report two novel *RMND1* likely pathogenic variants leading to the mildest, so far reported, *RMND1*-related phenotype that corresponds to PRLTS with renal involvement. It was identified in two adult siblings with a very similar clinical presentation. Our study highlights the importance of including *RMND1* to the list of PRLTS causative factors and directs attention to ovaries as yet another organ affected by RMND1 deficiency. Future functional studies could be helpful to clarify the molecular mechanisms underlying the differences in phenotype severity of *RMND1*-related disorders.

Author Contributions: Conceptualization, M.O. and D.O.; methodology, D.O., J.P., I.S., and H.S.; formal analysis, D.O., J.P., and I.S.; investigation, D.O., J.P., and I.S.; resources, M.O. and H.S.; writing—original draft preparation, M.O. and D.O.; writing—review and editing, J.P., I.S., and H.S.; visualization, D.O. and J.P.; supervision, M.O.; project administration, M.O.; funding acquisition, M.O. and H.S. All authors have read and agreed to the published version of the manuscript.

Funding: This work was funded by the National Science Centre Grant No. 2016/22/E/NZ5/00470 and the Institute of Physiology and Pathology of Hearing. The APC was funded by the Institute of Physiology and Pathology of Hearing.

Acknowledgments: We are grateful to the patients and their family for participation in this study.

Conflicts of Interest: The authors declare no conflict of interest.

References

1. Garcia-Diaz, B.; Barros, M.H.; Sanna-Cherchi, S.; Emmanuele, V.; Akman, H.O.; Ferreiro-Barros, C.C.; Horvath, R.; Tadesse, S.; El Gharaby, N.; DiMauro, S.; et al. Infantile encephaloneuromyopathy and defective mitochondrial translation are due to a homozygous RMND1 mutation. *Am. J. Hum. Genet.* **2012**, *91*, 729–736. [CrossRef] [PubMed]
2. Janer, A.; Antonicka, H.; Lalonde, E.; Nishimura, T.; Sasarman, F.; Brown, G.K.; Brown, R.M.; Majewski, J.; Shoubridge, E.A. An RMND1 Mutation causes encephalopathy associated with multiple oxidative phosphorylation complex deficiencies and a mitochondrial translation defect. *Am. J. Hum. Genet.* **2012**, *91*, 737–743. [CrossRef] [PubMed]
3. Janer, A.; van Karnebeek, C.D.; Sasarman, F.; Antonicka, H.; Al Ghamdi, M.; Shyr, C.; Dunbar, M.; Stockler-Ispiroglu, S.; Ross, C.J.; Vallance, H.; et al. RMND1 deficiency associated with neonatal lactic acidosis, infantile onset renal failure, deafness, and multiorgan involvement. *Eur. J. Hum. Genet.* **2015**, *23*, 1301–1307. [CrossRef]
4. Ng, Y.S.; Alston, C.L.; Diodato, D.; Morris, A.A.; Ulrick, N.; Kmoch, S.; Houstek, J.; Martinelli, D.; Haghighi, A.; Atiq, M.; et al. The clinical, biochemical and genetic features associated with RMND1-related mitochondrial disease. *J. Med. Genet.* **2016**, *53*, 768–775. [CrossRef] [PubMed]
5. Shayota, B.J.; Le, N.T.; Bekheirnia, N.; Rosenfeld, J.A.; Goldstein, A.C.; Moritz, M.; Bartholomew, D.W.; Pastore, M.T.; Xia, F.; Eng, C.; et al. Characterization of the renal phenotype in RMND1-related mitochondrial disease. *Mol. Genet. Genomic Med.* **2019**, *7*, e973. [CrossRef]
6. Demain, L.A.M.; Antunes, D.; O'Sullivan, J.; Bhaskar, S.S.; O'Keefe, R.T.; Newman, W.G. A known pathogenic variant in the essential mitochondrial translation gene RMND1 causes a Perrault-like syndrome with renal defects. *Clin. Genet.* **2018**, *94*, 276–277. [CrossRef]
7. Levey, A.S.; Stevens, L.A. Estimating GFR using the CKD Epidemiology Collaboration (CKD-EPI) creatinine equation: More accurate GFR estimates, lower CKD prevalence estimates, and better risk predictions. *Am. J. Kidney Dis.* **2010**, *55*, 622–627. [CrossRef]
8. Schmitz-Hubsch, T.; du Montcel, S.T.; Baliko, L.; Berciano, J.; Boesch, S.; Depondt, C.; Giunti, P.; Globas, C.; Infante, J.; Kang, J.S.; et al. Scale for the assessment and rating of ataxia: Development of a new clinical scale. *Neurology* **2006**, *66*, 1717–1720. [CrossRef]
9. Schmitz-Hubsch, T.; Coudert, M.; Bauer, P.; Giunti, P.; Globas, C.; Baliko, L.; Filla, A.; Mariotti, C.; Rakowicz, M.; Charles, P.; et al. Spinocerebellar ataxia types 1, 2, 3, and 6: Disease severity and nonataxia symptoms. *Neurology* **2008**, *71*, 982–989. [CrossRef]

10. Lohse, M.; Bolger, A.M.; Nagel, A.; Fernie, A.R.; Lunn, J.E.; Stitt, M.; Usadel, B. RobiNA: A user-friendly, integrated software solution for RNA-Seq-based transcriptomics. *Nucleic Acids Res.* **2012**, *40*, W622–W627. [CrossRef]
11. Li, H.; Durbin, R. Fast and accurate short read alignment with Burrows-Wheeler transform. *Bioinformatics* **2009**, *25*, 1754–1760. [CrossRef] [PubMed]
12. Faust, G.G.; Hall, I.M. SAMBLASTER: Fast duplicate marking and structural variant read extraction. *Bioinformatics* **2014**, *30*, 2503–2505. [CrossRef] [PubMed]
13. McKenna, A.; Hanna, M.; Banks, E.; Sivachenko, A.; Cibulskis, K.; Kernytsky, A.; Garimella, K.; Altshuler, D.; Gabriel, S.; Daly, M.; et al. The Genome Analysis Toolkit: A MapReduce framework for analyzing next-generation DNA sequencing data. *Genome Res.* **2010**, *20*, 1297–1303. [CrossRef] [PubMed]
14. Garrison, E.; Marth, G. Haplotype-based variant detection from short-read sequencing. *arXiv* **2012**, arXiv:1207.3907.
15. Poplin, R.; Chang, P.C.; Alexander, D.; Schwartz, S.; Colthurst, T.; Ku, A.; Newburger, D.; Dijamco, J.; Nguyen, N.; Afshar, P.T.; et al. A universal SNP and small-indel variant caller using deep neural networks. *Nat. Biotechnol.* **2018**, *36*, 983–987. [CrossRef]
16. Cibulskis, K.; Lawrence, M.S.; Carter, S.L.; Sivachenko, A.; Jaffe, D.; Sougnez, C.; Gabriel, S.; Meyerson, M.; Lander, E.S.; Getz, G. Sensitive detection of somatic point mutations in impure and heterogeneous cancer samples. *Nat. Biotechnol.* **2013**, *31*, 213–219. [CrossRef]
17. McLaren, W.; Gil, L.; Hunt, S.E.; Riat, H.S.; Ritchie, G.R.; Thormann, A.; Flicek, P.; Cunningham, F. The Ensembl Variant Effect Predictor. *Genome Biol.* **2016**, *17*, 122. [CrossRef]
18. Liu, X.; Wu, C.; Li, C.; Boerwinkle, E. dbNSFP v3.0: A One-Stop Database of Functional Predictions and Annotations for Human Nonsynonymous and Splice-Site SNVs. *Hum. Mutat.* **2016**, *37*, 235–241. [CrossRef]
19. Karczewski, K.J.; Francioli, L.C.; Tiao, G.; Cummings, B.B.; Alföldi, J.; Wang, Q.; Collins, R.L.; Laricchia, K.M.; Ganna, A.; Birnbaum, D.P.; et al. The mutational constraint spectrum quantified from variation in 141,456 humans. *bioRxiv* **2020**, *10*, 531210. [CrossRef]
20. Landrum, M.J.; Lee, J.M.; Riley, G.R.; Jang, W.; Rubinstein, W.S.; Church, D.M.; Maglott, D.R. ClinVar: Public archive of relationships among sequence variation and human phenotype. *Nucleic Acids Res.* **2014**, *42*, D980–D985. [CrossRef]
21. Stenson, P.D.; Ball, E.V.; Mort, M.; Phillips, A.D.; Shiel, J.A.; Thomas, N.S.; Abeysinghe, S.; Krawczak, M.; Cooper, D.N. Human Gene Mutation Database (HGMD): 2003 update. *Hum. Mutat.* **2003**, *21*, 577–581. [CrossRef] [PubMed]
22. Adzhubei, I.; Jordan, D.M.; Sunyaev, S.R. Predicting functional effect of human missense mutations using PolyPhen-2. *Curr. Protoc. Hum. Genet.* **2013**, *76*, 7–20. [CrossRef] [PubMed]
23. Kumar, P.; Henikoff, S.; Ng, P.C. Predicting the effects of coding non-synonymous variants on protein function using the SIFT algorithm. *Nat. Protoc.* **2009**, *4*, 1073–1081. [CrossRef]
24. Schwarz, J.M.; Cooper, D.N.; Schuelke, M.; Seelow, D. MutationTaster2: Mutation prediction for the deep-sequencing age. *Nat. Methods* **2014**, *11*, 361–362. [CrossRef] [PubMed]
25. Chun, S.; Fay, J.C. Identification of deleterious mutations within three human genomes. *Genome Res.* **2009**, *19*, 1553–1561. [CrossRef] [PubMed]
26. Kircher, M.; Witten, D.M.; Jain, P.; O'Roak, B.J.; Cooper, G.M.; Shendure, J. A general framework for estimating the relative pathogenicity of human genetic variants. *Nat. Genet.* **2014**, *46*, 310–315. [CrossRef] [PubMed]
27. Davydov, E.V.; Goode, D.L.; Sirota, M.; Cooper, G.M.; Sidow, A.; Batzoglou, S. Identifying a high fraction of the human genome to be under selective constraint using GERP++. *PLoS Comput. Biol.* **2010**, *6*, e1001025. [CrossRef] [PubMed]
28. Papadopoulos, J.S.; Agarwala, R. COBALT: Constraint-based alignment tool for multiple protein sequences. *Bioinformatics* **2007**, *23*, 1073–1079. [CrossRef] [PubMed]
29. Waterhouse, A.M.; Procter, J.B.; Martin, D.M.; Clamp, M.; Barton, G.J. Jalview Version 2–a multiple sequence alignment editor and analysis workbench. *Bioinformatics* **2009**, *25*, 1189–1191. [CrossRef]
30. Oza, A.M.; DiStefano, M.T.; Hemphill, S.E.; Cushman, B.J.; Grant, A.R.; Siegert, R.K.; Shen, J.; Chapin, A.; Boczek, N.J.; Schimmenti, L.A.; et al. Expert specification of the ACMG/AMP variant interpretation guidelines for genetic hearing loss. *Hum. Mutat.* **2018**, *39*, 1593–1613. [CrossRef]

31. Richards, S.; Aziz, N.; Bale, S.; Bick, D.; Das, S.; Gastier-Foster, J.; Grody, W.W.; Hegde, M.; Lyon, E.; Spector, E.; et al. Standards and guidelines for the interpretation of sequence variants: A joint consensus recommendation of the American College of Medical Genetics and Genomics and the Association for Molecular Pathology. *Genet. Med.* **2015**, *17*, 405–424. [CrossRef] [PubMed]
32. Levin, A.; Stevens, P.E.; Bilous, R.W.; Coresh, J.; De Francisco, A.L.M.; De Jong, P.E.; Griffith, K.E.; Hemmelgarn, B.R.; Iseki, K.; Lamb, E.J.; et al. Kidney disease: Improving global outcomes (KDIGO) CKD work group. KDIGO 2012 clinical practice guideline for the evaluation and management of chronic kidney disease. *Kidney Int. Suppl.* **2013**, *3*, 150. [CrossRef]
33. Tucker, E.J.; Rius, R.; Jaillard, S.; Bell, K.; Lamont, P.J.; Travessa, A.; Dupont, J.; Sampaio, L.; Dulon, J.; Vuillaumier-Barrot, S.; et al. Genomic sequencing highlights the diverse molecular causes of Perrault syndrome: A peroxisomal disorder (PEX6), metabolic disorders (CLPP, GGPS1), and mtDNA maintenance/translation disorders (LARS2, TFAM). *Hum. Genet.* **2020**. [CrossRef] [PubMed]
34. Baba, M.; Shimbo, T.; Horio, M.; Ando, M.; Yasuda, Y.; Komatsu, Y.; Masuda, K.; Matsuo, S.; Maruyama, S. Longitudinal Study of the Decline in Renal Function in Healthy Subjects. *PLoS ONE* **2015**, *10*, e0129036. [CrossRef] [PubMed]
35. Broenen, E.; Ranchin, B.; Besmond, C.; Freychet, C.; Fouilhoux, A.; Perouse de Montclos, T.; Ville, D.; Bacchetta, J. RMND1 mutations in two siblings: Severe renal hypoplasia but different levels of extrarenal abnormality severity: The ethics of decision making. *Arch. Pediatr.* **2019**, *26*, 377–380. [CrossRef]
36. Ravn, K.; Neland, M.; Wibrand, F.; Duno, M.; Ostergaard, E. Hearing impairment and renal failure associated with RMND1 mutations. *Am. J. Med. Genet. Part A* **2016**, *170*, 142–147. [CrossRef]
37. Parikh, S.; Karaa, A.; Goldstein, A.; Ng, Y.S.; Gorman, G.; Feigenbaum, A.; Christodoulou, J.; Haas, R.; Tarnopolsky, M.; Cohen, B.K.; et al. Solid organ transplantation in primary mitochondrial disease: Proceed with caution. *Mol. Genet. Metab.* **2016**, *118*, 178–184. [CrossRef]
38. Theunissen, T.E.; Szklarczyk, R.; Gerards, M.; Hellebrekers, D.M.; Mulder-Den Hartog, E.N.; Vanoevelen, J.; Kamps, R.; de Koning, B.; Rutledge, S.L.; Schmitt-Mechelke, T.; et al. Specific MRI Abnormalities Reveal Severe Perrault Syndrome due to CLPP Defects. *Front. Neurol.* **2016**, *7*, 203. [CrossRef]
39. Lerat, J.; Jonard, L.; Loundon, N.; Christin-Maitre, S.; Lacombe, D.; Goizet, C.; Rouzier, C.; Van Maldergem, L.; Gherbi, S.; Garabedian, E.N.; et al. An Application of NGS for Molecular Investigations in Perrault Syndrome: Study of 14 Families and Review of the Literature. *Hum. Mutat.* **2016**, *37*, 1354–1362. [CrossRef]
40. Dursun, F.; Mohamoud, H.S.; Karim, N.; Naeem, M.; Jelani, M.; Kirmizibekmez, H. A Novel Missense Mutation in the CLPP Gene Causing Perrault Syndrome Type 3 in a Turkish Family. *J. Clin. Res. Pediatr. Endocrinol.* **2016**, *8*, 472–477. [CrossRef]
41. Demain, L.A.; Urquhart, J.E.; O'Sullivan, J.; Williams, S.G.; Bhaskar, S.S.; Jenkinson, E.M.; Lourenco, C.M.; Heiberg, A.; Pearce, S.H.; Shalev, S.A.; et al. Expanding the Genotypic Spectrum of Perrault syndrome. *Clin. Genet.* **2017**, *91*, 302–312. [CrossRef] [PubMed]
42. Ahmed, S.; Jelani, M.; Alrayes, N.; Mohamoud, H.S.; Almramhi, M.M.; Anshasi, W.; Ahmed, N.A.; Wang, J.; Nasir, J.; Al-Aama, J.Y. Exome analysis identified a novel missense mutation in the CLPP gene in a consanguineous Saudi family expanding the clinical spectrum of Perrault Syndrome type-3. *J. Neurol. Sci.* **2015**, *353*, 149–154. [CrossRef] [PubMed]
43. Jenkinson, E.M.; Rehman, A.U.; Walsh, T.; Clayton-Smith, J.; Lee, K.; Morell, R.J.; Drummond, M.C.; Khan, S.N.; Naeem, M.A.; Rauf, B.; et al. Perrault syndrome is caused by recessive mutations in CLPP, encoding a mitochondrial ATP-dependent chambered protease. *Am. J. Hum. Genet.* **2013**, *92*, 605–613. [CrossRef] [PubMed]
44. Chatzispyrou, I.A.; Alders, M.; Guerrero-Castillo, S.; Zapata Perez, R.; Haagmans, M.A.; Mouchiroud, L.; Koster, J.; Ofman, R.; Baas, F.; Waterham, H.R.; et al. A homozygous missense mutation in ERAL1, encoding a mitochondrial rRNA chaperone, causes Perrault syndrome. *Hum. Mol. Genet.* **2017**, *26*, 2541–2550. [CrossRef] [PubMed]
45. Foley, A.R.; Zou, Y.; Dunford, J.E.; Rooney, J.; Chandra, G.; Xiong, H.; Straub, V.; Voit, T.; Romero, N.; Donkervoort, S.; et al. GGPS1 Mutations Cause Muscular Dystrophy/Hearing Loss/Ovarian Insufficiency Syndrome. *Ann. Neurol.* **2020**. [CrossRef] [PubMed]

46. Karstensen, H.G.; Rendtorff, N.D.; Hindbaek, L.S.; Colombo, R.; Stein, A.; Birkebaek, N.H.; Hartmann-Petersen, R.; Lindorff-Larsen, K.; Hojland, A.T.; Petersen, M.B.; et al. Novel HARS2 missense variants identified in individuals with sensorineural hearing impairment and Perrault syndrome. *Eur. J. Med. Genet.* **2020**, *63*, 103733. [CrossRef]
47. Pierce, S.B.; Chisholm, K.M.; Lynch, E.D.; Lee, M.K.; Walsh, T.; Opitz, J.M.; Li, W.; Klevit, R.E.; King, M.C. Mutations in mitochondrial histidyl tRNA synthetase HARS2 cause ovarian dysgenesis and sensorineural hearing loss of Perrault syndrome. *Proc. Natl. Acad. Sci. USA* **2011**, *108*, 6543–6548. [CrossRef]
48. Kim, M.J.; Kim, S.J.; Kim, J.; Chae, H.; Kim, M.; Kim, Y. Genotype and phenotype heterogeneity in perrault syndrome. *J. Pediatr. Adolesc. Gynecol.* **2013**, *26*, e25–e27. [CrossRef]
49. Pierce, S.B.; Walsh, T.; Chisholm, K.M.; Lee, M.K.; Thornton, A.M.; Fiumara, A.; Opitz, J.M.; Levy-Lahad, E.; Klevit, R.E.; King, M.C. Mutations in the DBP-deficiency protein HSD17B4 cause ovarian dysgenesis, hearing loss, and ataxia of Perrault Syndrome. *Am. J. Hum. Genet.* **2010**, *87*, 282–288. [CrossRef] [PubMed]
50. Lieber, D.S.; Hershman, S.G.; Slate, N.G.; Calvo, S.E.; Sims, K.B.; Schmahmann, J.D.; Mootha, V.K. Next generation sequencing with copy number variant detection expands the phenotypic spectrum of HSD17B4-deficiency. *BMC Med. Genet.* **2014**, *15*, 30. [CrossRef]
51. Chen, K.; Yang, K.; Luo, S.S.; Chen, C.; Wang, Y.; Wang, Y.X.; Li, D.K.; Yang, Y.J.; Tang, Y.L.; Liu, F.T.; et al. A homozygous missense variant in HSD17B4 identified in a consanguineous Chinese Han family with type II Perrault syndrome. *BMC Med. Genet.* **2017**, *18*, 91. [CrossRef] [PubMed]
52. Pierce, S.B.; Gersak, K.; Michaelson-Cohen, R.; Walsh, T.; Lee, M.K.; Malach, D.; Klevit, R.E.; King, M.C.; Levy-Lahad, E. Mutations in LARS2, encoding mitochondrial leucyl-tRNA synthetase, lead to premature ovarian failure and hearing loss in Perrault syndrome. *Am. J. Hum. Genet.* **2013**, *92*, 614–620. [CrossRef] [PubMed]
53. Solda, G.; Caccia, S.; Robusto, M.; Chiereghin, C.; Castorina, P.; Ambrosetti, U.; Duga, S.; Asselta, R. First independent replication of the involvement of LARS2 in Perrault syndrome by whole-exome sequencing of an Italian family. *J. Hum. Genet.* **2016**, *61*, 295–300. [CrossRef] [PubMed]
54. Kosaki, R.; Horikawa, R.; Fujii, E.; Kosaki, K. Biallelic mutations in LARS2 can cause Perrault syndrome type 2 with neurologic symptoms. *Am. J. Med. Genet. A* **2018**, *176*, 404–408. [CrossRef] [PubMed]
55. Carminho-Rodrigues, M.T.; Klee, P.; Laurent, S.; Guipponi, M.; Abramowicz, M.; Cao-van, H.; Guinand, N.; Paoloni-Giacobino, A. LARS2-Perrault syndrome: A new case report and literature review. *BMC Med. Genet.* **2020**, *21*, 109. [CrossRef] [PubMed]
56. Al-Jaroudi, D.; Enabi, S.; AlThagafi, M.S. Perrault syndrome with amenorrhea, infertility, Tarlov cyst, and degenerative disc. *Gynecol. Endocrinol.* **2019**, *35*, 1037–1039. [CrossRef]
57. Riley, L.G.; Rudinger-Thirion, J.; Frugier, M.; Wilson, M.; Luig, M.; Alahakoon, T.I.; Nixon, C.Y.; Kirk, E.P.; Roscioli, T.; Lunke, S.; et al. The expanding LARS2 phenotypic spectrum: HLASA, Perrault syndrome with leukodystrophy, and mitochondrial myopathy. *Hum. Mutat.* **2020**, *41*, 1425–1434. [CrossRef]
58. Pan, Z.; Xu, H.; Tian, Y.; Liu, D.; Liu, H.; Li, R.; Dou, Q.; Zuo, B.; Zhai, R.; Tang, W.; et al. Perrault syndrome: Clinical report and retrospective analysis. *Mol. Genet. Genomic Med.* **2020**, e1445. [CrossRef]
59. van der Knaap, M.S.; Bugiani, M.; Mendes, M.I.; Riley, L.G.; Smith, D.E.C.; Rudinger-Thirion, J.; Frugier, M.; Breur, M.; Crawford, J.; van Gaalen, J.; et al. Biallelic variants in LARS2 and KARS cause deafness and (ovario)leukodystrophy. *Neurology* **2019**, *92*, e1225–e1237. [CrossRef]
60. Cherot, E.; Keren, B.; Dubourg, C.; Carre, W.; Fradin, M.; Lavillaureix, A.; Afenjar, A.; Burglen, L.; Whalen, S.; Charles, P.; et al. Using medical exome sequencing to identify the causes of neurodevelopmental disorders: Experience of 2 clinical units and 216 patients. *Clin. Genet.* **2018**, *93*, 567–576. [CrossRef]
61. Gotta, F.; Lamp, M.; Geroldi, A.; Trevisan, L.; Origone, P.; Fugazza, G.; Fabbri, S.; Nesti, C.; Rubegni, A.; Morani, F.; et al. A novel mutation of Twinkle in Perrault syndrome: A not rare diagnosis? *Ann. Hum. Genet.* **2020**, *84*, 417–422. [CrossRef] [PubMed]
62. Oldak, M.; Ozieblo, D.; Pollak, A.; Stepniak, I.; Lazniewski, M.; Lechowicz, U.; Kochanek, K.; Furmanek, M.; Tacikowska, G.; Plewczynski, D.; et al. Novel neuro-audiological findings and further evidence for TWNK involvement in Perrault syndrome. *J. Transl. Med.* **2017**, *15*, 25. [CrossRef] [PubMed]
63. Dominguez-Ruiz, M.; Garcia-Martinez, A.; Corral-Juan, M.; Perez-Alvarez, A.I.; Plasencia, A.M.; Villamar, M.; Moreno-Pelayo, M.A.; Matilla-Duenas, A.; Menendez-Gonzalez, M.; Del Castillo, I. Perrault syndrome with neurological features in a compound heterozygote for two TWNK mutations: Overlap of TWNK-related recessive disorders. *J. Transl. Med.* **2019**, *17*, 290. [CrossRef] [PubMed]

64. Fekete, B.; Pentelenyi, K.; Rudas, G.; Gal, A.; Grosz, Z.; Illes, A.; Idris, J.; Csukly, G.; Domonkos, A.; Molnar, M.J. Broadening the phenotype of the TWNK gene associated Perrault syndrome. *BMC Med. Genet.* **2019**, *20*, 198. [CrossRef]
65. Morino, H.; Pierce, S.B.; Matsuda, Y.; Walsh, T.; Ohsawa, R.; Newby, M.; Hiraki-Kamon, K.; Kuramochi, M.; Lee, M.K.; Klevit, R.E.; et al. Mutations in Twinkle primase-helicase cause Perrault syndrome with neurologic features. *Neurology* **2014**, *83*, 2054–2061. [CrossRef]

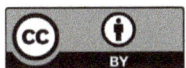

© 2020 by the authors. Licensee MDPI, Basel, Switzerland. This article is an open access article distributed under the terms and conditions of the Creative Commons Attribution (CC BY) license (http://creativecommons.org/licenses/by/4.0/).

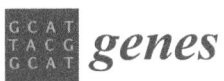

Article

Genetics of Hearing Impairment in North-Eastern Romania—A Cost-Effective Improved Diagnosis and Literature Review

Irina Resmerita [1,*], Romica Sebastian Cozma [2,*], Roxana Popescu [1], Luminita Mihaela Radulescu [2], Monica Cristina Panzaru [1], Lacramioara Ionela Butnariu [1], Lavinia Caba [1], Ovidiu-Dumitru Ilie [3], Eva-Cristiana Gavril [1], Eusebiu Vlad Gorduza [1] and Cristina Rusu [1]

[1] Department of Medical Genetics, Faculty of Medicine, "Grigore T. Popa" University of Medicine and Pharmacy, University Street, No 16, 700115 Iasi, Romania; roxana.popescu2014@gmail.com (R.P.); monica.panzaru@umfiasi.ro (M.C.P.); lacrybutnariu@gmail.com (L.I.B.); lavinia_zanet@yahoo.com (L.C.); evagavril@yahoo.com (E.-C.G.); vgord@mail.com (E.V.G.); abcrusu@gmail.com (C.R.)
[2] Department of Otorhinolaryngology, Faculty of Medicine, "Grigore T. Popa" University of Medicine and Pharmacy, University Street, No 16, 700115 Iasi, Romania; lmradulescu@yahoo.com
[3] Department of Biology, Faculty of Biology, "Alexandru Ioan Cuza" University, Carol I Avenue, No 20A, 700505 Iasi, Romania; ovidiuilie90@yahoo.com
* Correspondence: irina.resmerita@gmail.com or irina.resmerita@umfiasi.ro (I.R.); scozma2005@yahoo.com (R.S.C.); Tel.: +40-0741195689 (I.R.)

Received: 30 October 2020; Accepted: 12 December 2020; Published: 15 December 2020

Abstract: Background: We have investigated the main genetic causes for non-syndromic hearing impairment (NSHI) in the hearing impairment individuals from the North-Eastern Romania and proposed a cost-effective diagnosis protocol. Methods: MLPA followed by Sanger Sequencing were used for all 291 patients included in this study. Results: MLPA revealed abnormal results in 141 cases (48.45%): 57 (40.5%) were c.35delG homozygous, 26 (18.44%) were c.35delG heterozygous, 14 (9.93%) were compound heterozygous and 16 (11.35%) had other types of variants. The entire coding region of *GJB2* was sequenced and out of 150 patients with normal results at MLPA, 29.33% had abnormal results: variants in heterozygous state: c.71G>A (28%), c.457G>A (20%), c.269T>C (12%), c.109G>A (12%), c.100A>T (12%), c.551G>C (8%). Out of 26 patients with c.35delG in heterozygous state, 38.46% were in fact compound heterozygous. Conclusions: We identified two variants: c.109G>A and c.100A>T that have not been reported in any study from Romania. MLPA is an inexpensive, rapid and reliable technique that could be a cost-effective diagnosis method, useful for patients with hearing impairment. It can be adaptable for the mutation spectrum in every population and followed by Sanger sequencing can provide a genetic diagnosis for patients with different degrees of hearing impairment.

Keywords: hearing impairment; *GJB2*; NSHI; genetic screening; MLPA; cost-effective diagnosis

1. Introduction

Hearing impairment (HI) is the most common and heterogeneous sensory deficiency. It is defined by a unilateral or bilateral decrease in hearing acuity, more precisely a decrease in the hearing threshold in decibels (dB), at different frequencies. World Health Organization (WHO, Geneva, Switzerland) estimates that HI affects 466 million people around the world (6.1% of the world's population), of which 34 million children. It is considered that 1/1000 newborns have a form of congenital hearing impairment [1,2]

More than 50% of cases of deafness are due to genetic causes [3] out of which 67% are classified as non-syndromic hearing impairment (NSHI) (no clinical findings that define a recognizable syndrome are associated), whereas a specific syndrome can be identified in 33% of cases [4].

In the last 5 years, progress has been made in identifying new hearing impairment genetic causes, due to research and new technology. Approximately 121 loci for NSHI have been currently mapped: 49 autosomal dominant, 76 autosomal recessive and 5 X-linked [5].

GJB2 (NM_004004.5) or Gap Junction Protein β 2, situated on chromosome 13q12 (DFNB1 locus), is the most common cause of congenital hearing loss in many populations [6] including European and Mediterranean countries [7–9]. More than 150 different pathogenic variants in *GJB2* have been reported. The most frequent variant in the Caucasian populations is c.35delG, representing about 60% of all cases of NSHI [7,10–12].

GJB3 (Gap Junction Protein β 3) and *GJB6* (Gap Junction Protein β 6) are the next frequent genes that can cause hearing impairment but they are less common, with less than 10 mutations cited [13–15].

The aim of this study was to identify and investigate the main genetic causes for NSHI in the hearing impairment subjects from the North-Eastern Romania and to convince other specialties to advice for genetic testing and counseling. Subsequently we verified a possibility to use Multiplex Ligation-dependent Probe Amplification (MLPA) as a cost-effective diagnosis protocol for developing countries and as a first intention genetic method. Genetic screening is feasible, *GJB2* being accountable for a large proportion of NSHI.

MLPA is a technique that can analyze in a single reaction up to 50 DNA sequences and detect copy number variations of several human genes, including small intragenic rearrangements but also single-nucleotide polymorphisms or aberrant DNA methylation. To our knowledge, the studies of hearing loss in Romania are based on RFLP (restriction fragment length polymorphism), ARMS-PCR (amplification refractory mutation system-polymerase chain reaction) analysis and Sanger Sequencing. Our Genetic Centre has experience in MLPA for other pathologies since 2012, so we tried to implement it as a screening method for hearing impairment individuals.

In patients with hearing impairment, the diagnostic approach starts with personal medical history, physical examination and family history for at least three generations and should continue with genetic tests and appropriate management.

2. Materials and Methods

2.1. Ethical Compliance

The patients included in the study were registered under a numerical code in order to maintain anonymity. The use of the results was done according to a protocol approved by the Ethics Commission of "Grigore T. Popa" University of Medicine and Pharmacy Iasi (approval No. 14789) and the Ethics Commission of "Saint Mary" Emergency Children's Hospital Iasi (approval No. 681). Informed consent was signed by from patients, parents or legal guardians before beginning the research. All subjects included in this study were offered voluntary entrance.

2.2. Patient Recruitment

In the study (2015–2019), were enrolled 395 subjects with mild to profound and bilateral hearing impairment from the Iasi Regional Center for Medical Genetics and Audiology Department of Iasi Rehabilitation Clinical Hospital. All the subjects were clinically characterized by physical and auditory examinations. A number of 104 individuals were excluded from this study based on: syndromic or environmental/infectious etiology for hearing loss. The limitation of this study is that it investigates only the hearing loss subjects in order to assess the prevalence of certain type of mutations, so it does not include a control group.

2.3. Audiologic Assessment

Auditory functional assessment was performed only in the absence of the pathology of the middle ear, confirmed by otomicroscopy and wideband tympanometry. In cases identified with otitis media, the appropriate treatment was recommended and the child was rescheduled for repeated controls until the condition of the middle ear allowed audiological testing (normal otomicroscopy with wideband tympanogram of type A).

The audiological evaluation was adapted to the age and to the psycho-intellectual development of children. Thus, in children over 6 years of age, the auditory thresholds were measured by standard liminal tonal audiometry (air and bone conduction for 250 to 8000 Hz). In those under 6 years of age, as well as in some children over 6 years of age but who could not collaborate in subjective audiometric testing, the identification of hearing thresholds was done by objective audiological assessment of cross check type. The auditory steady state response and brainstem evoked response audiometry using insert headphones and distortion product otoacoustic emissions were measured in natural sleep. We performed visual reinforced audiometry or/and free field audiometric examination for subjective threshold confirmation in children who collaborated. In these cases, the conduction hearing loss was excluded based on normal otomicroscopy accompanied by type A wideband tympanometry. The audiologic evaluations were performed in soundproof rooms, using Interacoustics equipment (Equinox audiometer and Eclipse EP25). The audiologic follow-up was made periodically with the same methods adapted to each child's particularity (age and medical condition), mainly at 4-, 6- or 12-months intervals, in order to identify the dynamic evolution of hearing impairment and for the fitting of the conventional hearing aids. Children with progressive hearing loss received the indication for cochlear implantation when they were included in the category of severe or profound hearing loss.

All subjects had cranial computed tomography (CT) scan and none showed ear malformation.

2.4. Research Methodology

a. DNA genomic extraction

DNA was extracted from 3 mL of peripheral blood samples stored with EDTA agent, using Wizard Genomic DNA Purification Kit (Promega Corp., Madison, WI, USA).

b. MLPA

The probe mix P163 *GJB-WFS1-POU3F4* was used for the detection of deletions or duplications in the *GJB2*, *GJB3*, *GJB6*, *POU3F4* genes, genomic microdeletions upstream of *POU3F4* and the presence of six specific variants in the *GJB2* gene: c.313_326del14, c.235delC, c.167delT, c.101T>C and c.35delG.

The MLPA analysis was performed according to the manufacturer's protocol. Briefly, 100 nanograms of genomic DNA was denatured and hybridized with SALSA probes at 60 °C for approximately 17 h. PCR was performed after 15 min ligation at 54 °C, using Cy5 labeled primers. Fluorescent amplification products were separated based on their length by capillary electrophoresis in a CEQ 8000 GeXP Genetic Analysis System (Beckman Coulter, Brea, CA, USA) and the results were analyzed using Coffalyser.NET V9 program (MRC-Holland, Amsterdam, The Netherlands).

The probe ratio of deletion and duplication were fixed at 0.7 and 1.3 respectively.

Genomic regions of the *GJB2* gene were sequenced bidirectionally in heterozygous or normal individuals.

c. Sanger Sequencing

All samples were analyzed at the University of Medicine and Pharmacy "Grigore T. Popa" Iasi. The amplification using 125ng genomic DNA (25 μL reaction volume) was performed in a Sensoquest Thermocycler (Sensoquest, Göttingen, Germany), using Herculase II Fusion DNA Polymerase (Agilent Technologies, Santa Clara, CA, USA). PCR conditions included: initial denaturation (10 min at 95 °C), followed by 35 cycles of denaturation (30 s at 94 °C), annealing (30 s at 57 °C) and elongation (60 s at 72 °C), with a final elongation at 72 °C for 5 min, as described by M. RamShankar [16].

The sequencing was performed using primers previously described [16] and GenomeLab™ Dye Terminator Cycle Sequencing (DTCS) Quick Start kit (Beckman Coulter, Brea, CA, USA). A modified protocol was used with 10 µL reaction volume according to Azadan et al. [17]. The Agencourt system (Beckman-Coulter) was used to purify PCR amplicons (Agencourt AMPure XP, Brea, CA, USA) and sequencing products (Agencourt Cleanseq® system, Brea, CA USA). The final products were subsequently separated and detected on a CEQ 8000 GeXP Genetic Analysis System (Beckman-Coulter). Sequences were analyzed in both directions (forward and reverse) and compared with the NCBI reference sequence NM_004004, using Mega6 software. The variants were verified for pathogenicity in Mutation taster, ClinVar and PolyPhen for the evaluation of disease-causing potential of sequence alterations [18–20].

d. Statistical Analysis

Experiment results were analyzed in Excel and presented in descriptive statistics.

3. Results

A total sample of 291 patients from North-Eastern Romania were collected between 2015–2019. HI was reported to be congenital and without other accompanying clinical features. All patients included in this study showed different pathologic levels of auditory thresholds, from mild to profound bilateral hearing impairment. The patients' age ranged between 1 month to 52 years (median age 12.31).

Among the 291 probands, 74.6% (217/291) were sporadic cases of HI (simplex probands) (of which 15 with parental consanguinity) and 25.4% (74/291) had at least one first degree affected relative with bilateral HI (multiplex probands), of which 4 with parental consanguinity.

Mutations in *GJB2*, *GJB3*, *GJB6*, *POU3F4* and *WFS1* genes were analyzed by MLPA that revealed abnormal results in 141 cases (48.45%). Out of the total of 141 abnormal cases, 4 (2.84%) had variants in *WFS1* gene and 137 (97.16%) in *GJB2* gene: 57 (40.43%) were c.35delG homozygous, 26 (18.44%) were c.35delG heterozygous, 30 (21.28%) were compound heterozygous and 28 (19.86%) had other types of variants. No mutations were identified by MLPA in *GJB3*, *GJB6* and *POU3F4* genes.

Referring to the *WFS1* gene, all of the 4 patients with variants in this gene had exon 8 deletion (see Table 1). They had non-progressive mild to moderate hearing impairment and the age ranges from 15 to 20 years. We included these patients in a different study.

Table 1. Variants spectrum found in this study.

	Variants	Protein Change	Clinical Significance	Patients (n)
MLPA	c.35delG, rs80338939	p.Gly12Valfs	Pathogenic	97
	c.101T>C, rs35887622	p.Met34Thr	Pathogenic	19
	c.313_326del14, rs111033253	p.Lys105Glyfs	Pathogenic	12
	c.-23+1G>A, rs80338940	p.Trp3Ter	Pathogenic	6
	Del *WFS* 1-8		Pathogenic	4
	Del ex1 *GJB2*		Pathogenic	3
SANGER SEQUENCING	c.71G>A, rs104894396	p.Trp24Ter	Pathogenic	15
	c.551G>C, rs80338950	p.Arg184Pro	Pathogenic	4
	c.109G>A, rs72474224	p.Val37Ile	Pathogenic	3
	c.269T>C, rs8033894	p.Leu90Pro	Pathogenic	3
	c.100A>T, rs564084861	p.Met34Leu	Uncertain significance	3
	c.457G>A, rs111033186	p.Val153Ile	Likely benign	5
	c.380G>A, rs111033196	p.Arg127His	Benign	10
	c.39G>A	p.(=)	Benign	4
	c.341C>G	p.Glu114Gly	Benign	4
	c.79G>A, rs2274084	p.Val27Ile	Benign	6

Regarding the *GJB2* gene, the most common pathogenic variant in the Romanian population is c.35delG, found in 97 patients in our study (33.3%). Of these, 57 patients (58.76%) had the c.35delG variant in homozygous state, 26 (26.84%) in heterozygous state and 14 (14.4%) were compound heterozygous for 3 different 35delG/non-35delG variants.

The entire coding region of *GJB2* was sequenced in all individuals included in this study. Out of 26 patients with c.35delG variant in heterozygous state, 10 patients (38.46%) were in fact compound heterozygous. Among 150 patients with normal results at MLPA, 44 patients (29.33%) had abnormal results: 25 patients with variants in heterozygous state: 7 with c.71G>A (28%), 5 with c.457G>A (20%), 3 with c.269T>C (12%), 3 with c.109G>A (12%), 3 with c.100A>T (12%), 2 with c.551G>C (8%). All the patients with c.35delG in homozygous state were confirmed with Sanger Sequencing.

The *GJB2* variant spectrum found in this study is listed in Table 1.

Genotype-phenotype correlation was performed based on the distribution of the severity of HI in c.35delG and non-35delG genotype categories as shown in Table 2. Most cases had hearing loss before age 18. A small proportion of patients with mild hearing impairment showed a sequence variation in *GJB2*. Out of 18 patients with mild hearing loss, only 2 of them had c.35delG in homozygous state (diagnosed before age 4) and 4 patients had c.35delG in heterozygous state (diagnosed after the age 4). 81 patients had *GJB2* biallelic mutations and severe or profound hearing impairment: 20 (24.6%) of them had severe HI and c.35delG in homozygous state, 28 (34.5%) had profound HI and c.35delG in homozygous state, while 8 patients (9.87%) with severe HI had c.35delG in compound heterozygous state and 14 patients with profound HI had c.35delG in compound heterozygous state.

Table 2. Correlations of *GJB2* genotypes and severity of hearing loss.

Genotypes		No of Subjects	Mild (21–40 dB)	Moderate (41–70 dB)	Severe (71–90 dB)	Profound (>90 dB)
c.35delG Homozygous	c.35delG/c.35delG	57	2	7	20	28
c.35delG Heterozygous	c.35delG/wt	26	4	11	7	4
c.35delG Compound Heterozygous	c.35delG/c.101T>C	10	-	6	2	2
	c.35delG/c.313_326del14	6	-	1	2	3
	c.35delG/c.-23+1G>A	4	-	-	1	3
	c.35delG/c.71G>A	8	-	1	3	4
	c.35delG/c.551G>C	2	-	-	-	2
Non-35delG Compound Heterozygous	c.79G>A/c.380G>A	1	-	1	-	-
	c.79G>A/c.341C>G/C.380G>A	4	1	3	-	-
	c.79G>A/c.39G>A	4	2	2	-	-
Non-35delG Heterozygous	c.101T>C/wt	9	5	2	1	1
	c.71G>A/wt	7	-	5	1	1
	c.457G>A/wt	5	1	2	2	-
	c.313_326del14/wt	2	-	1	1	-
	c.269T>C	3	-	-	2	1
	c.109G>A/wt	3	-	-	2	1
	c.551G>C/wt	2	-	1	1	-
	c.380G>A/wt	2	2	-	-	-
	c.100A>T	3	2	1	-	-
Total		158	19	44	45	50

4. Discussion

Hearing impairment is one of the most heterogeneous conditions of considerable concern in medicine nowadays. Each population has a different etiologic profile based on ethnic, geographic, social and medical background. It is diagnosed in 1–2 of 1000 newborns [21], genetic factors are responsible to up to 2/3 of HI cases (70% non-syndromic and 30% syndromic deafness) [22]. The remaining one-third of cases can be caused by environmental and unidentified genetic factors.

The prevalence of *GJB2* gene mutations can vary according to ethnicity: more than 50% in the European population [23], 16% in China [24] and Iran [25], 9.6% in Mexican population [26] and 6.1% in Pakistan. Among the European population, the c.35delG variant represents 2/3 of the total mutations in the *GJB2* gene [27,28]. In other populations variants such as: c.235delC variant in Japanese and other Asian populations [29,30], c.167delT in the Ashkenazi Jews [31], c.71G>A in Indians and Roma [16,32] are prevalent.

Romania is a Latin country from Central-Eastern Europe and it is heterogenous from an ethnic point of view. The variant frequency and spectrum is different compared to other countries. The most important minorities in Romania are the Hungarian minority in North-West region, followed by Roma and other minorities.

We performed a genetic screening of *GJB2* gene (responsible for the major etiologies of hereditary hearing impairment among Romanians), *GJB3*, *GJB6*, *POU3F4* and *WFS1* genes. Genetic diagnosis was confirmed in 174 (59.7%) of the 291 patients with different degrees of hearing impairment, most of them being accounted for *GJB2* gene. This data is in accordance with the literature, *GJB2* mutations are frequent in all studied populations [13,14,33–38]. In some populations *GJB2* mutations are prevalent due to consanguineous marriages. In Turkey autosomal recessive inheritance is responsible for 76.9 % of the studied cases [39].

In this study we did not found any significant difference in the severity and evolution of hearing impairment when comparing the 74 multiplex probands with 217 simplex probands.

The c.35delG variant (rs80338939) is responsible for approximately 70% of autosomal recessive NSHI and is the most common cause of hearing loss in Caucasian populations [7,40]. The carrier rate is estimated to be the highest in Europe with a mean rate of 1.89% and a variation across countries with a higher rate of 2.48% in Southern Europe compared with 1.53% in Northern Europe [41]. This frequency was found also in hearing-impaired population from Hungary, Czech Republic, Poland and Austria, where c.35delG was prevalent [10,42–44]. In Romania there are relatively few data about the frequency and audiological features of *GJB2* gene sequence variants [45].

Because c.35delG is the most frequent variant in the coding region of the *GJB2* gene, it has become the first intention genetic investigation for patients with non-syndromic hearing loss.

In our study, the 35delG variant was present in 97 out of 291 (33.3%) patients with different degrees of hearing impairment. These results are in accordance with the findings previously reported in other Romanian and Central European studies [45,46]. All our patients with c.35delG variant were diagnosed by MLPA and confirmed with Sanger Sequencing of *GJB2* gene.

The study revealed that subjects with 35delG in homozygous state present more severe hearing impairment, compared with the 35delG/non-35delG compound heterozygotes. The subjects with two non-35delG variants have an even less degree of hearing impairment. This observation is in accordance with other studies which conclude that c.35delG in homozygous state is associated with a higher risk for severe hearing impairment [10,45,47–49].

The next frequent variant was c.101T>C (rs35887622), accounting for 19 out of 291 (6.5%) patients. In the Caucasian population the frequency of the c.101T>C variant was determined to be up to 6.5% [50] and was initially reported as a polymorphism. Different studies of *GJB2* have determined that the c.101T>C variant is more frequent in individuals with mid-west American, UK [51] and German [50] origins, in comparison with those with French, Spanish, Italian and Japanese origin. A possible explanation may be that these variants are found in an ancestral mutation event that occurred in UK or Ireland.

More than 50% of our patients with c.101T>C variant had moderate to profound hearing impairment. Also, at the time of the diagnosis, the age of the patients with c.101T>C was greater than the age of the patients with c.35delG. The results of a large study on the UK population affirmed that this variant is associated with mild/moderate HI [51]. The lower pathogenicity of the mutation that leads to later and milder manifestation of hearing impairment may sustain this finding. The majority of diagnosed cases with c.101T>C in our study were older than 18 years. One possible explanation can be that adults with mild forms of HI may not pursue audiology or genetic investigations. The progression of HI was found in few cases, because it was slow and long-term follow-up information was not possible.

The incomplete penetrance of c.101T>C variant was not confirmed because the study included only subjects with HI. The phenotype of the patients with hearing impairment was variable: the individuals with biallelic c.101T>C and c.35delG had moderate to profound hearing loss and the heterozygous c.101T>C had mild to moderate forms of hearing loss. No individuals with c.101T>C in homozygous state were found.

The c.313_326del14 variant (rs111033253), called in the past c.310del14, c.312del14 or c.314del14, truncates the *GJB2* gene and disrupts the integrity of connexons. In many European populations, this variant has been identified previously with a frequency of pathogenic alleles from 0.47% to 28.3% [8].

The frequency of the c.313_326del14, variant in our group of participants was another finding in our study. The genotype was found in 8 of 291 patients (2.75 % of pathogenic alleles). A number of 6 patients were compound heterozygous with moderate to severe hearing impairment and the age of diagnosis being under 18 years and 2 patients had c.313-326del14 in heterozygous state with mild to moderate hearing impairment.

The c.71G>A variant is the fourth most common in our study and it had over five times lower frequency than the c.35delG variant. This mutation, previously called W24X, was first described in a Pakistani family [52] and later on was also discovered in several Asian families [53–57]. This finding indicates that it is the predominating cause of HI in India [58,59] and is prevalent in the Roma population with autosomal recessive NSHI [60]. In this study, it was found only in Roma patients: 15 individuals of 291 (15.5%) had this variant: 8 were compound heterozygous with c.35delG and 7 were in heterozygous state.

The c.71G>A frequency in different Roma subgroups is variable: it ranges from 0.0% to 26.1% in Slovak subgroups [60] and up to 4.0% in Spanish subgroups [61]. This finding is a result of the social structure of the Romani people, since they are considered to be a conglomerate of genetically isolated founder populations, with a high degree of consanguinity [61].

Our data is not concordant with other Central European series or the study from North-Western Romania, where 35delG and c.71G>A were the most common mutations [46], one explanation being the fact that the c.71G>A is predominant in Roma populations and they experience more problems accessing health care, from financial constraints, mobility issues or simply because they do not speak Romanian language.

The findings in Roma population confirm the ethnic origin of this mutation. Due to the fact that the sample of Roma patients is small, we cannot compare with other studies. The degree of addressability to medical care of the Roma-population from North-Eastern Romania is even lower than in North-Western Romania.

Another result determined in the present study was the presence of c.-23+1G>A, rs80338940 formerly called IVS1+1G>A, which is a splice site mutation found in exon 1 and intron 1 of *GJB2* gene in patients with hearing impairment. The mutation (revealed for the first time in 1999 by Denoyelle et al. [62]) was determined to be compound heterozygous and allele frequency was determined as 1% [63,64]. In our study, this variant was found in 4 of 291 patients (1.37%). The c.−23+1G>A variant was found with c.35delG variant and the subjects had severe to profound forms of HI. Previous studies showed that the patients with c.35delG/c.−23+1G>A in compound heterozygous state showed moderate HI [65] and profound HI [66]. To date, to our knowledge, homozygotes for the c.−23+1G>A variant have not been reported.

In 6 patients of 291 included in the study were identified two variants: c.109G>A and c.100A>T that have not been reported in any study from Romania. Out of these, 3 had c.109G>A variant and presented the same pattern of HI (progressive, bilateral and profound to severe) while the other 3 had c.100A>T (non-progressive, moderate, bilateral hearing impairment).

Our results contribute to define the mutation spectrum in the Romanian individuals with hearing impairment. Despite the genetic heterogeneity of NSHI, 217 patients were diagnosed out of a cohort of 291 patients. MLPA confirmed the genetic diagnosis in 141 cases (48.45%). We selected for further study the patients to which the *GJB2* mutations did not explain their hearing impairment and the patients with variants in *WFS1* gene.

Regarding our second aim of the study, we concluded that MLPA can be used as first intention genetic test for patients with HI due to some advantages over the Sanger Sequencing method: it is time saving, has a low price for consumables, the initial investment is lower for the platform than for Sanger Sequencing, the interpretation is much faster and it could easily detect the number copies variation and most frequent pathogenic variants. A description of the advantages and disadvantages is presented in Table 3.

Table 3. Advantages and disadvantages for the methods used in this study [67,68].

Method	Advantages	Disadvantages
MLPA	Low costs Time efficient Free analysis software High throughput Can detect changes in the copy number, DNA methylation and known point mutation Adaptable and updated	Sensitive to impurities Not suitable for unknown point mutations
Sanger Sequencing	Suitable for unknown point mutations Comprehensive coverage to any desired region	High costs Time consuming Limited number of targets Sequence quality degrades after 700 to 900 bases

This is the first report of the utility of MLPA and Sanger sequencing of HI in Romania; the results show notable findings in comparison to other European populations. However, some limitations should be noted: the samples included in this study are not truly representative for the entire Romania as all samples were collected from individuals with different degrees of hearing impairment, born in North-Eastern Romania, we did not have access to all of the parental samples to confirm compound heterozygosity. Our results need further studies on larger patient groups, especially Roma-population, in order to estimate the real incidence of the disease and to make more accurate predictions about the genotype phenotype correlation in our population.

We recommend genetic investigations in all subjects with hearing impairment that cannot be explained by other factors. In our knowledge, this is the first report on the utility and cost-effective of genetic testing in a cohort of Romanian patients with congenital NSHI. Sanger sequencing for *GJB2* gene is feasible because this is a small gene, with only 2 exons and the costs are reasonable and extra equipment are not necessary.

The genetic diagnosis in hearing impairment is important for many reasons: allows us to determine the etiology of deafness, offers the possibility to provide genetic counseling and prenatal diagnosis and not at least, based on the genotype-phenotype correlation provides prognostic information and facilitates an adequate management.

5. Conclusions

In this study, 217 patients had pathogenic/likely pathogenic variants, 141 being confirmed by MLPA. We identified two variants: c.109G>A and c.100A>T that have not being reported in any study from Romania. The most common variant in our study is c.35delG followed by c.101T>C, c.313_326del14 and c.71G>A.

All of the patients had been confirmed with Sanger Sequencing, proving that MLPA can be a cost-effective diagnosis method, useful for every patient with hearing impairment. MLPA is an inexpensive, rapid and reliable technique that could help as first intention genetic test for every individual with NSHI. Moreover, it can be adaptable for the mutation spectrum in every population and can be followed by Sanger sequencing for *GJB2* gene in cases of normal results.

Author Contributions: Conceptualization: I.R. and C.R.; methodology: R.P., O.-D.I. and R.S.C.; software: O.-D.I., R.S.C. and R.P.; validation: E.V.G., R.S.C. and C.R.; formal analysis: M.C.P., L.C.; investigation: I.R., M.C.P., L.I.B., L.C., L.M.R.; resources: I.R., E.-C.G.; data curation: E.V.G., R.S.C., R.P.; writing—original draft preparation: I.R.; writing—review and editing, C.R., R.S.C., M.C.P., L.C., R.P. visualization: I.R., E.-C.G., R.S.C.; supervision: C.R., E.V.G. All authors researched the literature, discussed the findings, reviewed and approved the final manuscript. All authors have read and agreed to the published version of the manuscript.

Funding: This research received no external funding.

Acknowledgments: We thank all the patients who participated in this study.

Conflicts of Interest: The authors declare no conflict of interest.

References

1. World Health Organization. Deafness and Hearing Loss. Available online: https://www.who.int/health-topics/hearing-loss (accessed on 1 September 2020).
2. Berg, A.L.; Spitzer, J.B.; Towers, H.M.; Bartosiewicz, C.; Diamond, B.E. Newborn hearing screening in the NICU: Profile of failed auditory brainstem response/passed otoacoustic emission. *Pediatrics* **2005**, *116*, 933–938. [CrossRef] [PubMed]
3. D'Aguillo, C.; Bressler, S.; Yan, D.; Mittal, R.; Fifer, R.; Blanton, S.H.; Liu, X. Genetic screening as an adjunct to universal newborn hearing screening: Literature review and implications for non-congenital pre-lingual hearing loss. *Int. J. Audiol.* **2019**, *58*, 834–850. [CrossRef] [PubMed]
4. Gorlin, R.J.; Gorlin, R.J.; Toriello, H.V.; Cohen, M.M. *Hereditary Hearing Loss and Its Syndromes*; Oxford University Press: New York, NY, USA, 1995.
5. Van Camp, G.S.R. Hereditary Hearing Loss Homepage. Available online: https://hereditaryhearingloss.org (accessed on 31 August 2020).
6. Putcha, G.V.; Bejjani, B.A.; Bleoo, S.; Booker, J.K.; Carey, J.C.; Carson, N.; Das, S.; Dempsey, M.A.; Gastier-Foster, J.M.; Greinwald, J.H., Jr.; et al. A multicenter study of the frequency and distribution of GJB2 and GJB6 mutations in a large North American cohort. *Genet. Med.* **2007**, *9*, 413–426. [CrossRef] [PubMed]
7. Koohiyan, M. Genetics of Hereditary Hearing Loss in the Middle East: A Systematic Review of the Carrier Frequency of the GJB2 Mutation (35delG). *Audiol. Neurootol.* **2019**, *24*, 161–165. [CrossRef]
8. Mikstiene, V.; Jakaitiene, A.; Byckova, J.; Gradauskiene, E.; Preiksaitiene, E.; Burnyte, B.; Tumiene, B.; Matuleviciene, A.; Ambrozaityte, L.; Uktveryte, I.; et al. The high frequency of GJB2 gene mutation c.313_326del14 suggests its possible origin in ancestors of Lithuanian population. *BMC Genet.* **2016**, *17*, 45. [CrossRef]
9. Carlsson, P.I.; Karltorp, E.; Carlsson-Hansen, E.; Ahlman, H.; Moller, C.; Vondobeln, U. GJB2 (Connexin 26) gene mutations among hearing-impaired persons in a Swedish cohort. *Acta Otolaryngol.* **2012**, *132*, 1301–1305. [CrossRef]
10. Bouzaher, M.H.; Worden, C.P.; Jeyakumar, A. Systematic Review of Pathogenic GJB2 Variants in the Latino Population. *Otol. Neurotol.* **2020**, *41*, e182–e191. [CrossRef]
11. Koohiyan, M.; Koohian, F.; Azadegan-Dehkordi, F. GJB2-related hearing loss in central Iran: Review of the spectrum and frequency of gene mutations. *Ann. Hum. Genet.* **2020**, *84*, 107–113. [CrossRef]
12. Figueroa-Ildefonso, E.; Bademci, G.; Rajabli, F.; Cornejo-Olivas, M.; Villanueva, R.D.C.; Badillo-Carrillo, R.; Inca-Martinez, M.; Neyra, K.M.; Sineni, C.; Tekin, M. Identification of Main Genetic Causes Responsible for Non-Syndromic Hearing Loss in a Peruvian Population. *Genes* **2019**, *10*, 581. [CrossRef]
13. Kucuk Kurtulgan, H.; Altuntas, E.E.; Yildirim, M.E.; Ozdemir, O.; Bagci, B.; Sezgin, I. The Analysis of GJB2, GJB3 and GJB6 Gene Mutations in Patients with Hereditary Non-Syndromic Hearing Loss Living in Sivas. *J. Int. Adv. Otol.* **2019**, *15*, 373–378. [CrossRef]
14. Naddafnia, H.; Noormohammadi, Z.; Irani, S.; Salahshoorifar, I. Frequency of GJB2 mutations, GJB6-D13S1830 and GJB6-D13S1854 deletions among patients with non-syndromic hearing loss from the central region of Iran. *Mol. Genet. Genomic Med.* **2019**, *7*, e00780. [CrossRef] [PubMed]

15. Sun, S.; Niu, L.; Tian, J.; Chen, W.; Li, Y.; Xia, N.; Jyu, C.; Chen, X.; Zhang, C.; Lan, X. Analysis of GJB2, SLC26A4, GJB3 and 12S rRNA gene mutations among patients with nonsyndromic hearing loss from eastern Shandong. *Zhonghua Yi Xue Yi Chuan Xue Za Zhi* **2019**, *36*, 433–438. [CrossRef] [PubMed]
16. RamShankar, M.; Girirajan, S.; Dagan, O.; Ravi Shankar, H.M.; Jalvi, R.; Rangasayee, R.; Avraham, K.B.; Anand, A. Contribution of connexin26 (GJB2) mutations and founder effect to non-syndromic hearing loss in India. *J. Med. Genet.* **2003**, *40*, e68. [CrossRef] [PubMed]
17. Azadan, R.J.; Fogleman, J.C.; Danielson, P.B. Capillary electrophoresis sequencing: Maximum read length at minimal cost. *Biotechniques* **2002**, *32*, 24–28. [CrossRef] [PubMed]
18. Schwarz, J.M.; Rodelsperger, C.; Schuelke, M.; Seelow, D. MutationTaster evaluates disease-causing potential of sequence alterations. *Nat. Methods* **2010**, *7*, 575–576. [CrossRef] [PubMed]
19. Schwarz, J.M.; Cooper, D.N.; Schuelke, M.; Seelow, D. MutationTaster2: Mutation prediction for the deep-sequencing age. *Nat. Methods* **2014**, *11*, 361–362. [CrossRef] [PubMed]
20. National Center for Biotechnology Information ClinVar. Available online: https://www.ncbi.nlm.nih.gov/clinvar/ (accessed on 2 September 2020).
21. Schmuziger, N.; Veraguth, D.; Probst, R. Universal newborn hearing screening—A silent revolution. *Praxis* **2008**, *97*, 1015–1021. [CrossRef]
22. Shearer, A.E.; Hildebrand, M.S.; Smith, R.J.H. Hereditary Hearing Loss and Deafness Overview GeneReviews ((R)). Available online: https://www.ncbi.nlm.nih.gov/pubmed/20301607 (accessed on 2 September 2020).
23. Kenneson, A.; Van Naarden Braun, K.; Boyle, C. GJB2 (connexin 26) variants and nonsyndromic sensorineural hearing loss: A HuGE review. *Genet. Med.* **2002**, *4*, 258–274. [CrossRef]
24. Liu, X.Z.; Xia, X.J.; Ke, X.M.; Ouyang, X.M.; Du, L.L.; Liu, Y.H.; Angeli, S.; Telischi, F.F.; Nance, W.E.; Balkany, T.; et al. The prevalence of connexin 26 (GJB2) mutations in the Chinese population. *Hum. Genet.* **2002**, *111*, 394–397. [CrossRef]
25. Ghasemnejad, T.; Shekari Khaniani, M.; Zarei, F.; Farbodnia, M.; Mansoori Derakhshan, S. An update of common autosomal recessive non-syndromic hearing loss genes in Iranian population. *Int. J. Pediatr. Otorhinolaryngol.* **2017**, *97*, 113–126. [CrossRef]
26. Loeza-Becerra, F.; Rivera-Vega Mdel, R.; Martinez-Saucedo, M.; Gonzalez-Huerta, L.M.; Urueta-Cuellar, H.; Berrruecos-Villalobos, P.; Cuevas-Covarrubias, S. Particular distribution of the GJB2/GJB6 gene mutations in Mexican population with hearing impairment. *Int. J. Pediatr. Otorhinolaryngol.* **2014**, *78*, 1057–1060. [CrossRef] [PubMed]
27. Van Laer, L.; Coucke, P.; Mueller, R.F.; Caethoven, G.; Flothmann, K.; Prasad, S.D.; Chamberlin, G.P.; Houseman, M.; Taylor, G.R.; Van de Heyning, C.M.; et al. A common founder for the 35delG GJB2 gene mutation in connexin 26 hearing impairment. *J. Med. Genet.* **2001**, *38*, 515–518. [CrossRef]
28. Gasparini, P.; Rabionet, R.; Barbujani, G.; Melchionda, S.; Petersen, M.; Brondum-Nielsen, K.; Metspalu, A.; Oitmaa, E.; Pisano, M.; Fortina, P.; et al. High carrier frequency of the 35delG deafness mutation in European populations. Genetic Analysis Consortium of GJB2 35delG. *Eur. J. Hum. Genet.* **2000**, *8*, 19–23. [CrossRef] [PubMed]
29. Shinagawa, J.; Moteki, H.; Nishio, S.Y.; Noguchi, Y.; Usami, S.I. Haplotype Analysis of GJB2 Mutations: Founder Effect or Mutational Hot Spot? *Genes* **2020**, *11*, 250. [CrossRef] [PubMed]
30. Ohtsuka, A.; Yuge, I.; Kimura, S.; Namba, A.; Abe, S.; Van Laer, L.; Van Camp, G.; Usami, S. GJB2 deafness gene shows a specific spectrum of mutations in Japan, including a frequent founder mutation. *Hum. Genet.* **2003**, *112*, 329–333. [CrossRef] [PubMed]
31. Dong, J.; Katz, D.R.; Eng, C.M.; Kornreich, R.; Desnick, R.J. Nonradioactive detection of the common Connexin 26 167delT and 35delG mutations and frequencies among Ashkenazi Jews. *Mol. Genet. Metab.* **2001**, *73*, 160–163. [CrossRef]
32. Safka Brozkova, D.; Varga, L.; Uhrova Meszarosova, A.; Slobodova, Z.; Skopkova, M.; Soltysova, A.; Ficek, A.; Jencik, J.; Lastuvkova, J.; Gasperikova, D.; et al. Variant c.2158-2A>G in MANBA is an important and frequent cause of hereditary hearing loss and β-mannosidosis among the Czech and Slovak Roma population-evidence for a new ethnic-specific variant. *Orphanet. J. Rare Dis.* **2020**, *15*, 222. [CrossRef]

33. Kecskemeti, N.; Szonyi, M.; Gaborjan, A.; Kustel, M.; Milley, G.M.; Suveges, A.; Illes, A.; Kekesi, A.; Tamas, L.; Molnar, M.J.; et al. Analysis of GJB2 mutations and the clinical manifestation in a large Hungarian cohort. *Eur. Arch. Otorhinolaryngol.* **2018**, *275*, 2441–2448. [CrossRef]
34. Bonyadi, M.J.; Fotouhi, N.; Esmaeili, M. Spectrum and frequency of GJB2 mutations causing deafness in the northwest of Iran. *Int. J. Pediatr. Otorhinolaryngol.* **2014**, *78*, 637–640. [CrossRef]
35. Bliznets, E.A.; Marcul, D.N.; Khorov, O.G.; Markova, T.G.; Poliakov, A.V. The mutation spectrum of the GJB2 gene in Belarussian patients with hearing loss. Results of pilot genetic screening of hearing impairment in newborns. *Genetika* **2014**, *50*, 214–221. [PubMed]
36. Teek, R.; Kruustuk, K.; Zordania, R.; Joost, K.; Reimand, T.; Mols, T.; Oitmaa, E.; Kahre, T.; Tonisson, N.; Ounap, K. Prevalence of c.35delG and p.M34T mutations in the GJB2 gene in Estonia. *Int. J. Pediatr. Otorhinolaryngol.* **2010**, *74*, 1007–1012. [CrossRef] [PubMed]
37. Xiong, Y.; Zhong, M.; Chen, J.; Yan, Y.L.; Lin, X.F.; Li, X. Effect of GJB2 235delC and 30-35delG genetic polymorphisms on risk of congenital deafness in a Chinese population. *Genet. Mol. Res.* **2017**, *16*. [CrossRef] [PubMed]
38. Barashkov, N.A.; Pshennikova, V.G.; Posukh, O.L.; Teryutin, F.M.; Solovyev, A.V.; Klarov, L.A.; Romanov, G.P.; Gotovtsev, N.N.; Kozhevnikov, A.A.; Kirillina, E.V.; et al. Spectrum and Frequency of the GJB2 Gene Pathogenic Variants in a Large Cohort of Patients with Hearing Impairment Living in a Subarctic Region of Russia (the Sakha Republic). *PLoS ONE* **2016**, *11*, e0156300. [CrossRef]
39. Tekin, M.; Arici, Z.S. Genetic epidemiological studies of congenital/prelingual deafness in Turkey: Population structure and mating type are major determinants of mutation identification. *Am. J. Med. Genet. A* **2007**, *143*, 1583–1591. [CrossRef] [PubMed]
40. Felix, F.; Zallis, M.G.; Tomita, S.; Baptista, M.M.; Ribeiro, M.G. Evaluation of the presence of the 35delG mutation in patients with severe to profound hearing loss based on ethnicity. *Rev. Laryngol. Otol. Rhinol.* **2014**, *135*, 171–174.
41. Mahdieh, N.; Rabbani, B.; Wiley, S.; Akbari, M.T.; Zeinali, S. Genetic causes of nonsyndromic hearing loss in Iran in comparison with other populations. *J. Hum. Genet.* **2010**, *55*, 639–648. [CrossRef] [PubMed]
42. Toth, T.; Kupka, S.; Haack, B.; Riemann, K.; Braun, S.; Fazakas, F.; Zenner, H.P.; Muszbek, L.; Blin, N.; Pfister, M.; et al. GJB2 mutations in patients with non-syndromic hearing loss from Northeastern Hungary. *Hum. Mutat.* **2004**, *23*, 631–632. [CrossRef]
43. Ramsebner, R.; Volker, R.; Lucas, T.; Hamader, G.; Weipoltshammer, K.; Baumgartner, W.D.; Wachtler, F.J.; Kirschhofer, K.; Frei, K. High incidence of GJB2 mutations during screening of newborns for hearing loss in Austria. *Ear. Hear.* **2007**, *28*, 298–301. [CrossRef]
44. Oldak, M.; Lechowicz, U.; Pollak, A.; Ozieblo, D.; Skarzynski, H. Overinterpretation of high throughput sequencing data in medical genetics: First evidence against TMPRSS3/GJB2 digenic inheritance of hearing loss. *J. Transl. Med.* **2019**, *17*, 269. [CrossRef]
45. Lazar, C.; Popp, R.; Trifa, A.; Mocanu, C.; Mihut, G.; Al-Khzouz, C.; Tomescu, E.; Figan, I.; Grigorescu-Sido, P. Prevalence of the c.35delG and p.W24X mutations in the GJB2 gene in patients with nonsyndromic hearing loss from North-West Romania. *Int. J. Pediatr. Otorhinolaryngol.* **2010**, *74*, 351–355. [CrossRef]
46. Sansovic, I.; Knezevic, J.; Musani, V.; Seeman, P.; Barisic, I.; Pavelic, J. GJB2 mutations in patients with nonsyndromic hearing loss from Croatia. *Genet. Test Mol. Biomark.* **2009**, *13*, 693–699. [CrossRef]
47. Leclere, J.C.; Le Gac, M.S.; Le Marechal, C.; Ferec, C.; Marianowski, R. GJB2 mutations: Genotypic and phenotypic correlation in a cohort of 690 hearing-impaired patients, toward a new mutation? *Int. J. Pediatr. Otorhinolaryngol.* **2017**, *102*, 80–85. [CrossRef]
48. Doria, M.; Neto, A.P.; Santos, A.C.; Barros, H.; Fernandes, S.; Moura, C.P. Prevalence of 35delG and Met34Thr GJB2 variants in Portuguese samples. *Int. J. Pediatr. Otorhinolaryngol.* **2015**, *79*, 2187–2190. [CrossRef] [PubMed]
49. Tlili, A.; Al Mutery, A.; Kamal Eddine Ahmad Mohamed, W.; Mahfood, M.; Hadj Kacem, H. Prevalence of GJB2 Mutations in Affected Individuals from United Arab Emirates with Autosomal Recessive Nonsyndromic Hearing Loss. *Genet. Test Mol. Biomark.* **2017**, *21*, 686–691. [CrossRef] [PubMed]

50. Zoll, B.; Petersen, L.; Lange, K.; Gabriel, P.; Kiese-Himmel, C.; Rausch, P.; Berger, J.; Pasche, B.; Meins, M.; Gross, M.; et al. Evaluation of Cx26/GJB2 in German hearing impaired persons: Mutation spectrum and detection of disequilibrium between M34T (c.101T>C) and -493del10. *Hum. Mutat.* **2003**, *21*, 98. [CrossRef]
51. Hall, A.; Pembrey, M.; Lutman, M.; Steer, C.; Bitner-Glindzicz, M. Prevalence and audiological features in carriers of GJB2 mutations, c.35delG and c.101T>C (p.M34T), in a UK population study. *BMJ Open* **2012**, *2*. [CrossRef] [PubMed]
52. Lench, N.J.; Markham, A.F.; Mueller, R.F.; Kelsell, D.P.; Smith, R.J.; Willems, P.J.; Schatteman, I.; Capon, H.; Van De Heyning, P.J.; Van Camp, G. A Moroccan family with autosomal recessive sensorineural hearing loss caused by a mutation in the gap junction protein gene connexin 26 (GJB2). *J. Med. Genet.* **1998**, *35*, 151–152. [CrossRef] [PubMed]
53. Green, G.E.; Scott, D.A.; McDonald, J.M.; Woodworth, G.G.; Sheffield, V.C.; Smith, R.J. Carrier rates in the midwestern United States for GJB2 mutations causing inherited deafness. *JAMA* **1999**, *281*, 2211–2216. [CrossRef] [PubMed]
54. Kudo, T.; Ikeda, K.; Oshima, T.; Kure, S.; Tammasaeng, M.; Prasansuk, S.; Matsubara, Y. GJB2 (connexin 26) mutations and childhood deafness in Thailand. *Otol. Neurotol.* **2001**, *22*, 858–861. [CrossRef]
55. Rickard, S.; Kelsell, D.P.; Sirimana, T.; Rajput, K.; MacArdle, B.; Bitner-Glindzicz, M. Recurrent mutations in the deafness gene GJB2 (connexin 26) in British Asian families. *J. Med. Genet.* **2001**, *38*, 530–533. [CrossRef]
56. Dahl, H.H.; Tobin, S.E.; Poulakis, Z.; Rickards, F.W.; Xu, X.; Gillam, L.; Williams, J.; Saunders, K.; Cone-Wesson, B.; Wake, M. The contribution of GJB2 mutations to slight or mild hearing loss in Australian elementary school children. *J. Med. Genet.* **2006**, *43*, 850–855. [CrossRef] [PubMed]
57. Bazazzadegan, N.; Nikzat, N.; Fattahi, Z.; Nishimura, C.; Meyer, N.; Sahraian, S.; Jamali, P.; Babanejad, M.; Kashef, A.; Yazdan, H.; et al. The spectrum of GJB2 mutations in the Iranian population with non-syndromic hearing loss—A twelve year study. *Int. J. Pediatr. Otorhinolaryngol.* **2012**, *76*, 1164–1174. [CrossRef]
58. Mahdieh, N.; Mahmoudi, H.; Ahmadzadeh, S.; Bakhtiyari, S. GJB2 mutations in deaf population of Ilam (Western Iran): A different pattern of mutation distribution. *Eur. Arch. Otorhinolaryngol.* **2016**, *273*, 1161–1165. [CrossRef] [PubMed]
59. Mishra, S.; Pandey, H.; Srivastava, P.; Mandal, K.; Phadke, S.R. Connexin 26 (GJB2) Mutations Associated with Non-Syndromic Hearing Loss (NSHL). *Indian J. Pediatr.* **2018**, *85*, 1061–1066. [CrossRef] [PubMed]
60. Minarik, G.; Ferak, V.; Ferakova, E.; Ficek, A.; Polakova, H.; Kadasi, L. High frequency of GJB2 mutation W24X among Slovak Romany (Gypsy) patients with non-syndromic hearing loss (NSHL). *Gen. Physiol. Biophys.* **2003**, *22*, 549–556. [PubMed]
61. Bouwer, S.; Angelicheva, D.; Chandler, D.; Seeman, P.; Tournev, I.; Kalaydjieva, L. Carrier rates of the ancestral Indian W24X mutation in GJB2 in the general Gypsy population and individual subisolates. *Genet. Test.* **2007**, *11*, 455–458. [CrossRef]
62. Denoyelle, F.; Marlin, S.; Weil, D.; Moatti, L.; Chauvin, P.; Garabedian, E.N.; Petit, C. Clinical features of the prevalent form of childhood deafness, DFNB1, due to a connexin-26 gene defect: Implications for genetic counselling. *Lancet* **1999**, *353*, 1298–1303. [CrossRef]
63. Del Castillo, F.J.; Rodriguez-Ballesteros, M.; Alvarez, A.; Hutchin, T.; Leonardi, E.; de Oliveira, C.A.; Azaiez, H.; Brownstein, Z.; Avenarius, M.R.; Marlin, S.; et al. A novel deletion involving the connexin-30 gene, del(GJB6-d13s1854), found in trans with mutations in the GJB2 gene (connexin-26) in subjects with DFNB1 non-syndromic hearing impairment. *J. Med. Genet.* **2005**, *42*, 588–594. [CrossRef]
64. Shahin, H.; Walsh, T.; Sobe, T.; Lynch, E.; King, M.C.; Avraham, K.B.; Kanaan, M. Genetics of congenital deafness in the Palestinian population: Multiple connexin 26 alleles with shared origins in the Middle East. *Hum. Genet.* **2002**, *110*, 284–289. [CrossRef]
65. Cryns, K.; Orzan, E.; Murgia, A.; Huygen, P.L.; Moreno, F.; del Castillo, I.; Chamberlin, G.P.; Azaiez, H.; Prasad, S.; Cucci, R.A.; et al. A genotype-phenotype correlation for GJB2 (connexin 26) deafness. *J. Med. Genet.* **2004**, *41*, 147–154. [CrossRef]
66. Da Silva-Costa, S.M.; Coeli, F.B.; Lincoln-de-Carvalho, C.R.; Marques-de-Faria, A.P.; Kurc, M.; Pereira, T.; Pomilio, M.C.; Sartorato, E.L. Screening for the GJB2 c.-3170 G>A (IVS 1+1 G>A) mutation in Brazilian deaf individuals using multiplex ligation-dependent probe amplification. *Genet. Test. Mol. Biomark.* **2009**, *13*, 701–704. [CrossRef] [PubMed]

67. Homig-Holzel, C.; Savola, S. Multiplex ligation-dependent probe amplification (MLPA) in tumor diagnostics and prognostics. *Diagn. Mol. Pathol.* **2012**, *21*, 189–206. [CrossRef] [PubMed]
68. Veldhuisen, B.; van der Schoot, C.E.; de Haas, M. Multiplex ligation-dependent probe amplification (MLPA) assay for blood group genotyping, copy number quantification and analysis of RH variants. *Immunohematology* **2015**, *31*, 58–61. [PubMed]

Publisher's Note: MDPI stays neutral with regard to jurisdictional claims in published maps and institutional affiliations.

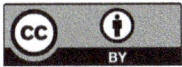 © 2020 by the authors. Licensee MDPI, Basel, Switzerland. This article is an open access article distributed under the terms and conditions of the Creative Commons Attribution (CC BY) license (http://creativecommons.org/licenses/by/4.0/).

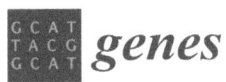

Article

*GJB*2 and *GJB*6 Genetic Variant Curation in an Argentinean Non-Syndromic Hearing-Impaired Cohort

Paula Buonfiglio [1], Carlos D. Bruque [2,3], Leonela Luce [4,5], Florencia Giliberto [4,5], Vanesa Lotersztein [6], Sebastián Menazzi [7], Bibiana Paoli [8], Ana Belén Elgoyhen [1,9] and Viviana Dalamón [1,*]

1. Laboratorio de Fisiología y Genética de la Audición, Instituto de Investigaciones en Ingeniería Genética y Biología Molecular "Dr. Héctor N. Torres", Consejo Nacional de Investigaciones Científicas y Técnicas—INGEBI/CONICET, C1428ADN Ciudad Autónoma de Buenos Aires, Argentina; paulabuonfiglio@gmail.com (P.B.); abelgoyhen@gmail.com (A.B.E.)
2. Centro Nacional de Genética Médica, ANLIS-Malbrán, C1425 Ciudad Autónoma de Buenos Aires, Argentina; bruquecarlos@gmail.com
3. Instituto de Biología y Medicina Experimental, Consejo Nacional de Investigaciones Científicas y Técnicas—IBYME/CONICET, C1428ADN Ciudad Autónoma de Buenos Aires, Argentina
4. Laboratorio de Distrofinopatías, Cátedra de Genética, Facultad de Farmacia y Bioquímica, Universidad de Buenos Aires, C1113AAD Ciudad Autónoma de Buenos Aires, Argentina; leonelaluce@gmail.com (L.L.); gilibertoflor@gmail.com (F.G.)
5. Instituto de Inmunología, Genética y Metabolismo—INIGEM/CONICET, Universidad de Buenos Aires, C1113AAD Ciudad Autónoma de Buenos Aires, Argentina
6. Servicio de Genética, Hospital Militar Central "Dr. Cosme Argerich", C1426 Ciudad Autónoma de Buenos Aires, Argentina; vlotersztein@yahoo.com.ar
7. Servicio de Genética, Hospital de Clínicas "José de San Martín", C1120AAR Ciudad Autónoma de Buenos Aires, Argentina; smenazzi@gmail.com
8. Servicio de Otorrinolaringología Infantil, Hospital de Clínicas "José de San Martín", C1120AAR Ciudad Autónoma de Buenos Aires, Argentina; bibianapaoli@uolsinectis.com.ar
9. Departamento de Farmacología, Facultad de Medicina, Universidad de Buenos Aires, C1121ABG Ciudad Autónoma de Buenos Aires, Argentina
* Correspondence: vividalamon@gmail.com; Tel.: +54-11-47832871

Received: 18 September 2020; Accepted: 13 October 2020; Published: 21 October 2020

Abstract: Genetic variants in *GJB*2 and *GJB*6 genes are the most frequent causes of hereditary hearing loss among several deaf populations worldwide. Molecular diagnosis enables proper genetic counseling and medical prognosis to patients. In this study, we present an update of testing results in a cohort of Argentinean non-syndromic hearing-impaired individuals. A total of 48 different sequence variants were detected in genomic DNA from patients referred to our laboratory. They were manually curated and classified based on the American College of Medical Genetics and Genomics/Association for Molecular Pathology ACMG/AMP standards and hearing-loss-gene-specific criteria of the ClinGen Hearing Loss Expert Panel. More than 50% of sequence variants were reclassified from their previous categorization in ClinVar. These results provide an accurately interpreted set of variants to be taken into account by clinicians and the scientific community, and hence, aid the precise genetic counseling to patients.

Keywords: *GJB*2; *GJB*6; genetic variants; curation; hearing loss; argentina

1. Introduction

Congenital hearing loss (HL) is the most common sensory disorder that affects approximately 1–2 of 1000 infants, with 50% of cases resulting from genetic factors [1]. In 70–80% of neonates who fail newborn hearing screening, no other distinguishing physical findings are present and the HL is classified as non-syndromic. The majority of non-syndromic cases are of autosomal recessive inheritance (80%), 12–15% autosomal dominant, 1–5% X-linked and 1–5% mitochondrial [2]. In general, autosomal recessive loci are related to a prelingual HL, while autosomal dominant loci to a postlingual HL phenotype [3]. A large number of genes are involved in hereditary HL. To date, a total of 121 non-syndromic causative genes have been described: 76 of recessive inheritance, 49 of dominant inheritance and five X-linked (some genes can cause recessive and dominant hearing impairment) [4]. This landscape illustrates the auditory system complexity, comprising a large number of proteins, which together participate in hearing physiology and development [5].

Despite the wide genetic heterogeneity of hearing impairment, the most commonly mutated genes in severe to profound autosomal recessive non-syndromic hearing loss (ARNSHL) are *GJB2* and *GJB6* (encoding connexin-26 and 30, respectively), accounting for nearly 50% of the cases in most populations around the Mediterranean Sea [6–11]. *GJB2* and *GJB6* (DFNB1) genes are part of a gene family that encode gap-junction proteins. It is well demonstrated that they are expressed in cochlear supporting cells, with a role in endolymph potassium recycling, inositol triphosphate (IP3) transfer and diffusion of different metabolites [12,13]. Connexins (Cx) are formed of four transmembrane domains, two extracellular loops and three cytoplasmic domains: the amino-terminus, a cytoplasmic loop and the carboxy-terminus domain [13].

Both *GJB2* and *GJB6* are located in chromosome 13q12. The *GJB2* gene comprises two exons and the coding region is completely contained in the second exon, leading to a 2290-nucleotide mRNA (GeneBank: NM_004004.6). On the other hand, the *GJB6* gene consists of five exons and the last one contains the entire coding sequence which is transcribed to a 2110 bp mRNA (GeneBank: NM_006783.4). In general, mutations which produce a loss of gap-junction channel function are related to non-syndromic ARSHL [14–16].

The most frequent mutation in *GJB2* is c.35delG in the Caucasian population [7,9,17–19]. In addition, there are more than 300 pathogenic variants identified in *GJB2* (Deafness Variation Database) [20]. In the case of *GJB6*, two large deletions of 309 and 232-kb, del(*GJB6*-D13S1830) and del(*GJB6*-D13S1854), respectively, in the 5′ region of the gene, along with other rarer and less studied deletions, have been described [10,21–25]. Previous studies have demonstrated that different cohorts of Argentinean patients carry similar frequent genetic variants in *GJB2* and *GJB6* [26–31].

Identifying the genetic etiology of hearing impairment can provide proper counseling, clinical management and accurate estimation of deafness odds recurrence within a family [29,30]. Moreover, molecular diagnosis contributes with valuable prognosis information: DFNB1-hearing loss is not related to other phenotypic symptoms nor to significant hearing loss progression over time, and in general, it is related to a congenital profound bilateral hearing loss [32]. Affected probands carrying two truncating/nonsense variants in *GJB2* present a more severe degree of hearing loss than those who carry two missense variants [18,28,33,34]. Furthermore, patients with *GJB2* genetic variants present excellent outcomes in speech perception/production skills after cochlear implantation [35–37]. Therefore, correct interpretation of the phenotypic consequences of genetic variants is crucial in genetic diagnosis, since discrepancies in sequence variant interpretation and classification has been reported to lead to serious impact in patient health maintenance [38–40]. Thus, the American College of Medical Genetics and Genomics (ACMG) and the Association for Molecular Pathology (AMP) has developed guidelines for clinical interpretation of genetic variants [41]. In addition, the ClinGen Hearing Loss Clinical Domain Working Group (HLWG) has adapted the ACMG/AMP guidelines for the classification of genetic variants in the hearing loss framework [28,42].

In the present study we aimed to identify causative mutations in *GJB2* and *GJB6* genes in Argentinean non-syndromic hearing-impaired patients and report an update of allele and genotype frequencies. Furthermore, we performed a thorough manual curation of sequence variants according to ACMG/AMP standards and applied rigorously the latest hearing loss gene-specific criteria of the ClinGen Hearing Loss Expert Panel (HL-EP) [41,42]. These findings clearly highlight the importance of genetic studies with the appropriate comprehensive analysis by experts in the field, with the goal of providing an accurate molecular diagnosis, and consequently, precise genetic counseling to the patients.

2. Materials and Methods

2.1. Part A: Identification of Variants in an Argentinean Cohort

2.1.1. Patients

This study includes a total of 600 Argentinean non-related patients (290 females and 310 males) with non-syndromic sensorineural hearing loss. Clinical evaluation was performed by a clinical geneticist and included: personal history, physical examination, audiometric information, age of hearing impairment onset, hearing thresholds, pedigree and genetic assessment. For each patient, a complete medical history was obtained to exclude the possibility of environmental causes of hearing impairment (e.g., ototoxic drugs, infectious diseases, acoustic trauma). All subjects gave their informed consent for inclusion before they participated in the study. The study was conducted in accordance with the Declaration of Helsinki, and the protocol was approved by the Ethics Committee of Administración Nacional de Laboratorios e Institutos de Salud (ANLIS) (1912–2018). The workflow is summarized in Figure 1A.

A total of 477 sporadic and 123 familial cases (80% and 20%, respectively) were sequentially referred to the Laboratory of Physiology and Genetic of Hearing, INGEBI, in Buenos Aires, Argentina from 2004 to March 2020. Familial cases were of a dominant and recessive form of inheritance (59 and 64/123). All patients were analyzed by an ear-nose-throat (ENT) specialist using standard methods. The severity of deafness was classified considering the following thresholds in decibels: mild (20 to 39 dB), moderate (40 to 69 dB), severe (70 to 89 dB) and profound (90 dB). The patient's deafness severity was defined by the ear with the minor degree of hearing loss. Complete audiological history data were compiled from affected subjects in case of need. Overall, 479 of patients (47%) exhibited prelingual HL, while 121 (20%) a postlingual phenotype. The severity of HL was: 102 moderate, 106 severe and 392 profound. A total of 69 patients were cochlear implanted. This prospective study (2004–2020) includes data previously reported in Dalamón et al. 2013 ($n = 476$ patients), but that was not curated following HL-EP standards.

2.1.2. Samples

Genomic DNA was isolated from whole blood samples extracted with 5% ethylene-diamine tetraacetic acid (EDTA) (Sigma-Aldrich, St. Louis, MO, USA) using the cetyltrimethyl-ammonium bromide (CTAB) (Sigma-Aldrich, St. Louis, MO, USA) method [43]. DNA concentration and quality were measured by absorbance at 260 nm and by the A260 nm/A280 nm and A260 nm/A230 nm ratios, respectively (NanoDrop™) (Thermo Fisher Scientific, Wilmington, NC, USA). All samples were stored at −20 °C.

2.1.3. *GJB2/GJB6* Molecular Studies

Genetic variants in *GJB2* were studied by direct sequencing of the coding exon 2, non-coding exon 1 and intronic boundaries. The splice site variants c.-23+1G>A and c.-22-2A>C were included in the screening. Primers, protocols and cycling programs used were as previously reported [28]. Bidirectional DNA sequencing was performed on an automatic sequencer (3730xl DNA Analyzer, Applied Biosystems, Foster City, CA, USA). Sequences obtained were analyzed by CodonCodeAligner program [44] and the BLAST NCBI interface (Basic local alignment search tool) [45] using the consensus sequence of *GJB2* gene (GeneBank

NG_008358.1). To examine the large deletions in *GJB6*:del(*GJB6*-D13S1830) and del(*GJB6*-D13S1854), a GAP-PCR and subsequent analysis were performed according to reported protocols [10,21].

2.1.4. Data Analysis

In order to establish a genotype/phenotype correlation, presumably pathogenic identified *GJB2* allele variants were classified as truncating (T) and non-truncating (NT) mutations [46]. Truncating mutations are loss-of-function (LoF) and include nonsense variants, insertions, deletions and duplications that introduce a shift in reading frame leading to a premature termination of protein translation, as well as the donor splice-site variant c.-23+1G>A leading to non-functional mRNA. Both del(*GJB6*-D13S1830) and del(*GJB6*-D13S1854) were also classified as truncating, because they lead to a nearly complete absence of Cx26 protein expression [10,47,48]. The group of non-truncating variants consists of missense variants (leading to amino acid substitutions) and the in-frame deletion (delGlu120). The acceptor splice-site variant c.-22-2A>C was defined as non-truncating since a residual expression of the wild type transcript due to the activation of an alternative acceptor splice site has been reported [49]. A chi square statistical analysis was performed in order to analyze the differences between groups.

2.2. Part B: Curation of Variants

GJB2-*GJB6* Variant Curation

Manual curation of variants required information gathered from: population data, genotypes, segregation, phenotypic features and functional and experimental data of the reported variants. Nomenclature of sequence variants identified were achieved according to HGVS standards [50] and manually revised with the Mutalyzer name-checker tool [51]. Computational and predictive evidence was performed in silico through diverse strategies according to the type of variant analyzed: missense variants with REVEL [52] and Combined Annotation Dependent Depletion (CADD) [53] tools, splice site and silent variants with Human Splicing Finder [54] and MaxEntScan softwares [55] and loss of function variants (nonsense, frameshift and canonical splice site) following the ACMG/AMP recommendations [56]. REVEL, CADD and MaxEntScan scores were determined with the Variant Effect Predictor tool [57].

Reports in PubMed, as well as internal data from our laboratory, and seven different databases were used: 1. gnomAD [58], 2. dbSNP [59], 3. NHLBI-ESP's EVS [60], 4. ClinVar [61], 5. LOVD [62], 6. Deafness Variation Database (DVD) [20] and 7. Database of Genomics Variants [63,64]. Variant filtering allele frequency was calculated by using inverse allele frequency [65]. More than 250 publications from PubMed were revised up to June 2020 to validate genetic variant interpretation. Clinical histories of patients were used to provide further information regarding segregation analysis and phenotypic features.

Collected information was manually assessed in order to organize and score the strength of evidence. Genetic variants were interpreted according to ACMG/AMP guidelines [41] and hearing loss gene specific criteria of the ClinGen HL-EP [42]. The final criteria score was manually assigned through the Varsome tool [66] in order to obtain the variant classification. Members of the Laboratory of Physiology and Genetics of Hearing discussed and reviewed final variant classification. A summary of information to be used by clinicians concerning variant specific criteria is detailed in Supplementary Table S1.

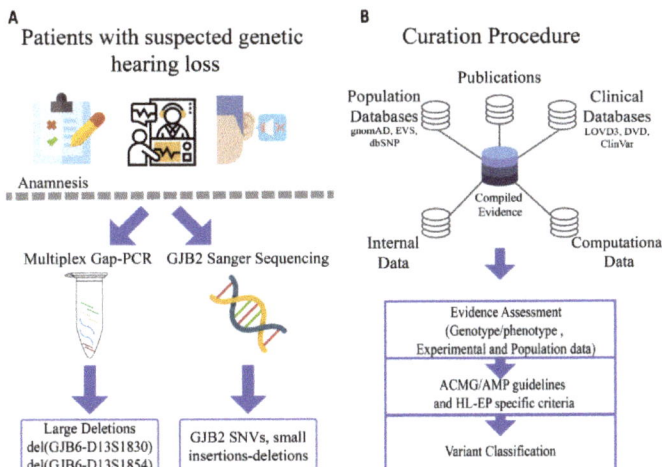

Figure 1. General workflow of this study. (**A**): Molecular screening of patients. Some icons were obtained from flaticon webpage [67]. (**B**): Variant curation process.

3. Results

3.1. General Genetic Findings

GJB2 and *GJB6* single nucleotide variants (SNVs) and deletions del(*GJB6*-D13S1830) and del(*GJB6*-D13S1854) were studied in 600 NSHL Argentinean patients by Sanger Sequencing and GAP-PCR, respectively. Overall, 48 different sequence variants were identified in the 1200 alleles tested from the entire cohort of patients. The most frequent mutated alleles detected were: c.35delG (9.1%), p.Val27Ile (8.3%), p.Met34Thr (1.5%), c.167delT (1.16%) and the del(*GJB6*-D13S1830) (0.99%), followed by p.Val37Ile, p.(Glu47*), p.Arg143Trp, p.(Lys168Arg) and del(*GJB6*-D13S1854) with frequencies from 0.83% to 0.4%. Other variants were found less than five times in the cohort; their specific allele frequency is detailed hereafter.

A total of 229 patients, representing 38% of the studied cohort, exhibited genetic variants in *GJB2/GJB6*, either in heterozygous (n = 117) or homozygous states, two different variants in the same gene, or *GJB6* deletions in combination with *GJB2* variants. Familial segregation was performed in 36/97 cases, confirming the in trans occurrence. All other genotypes involving two known causative variants were presumed of biallelic inheritance. A total of 42 diverse biallelic genotypes were identified (Figure 2). The most prevalent genotype detected was the homozygous c.(35delG) variant (33.3% of the biallelic mutations), followed by the compound heterozygous c.(35delG);(167delT) (8.33%). Genotype (*GJB2*:c.35delG);(*GJB6*:del(*GJB6*-D13S1830)) and (*GJB2*:c.35delG);(*GJB6*:del(*GJB6*-D13S1854)) were detected in 5.2% and 4.16% of hearing-impaired individuals, respectively. Compound heterozygous involving one of the large deletions in *GJB6* accounted for the 15.6% of the total detected genotypes (15/96).

Biallelic causative mutations were found in 36% of ARNSHL familial cases (23/64) and 15.5% of sporadic ones (74/477). Overall, 38.5% of the cases were compound heterozygous for the c.(35delG) variant in trans with different mutations, and other 30.2% carried two different non-35delG variants.

Additionally, two patients carried the mutations p.Arg75Trp and p.Arg75Gln with a dominant mode of inheritance. A summary of genotypes, phenotypes and segregation is detailed in Supplementary Table S2.

3.2. Genotype-Phenotype Characterization

In order to correlate the identified genotypes with audiological features, we categorized the genetic variants as truncating (T) or non-truncating (NT). The variants of the 97 positively genotyped patients with biallelic recessive *GJB2*, dominant *GJB2* and/or compound *GJB2/GJB6* variants were correlated with their HL severity (moderate, severe, profound).

A total of 42 different genotypes were categorized: 11 homozygous truncating (T/T), 23 heterozygous truncating/non-truncating (T/NT), six homozygous non-truncating (NT/NT) and two autosomal dominant NT (AD). Distribution of genotypes/phenotypes and relative frequencies of the degree of HL in the three groups are shown in Figure 2.

Biallelic T/T genotypes were mostly related to a worse degree of hearing impairment, since 83% of those patients exhibited profound HL, 12% severe and 5% moderate HL. In contrast, biallelic NT/NT genotypes showed a milder degree of hearing impairment since 60% of these cases had moderate HL and 20% severe/profound HL. Compound heterozygous T/NT genotypes ranged from moderate to profound with no clear trends: 43% with profound HL, 18% severe HL and 39% moderate HL (Figure 2 inner box). There were significant differences among the three groups, with X^2 testing ($p < 0.0001$).

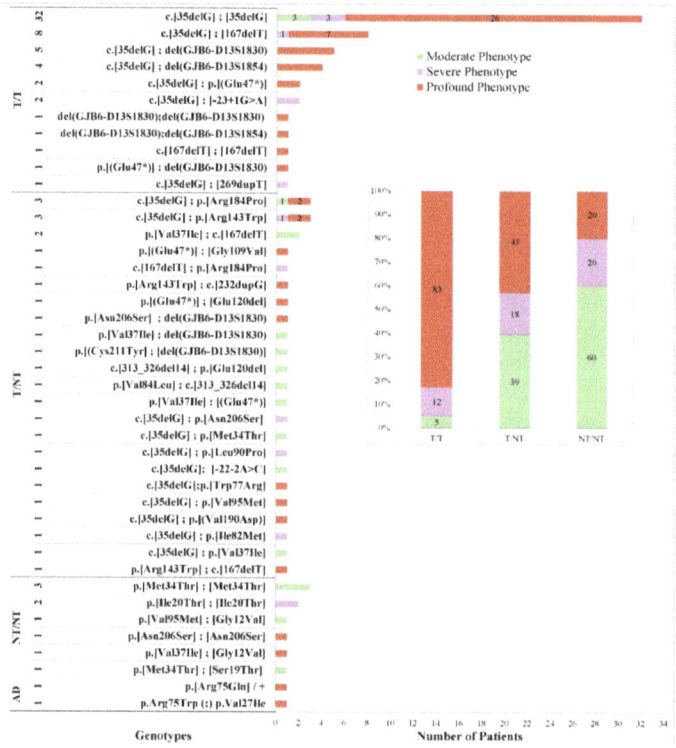

Figure 2. Distribution of Genotypes and Phenotypes of Patients. Moderate phenotype is shown in green, severe in violet and profound in red. The total number of each genotype is listed on the left together with its categorization: biallelic truncating (T/T), compound heterozygous truncating/non-truncating (T/NT) and biallelic non-truncating (NT/NT). Nomenclature was performed following HGVS recommendations; however, some variants keep the old annotation due to their common use in literature. In the inner box: Relative frequencies of the degree of HL in the three groups of genotypes. Biallelic T/T genotypes were mostly related to a worse degree of hearing impairment, since 83% of those patients exhibited profound HL. There were significant differences among the three groups, with X^2 testing ($p < 0.0001$).

3.3. Variant Curation

In order to further analyze and validate the identified variants, we performed a manual revision of available evidence following the Guidelines and recommendations of the ACMG/AMP and The ClinGen Hearing loss Expert Panel.

A total of 48 sequence variants were identified in *GJB2* and *GJB6* in our study cohort and 44 were manually curated, since four variants had been already curated as pathogenic by the HL-EP group: c.35delG, p.Met34Thr, p.Val37Ile and c.167delT. Variant c.-22-2A>C was reported as Variant of Unknown Significance (VUS) by the HL-EP group but was reclassified with new available information in this work explained further below.

From the total of variants analyzed, 23 were classified as pathogenic (P), three likely pathogenic (LP), nine uncertain significance (VUS), four likely benign (LB) and five benign (B). The final classification of the 44 variants and their general information is shown in Table 1.

Table 1. Curated Variants. A total of 48 sequence variants were identified in *GJB2* and *GJB6* and 44 were manually curated, since four variants had been already curated by the HL-EP group (with asterisk). In bold format are remarked the 27 variants evaluated in this study that changed their previous category submitted in ClinVar, based on the specific criteria applied during the curation procedure.

Nucleotide Change	Protein Variant	Mutated Alleles/ Total Alleles Tested (Percentage)	Reference	ClinVar	Final Classification (ACMG/AMP HL-EP)	Rules Applied
c.-23+1G>A	-	2/1200 (0.16%)	[68]	Pathogenic	Pathogenic	PM2, PVS1, PM3_VS, PS3_P
c.-22-12C>T	-	1/1200 (0.083%)	[69]	Benign	Benign	BA1, BP4
c.-22-2A>C	-	1/1200 (0.083%)	[70]	VUS *	**Likely Pathogenic**	PM3_M, PP1_S, PS3_P, BS1.
c.-15C>T	-	1/1200 (0.083%)	[69]	Benign/ Likely Benign	**Benign**	BA1, BP4
c.23C>T	p.Thr8Met	1/1200 (0.083%)	[71]	Conflicting Interpretation	**VUS**	PM2_P, PS3_P, PM3
c.24G>A	p.(Thr8=)	1/1200 (0.083%)	[72]	Conflicting Interpretation	**VUS**	PP3, PM2
c.29T>C	p.Leu10Pro	1/1200 (0.083%)	[73]	absent	**VUS**	PM2, PP3, PS3_M
c.35G>T	p.Gly12Val	2/1200 (0.16%)	[74]	Pathogenic/ Likely Pathogenic	**Pathogenic**	PM2_M, PM3_VS, PP3, PS3_M
c.35delG	p.Gly12Valfs*2	111/1200 (9.25%)	[75]	Pathogenic *	Pathogenic	already curated by HL-EP
c.56G>C	p.Ser19Thr	1/1200 (0.083%)	[74]	Likely Pathogenic	**Pathogenic**	PM2, PM3_VS, PP1_M, PS3_M
c.59T>C	p.Ile20Thr	4/1200 (0.34%)	[76]	Pathogenic/ Likely Pathogenic	**Pathogenic**	PM2, PM3, PP1_P, PP3, PS3_M
c.79G>A	p.Val27Ile	100/1200 (8.34%)	[77]	Benign	Benign	BA1, BP2, BS3_P
c.101T>C	p.Met34Thr	19/1200 (1.58%)	[78]	Pathogenic *	Pathogenic	already curated by HL-EP
c.109G>A	p.Val37Ile	10/1200 (0.84%)	[77]	Pathogenic *	Pathogenic	already curated by HL-EP
c.139G>T	p.(Glu47*)	6/1200 (0.5%)	[79]	Pathogenic	Pathogenic	PVS1, PM2_P, PM3_VS
c.167delT	p.Leu56Argfs*81	14/1200 (1.16%)	[75]	Pathogenic *	Pathogenic	already curated by HL-EP

Table 1. Cont.

Nucleotide Change	Protein Variant	Mutated Alleles/ Total Alleles Tested (Percentage)	Reference	ClinVar	Final Classification (ACMG/AMP HL-EP)	Rules Applied
c.223C>T	p.Arg75Trp	1/1200 (0.083%)	[80]	Pathogenic	Pathogenic	PM2, PS2_VS, PP1_P, PP3, PS3
c.224G>A	p.Arg75Gln	1/1200 (0.083%)	[81]	Pathogenic	Pathogenic	PM2, PS4_M, PP1_M, PM5, PP3, PS3_M
c.229T>C	p.Trp77Arg	1/1200 (0.083%)	[82]	Pathogenic	Pathogenic	PM2_P, PM3_VS, PP3, PS3_M
c.232dupG	p.(Ala78Glyfs*24)	1/1200 (0.083%)	[83]	Likely Pathogenic	**Pathogenic**	PM2, PVS1, PM3
c.232G>T	p.(Ala78Ser)	1/1200 (0.083%)	[28]	absent	**VUS**	PM2, PP3, PM5
c.246C>G	p.Ile82Met	1/1200 (0.083%)	[84]	Likely Pathogenic	**Pathogenic**	PM2, PP1_M, PM3_VS, PP3, PS3_M
c.249C>G	p.Phe83Leu	2/1200 (0.16%)	[85]	Benign/ Likely Benign	**Likely Benign**	BS1_P, BP2, BS3_P
c.250G>C	p.Val84Leu	1/1200 (0.083%)	[77]	Pathogenic/ Likely Pathogenic	**Pathogenic**	PM2, PP3, PM3_VS, PP1_P
c.269T>C	p.Leu90Pro	3/1200 (0.25%)	[68]	Conflicting Interpretation	**Pathogenic**	BS1_P, PP3, PM3_VS, PS3_M
c.269dup	p.(Val91Serfs*11)	1/1200 (0.083%)	[68]	Pathogenic	Pathogenic	PM2, PVS1, PM3_VS, PP1_M
c.283G>A	p.(Val95Met)	2/1200 (0.16%)	[77]	Pathogenic/ Likely Pathogenic	**Pathogenic**	PM2, PM3_VS, PP1_P, PP3
c.313_326del14	p.(Lys105Glyfs*5)	2/1200 (0.16%)	[79]	Pathogenic	Pathogenic	PM2_P, PVS1, PM3_VS.
c.326G>T	p.Gly109Val	1/1200 (0.083%)	[86]	absent	**Likely Pathogenic**	PM2, PM3, PS3_M
c.334_335delAA	p.(Lys112Glufs*2)	2/1200 (0.16%)	[77]	Pathogenic /Likely Pathogenic	**Pathogenic**	PM2, PVS1, PM3_VS, PP1_M
c.358_360delGAG	p.Glu120del	2/1200 (0.16%)	[79]	Pathogenic	Pathogenic	PM2_P, PM4, PM3_VS, PS3_M
c.380G>A	p.Arg127His	1/1200 (0.083%)	[87]	Conflicting Interpretation	**Benign**	BA1, BS2, BS4, PM3_P
c.384C>T	p.(Ile128=)	1/1200 (0.083%)	[75]	Likely Benign	Likely Benign	PM2, BP2, BP4, BP7
c.385G>A	p.(Glu129Lys)	1/1200 (0.083%)	[71]	Conflicting Interpretation	**VUS**	PM2, PM3
c.427C>T	p.Arg143Trp	5/1200 (0.42%)	[88]	Pathogenic	Pathogenic	PM2_P, PM3_VS, PP1_P
c.439G>A	p.(Glu147Lys)	1/1200 (0.083%)	[89]	Pathogenic/ Likely Pathogenic	**Pathogenic**	PM2, PM3_VS, PP1_Mod, PP3
c.457G>A	p.Val153Ile	3/1200 (0.25%)	[90]	Benign/ Likely Benign	**Benign**	BA1, BS2
c.478G>A	p.(Gly160Ser)	2/1200 (0.16%)	[85]	Conflicting Interpretation	**Likely Benign**	BS1_P, PP3, BP2, PM3
c.487A>G	p.Met163Val	2/1200 (0.16%)	[90]	VUS	VUS	PM2_P, PP3, PS3_M, BS2
c.487A>C	p.Met163Leu	1/1200 (0.083%)	[91]	Pathogenic	**VUS**	PM2, PS3_P
c.503A>G	p.(Lys168Arg)	5/1200 (0.42%)	[92]	Conflicting Interpretation	**VUS**	PM2_P, PP3

Table 1. Cont.

Nucleotide Change	Protein Variant	Mutated Alleles/ Total Alleles Tested (Percentage)	Reference	ClinVar	Final Classification (ACMG/AMP HL-EP)	Rules Applied
c.551G>C	p.Arg184Pro	4/1200 (0.34%)	[79]	Conflicting Interpretation	**Pathogenic**	PM2, PM3_VS, PP3, PS3_M
c.569T>A	p.(Val190Asp)	1/1200 (0.083%)	[28]	absent	**VUS**	PM2, PM3, PP3
c.617A>G	p.Asn206Ser	4/1200 (0.34%)	[90]	Pathogenic	**Pathogenic**	PM2_P, PP3, PP1_M, PM3_VS, PS3_M
c.632G>A	p.(Cys211Tyr)	1/1200 (0.083%)	[28]	absent	**Likely Pathogenic**	PM2, PM3, PP3, PP1_P
c.*1C>T (3'UTR)	-	2/1200 (0.16%)	[93]	Conflicting Interpretation	**Likely Benign**	BS1_P, BP4
del(GJB6-D13S1830)	-	12/1200 (1%)	[10]	Pathogenic	**Pathogenic**	PS3, PS4, PM2_P, PM3_VS
del(GJB6-D13S1854)	-	5/1200 (0.42%)	[21]	Pathogenic	**Pathogenic**	PM2, PS3, PS4, PM3_VS

Genetic variants' distribution spanned the entire length of Cx26 and involved almost all protein domains (Figure 3).

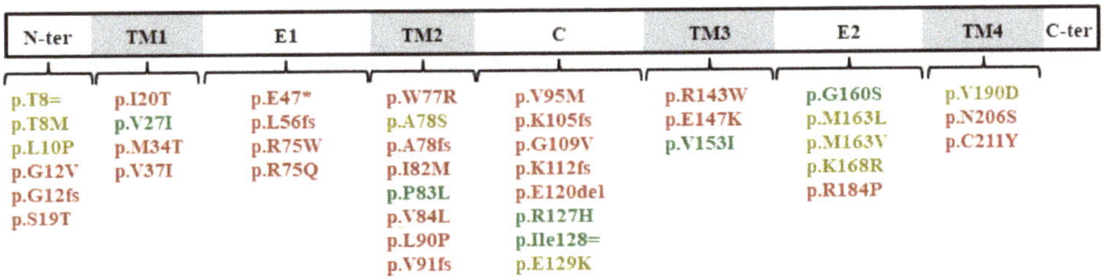

Figure 3. Distribution of coding genetic variants in connexin 26. Different colors refer to their classification after the curation process. Pathogenic and likely pathogenic variants are in red; benign and likely benign in green; uncertain significance in yellow.

Interestingly, based on the specific criteria applied during our curation procedure, 59% of sequence variants evaluated in this study changed their previous category submitted to ClinVar: 36% with considerable re-interpretation and 23% with resolution of similar categories (for instance, P/LP submission for p.Gly12Val variant was confirmed as pathogenic or B/LB submission for p.Val153Ile variant was classified as benign) (Figure 4).

After the curation procedure, the pathogenic final classification represented a total of 23 variants, of which 11 changed their previous status in ClinVar, and 12 remained in the same category (Figure 4). In addition, nine variants previously considered as conflicting interpretation of pathogenicity were reclassified as: pathogenic (two cases), benign or likely benign (three cases) and uncertain significance (four cases). The c.269T>C, p.Leu90Pro and c.551G>C, p.Arg184Pro variants were reinterpreted as pathogenic, since both mutations had strong evidence concerning allelic data (PM3_VeryStrong) and functional studies demonstrating a deleterious effect (PS3). The c.380G>A, p.(Arg127His); c.478G>A, p.(Gly160Ser) and the 3'UTR variant c.*1C>T were reclassified to likely benign and benign mostly based on their high population frequencies (BA1 and BS1 rules). The last four variants with conflicting interpretations in ClinVar: c.23C>T, p.Thr8Met; c.24G>A, p.(Thr8=); c.385G>A, p.(Glu129Lys); c.503A>G, p.(Lys168Arg), were reclassified as being of uncertain significance since available information was not sufficient to determine their pathogenicity. The c.487A>C, p.Met163Leu variant listed in ClinVar as pathogenic for dominant HL, was reinterpreted in this work as being of uncertain significance, due to the lack of strong evidence: absent in population database (PM2), low REVEL score, functional study with only supporting evidence (PS3_P) and only reported three times (PS4_P).

Remarkably, we propose that the splice site variant c.-22-2A>C interpreted as being of uncertain significance by the HL-EP group should be reclassified as likely pathogenic according to new uncovered data. Thus, due to the usage of an alternative variant nomenclature c.-24A>C (not HGVS), a previous report by [70] had not been taken into account for variant classification. After consultation with the author [70], correct nomenclature was confirmed, thus, the allelic data of the report was considered, strengthening the PM3 criteria, and hence, the variant pathogenicity. Final classification and comment on clinical significance for each variant was submitted to ClinVar.

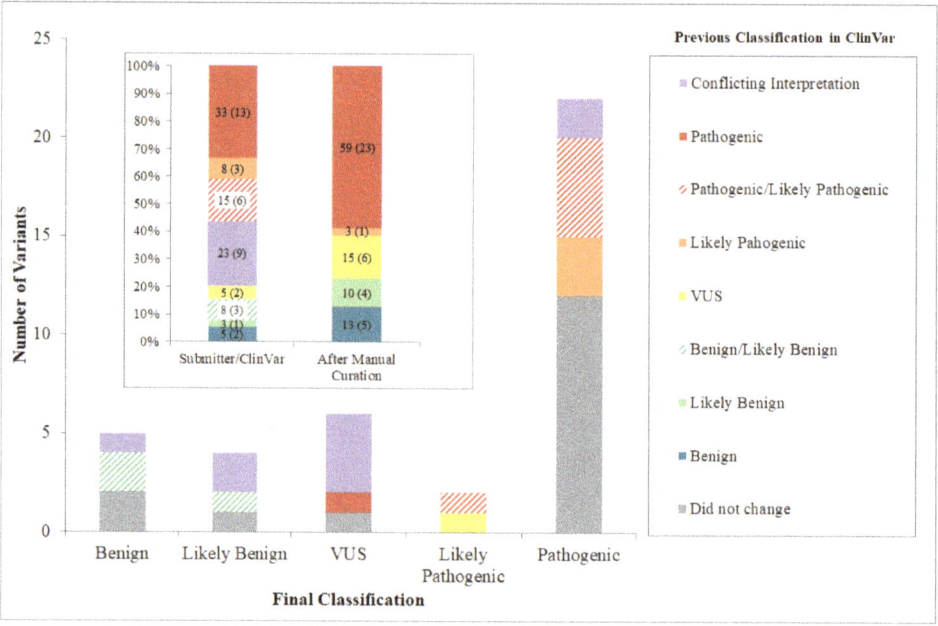

Figure 4. Final *GJB2* and *GJB6* variant classification. The height of each bar represents the number of variants for each classification. The colored segments of each bar represent previous classification in ClinVar. As a result of the curation process 59% of sequence variants changed their previous category submitted to ClinVar. The inner box shows the comparison of the 44 variant classifications between ClinVar submitters (from the original ACMG/AMP criteria) versus applying HL-EP specifications, demonstrating a reduction of "conflicting interpretation" and the increase of "pathogenic" categories. The number of variants for each interpretation is in brackets.

The most frequently applied rules were PM2 and PM3 (20% each), corresponding to population and allelic data, respectively, followed by the PS3 standard, which included functional studies demonstrating a deleterious effect (12%) (Figure 5A). The frequency of rules used among the three main categories (B/LB, VUS and LP/P) is shown in Figure 5B. In this regard, PM3_VeryStrong and PM2 rules together with computational evidence suggesting a damaging impact of the mutation to the protein (PP3) and deleterious effect demonstrated by functional assays (PS3) were the most frequent criteria applied, particularly for the classification of pathogenic and likely pathogenic variants. High frequency of variants in the general populations (BA1), neutral impact predicted by in silico analysis (BP4) and allelic data (BP2) were associated with benign or likely benign categories. In the case of variants interpreted as uncertain significance, damaging computational evidence was almost always applied along with low frequency in the general population. However, this evidence was not strong enough to determine its pathogenicity. Complete information about the criteria applied and variant interpretation is detailed in Supplementary Table S3.

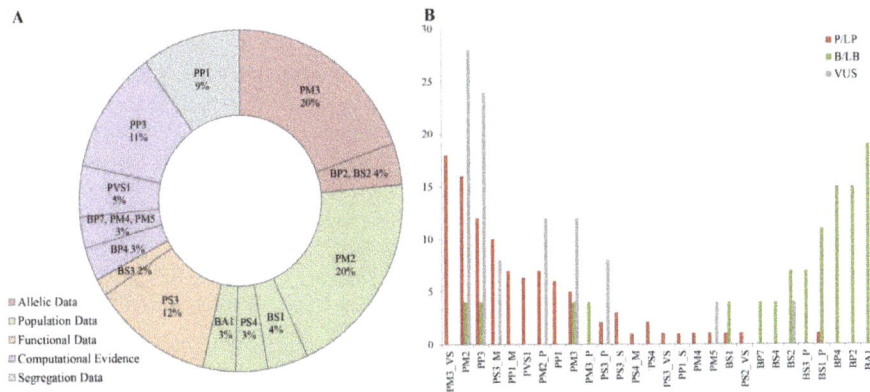

Figure 5. Frequency of rules applied during curation procedure. (**A**). PM2 and PM3 were the most frequently criteria applied (corresponding to population and allelic data), along with the PS3 rule, which included functional studies demonstrating a deleterious effect. (**B**). ACMG/AMP and HL-EP rules correspondence with final classification. Red, grey and green colors indicate the final variant interpretation (P/LP, B/LB and VUS) when the rule was applied. Some criteria demonstrate a bigger weight in the classification of variants. Rules applied with a modified strength are denoted by the rule followed by _P for Supporting, _M for Moderate, _S for Strong, and _VS for Very Strong.

4. Discussion

Autosomal Recessive Non-Syndromic Hearing Loss (ARNSHL) is a heterogeneous condition that affects millions of individuals worldwide. Genetic variants in *GJB2* and *GJB6* genes are the most prevalent genetic causes of HL among several populations, and consequently, are the focus of universal newborn hearing screening programs [77,94,95]. Identifying mutations in those genes becomes crucial in molecular strategy approaches, as they provide valuable prognostic information for medical intervention. This study provides an update and extension of our previous reports and states that sequence variants in *GJB2* and *GJB6* genes are frequent in Argentinean patients with non-syndromic sensorineural HL [26–28,96].

Molecular diagnosis due to *GJB2* and *GJB6* variants was more successful in family cases with ARNSHL than in sporadic ones (36% vs. 15.5%). As reported previously, our data confirms c.35delG as the most frequent *GJB2* mutation causing non-syndromic hearing loss in the Argentinean population with a prevalence of 9.25% of the detected *GJB2*-mutated alleles [26–28,30]. These results are in concordance with Caucasian population frequencies [73,75,87,97]. On the other hand, since 26/98 (26.5%) genotyped patients resulted in *GJB2* compound heterozygous for non-c.35delG alleles, appropriate molecular diagnosis requires the complete sequencing of the gene including the untranslated exon 1. Interestingly, both dominant mutations in *GJB2* were detected in the same protein residue (Arg75) and led to a profound HL phenotype, in accordance with the dominant negative effect of the two variants demonstrated by functional studies [98–100]. Of note, both variants del(*GJB6*-D13S1830) and del(*GJB6*-D13S1854) accounted for 15.3% of genotyped patients, which resulted in similar frequencies reported in Spain but greater than other European countries [6–8,21,97,101–103]. Our cohort of patients exhibited non-syndromic moderate-to-profound hearing loss due to biallelic *GJB2* mutations and compound *GJB2/GJB6* mutations. In accordance with previous studies truncating variants were mostly related to profound HL, while non-truncating variants to a milder degree of hearing impairment, reinforcing the notion that inactivating variants lead to a severe degree of HL [8,34,46,97].

Regarding variant curation, allelic and population data along with computational evidence were the most used information in variant assessment. The PM3 and PM2 rules accounted for 20% each of the total parameters applied. The PM3 criteria gathers the information regarding the compound heterozygous variants in HL patients. Since *GJB2* variants are mostly related to an autosomal recessive mode of inheritance, the identification of a second mutation resulted essential and conclusive in variant interpretation. In addition, the absence or low frequency of the sequence variant in the general population (defined by PM2 rule) represented an important evidence during data analysis.

The curation of variants performed in the present work highlights the importance of specialized guidelines to analyze and interpret variants for the clinical use of databases. Moreover, it indicates the need of scientific community interaction and data sharing to avoid or reduce difficulties in variant curation [104,105]. Manual curation, although time consuming is strictly needed, as shown for the p.Met163Leu variant, which was originally interpreted as pathogenic for autosomal dominant HL by one submitter, and now reclassified to uncertain significance. An additional example is that of the splice site variant c.-22-2A>C, classified as of uncertain significance and now reinterpreted to likely pathogenic as a result of the clarification of nomenclature issues, and hence, strengthening the criteria applied. Likewise, more than half of the mutations were reclassified after the curation procedure, and satisfyingly, this reduced the number of "conflicting interpretation" categorization submitted to ClinVar.

In summary, the present work provides a set of variants that lead to hearing loss with an accurate interpretation of their phenotypic consequence. Moreover, it demonstrates the importance of a comprehensive analysis of sequence data performed by experts in the hearing field in order to provide reliable data to be used by clinicians in patient diagnosis and genetic counseling.

Supplementary Materials: The following are available online at http://www.mdpi.com/2073-4425/11/10/1233/s1, Table S1: Summary of HL-EP specifications, Table S2: Summary of genotypes detected and Table S3: Curated variants procedure.

Author Contributions: P.B. performed the molecular genetic studies and curation of variants and wrote the manuscript. C.D.B. contributed with graphic design and variant curation. L.L. and F.G. contributed with bioinformatic analysis. V.L., S.M. and B.P. recruited patients and acquired the clinical data. A.B.E. raised funding and assured the general supervision of the research group. V.D. designed the genetic study and wrote the manuscript. All authors have read and agreed to the published version of the manuscript.

Funding: This study was supported by an International Research Scholar grant from the Grand Prix Fondation Pour L'Audition and from the "Agencia Nacional de Promoción Científica y Tecnológica" PICT-2018-00539 to A.B.E., and a grant for Medical Research from Fundación Alberto J. Roemmers to P.B.

Acknowledgments: We acknowledge Ezequiel Surace for proofreading the manuscript carefully and Bruno de Brasi for their comments and suggestions that have greatly helped in improving the quality of the report. Paula Buonfiglio is a CONICET fellow. We thank all families for their kind contribution to this study.

Conflicts of Interest: The authors declare no conflict of interest.

References

1. Morton, C.C.; Nance, W.E. Newborn hearing screening—A silent revolution. *N. Engl. J. Med.* **2006**, *354*, 2151–2164. [CrossRef]
2. Morton, N.E. Genetic Epidemiology of Hearing Impairment. *Ann. N. Y. Acad. Sci.* **1991**, *630*, 16–31. [CrossRef] [PubMed]
3. Shearer, A.E.; Hildebrand, M.S.; Smith, R.J.H. Hereditary Hearing Loss and Deafness Overview. In *GeneReviews*; Adam, M.P., Ardinger, H.H., Pagon, R.A., Wallace, S.E., Bean, L.J.H., Stephens, K., Amemiya, A., Eds.; University of Washington, Seattle: Seattle, WA, USA, 1999.
4. Van Camp, G.; Smith, R.J.H. Hereditary Hearing Loss Homepage. Available online: https://hereditaryhearingloss.org (accessed on 16 October 2020).

5. Richardson, G.P.; de Monvel, J.B.; Petit, C. How the Genetics of Deafness Illuminates Auditory Physiology. *Annu. Rev. Physiol.* **2011**, *73*, 311–334. [CrossRef] [PubMed]
6. Cama, E.; Melchionda, S.; Palladino, T.; Carella, M.; Santarelli, R.; Genovese, E.; Benettazzo, F.; Zelante, L.; Arslan, E. Hearing loss features in GJB2 biallelic mutations and GJB2/GJB6 digenic inheritance in a large Italian cohort. *Int. J. Audiol.* **2009**, *48*, 12–17. [CrossRef] [PubMed]
7. Del Castillo, I.; Moreno-Pelayo, M.A.; Del Castillo, F.J.; Brownstein, Z.; Marlin, S.; Adina, Q.; Cockburn, D.J.; Pandya, A.; Siemering, K.R.; Chamberlin, G.P.; et al. Prevalence and evolutionary origins of the del(GJB6-D13S1830) mutation in the DFNB1 locus in hearing-impaired subjects: A multicenter study. *Am. J. Hum. Genet.* **2003**, *73*, 1452–1458. [CrossRef]
8. Feldmann, D.; Denoyelle, F.; Chauvin, P.; Garabédian, E.-N.; Couderc, R.; Odent, S.; Joannard, A.; Schmerber, S.; Delobel, B.; Leman, J.; et al. Large deletion of the GJB6 gene in deaf patients heterozygous for the GJB2 gene mutation: Genotypic and phenotypic analysis. *Am. J. Med. Genet. A* **2004**, *127A*, 263–267. [CrossRef] [PubMed]
9. Pampanos, A.; Economides, J.; Iliadou, V.; Neou, P.; Leotsakos, P.; Voyiatzis, N.; Eleftheriades, N.; Tsakanikos, M.; Antoniadi, T.; Hatzaki, A.; et al. Prevalence of GJB2 mutations in prelingual deafness in the Greek population. *Int. J. Pediatr. Otorhinolaryngol.* **2002**, *65*, 101–108. [CrossRef]
10. del Castillo, I.; Villamar, M.; Moreno-Pelayo, M.A.; del Castillo, F.J.; Alvarez, A.; Tellería, D.; Menéndez, I.; Moreno, F. A deletion involving the connexin 30 gene in nonsyndromic hearing impairment. *N. Engl. J. Med.* **2002**, *346*, 243–249. [CrossRef]
11. Hilgert, N.; Smith, R.J.H.; Van Camp, G. Forty-six genes causing nonsyndromic hearing impairment: Which ones should be analyzed in DNA diagnostics? *Mutat. Res.* **2009**, *681*, 189–196. [CrossRef]
12. Rabionet, R.; Gasparini, P.; Estivill, X. Molecular genetics of hearing impairment due to mutations in gap junction genes encoding beta connexins. *Hum. Mutat.* **2000**, *16*, 190–202. [CrossRef]
13. Meşe, G.; Richard, G.; White, T.W. Gap Junctions: Basic Structure and Function. *J. Investig. Dermatol.* **2007**, *127*, 2516–2524. [CrossRef] [PubMed]
14. Bruzzone, R.; Veronesi, V.; Gomès, D.; Bicego, M.; Duval, N.; Marlin, S.; Petit, C.; D'Andrea, P.; White, T.W. Loss-of-function and residual channel activity of connexin26 mutations associated with non-syndromic deafness. *FEBS Lett.* **2003**, *533*, 79–88. [CrossRef]
15. Palmada, M.; Schmalisch, K.; Böhmer, C.; Schug, N.; Pfister, M.; Lang, F.; Blin, N. Loss of function mutations of the GJB2 gene detected in patients with DFNB1-associated hearing impairment. *Neurobiol. Dis.* **2006**, *22*, 112–118. [CrossRef] [PubMed]
16. White, T.W. Functional analysis of human Cx26 mutations associated with deafness. *Brain Res. Rev.* **2000**, *32*, 181–183. [CrossRef]
17. Gasparini, P.; the Genetic Analysis Consortium of GJB235delG; Rabionet, R.; Barbujani, G.; Melchionda, S.; Petersen, M.; Brøndum-Nielsen, K.; Metspalu, A.; Oitmaa, E.; Pisano, M.; et al. High carrier frequency of the 35delG deafness mutation in European populations. *Eur. J. Hum. Genet.* **2000**, *8*, 19–23. [CrossRef]
18. Cryns, K. A genotype-phenotype correlation for GJB2 (connexin 26) deafness. *J. Med. Genet.* **2004**, *41*, 147–154. [CrossRef]
19. Lucotte, G. High prevalences of carriers of the 35delG mutation of connexin 26 in the Mediterranean area. *Int. J. Pediatri. Otorhinolaryngol.* **2007**, *71*, 741–746. [CrossRef]
20. Azaiez, H.; Booth, K.T.; Ephraim, S.S.; Crone, B.; Black-Ziegelbein, E.A.; Marini, R.J.; Eliot Shearer, A.; Sloan-Heggen, C.M.; Kolbe, D.; Casavant, T.; et al. Genomic Landscape and Mutational Signatures of Deafness-Associated Genes. *Am. J. Hum. Genet.* **2018**, *103*, 484–497. [CrossRef]
21. del Castillo, F.J. A novel deletion involving the connexin-30 gene, del(GJB6-d13s1854), found in trans with mutations in the GJB2 gene (connexin-26) in subjects with DFNB1 non-syndromic hearing impairment. *J. Med. Genet.* **2005**, *42*, 588–594. [CrossRef]
22. Wilch, E.; Azaiez, H.; Fisher, R.A.; Elfenbein, J.; Murgia, A.; Birkenhäger, R.; Bolz, H.; Da Silva-Costa, S.M.; Del Castillo, I.; Haaf, T.; et al. A novel DFNB1 deletion allele supports the existence of a distant cis-regulatory region that controls GJB2 and GJB6 expression. *Clin. Genet.* **2010**, *78*, 267–274. [CrossRef] [PubMed]
23. Feldmann, D.; Le Maréchal, C.; Jonard, L.; Thierry, P.; Czajka, C.; Couderc, R.; Ferec, C.; Denoyelle, F.; Marlin, S.; Fellmann, F. A new large deletion in the DFNB1 locus causes nonsyndromic hearing loss. *Eur. J. Med. Genet.* **2009**, *52*, 195–200. [CrossRef]

24. Bliznetz, E.A.; Makienko, O.N.; Okuneva, E.G.; Markova, T.G.; Polyakov, A.V. New recurrent large deletion, encompassing both GJB2 and GB6 genes, results in isolated sensorineural hearing impairment with autosomal recessive mode of inheritance. *Russ. J. Genet.* **2014**, *50*, 415–420. [CrossRef]
25. Tayoun, A.N.A.; Abou Tayoun, A.N.; Mason-Suares, H.; Frisella, A.L.; Bowser, M.; Duffy, E.; Mahanta, L.; Funke, B.; Rehm, H.L.; Amr, S.S. Targeted Droplet-Digital PCR as a Tool for Novel Deletion Discovery at the DFNB1 Locus. *Hum. Mutat.* **2016**, *37*, 119–126. [CrossRef] [PubMed]
26. Dalamón, V.; Lotersztein, V.; Béhèran, A.; Lipovsek, M.; Diamante, F.; Pallares, N.; Francipane, L.; Frechtel, G.; Paoli, B.; Mansilla, E.; et al. GJB2 and GJB6 Genes: Molecular Study and Identification of Novel GJB2 Mutations in the Hearing-Impaired Argentinean Population. *Audiol. Neurotol.* **2010**, *15*, 194–202. [CrossRef] [PubMed]
27. Dalamón, V.; Béhèran, A.; Diamante, F.; Pallares, N.; Diamante, V.; Elgoyhen, A.B. Prevalence of GJB2 mutations and the del(GJB6-D13S1830) in Argentinean non-syndromic deaf patients. *Hear. Res.* **2005**, *207*, 43–49. [CrossRef] [PubMed]
28. Dalamón, V.; Florencia Wernert, M.; Lotersztein, V.; Craig, P.O.; Diamante, R.R.; Barteik, M.E.; Curet, C.; Paoli, B.; Mansilla, E.; Elgoyhen, A.B. Identification of four novel connexin 26 mutations in non-syndromic deaf patients: Genotype-phenotype analysis in moderate cases. *Mol. Biol. Rep.* **2013**, *40*, 6945–6955. [CrossRef] [PubMed]
29. Gravina, L.P.; Foncuberta, M.E.; Estrada, R.C.; Barreiro, C.; Chertkoff, L. Carrier frequency of the 35delG and A1555G deafness mutations in the Argentinean population. *Int. J. Pediatri. Otorhinolaryngol.* **2007**, *71*, 639–643. [CrossRef]
30. Gravina, L.P.; Foncuberta, M.E.; Prieto, M.E.; Garrido, J.; Barreiro, C.; Chertkoff, L. Prevalence of DFNB1 mutations in Argentinean children with non-syndromic deafness. Report of a novel mutation in GJB2. *Int. J. Pediatr. Otorhinolaryngol.* **2010**, *74*, 250–254. [CrossRef]
31. Reynoso, R.A.; Hendl, S.; Barteik, M.E.; Curet, C.A.; Nicemboin, L.; Moreno Barral, J.; Rodríguez Ballesteros, M.; Del Castillo, I.; Moreno, F. Genetic study of hearing loss in families from Argentina. *Rev. Fac. Cien. Med. Univ. Nac. Cordoba* **2004**, *61*, 13–19.
32. Smith, R.J.H.; Jones, M.K.N. Nonsyndromic Hearing Loss and Deafness, DFNB1. 28 September 1998 [Updated 18 August 2016]. In *GeneReviews®*; Adam, M.P.; Ardinger, H.H.; Pagon, R.A.; Wallace, S.E.; Bean, L.J.H.; Stephens, K., Amemiya, A., Eds.; University of Washington, Seattle: Seattle, WA, USA, 1993. [PubMed]
33. D'Andrea, P.; Veronesi, V.; Bicego, M.; Melchionda, S.; Zelante, L.; Di Iorio, E.; Bruzzone, R.; Gasparini, P. Hearing loss: Frequency and functional studies of the most common connexin26 alleles. *Biochem. Biophys. Res. Commun.* **2002**, *296*, 685–691. [CrossRef]
34. Azaiez, H.; Parker Chamberlin, G.; Fischer, S.M.; Welp, C.L.; Prasad, S.D.; Thomas Taggart, R.; del Castillo, I.; Van Camp, G.; Smith, R.J.H. GJB2: The spectrum of deafness-causing allele variants and their phenotype. *Hum. Mutat.* **2004**, *24*, 305–311. [CrossRef]
35. Green, G.E.; Scott, D.A.; McDonald, J.M.; Teagle, H.F.B.; Tomblin, B.J.; Spencer, L.J.; Woodworth, G.G.; Knutson, J.F.; Gantz, B.J.; Sheffield, V.C.; et al. Performance of cochlear implant recipients withGJB2-related deafness. *Am. J. Med. Genet.* **2002**, *109*, 167–170. [CrossRef] [PubMed]
36. Bauer, P.W.; Geers, A.E.; Brenner, C.; Moog, J.S.; Smith, R.J.H. The Effect of GJB2 Allele Variants on Performance After Cochlear Implantation. *Laryngoscope* **2003**, *113*, 2135–2140. [CrossRef]
37. Usami, S.-I.; Nishio, S.-Y.; Moteki, H.; Miyagawa, M.; Yoshimura, H. Cochlear Implantation from the Perspective of Genetic Background. *Anat. Rec.* **2020**, *303*, 563–593. [CrossRef]
38. Amendola, L.M.; Jarvik, G.P.; Leo, M.C.; McLaughlin, H.M.; Akkari, Y.; Amaral, M.D.; Berg, J.S.; Biswas, S.; Bowling, K.M.; Conlin, L.K.; et al. Performance of ACMG-AMP Variant-Interpretation Guidelines among Nine Laboratories in the Clinical Sequencing Exploratory Research Consortium. *Am. J. Hum. Genet.* **2016**, *99*, 247. [CrossRef] [PubMed]
39. Booth, K.T.; Kahrizi, K.; Babanejad, M.; Daghagh, H.; Bademci, G.; Arzhangi, S.; Zareabdollahi, D.; Duman, D.; El-Amraoui, A.; Tekin, M.; et al. Variants in CIB2 cause DFNB48 and not USH1J. *Clin. Genet.* **2018**, *93*, 812–821. [CrossRef]
40. Harrison, S.M.; Dolinsky, J.S.; Knight Johnson, A.E.; Pesaran, T.; Azzariti, D.R.; Bale, S.; Chao, E.C.; Das, S.; Vincent, L.; Rehm, H.L. Clinical laboratories collaborate to resolve differences in variant interpretations submitted to ClinVar. *Genet. Med.* **2017**, *19*, 1096–1104. [CrossRef]

41. Richards, S.; Aziz, N.; Bale, S.; Bick, D.; Das, S.; Gastier-Foster, J.; Grody, W.W.; Hegde, M.; Lyon, E.; Spector, E.; et al. Standards and guidelines for the interpretation of sequence variants: A joint consensus recommendation of the American College of Medical Genetics and Genomics and the Association for Molecular Pathology. *Genet. Med.* **2015**, *17*, 405–423. [CrossRef]
42. Oza, A.M.; DiStefano, M.T.; Hemphill, S.E.; Cushman, B.J.; Grant, A.R.; Siegert, R.K.; Shen, J.; Chapin, A.; Boczek, N.J.; Schimmenti, L.A.; et al. Expert specification of the ACMG/AMP variant interpretation guidelines for genetic hearing loss. *Hum. Mutat.* **2018**, *39*, 1593–1613. [CrossRef]
43. Murray, M.G.; Thompson, W.F. Rapid isolation of high molecular weight plant DNA. *Nucleic Acids Res.* **1980**, *8*, 4321–4326. [CrossRef]
44. Sequence Assembly and Alignment Software-CodonCode. Available online: https://www.codoncode.com/ (accessed on 16 October 2020).
45. Altschul, S.F.; Gish, W.; Miller, W.; Myers, E.W.; Lipman, D.J. Basic local alignment search tool. *J. Mol. Biol.* **1990**, *215*, 403–410. [CrossRef]
46. Snoeckx, R.L.; Huygen, P.L.M.; Feldmann, D.; Marlin, S.; Denoyelle, F.; Waligora, J.; Mueller-Malesinska, M.; Pollak, A.; Ploski, R.; Murgia, A.; et al. GJB2 Mutations and Degree of Hearing Loss: A Multicenter Study. *Am. J. Hum. Genet.* **2005**, *77*, 945–957. [CrossRef] [PubMed]
47. Shahin, H.; Walsh, T.; Sobe, T.; Lynch, E.; King, M.-C.; Avraham, K.B.; Kanaan, M. Genetics of congenital deafness in the Palestinian population: Multiple connexin 26 alleles with shared origins in the Middle East. *Hum. Genet.* **2002**, *110*, 284–289. [CrossRef] [PubMed]
48. Del Castillo, F.J.; Del Castillo, I. DFNB1 Non-syndromic Hearing Impairment: Diversity of Mutations and Associated Phenotypes. *Front. Mol. Neurosci.* **2017**, *10*, 428. [CrossRef]
49. Gandía, M.; Del Castillo, F.J.; Rodríguez-Álvarez, F.J.; Garrido, G.; Villamar, M.; Calderón, M.; Moreno-Pelayo, M.A.; Moreno, F.; del Castillo, I. A novel splice-site mutation in the GJB2 gene causing mild postlingual hearing impairment. *PLoS ONE* **2013**, *8*, e73566. [CrossRef] [PubMed]
50. den Dunnen, J.T.; Dalgleish, R.; Maglott, D.R.; Hart, R.K.; Greenblatt, M.S.; McGowan-Jordan, J.; Roux, A.-F.; Smith, T.; Antonarakis, S.E.; Taschner, P.E.M. HGVS Recommendations for the Description of Sequence Variants: 2016 Update. *Hum. Mutat.* **2016**, *37*, 564–569. [CrossRef]
51. Wildeman, M.; van Ophuizen, E.; den Dunnen, J.T.; Taschner, P.E.M. Improving sequence variant descriptions in mutation databases and literature using the Mutalyzer sequence variation nomenclature checker. *Hum. Mutat.* **2008**, *29*, 6–13. [CrossRef]
52. Ioannidis, N.M.; Rothstein, J.H.; Pejaver, V.; Middha, S.; McDonnell, S.K.; Baheti, S.; Musolf, A.; Li, Q.; Holzinger, E.; Karyadi, D.; et al. REVEL: An Ensemble Method for Predicting the Pathogenicity of Rare Missense Variants. *Am. J. Hum. Genet.* **2016**, *99*, 877–885. [CrossRef]
53. Rentzsch, P.; Witten, D.; Cooper, G.M.; Shendure, J.; Kircher, M. CADD: Predicting the deleteriousness of variants throughout the human genome. *Nucleic Acids Res.* **2019**, *47*, D886–D894. [CrossRef]
54. Desmet, F.-O.; Hamroun, D.; Lalande, M.; Collod-Béroud, G.; Claustres, M.; Béroud, C. Human Splicing Finder: An online bioinformatics tool to predict splicing signals. *Nucleic Acids Res.* **2009**, *37*, e67. [CrossRef] [PubMed]
55. Yeo, G.; Burge, C.B. Maximum entropy modeling of short sequence motifs with applications to RNA splicing signals. *Burge. J. Comput. Biol.* **2004**, *11*, 377–394.
56. Abou Tayoun, A.N.; Pesaran, T.; DiStefano, M.T.; Oza, A.; Rehm, H.L.; Biesecker, L.G.; Harrison, S.M.; ClinGen Sequence Variant Interpretation Working Group (ClinGen SVI). Recommendations for interpreting the loss of function PVS1 ACMG/AMP variant criterion. *Hum. Mutat.* **2018**, *39*, 1517–1524. [CrossRef]
57. Shamsani, J.; Kazakoff, S.H.; Armean, I.M.; McLaren, W.; Parsons, M.T.; Thompson, B.A.; O'Mara, T.A.; Hunt, S.E.; Waddell, N.; Spurdle, A.B. A plugin for the Ensembl Variant Effect Predictor that uses MaxEntScan to predict variant spliceogenicity. *Bioinformatics* **2019**, *35*, 2315–2317. [CrossRef] [PubMed]
58. Karczewski, K.J.; Francioli, L.C.; Tiao, G.; Cummings, B.B.; Alföldi, J.; Wang, Q.; Collins, R.L.; Laricchia, K.M.; Ganna, A.; Birnbaum, D.P.; et al. The mutational constraint spectrum quantified from variation in 141,456 humans. *Nature* **2020**, *581*, 434–443. [CrossRef] [PubMed]
59. Sherry, S.T. dbSNP: The NCBI database of genetic variation. *Nucleic Acids Res.* **2001**, *29*, 308–311. [CrossRef]
60. Exome Variant Server, NHLBI GO Exome Sequencing Project (ESP), Seattle, WA. Available online: http://evs.gs.washington.edu/EVS/ (accessed on 16 October 2020).

61. Landrum, M.J.; Lee, J.M.; Benson, M.; Brown, G.R.; Chao, C.; Chitipiralla, S.; Gu, B.; Hart, J.; Hoffman, D.; Jang, W.; et al. ClinVar: Improving access to variant interpretations and supporting evidence. *Nucleic Acids Res.* **2018**, *46*, D1062–D1067. [CrossRef]
62. Fokkema, I.F.A.C.; Ivo, F.A.; Taschner, P.E.M.; Schaafsma, G.C.P.; Celli, J.; Laros, J.F.J.; den Dunnen, J.T. LOVD v.2.0: The next generation in gene variant databases. *Hum. Mutat.* **2011**, *32*, 557–563. [CrossRef]
63. MacDonald, J.R.; Ziman, R.; Yuen, R.K.C.; Feuk, L.; Scherer, S.W. The Database of Genomic Variants: A curated collection of structural variation in the human genome. *Nucleic Acids Res.* **2014**, *42*, D986–D992. [CrossRef]
64. EMBL-EBI Database of Genomic Variants Archive. Available online: https://www.ebi.ac.uk/dgva/ (accessed on 16 October 2020).
65. Frequency Filter. Available online: https://www.cardiodb.org/allelefrequencyapp/ (accessed on 16 October 2020).
66. Kopanos, C.; Tsiolkas, V.; Kouris, A.; Chapple, C.E.; Aguilera, M.A.; Meyer, R.; Massouras, A. VarSome: The human genomic variant search engine. *Bioinformatics* **2019**, *35*, 1978–1980. [CrossRef]
67. 6601 Free Vector Icons of Webpage. Available online: https://www.flaticon.com/free-icons/webpage (accessed on 16 October 2020).
68. Denoyelle, F.; Marlin, S.; Weil, D.; Moatti, L.; Chauvin, P.; Garabédian, E.N.; Petit, C. Clinical features of the prevalent form of childhood deafness, DFNB1, due to a connexin-26 gene defect: Implications for genetic counselling. *Lancet* **1999**, *353*, 1298–1303. [CrossRef]
69. Gasmelseed, N.M.A.; Schmidt, M.; Magzoub, M.M.A.; Macharia, M.; Elmustafa, O.M.; Ototo, B.; Winkler, E.; Ruge, G.; Horstmann, R.D.; Meyer, C.G. Low frequency of deafness-associated GJB2 variants in Kenya and Sudan and novel GJB2 variants. *Hum. Mutat.* **2004**, *23*, 206–207. [CrossRef] [PubMed]
70. Sansović, I.; Knezević, J.; Musani, V.; Seeman, P.; Barisić, I.; Pavelić, J. GJB2 mutations in patients with nonsyndromic hearing loss from Croatia. *Genet. Test. Mol. Biomark.* **2009**, *13*, 693–699. [CrossRef]
71. Kenna, M.A.; Wu, B.L.; Cotanche, D.A.; Korf, B.R.; Rehm, H.L. Connexin 26 studies in patients with sensorineural hearing loss. *Arch. Otolaryngol. Head Neck Surg.* **2001**, *127*, 1037–1042. [CrossRef] [PubMed]
72. Matos, T.D.; Simões-Teixeira, H.; Caria, H.; Gonçalves, A.C.; Chora, J.; Correia, M.D.C.; Moura, C.; Rosa, H.; Monteiro, L.; O'Neill, A.; et al. Spectrum and frequency of GJB2 mutations in a cohort of 264 Portuguese nonsyndromic sensorineural hearing loss patients. *Int. J. Audiol.* **2013**, *52*, 466–471. [CrossRef]
73. Pandya, A.; Arnos, K.S.; Xia, X.J.; Welch, K.O.; Blanton, S.H.; Friedman, T.B.; Garcia Sanchez, G.; Liu MD, X.Z.; Morell, R.; Nance, W.E. Frequency and distribution of GJB2 (connexin 26) and GJB6 (connexin 30) mutations in a large North American repository of deaf probands. *Genet. Med.* **2003**, *5*, 295–303. [CrossRef] [PubMed]
74. Rabionet, R.; Zelante, L.; López-Bigas, N.; D'Agruma, L.; Melchionda, S.; Restagno, G.; Arbonés, M.L.; Gasparini, P.; Estivill, X. Molecular basis of childhood deafness resulting from mutations in the GJB2 (connexin 26) gene. *Hum. Genet.* **2000**, *106*, 40–44.
75. Zelante, L.; Gasparini, P.; Estivill, X.; Melchionda, S.; D'Agruma, L.; Govea, N.; Milá, M.; Monica, M.D.; Lutfi, J.; Shohat, M.; et al. Connexin26 mutations associated with the most common form of non-syndromic neurosensory autosomal recessive deafness (DFNB1) in Mediterraneans. *Hum. Mol. Genet.* **1997**, *6*, 1605–1609. [CrossRef]
76. Löffler, J.; Nekahm, D.; Hirst-Stadlmann, A.; Günther, B.; Menzel, H.J.; Utermann, G.; Janecke, A.R. Sensorineural hearing loss and the incidence of Cx26 mutations in Austria. *Eur. J. Hum. Genet.* **2001**, *9*, 226–230. [CrossRef]
77. Kelley, P.M.; Harris, D.J.; Comer, B.C.; Askew, J.W.; Fowler, T.; Smith, S.D.; Kimberling, W.J. Novel mutations in the connexin 26 gene (GJB2) that cause autosomal recessive (DFNB1) hearing loss. *Am. J. Hum. Genet.* **1998**, *62*, 792–799. [CrossRef]
78. Kelsell, D.P.; Dunlop, J.; Stevens, H.P.; Lench, N.J.; Liang, J.N.; Parry, G.; Mueller, R.F.; Leigh, I.M. Connexin 26 mutations in hereditary non-syndromic sensorineural deafness. *Nature* **1997**, *387*, 80–83. [CrossRef]
79. Denoyelle, F.; Weil, D.; Maw, M.A.; Wilcox, S.A.; Lench, N.J.; Allen-Powell, D.R.; Osborn, A.H.; Dahl, H.H.; Middleton, A.; Houseman, M.J.; et al. Prelingual deafness: High prevalence of a 30delG mutation in the connexin 26 gene. *Hum. Mol. Genet.* **1997**, *6*, 2173–2177. [CrossRef]
80. Richard, G.; White, T.W.; Smith, L.E.; Bailey, R.A.; Compton, J.G.; Paul, D.L.; Bale, S.J. Functional defects of Cx26 resulting from a heterozygous missense mutation in a family with dominant deaf-mutism and palmoplantar keratoderma. *Hum. Genet.* **1998**, *103*, 393–399. [CrossRef] [PubMed]

81. Uyguner, O.; Tukel, T.; Baykal, C.; Eris, H.; Emiroglu, M.; Hafiz, G.; Ghanbari, A.; Baserer, N.; Yuksel-Apak, M.; Wollnik, B. The novel R75Q mutation in the GJB2 gene causes autosomal dominant hearing loss and palmoplantar keratoderma in a Turkish family. *Clin. Genet.* **2002**, *62*, 306–309. [CrossRef] [PubMed]
82. Carrasquillo, M.M.; Zlotogora, J.; Barges, S.; Chakravarti, A. Two different connexin 26 mutations in an inbred kindred segregating non-syndromic recessive deafness: Implications for genetic studies in isolated populations. *Hum. Mol. Genet.* **1997**, *6*, 2163–2172. [CrossRef]
83. Putcha, G.V.; Bejjani, B.A.; Bleoo, S.; Booker, J.K.; Carey, J.C.; Carson, N.; Das, S.; Dempsey, M.A.; Gastier-Foster, J.M.; Greinwald, J.H., Jr.; et al. A multicenter study of the frequency and distribution of GJB2 and GJB6 mutations in a large North American cohort. *Genet. Med.* **2007**, *9*, 413–426. [CrossRef]
84. Kupka, S.; Braun, S.; Aberle, S.; Haack, B.; Ebauer, M.; Zeissler, U.; Zenner, H.-P.; Blin, N.; Pfister, M. Frequencies of GJB2 mutations in German control individuals and patients showing sporadic non-syndromic hearing impairment. *Hum. Mutat.* **2002**, *20*, 77–78. [CrossRef] [PubMed]
85. Scott, D.A.; Kraft, M.L.; Carmi, R.; Ramesh, A.; Elbedour, K.; Yairi, Y.; Srisailapathy, C.R.; Rosengren, S.S.; Markham, A.F.; Mueller, R.F.; et al. Identification of mutations in the connexin 26 gene that cause autosomal recessive nonsyndromic hearing loss. *Hum. Mutat.* **1998**, *11*, 387–394. [CrossRef]
86. Dalamón, V.; Loterszstein, V.; Lipovsek, M.; Bèherán, A.; Mondino, M.E.; Diamante, F.; Pallares, N.; Diamante, V.; Elgoyhen, A.B. Performance of speech perception after cochlear implantation in DFNB1 patients. *Acta Otolaryngol.* **2009**, *129*, 395–398. [CrossRef]
87. Estivill, X.; Fortina, P.; Surrey, S.; Rabionet, R.; Melchionda, S.; D'Agruma, L.; Mansfield, E.; Rappaport, E.; Govea, N.; Milà, M.; et al. Connexin-26 mutations in sporadic and inherited sensorineural deafness. *Lancet* **1998**, *351*, 394–398. [CrossRef]
88. Brobby, G.W.; Müller-Myhsok, B.; Horstmann, R.D. Connexin 26 R143W mutation associated with recessive nonsyndromic sensorineural deafness in Africa. *N. Engl. J. Med.* **1998**, *338*, 548–550. [CrossRef]
89. Frei, K.; Lucas, T.; Ramsebner, R.; Schöfer, C.; Baumgartner, W.-D.; Weipoltshammer, K.; Erginel-Unaltuna, N.; Wachtler, F.J.; Kirschhofer, K. A novel connexin 26 mutation associated with autosomal recessive sensorineural deafness. *Audiol. Neurootol.* **2004**, *9*, 47–50. [CrossRef] [PubMed]
90. Marlin, S.; Garabédian, E.N.; Roger, G.; Moatti, L.; Matha, N.; Lewin, P.; Petit, C.; Denoyelle, F. Connexin 26 gene mutations in congenitally deaf children: Pitfalls for genetic counseling. *Arch. Otolaryngol. Head Neck Surg.* **2001**, *127*, 927–933. [CrossRef] [PubMed]
91. Matos, T.D.; Caria, H.; Simões-Teixeira, H.; Aasen, T.; Dias, O.; Andrea, M.; Kelsell, D.P.; Fialho, G. A novel M163L mutation in connexin 26 causing cell death and associated with autosomal dominant hearing loss. *Hear. Res.* **2008**, *240*, 87–92. [CrossRef] [PubMed]
92. Samanich, J.; Lowes, C.; Burk, R.; Shanske, S.; Lu, J.; Shanske, A.; Morrow, B.E. Mutations in GJB2, GJB6, and mitochondrial DNA are rare in African American and Caribbean Hispanic individuals with hearing impairment. *Am. J. Med. Genet. A* **2007**, *143A*, 830–838. [CrossRef]
93. Frei, K.; Ramsebner, R.; Lucas, T.; Hamader, G.; Szuhai, K.; Weipoltshammer, K.; Baumgartner, W.-D.; Wachtler, F.J.; Kirschhofer, K. GJB2 mutations in hearing impairment: Identification of a broad clinical spectrum for improved genetic counseling. *Laryngoscope* **2005**, *115*, 461–465. [CrossRef]
94. Oliveira, C.A.; Maciel-Guerra, A.T.; Sartorato, E.L. Deafness resulting from mutations in the GJB2 (connexin 26) gene in Brazilian patients. *Clin. Genet.* **2002**, *61*, 354–358. [CrossRef] [PubMed]
95. Morell, R.J.; Kim, H.J.; Hood, L.J.; Goforth, L.; Friderici, K.; Fisher, R.; Van Camp, G.; Berlin, C.I.; Oddoux, C.; Ostrer, H.; et al. Mutations in the Connexin 26 Gene (GJB2) among Ashkenazi Jews with Nonsyndromic Recessive Deafness. *N. Engl. J. Med.* **1998**, *339*, 1500–1505. [CrossRef]
96. Dalamon, V.; Fiori, M.C.; Figueroa, V.A.; Oliva, C.A.; del Rio, R.; Gonzalez, W.; Canan, J.; Elgoyhen, A.B.; Altenberg, G.A.; Retamal, M.A. Gap-junctional channel and hemichannel activity of two recently identified connexin 26 mutants associated with deafness. *Pflügers Arch. Eur. J. Physiol.* **2016**, *468*, 909–918. [CrossRef]
97. Primignani, P.; Trotta, L.; Castorina, P.; Lalatta, F.; Sironi, F.; Radaelli, C.; Degiorgio, D.; Curcio, C.; Travi, M.; Ambrosetti, U.; et al. Analysis of the GJB2 and GJB6 Genes in Italian Patients with Nonsyndromic Hearing Loss: Frequencies, Novel Mutations, Genotypes, and Degree of Hearing Loss. *Genet. Test. Mol. Biomark.* **2009**, *13*, 209–217. [CrossRef]
98. Kudo, T. Transgenic expression of a dominant-negative connexin26 causes degeneration of the organ of Corti and non-syndromic deafness. *Hum. Mol. Genet.* **2003**, *12*, 995–1004. [CrossRef] [PubMed]

99. Marziano, N.K. Mutations in the gene for connexin 26 (GJB2) that cause hearing loss have a dominant negative effect on connexin 30. *Hum. Mol. Genet.* **2003**, *12*, 805–812. [CrossRef]
100. Piazza, V.; Beltramello, M.; Menniti, M.; Colao, E.; Malatesta, P.; Argento, R.; Chiarella, G.; Gallo, L.V.; Catalano, M.; Perrotti, N.; et al. Functional analysis of R75Q mutation in the gene coding for Connexin 26 identified in a family with nonsyndromic hearing loss. *Clin. Genet.* **2005**, *68*, 161–166. [CrossRef] [PubMed]
101. Neocleous, V.; Aspris, A.; Shahpenterian, V.; Nicolaou, V.; Panagi, C.; Ioannou, I.; Kyamides, Y.; Anastasiadou, V.; Phylactou, L.A. High Frequency of 35delG GJB2 Mutation and Absence of del(GJB6-D13S1830) in Greek Cypriot Patients with Nonsyndromic Hearing Loss. *Genet. Test.* **2006**, *10*, 285–289. [CrossRef] [PubMed]
102. Günther, B.; Steiner, A.; Nekahm-Heis, D.; Albegger, K.; Zorowka, P.; Utermann, G.; Janecke, A. The 342-kb deletion inGJB6is not present in patients with non-syndromic hearing loss from Austria. *Hum. Mutat.* **2003**, *22*, 180. [CrossRef]
103. Uyguner, O.; Emiroglu, M.; Uzumcu, A.; Hafiz, G.; Ghanbari, A.; Baserer, N.; Yuksel-Apak, M.; Wollnik, B. Frequencies of gap- and tight-junction mutations in Turkish families with autosomal-recessive non-syndromic hearing loss. *Clin. Genet.* **2003**, *64*, 65–69. [CrossRef]
104. Pandey, K.R.; Maden, N.; Poudel, B.; Pradhananga, S.; Sharma, A.K. The Curation of Genetic Variants: Difficulties and Possible Solutions. *Genom. Proteom. Bioinform.* **2012**, *10*, 317–325. [CrossRef]
105. Fokkema, I.F.A.C.; Ivo, F.A.; Velde, K.J.; Slofstra, M.K.; Ruivenkamp, C.A.L.; Vogel, M.J.; Pfundt, R.; Blok, M.J.; Lekanne Deprez, R.H.; Waisfisz, Q.; et al. Dutch genome diagnostic laboratories accelerated and improved variant interpretation and increased accuracy by sharing data. *Hum. Mutat.* **2019**, *40*, 2230–2238. [CrossRef]

Publisher's Note: MDPI stays neutral with regard to jurisdictional claims in published maps and institutional affiliations.

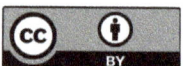

© 2020 by the authors. Licensee MDPI, Basel, Switzerland. This article is an open access article distributed under the terms and conditions of the Creative Commons Attribution (CC BY) license (http://creativecommons.org/licenses/by/4.0/).

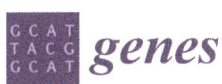

Article

High Rates of Three Common *GJB2* Mutations c.516G>C, c.-23+1G>A, c.235delC in Deaf Patients from Southern Siberia Are Due to the Founder Effect

Marina V. Zytsar [1], Marita S. Bady-Khoo [2], Valeriia Yu. Danilchenko [1], Ekaterina A. Maslova [1,3], Nikolay A. Barashkov [4,5], Igor V. Morozov [3,6], Alexander A. Bondar [6] and Olga L. Posukh [1,3,*]

[1] Federal Research Center Institute of Cytology and Genetics, Siberian Branch of the Russian Academy of Sciences, 630090 Novosibirsk, Russia; zytzar@bionet.nsc.ru (M.V.Z.); danilchenko_valeri@mail.ru (V.Y.D.); maslova@bionet.nsc.ru (E.A.M.)
[2] Perinatal Center of the Republic of Tyva, 667000 Kyzyl, Russia; marita.badyhoo@mail.ru
[3] Novosibirsk State University, 630090 Novosibirsk, Russia; Mor@niboch.nsc.ru
[4] Yakut Scientific Centre of Complex Medical Problems, 677019 Yakutsk, Russia; barashkov2004@mail.ru
[5] M.K. Ammosov North-Eastern Federal University, 677027 Yakutsk, Russia
[6] Institute of Chemical Biology and Fundamental Medicine, Siberian Branch of the Russian Academy of Sciences, 630090 Novosibirsk, Russia; alex.bondar@mail.ru
* Correspondence: posukh@bionet.nsc.ru

Received: 16 June 2020; Accepted: 17 July 2020; Published: 21 July 2020

Abstract: The mutations in the *GJB2* gene (13q12.11, MIM 121011) encoding transmembrane protein connexin 26 (Cx26) account for a significant portion of hereditary hearing loss worldwide. Earlier we found a high prevalence of recessive *GJB2* mutations c.516G>C, c.-23+1G>A, c.235delC in indigenous Turkic-speaking Siberian peoples (Tuvinians and Altaians) from the Tyva Republic and Altai Republic (Southern Siberia, Russia) and proposed the founder effect as a cause for their high rates in these populations. To reconstruct the haplotypes associated with each of these mutations, the genotyping of polymorphic genetic markers both within and flanking the *GJB2* gene was performed in 28 unrelated individuals homozygous for c.516G>C (n = 18), c.-23+1G>A (n = 6), or c.235delC (n = 4) as well as in the ethnically matched controls (62 Tuvinians and 55 Altaians) without these mutations. The common haplotypes specific for mutations c.516G>C, c.-23+1G>A, or c.235delC were revealed implying a single origin of each of these mutations. The age of mutations estimated by the DMLE+ v2.3 software and the single marker method is discussed in relation to ethnic history of Tuvinians and Altaians. The data obtained in this study support a crucial role of the founder effect in the high prevalence of *GJB2* mutations c.516G>C, c.-23+1G>A, c.235delC in indigenous populations of Southern Siberia.

Keywords: hearing loss; *GJB2*; founder effect; STR and SNP haplotypes; mutation age; Tuvinians; Altaians; Southern Siberia

1. Introduction

Mutations in the *GJB2* gene (gap junction protein, beta-2, 13q12.11, MIM 121011) encoding transmembrane protein connexin 26 (Cx26) lead to nonsyndromic autosomal recessive deafness 1A (DFNB1A, MIM 220290) which is the most common form of hereditary hearing loss in many populations [1]. High prevalence of the *GJB2*-associated deafness makes the *GJB2* gene testing essential for the establishment of genetic diagnosis of hearing loss.

Over 400 deafness-associated variations in *GJB2* have been reported in the Human Gene Mutation Database (http://www.hgmd.cf.ac.uk) [2]. Specific ethno-geographic prevalence patterns were found for many of them [3–5]. For instance, variant c.35delG (p.Gly12Valfs*2) is prevalent in deaf patients of Caucasian origin [3,6]; c.235delC (p.Leu79Cysfs*3) is common in some Asian populations [4,7–14];

c.167delT (p.Leu56Argfs*26) is frequent in Ashkenazi Jews [15,16]; c.427C>T (p.Arg143Trp) is specific for population of Ghana (West Africa) and Peru (South America) [17,18]; c.71G>A (p.Trp24*) is widely spread in Indians and European Gypsies [19–21]; c.109G>A (p.Val37Ile) prevails in populations of Southeast Asia [5]; the splice donor variant c.-23+1G>A was found in many populations worldwide but extremely high prevalence of c.-23+1G>A was detected among Yakuts (Eastern Siberia, Russia) [22]; c.131G>A (p.Trp44*) was found with high frequency among descendants of ancestral Mayan population in Guatemala [23].

High prevalence of some major *GJB2* mutations in certain populations was explained by the founder effect as evidenced by conservation of haplotypes with closely linked markers. In some cases, analysis of genetic background of these mutations allowed to elucidate their approximate age and a presumable region of origin. The key role of the founder effect in prevalence of mutation c.35delG was established in numerous studies by analysis of the c.35delG-bearing haplotypes: this mutation first appeared approximately 10000–14000 years ago in the Middle East and/or the Mediterranean and then spread by human migrations throughout Europe and worldwide [24–36]. The conservation of haplotype bearing mutation c.167delT found in Ashkenazi Jews suggests a single origin of this mutation which began to spread since a presumed Ashkenazi population bottleneck [15,16]. Haplotype analysis of genetic markers flanking the *GJB2* gene showed that a high rate of mutation c.71G>A (p.Trp24*) common for Indians is most probably due to the founder effect, and the age of this mutation was calculated as 7880 years [20]. Contribution of the founder effect in extremely high rate of mutation c.-23+1G>A among Yakuts (Eastern Siberia, Russia) was evidenced by the c.-23+1G>A haplotype analysis, and the age of this mutation was estimated at approximately 800 years [22]. Common haplotype was established for specific mutation c.131G>A (p.Trp44*) found in individuals from Guatemala suggesting a single founder from ancestral Mayan population [23]. The founder effect was also suggested in high prevalence of mutation c.235delC in East Asians (China, Japan, Korea), Mongolians (Mongolia), and Altaians (Southern Siberia, Russia) but there were only a few studies of the c.235delC-bearing haplotypes to support this hypothesis [8,9,14,37–39]. Additionally, Yan et al. (2003) proposed that c.235delC has probably derived from a founder mutation approximately 11500 years ago in the Lake Baikal region and spread to some Asian regions through subsequent migrations [38]. A haplotype block specific to East Asians with the c.109G>A (p.Val37Ile) mutation was found among deaf patients of Chinese, Japanese, Vietnamese, and Philippines ancestry and the age of p.Val37Ile in this Asian cohort was estimated at approximately 300 generations [40]. Shinagawa et al. (2020) confirmed the founder effect in origin of six *GJB2* mutations frequently observed in Japanese hearing loss patients (c.235delC, p.Val37Ile, p.[Gly45Glu;Tyr136*], p.Arg143Trp, c.176_191del, and c.299_300delAT) and estimated the year at which each mutation occurred: c.235delC—around 6500 years ago, p.[Gly45Glu;Tyr136*]—around 6000 years ago, p.Arg143Trp—around 6500 years ago, c.176_191del—around 4000 years ago, c.299_300delAT—around 7700 years ago, and p.Val37Ile - around 14500 or 5000 years ago [39].

In our recent study, we evaluated the spectrum and frequency of the *GJB2* gene variants in a large cohort of deaf Tuvinian patients and the ethnically matched controls from the Tyva Republic (Southern Siberia, Russia) [41]. A striking finding was a high prevalence of rare specific variant c.516G>C (p.Trp172Cys) in the *GJB2* gene accounting for 62.9% of all mutant *GJB2* alleles found in Tuvinian patients and having carrier frequency of 3.8% in controls. Other frequent *GJB2* mutations found in Tuvinian patients were c.-23+1G>A (27.6%) and c.235delC (5.2%). The c.235delC was previously found as a major *GJB2* mutation in Altaians living in the Altai Republic (Southern Siberia, Russia) neighboring the Tyva Republic [10]. In our recent study on enlarged cohort of Altaian deaf patients, the proportion of c.235delC, c.516G>C, and c.-23+1G>A among all mutant *GJB2* alleles found in Altaian patients was estimated as 51.9%, 29.6%, and 14.8%, respectively [42].

High rate of three *GJB2* mutations c.516G>C, c.-23+1G>A, and c.235delC in Tuvinians and Altaians implies a crucial role of the founder effect in their prevalence in indigenous populations of Southern Siberia. In this study we test a presumable common origin of each of these *GJB2* mutations by analysis of haplotypes bearing c.516G>C, c.-23+1G>A, and c.235delC.

2. Materials and Methods

2.1. Subjects

The pathogenic contribution of the *GJB2* mutations to deafness and their carrier frequencies were evaluated in our preliminary studies in indigenous populations of Southern Siberia (Tuvinians and Altaians) and three *GJB2* mutations (c.516G>C, c.-23+1G>A, c.235delC) were found to be common [10,41,42]. For the analysis of haplotypes bearing these mutations, we recruited in total 28 unrelated deaf patients who were homozygous for c.516G>C (seventeen Tuvinians and one Altaian), for c.-23+1G>A (six Tuvinians) or for c.235delC (four Altaians). The ethnically matched control samples were represented by 117 unrelated healthy individuals without mutations c.516G>C, c.-23+1G>A, and c.235delC (62 Tuvinians and 55 Altaians).

The study was conducted in accordance with the Declaration of Helsinki, and the protocol was approved by the Bioethics Commission at the Institute of Cytology and Genetics SB RAS, Novosibirsk, Russia (Protocol No. 9, 24 April 2012).

2.2. STRs and SNPs Genotyping

To determine common haplotypes for each of three major *GJB2* mutations c.516G>C, c.-23+1G>A, c.235delC, we performed genotyping of seven Short Tandem Repeats (D13S1316, D13S141, D13S175, D13S1853, D13S143, D13S1275, D13S292) flanking the *GJB2* gene and nine Single Nucleotide Polymorphisms (rs747931, rs5030700, rs3751385, rs2274083, rs2274084, rs1411911768, rs9552101, rs117685390, rs877098) intragenic and flanking the *GJB2* gene both in 28 unrelated deaf patients homozygous for c.516G>C, c.-23+1G>A, or c.235delC and in 117 unrelated healthy individuals (62 Tuvinians and 55 Altaians) who were negative for these mutations. The location of analyzed genetic markers on chromosome 13 is presented in Figure 1. Two additional SNPs (rs11147592, rs9509086) were genotyped in homozygous patients only. The total length of the region flanked by distal markers D13S1316 (centromeric) and D13S292 (telomeric) was approximately 3.5 Mb. All primers and genotyping methods are summarized in Supplementary Table S1. Fragment analysis and Sanger sequencing were performed in the SB RAS Genomics Core Facility (Institute of Chemical Biology and Fundamental Medicine SB RAS, Novosibirsk, Russia).

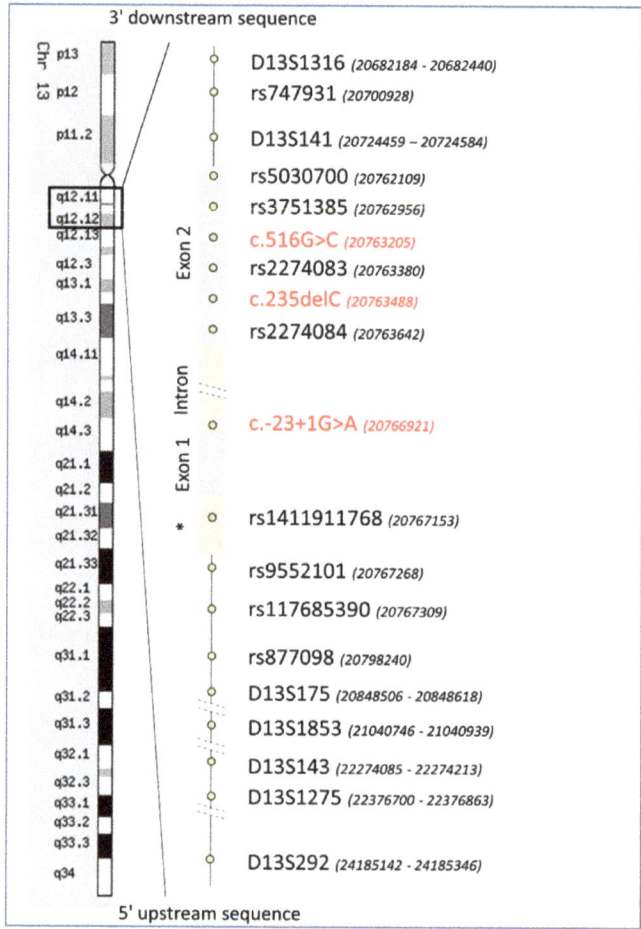

Figure 1. Schematic presentation of the *GJB2* gene structure and localization of genetic markers (seven STRs and nine SNPs) which were used for the reconstruction of haplotypes for *GJB2* mutations c.516G>C, c.-23+1G>A, and c.235delC. These mutations are marked by red color. *—basal (core) promoter (128 bp). Positions of genetic markers (shown in brackets) were defined according to GRCh37.p13 Genome Assembly (https://www.ncbi.nlm.nih.gov/assembly/GCA_000001405.14).

2.3. Reconstruction of STR and SNP Haplotypes

The reconstruction of the founder haplotypes from STRs and SNPs genotyping data and analysis of their frequencies were performed using Expectation–Maximization (EM) algorithm of the Arlequin 3.5.2.2 software [43]. The boundaries of haplotypes for each of three *GJB2* mutations were determined by observed linkage disequilibrium between the marker alleles and each mutation according to equation $\delta = (Pd-Pn)/(1-Pn)$, where δ is the measure of linkage disequilibrium, Pd is the marker allele frequency among mutant chromosomes, Pn is the frequency of the same allele among normal chromosomes [44].

2.4. Estimation of Mutations Age

Estimation of a mutation age is based on the expected decay of linkage disequilibrium between the mutation and alleles of surrounding genetic markers due to recombination ("genetic clock" concept).

We applied two approaches for estimating the age of mutations c.516G>C, c.-23+1G>A, and c.235delC. The first was the DMLE+ v2.3 software method (Disequilibrium Mapping using maximum-Likelihood Estimation, DMLE+: http://dmle.org/) [45] which is based on multiple linked marker loci and uses the Markov Chain Monte Carlo algorithm for Bayesian estimation of the mutation age. The second, used when appropriate, was the single marker method based on intra-allelic variation of a single marker [46]. For calculation the mutation age by the DMLE+ software, the demographic parameters (population size, population growth rate, and proportion of population sampled) are required in addition to the haplotype data and the map distances among marker loci and mutations. Since population growth rates for Tuvinian and Altaian populations could not be reliably estimated because of very limited knowledge of demographic variation of these populations along their history, we analyzed the haplotype data using several plausible growth rates: 0.05, 0.1, and 0.2. The parameter "proportion of population sampled" for each of three mutations (c.516G>C, c.-23+1G>A, c.235delC) was calculated on the basis of our previous data [10,41,42]. The contemporary population sizes for Tuvinians and Altaians according to the 2010 census were 249299 and 68814 peoples, respectively.

The estimation of the mutation age by the single marker method was performed using algorithm proposed by [46]:

$$g = \log[1 - Q/(1 - Pn)]/\log(1 - \Theta) \quad (1)$$

where g is the number of generations passed from the moment of the mutation appearance to the present; Q is the share of mutant chromosomes unlinked with the founder haplotype; Pn is the population frequency of allele included in the founder haplotype, and Θ is the recombinant fraction calculated from physical distance between marker and mutation (under the assumption that 1 cM = 1000 kb). To avoid possible underestimation of a mutation age as suggested by [47–49], we also applied the Luria-Delbrück correction [50] which takes into account the demographic parameters:

$$g_c = g + g_0 \quad (2)$$

$$g_0 = -(1/d) \ln(\Theta f_d) \quad (3)$$

where d is population growth rate, also assuming $f_d = e^d/(e^d - 1)$ and $f_d \approx 1/d$ at small d values [47].

The duration of one generation (g) was considered to be 25 years.

2.5. Statistical Analysis

Two-tailed Fisher's exact test with significance level of $p < 0.05$ was applied to compare allele frequencies between patients and controls.

3. Results

We assumed that the high prevalence of *GJB2* mutations c.516G>C (p.Trp172Cys), c.-23+1G>A, c.235delC in Tuvinians and Altaians is a consequence of the founder effect. To test whether all carriers of each of these mutations share a common haplotype, we performed genotyping of polymorphic genetic markers both intragenic and flanking *GJB2* gene (nine SNPs and seven STRs) in 28 unrelated individuals homozygous for c.516G>C (n = 18), c.-23+1G>A (n = 6), or c.235delC (n = 4) as well as in ethnically matched controls (62 Tuvinians and 55 Altaians). The choice of analyzed genetic markers was based on their physical location, their variability in Asian populations, and the availability of previously published data for other populations. Results of the STRs and the SNPs genotyping are summarized in Supplementary Table S2.

3.1. STR Haplotypes

Data on genotyping of seven STR markers (D13S1316, D13S141, D13S175, D13S1853, D13S143, D13S1275, D13S292) flanking the *GJB2* gene and encompassing approximately 3.5 Mb (Figure 1) were used to reconstruct STR haplotypes both in deaf patients homozygous for each *GJB2* mutations (c.516G>C, c.-23+1G>A or c.235delC) and in the ethnically matched controls. The boundaries of the shared STR haplotypes were determined by observed linkage disequilibrium between STR alleles and each mutation.

Three different haplotypes formed by specific alleles of five STRs (D13S1316, D13S141, D13S175, D13S1853, D13S143) with a length of approximately 1.6 Mb were found to be associated with mutation c.516G>C (Table 1) in Tuvinian patients and 39 STR haplotypes were reconstructed in Tuvinian control sample (data not shown). The 269-124-105-204-125 haplotype was the most common (67.9%) among mutant chromosomes bearing c.516G>C, while the frequency of this haplotype in normal chromosomes (1.6%) was significantly lower ($p < 10^{-14}$) (Table 1).

Table 1. The frequencies of common STR haplotypes found among the chromosomes bearing c.516G>C, c.-23+1G>A, c.235delC in comparison with the normal chromosomes.

Haplotypes *	Frequency of Haplotypes		x^2	p
	Mutant Chromosomes	Normal Chromosomes		
Haplotypes for c.516G>C: D13S1316-D13S141-D13S175-D13S1853-D13S143 (~ 1.6 Mb)				
269-124-105-204-125	0.6786	0.0161	79	$<10^{-14}$
267-124-105-204-125	0.2857	0.2979	0.0093	0.5462
269-124-105-204-129	0.0357	0	0.67	0.1842
other haplotypes	0	0.6860	-	-
Haplotypes for c.-23+1G>A: D13S141-D13S175-D13S1853-D13S143-D13S1275-D13S292 (~ 3.5 Mb)				
124-105-204-125-208-209	0.8333	0.0538	53	$<10^{-8}$
124-105-204-125-202-211	0.0833	0.0108	0.66	0.1695
124-105-204-125-210-209	0.0833	0.0472	0.011	0.4586
other haplotypes	0	0.8882	-	-
Haplotypes for c.235delC: D13S1316-D13S141-D13S175-D13S1853-D13S143-D13S1275 (~ 1.7 Mb)				
267-124-105-204-125-210	1.0	0	103	$<10^{-11}$
other haplotypes	0	1.0	-	-

* The most common haplotypes are shown in bold.

Significant linkage disequilibrium was found between mutation c.-23+1G>A and the specific alleles of six STRs (D13S141, D13S175, D13S1853, D13S143, D13S1275, D13S292) encompassing approximately 3.5 Mb long chromosome region. Three and sixty-eight STR haplotypes were reconstructed in Tuvinian patients homozygous for c.-23+1G>A (Table 1) and in Tuvinian controls (data not shown), respectively. Significant differences ($p < 10^{-8}$) were observed between frequency of the 124-105-204-125-208-209 haplotype predominantly found among all mutant chromosomes with c.-23+1G>A (83.3%) and its frequency among normal chromosomes in Tuvinian controls (5.4%) (Table 1).

The only haplotype found in all mutant chromosomes with c.235delC (Altaian patients) was 267-124-105-204-125-210 (D13S1316-D13S141-D13S175-D13S1853-D13S143-D13S1275) flanked by markers D13S1316 and D13S1275 (~ 1.7 Mb), whereas this haplotype was not detected on normal chromosomes in Altaian control sample ($p < 10^{-11}$) (Table 1).

3.2. SNP Haplotypes

To thoroughly analyze the structure of haplotypes associated with specific *GJB2* mutations, we have genotyped nine SNPs: four SNPs flanking *GJB2* gene (rs747931, rs9552101, rs117685390, rs877098) and five intragenic SNPs (rs5030700, rs3751385, rs2274083, rs2274084, rs1411911768) (Figure 1) in patients homozygous for c.516G>C, c.-23+1G>A, or c.235delC and in the ethnically matched controls.

Significant linkage disequilibrium was observed between each of three *GJB2* mutations and certain alleles of all analyzed SNPs.

The only haplotype T-C-C-A-G-T-G-T-C (rs747931-rs5030700-rs3751385-rs2274083-rs2274084-rs1411911768-rs9552101-rs117685390-rs877098) was found on all (100%) mutant chromosomes with c.516G>C in Tuvinian patients in contrast with normal chromosomes in Tuvinian controls where 24 different SNP haplotypes were reconstructed (data not shown) and frequency of haplotype T-C-C-A-G-T-G-T-C was estimated to be 2.17% ($p < 10^{-26}$) (Table 2).

Table 2. The frequencies of common SNP haplotypes found among the chromosomes bearing c.516G>C, c.-23+1G>A, c.235delC in comparison with the normal chromosomes.

Haplotypes *	Frequency of Haplotypes		x^2	p
	Mutant Chromosomes	Normal Chromosomes		
Haplotypes for c.516G>C:				
rs747931-rs5030700-rs3751385-rs2274083-rs2274084-rs1411911768-rs9552101-rs117685390-rs877098				
T-C-C-A-G-T-G-T-C	1	0.0217	120	$<10^{-26}$
other haplotypes	0	0.9783	-	-
Haplotypes for c.-23+1G>A:				
rs747931-rs5030700-rs3751385-rs2274083-rs2274084-rs1411911768-rs9552101-rs117685390-rs877098				
C-C-C-A-G-C-G-T-C	0.9167	0.0532	64	$<10^{-10}$
C-C-C-A-G-C-G-T-T	0.0833	0.1540	0.047	0.4488
other haplotypes	0	0.7928	-	-
Haplotypes for c.235delC:				
rs747931-rs5030700-rs3751385-rs2274083-rs2274084-rs1411911768-rs9552101-rs117685390-rs877098				
T-C-C-A-G-C-G-T-T	1	0.1587	26	1
other haplotypes	0	0.8413	-	-

* The most frequent haplotypes are shown in bold. The SNP alleles specific for the common SNP haplotypes are highlighted by frames.

Two SNP haplotypes were present in Tuvinian patients homozygous for c.-23+1G>A, while 26 different SNP haplotypes were reconstructed in the Tuvinian controls (data not shown). The C-C-C-A-G-C-G-T-C haplotype was predominant in Tuvinian patients (91.7%), while its frequency in the Tuvinian controls was 5.3% ($p < 10^{-10}$) (Table 2).

Only one SNP haplotype T-C-C-A-G-C-G-T-T was found in Altaian patients homozygous for c.235delC, while 22 different SNP haplotypes were identified in Altaian controls (data not shown). This haplotype was the second by frequency in the Altaian control sample and differences found between its frequency in Altaian patients (100%) and controls (15.9%) were insignificant (Table 2).

Comparative analysis of SNP haplotypes associated with each of three *GJB2* mutations (c.516G>C, c.-23+1G>A, or c.235delC) revealed three SNPs (rs747931, rs1411911768, and rs877098), whose allelic compositions clearly define the specificity of each of these haplotypes. Two of these SNPs, rs747931 and rs877098, are located distantly from the *GJB2* gene, while rs1411911768 is located in basal (core) promoter region (128 bp) of the *GJB2* gene (Figure 1). Allele T of rs1411911768 included in the common haplotype associated with c.516G>C in Tuvinian patients was present in all corresponding mutant chromosomes, while it was absent in common haplotypes for mutations c.-23+1G>A and c.235delC (Table 2). Allele C of rs747931 was detected in both c.-23+1G>A-associated haplotypes found in Tuvinian patients but it was absent in haplotypes associated with c.516G>C or c.235delC (Table 2). Variant T of rs877098 was only found in c.235delC haplotype in Altaian patients and in more rare c.-23+1G>A haplotype in Tuvinian patients, and it was absent in c.516G>C haplotype (Table 2).

Thus, the unique allelic combination of three SNPs (rs747931- // -rs1411911768- // -rs877098) was found for each of the three most frequent SNP haplotypes bearing *GJB2* mutations: T-T-C for c.516G>C, C-C-C—for c.-23+1G>A, and T-C-T—for c.235delC.

3.3. Age of Mutations c.516G>C, c.-23+1G>A, and c.235delC

The common haplotypes found for each of the mutations c.516G>C, c.-23+1G>A, or c.235delC prevailing in indigenous peoples of Southern Siberia imply that each of them had descended from a single ancestor. We estimated the numbers of generations (g) and years (in assumption that g = 25 years) passed from the common ancestral mutation event for each of these mutations assuming several population growth rates (0.05, 0.1, and 0.2) by the DMLE+ v2.3 program, which is sensitive to demographic parameters, and based on an analysis of multiple linked marker loci included in appropriate haplotype [45]. The single marker method for the estimation of the mutation age is based on the linkage disequilibrium and the recombination fraction observed for the alleles of surrounding genetic markers [46]. This approach implies analysis of alleles of the most distal markers which manifest significant linkage disequilibrium, while marker alleles with complete linkage disequilibrium (all disease chromosomes carried the same allele) are considered to be uninformative [51].

The DMLE+ program yielded the following estimations of the age of mutation c.516G>C: 91–180 generations (2275–4500 years) with d = 0.05, 57–106 generations (1425–2650 years) with d = 0.1 and 31–55 generations (775–1375 years) with d = 0.2 (Table 3). For c.516G>C age estimation by the single marker method we used allele (125) of the distal STR marker D13S143 found in high linkage disequilibrium with c.516G>C (Supplementary Table S2) that resulted in 27 generations passed from the origin of c.516G>C (675 years). After the Luria–Delbrück correction allowing to avoid possible underestimation of a mutation age due to demographic parameters [47–49], the age of c.516G>C increased at all population growth rates (d = 0.05, 0.1 or 0.2): 51 generations (1275 years), 46 generations (1150 years), 40 generations (1000 years), respectively.

Table 3. Summarized results of the c.516G>C, c.-23+1G>A, c.235delC dating by the DMLE+ program.

Mutation	d	g (95% CI)	Age (95% CI)
c.516G>C	0.05	91–180	2275–4500 years
	0.1	57–106	1425–2650 years
	0.2	31–55	775–1375 years
c.-23+1G>A	0.05	73–164	1825–4100 years
	0.1	42–91	1050–2275 years
	0.2	29–54	725–1350 years
c.235delC	0.05	45–126	1125–3150 years
	0.1	34–79	850–1975 years
	0.2	22–46	550–1150 years

d—population growth rate; g—the number of generations; the age of mutation was calculated as g × 25 years.

The DMLE+ estimations of the age of mutation c.-23+1G>A with different d (d = 0.05, 0.1, and 0.2) gave 73–164 generations (1825–4100 years), 42–91 generations (1050–2275 years), and 29–54 generations (725–1350 years), respectively (Table 3). When the age of c.-23+1G>A was estimated by the single marker method using allele (209) of the most distal marker D13S292 (more than 3.4 Mb from c.-23+1G>A), the age of c.-23+1G>A was drastically reduced to 4 generations (100 years) or 14–17 generations (350–425 years) after the Luria–Delbrück correction at various d (0.05, 0.1 and 0.2).

We were not able to estimate the age of c.235delC using the single marker method because of the lack of recombination in all markers included in STR and SNP haplotypes observed for c.235delC. Nevertheless, by using the DMLE+ program, the variations of the age of c.235delC were reasonably consistent, being 45–126 generations (1125–3150 years), 34–79 generations (850–1975 years), and 22–46 generations (550–1150 years) with d = 0.05, 0.1, and 0.2, respectively (Table 3).

4. Discussion

We found three *GJB2* mutations, c.516G>C, c.-23+1G>A, and c.235delC to be predominant in deaf Tuvinian and Altaian patients [10,41,42]. Tuvinians and Altaians are the indigenous Turkic-speaking populations of two neighboring federal subjects of the Russian Federation, the Tyva Republic (Tuva) and the Altai Republic, respectively, which are located in Southern Siberia. The Tyva Republic is bordered by Mongolia in the south and the east, whereas the Republic of Altai is bordered by Mongolia in the southeast, China in the south, and Kazakhstan in the southwest.

4.1. Ethnic History of Tuvinians and Altaians

Tuvinians (Tuvans) live mainly in the Tyva Republic in Russia (249299 people in total according to the 2010 census), though relatively small groups of Tuvinians also live in the northern part of Mongolia and in the Xinjiang Uygur Autonomous Region of China [52,53]. Tuvinians are one of the most ancient Turkic-speaking peoples inhabiting Central Asia and the Sayan-Altai region. The name "Tuva" probably originates from a Samoyedic tribe (referred to the VII century Chinese sources as "Dubo" or "Tupo") that populated the upper Yenisei river region. The location of Tuva in the geographical center of the Asian continent had a significant impact on the formation of its population because of the relations with residents of neighboring regions. At different times, Tuva was at the periphery of a powerful state of Huns (II century BC–I century AD) or was incorporated in the Ancient Turkic Khaganate (VI–VIII centuries), in the Uyghur Khaganate (VIII–IX centuries), in the Yenisei Kyrgyz Khaganate (IX–XII centuries), and also in the Mongol Empire (XIII–XIV centuries), which played an outstanding role in the history of the nomadic civilization and the ethno-political development of Central Asia and the Sayan-Altai region. These historical events had a certain impact on the consolidation of ancestral Tuvinian tribes and, ultimately, on their formation into a single ethnic group. At the end of the XIII–XIV centuries, the ethnic composition of Tuva population already included those groups that took part in the formation of the Tuvinian people: descendants of different Turkic-, Mongolic-, Ket-, and Samoyedic-speaking tribes [54,55].

The Altaians, indigenous inhabitants of the Altai Republic (68814 people in total according to the 2010 census), belong to two main ethnic groups originated from several ancient Turkic-speaking tribes: Southern Altaians (Altai-kizhi, Teleut, and Telengit) and Northern Altaians (Chelkan, Kumandin, and Tubalar) [56]. Southern Altaian language belongs to the Kipchak branch of Turkic language family whereas the Northern Altai languages are greater influenced by Samoyedic, Yeniseian, and Ugric languages. In the past, the Altai region, as well as Tuva, was conquered or influenced by powerful Turkic Khaganates as well as the Mongol Empire [56].

Thus, archaeological, linguistic, anthropological, and historical evidences indicate similarities in the ethnogenesis of Turkic-speaking Tuvinian and Altaians.

4.2. Common Haplotypes for c.516G>C, c.-23+1G>A, and c.235delC

High rate of the *GJB2* mutations (c.516G>C, c.-23+1G>A, and c.235delC) in Tuvinians and Altaians implies a crucial role of the founder effect in their prevalence. Analysis of the genetic markers (seven STRs and nine SNPs intragenic and flanking the *GJB2* gene) surrounding mutations c.516G>C, c.-23+1G>A, and c.235delC revealed common haplotypes for each mutation, spanning ~ 1.6 Mb, ~3.5 Mb, and ~ 1.7 Mb, respectively (Figure 2). Moreover, we found the unique allelic combinations of three SNPs (rs747931- // -rs1411911768- // -rs877098) that were highly specific for each of the most frequent haplotypes bearing *GJB2* mutations (T-T-C for c.516G>C, C-C-C for c.-23+1G>A, and T-C-T for c.235delC). These combinations were absent or sufficiently less common in the control samples that allows to use them as additional markers for identification of major *GJB2* mutations in indigenous populations of Siberia.

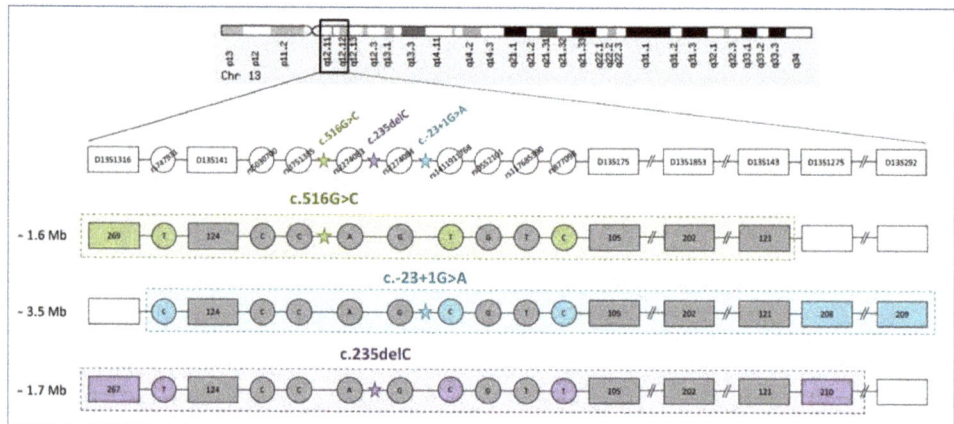

Figure 2. Schematic presentation of three common haplotypes bearing the *GJB2* mutations c.516G>C, c.-23+1G>A, or c.235delC. Locations of *GJB2* mutations and used genetic markers (seven STRs and nine SNPs) are shown at the top of the scheme. The STRs are indicated by rectangles, the SNPs - by circles. Founder haplotypes bearing mutations c.516G>C, c.-23+1G>A, c.235delC (spanning ~ 1.6 Mb, ~ 3.5 Mb, and ~ 1.7 Mb, respectively) are highlighted in dotted blocks. Identical alleles of genetic markers included in the haplotypes for each of *GJB2* mutations are shown in gray, while the alleles specific for corresponding mutations are indicated by different colors.

4.3. The c.516G>C Mutation

The *GJB2* variant c.516G>C (p.Trp172Cys, rs1302739538) accounts for 62.9% and 29.6% of all mutant *GJB2* alleles detected in deaf Tuvinian and Altaian patients, respectively, and the carrier frequencies of c.516G>C are 3.8% and 0.5% in the corresponding ethnically matched controls [41,42]. The c.516G>C substitution leads to a replacement of an aromatic non-polar tryptophan with a small polar cysteine at conservative amino acid position 172 (p.Trp172Cys) in the second extracellular loop of protein connexin 26 (Cx26). The c.516G>C meets the main criteria to be classified as pathogenic for autosomal recessive hearing loss based on the ACMG/AMP criteria [57] as specified by the Hearing Loss Expert Panel [58]. In our recent study [41], we suggested that this very rare *GJB2* mutation is endemic for Tuvinians living in the Republic of Tuva, since besides them c.516G>C was only found in Altaians from neighboring the Altai Republic (with less frequency) and in one deaf patient from Mongolia [59], and nowhere else in the world.

In this study, we obtained convincing evidence supporting the origin of mutation c.516G>C from a single ancestor. The common STR haplotype spanning about 1.6 Mb as well as the common internal SNP haplotype were identified in most of *GJB2* alleles carrying c.516G>C, and their frequencies in patients homozygous for c.516G>C were significantly different from controls. Interesting finding was a strong (100%) association of c.516G>C mutation with very rare allele T (A) of intragenic rs1411911768 (dbSNP: MAF A = 0.00002/3 TOPMED), which was found in Tuvinian and Altaian controls with sufficiently lower frequency (0.0565 and 0.0182, respectively) (Supplementary Table S2). We speculate that c.516G>C mutation could initially have arisen on the chromosome bearing rare allele of rs1411911768 in ancestors of these indigenous peoples (rather in Tuvinians, among whom c.516G>C is more prevalent) and reached current high prevalence as a result of the founder effect. The age of c.516G>C based on the single marker method was estimated to be 675 years or 1000–1275 years after the Luria–Delbrück correction, whereas the dating of this event by the DMLE+ program led to wide time ranges (2275–4500, 1425–2650, or 775–1375 years ago) with different population growth rates (d = 0.05, 0.1, or 0.2, respectively). We tend to think that c.516G>C is rather a relatively "young" mutation since a fast population growth was probably intrinsic to Tuvinians in the past because of a traditionally large family size observed in contemporary Tuvinians. In addition, the prevalence of this mutation is very restricted. The most plausible scenario suggests that c.516G>C has arisen in the territory of Tuva as the result of a unique event after main formation of the Tuvinian ethnic group (which took place at the end of the XIII–XIV centuries) and then spread into the neighboring territory of Altai. Taking into account the complexity of ethnic history of Tuvinians, it remains unclear, who actually were the c.516G>C founders—different ancient Turkic- or Mongolic-speaking groups or other aboriginal peoples who lived there. The introduction of c.516G>C into Tuva territory with migration flows of ancient Mongolic-speaking groups is not consistent with the finding of c.516G>C in only one deaf patient from Mongolia [14,59] as well as with its absence in Mongolian patients living in China [60,61]. It is known that several nomadic Tuvinian groups roamed in the past across the territories of Tuva and Mongolia had remained in Mongolia when Tuva was separated from Mongolia to become under Russian protectorate after the breakup of the Qing Empire in 1911–1912 [54,55]. Since the ethnicity of examined deaf patients was not reported in the study by Tekin et al. [59], the question about the origin of c.516G>C in Mongolia remains open.

4.4. The c.-23+1G>A Mutation

The proportion of the splice donor site mutation c.-23+1G>A reaches 27.6% of all mutant *GJB2* alleles in Tuvinian deaf patients [41] and 14.8% in Altaian patients [42]. Splice donor site *GJB2* variant c.-23+1G>A has been detected among deaf patients of different origin around the world [14,22,59,62–67]. The extremely high prevalence of c.-23+1G>A (up to 92.2% of all mutant *GJB2* alleles found in patients and carrier frequency reaching of 10.2%) observed in Yakuts, indigenous Turkic-speaking people living in the subarctic region of Russia (the Sakha Republic, Eastern Siberia), was explained by the founder effect in an isolated population and a probable selective advantage for the c.-23+1G>A heterozygotes in severe subarctic climate [22,67,68]. The c.-23+1G>A is also the most common mutation in deaf Mongolian patients from Mongolia [14,59].

To our knowledge, the haplotypes bearing c.-23+1G>A were analyzed only in a few studies [14,22,59,69]. Tekin et al. (2010) suggested diverse origins of c.-23+1G>A based on multiple c.-23+1G>A-associated haplotypes found in comparative analysis of seven Mongolian and three Anatolian Turkish c.-23+1G>A homozygous patients [59]. However, despite the fact that several different haplotypes were found to be associated with c.-23+1G>A in Mongolians, a single conserved haplotype (which appears to be a common haplotype in Mongolia) was identified in Turkish homozygous patients suggesting a single common ancestor with an intervening population bottleneck in the Turkish branch [59]. Barashkov et al. (2011) revealed the common origin of c.-23+1G>A in Yakuts (Eastern Siberia) by the reconstruction of 140 haplotypes bearing this mutation using eight polymorphic microsatellite markers flanking the *GJB2* gene and two intragenic SNP markers [22]. These findings are consistent with the founder effect hypothesis and support a common Central Asian origin of c.-23+1G>A since the Turkic-speaking ancestors of Yakuts migrated to the Eastern part of Siberia from their initial settlement in the Baikal Lake area under pressure of the Mongol expansion in XI - XIII centuries AD [70]. Solovyev et al. (2017) analyzed the c.-23+1G>A haplotypes in the sample of Yakut, Evenk, Russian, and Tuvinian deaf patients homozygous for c.-23+1G>A by using the same panel of SNPs (rs2313477, rs11841024, rs4769974, rs7994748, rs7987144, rs5030702, and rs1932429) as reported in the study by Tekin et al. [59] and revealed the reduced c.-23+1G>A haplotype diversity in the analyzed sample when compared with the haplotypes in Mongolians [69]. Interesting, that almost all examined patients (except one Yakut patient) in this study were homozygous for the allele T of intronic rs7994748 (*GJB2*) that is consistent with the studies by Grillo et al. (2015) and by Parzefall et al. (2017) in which the association of this rs7994748 allele with hearing loss was presumed [71,72]. In the study by Erdenechuluun et al. (2018) where five SNPs (rs747931, rs3751385, rs11147592, rs9509086, and rs9552102) were used for the c.-23+1G>A haplotype analysis in six Mongolian deaf patients, two c.-23+1G>A haplotypes were identified: major haplotype G-G-C-T-A (9/12 chromosomes) and a minor haplotype A-G-C-T-A (3/12 chromosomes) [14].

Our data on the common STR and SNP haplotypes for c.-23+1G>A found in Tuvinians evidence a single origin of this mutation and suggest the founder effect in its high prevalence in the Tyva Republic and neighboring territory of the Altai Republic. Based on the ethnic history of Tuvinians who experienced repeated influence of Mongolians at various stages of their ethnic formation [54,55], we speculate that c.-23+1G>A mutation can be introduced into Tuva by ancient Mongolic-speaking groups which were subsequently assimilated by the indigenous population of this region and then spread in Siberia by the migration flows. Our estimation of the c.-23+1G>A age yielded a wide range of 725–4100 years ago. This uncertainty could be probably attributed to a small size of the examined sample and an unclear population growth rate of Tuvinians in the past. Nevertheless, this estimation is consistent with previously reported age of c.-23+1G>A in the Sakha Republic (Yakutia) presumably introduced by Turkic-speaking ancestors of Yakuts approximately 800 years ago [22] further confirmed by the observed similarity of allelic composition of the common STR haplotypes in Tuvinian and Yakut patients homozygous for c.-23+1G>A (data not shown). Thus, our data support a proposed common Central Asian origin of mutation c.-23+1G>A and its further expansion defined by a specific population bottleneck at least throughout Siberia though further extensive studies in many populations are required to clarify this issue.

4.5. The c.235delC Mutation

High prevalence of c.235delC mutation was found in our previous study in the Altai Republic [10] and was later confirmed in an extended cohort of Altaian deaf patients since alleles with c.235delC accounted for 51.9% of all mutant *GJB2* alleles found in patients and the carrier frequency of c.235delC reached 3.7% in Altaian population sample [42].

According to numerous studies, c.235delC mutation prevails in patients with hearing loss in Asian populations (China, Japan, Mongolia, Korea) [4,7–9,11,12,14,37,59,62]. The founder effect, implying the origin of c.235delC from a common ancestor, was suggested for the explanation of high prevalence of c.235delC in Asia. Several studies focusing on the analysis of the haplotypes bearing c.235delC confirmed this hypothesis despite the certain differences between the sets of used genetic markers [8,9,14,37–39]. Based on the STR and SNP analysis, we found only one haplotype associated with c.235delC in Altaian homozygous patients. It is worth noting that some SNPs included in c.235delC-associated haplotype in Altaians overlap with the SNP markers analyzed in other studies and alleles observed coincide with the ones found in Asian patients having c.235delC [9,14,37–39]. We suggest that these findings are in favor of a common c.235delC-associated haplotype at least among Altaians, Mongolians, Chinese, and Japanese and accordingly, in favor of the origin of c.235delC from one ancestor. Additional studies using a unified panel of markers are needed to clarify the question.

As for the age of c.235delC, as far as we know, this issue was elucidated in only two studies [38,39]. In the study by Yan et al. seven SNPs flanking this mutation were analyzed in deaf patients (in a total of 26 homozygotes and 19 heterozygotes for c.235delC) from various regions of Asia (China, Japan, Korea, Mongolia) and association of c.235delC with one core haplotype A-G-A-C (SNP2-V27I-E114G-SNP1), with a length of approximately 2.6 kb, was discovered [38]. The allele T of the most distant marker SNP6 (rs747931) located at ~ 63 kb from c.235delC was used to evaluate the mutation age resulting in 460 generations or approximately 11500 years (assuming 25 years per generation). Yan et al. speculated that c.235delC might have arisen in the Baikal area and then spread to Mongolia, China, Korea, and Japan through subsequent migration [38]. In recent study by Shinagawa et al. the c.235delC-associated haplotypes were analyzed in total of 20 Japanese patients homozygous for c.235delC [39]. Based on observed linkage disequilibrium for 5'SNP6 (rs4769920) located at ~ 265 kb from c.235delC, the occurrence of c.235delC mutation was estimated around 6500 years ago [39]. Notably, the single marker method was applied for c.235delC age estimation in both studies [38,39], while we could not estimate the age of c.235delC by this method due to the lack of recombination in c.235delC haplotype in Altaian patients. Our estimation by the DMLE+ led to the lower values of the age of c.235delC (22–126 generations or 550–3150 years at the different population growth rates). Although we do not exclude that c.235delC is really "younger" in Altaians in comparison with the data from these studies [38,39], these differences are more likely due to different methods of the age estimation, the panels of used genetic markers, the sample sizes, as well as uncertainty in growth rates of Altaian population along their history. Additionally, our data are based on the limited population of Southern Siberia (Altaians) whereas, for example, in the study by Yan et al. (2003) the samples from various countries (Mongolia, China, Japan, and Korea) were analyzed.

5. Conclusions

The common haplotypes specific for *GJB2* mutations c.516G>C, c.-23+1G>A, and c.235delC imply a single origin for each of them. A crucial role of the founder effect in high prevalence of these mutations in indigenous populations of Southern Siberia was established.

Supplementary Materials: The following are available online at http://www.mdpi.com/2073-4425/11/7/833/s1, Table S1: Primer sequences and methods for STRs and SNPs genotyping. Table S2: The allelic frequencies of STRs (D13S1316, D13S141, D13S175, D13S1853, D13S143, D13S1275, D13S292) and SNPs (rs747931, rs5030700, rs3751385, rs2274083, rs2274084, rs1411911768, rs9552101, rs117685390, rs877098) in deaf patients homozygous for mutations c.516G>C, c.-23+1G>A or c.235delC and in the control samples (Tuvinians and Altaians).

Author Contributions: Conceptualization, O.L.P.; methodology, M.V.Z., O.L.P, I.V.M., A.A.B.; formal analysis, M.V.Z., V.Y.D., E.A.M., M.S.B.-K., I.V.M., A.A.B.; investigation, M.V.Z., V.Y.D., E.A.M., M.S.B.-K., I.V.M., A.A.B.; resources, O.L.P. and M.S.B.-K.; data curation, O.L.P. and M.S.B.-K.; writing—original draft preparation, M.V.Z., O.L.P., V.Y.D., E.A.M.; writing—review and editing, M.V.Z., O.L.P., V.Y.D., E.A.M., N.A.B., M.S.B.-K.; I.V.M., A.A.B.; supervision, O.L.P.; funding acquisition, O.L.P., M.V.Z., N.A.B. All authors have read and agreed to the published version of the manuscript.

Funding: This work was supported by the Budget Projects of Institute of Cytology and Genetics SB RAS: #0324-2019-0041 (to O.L.P.), #0259-2019-0009 (to M.V.Z. and V.Y.D.); by the Project of the Ministry of Science and Higher Education of the Russian Federation (basic part of funding to M.K. Ammosov North-Eastern Federal University #FSRG-2020-0016) (to N.A.B.); by the RFBR grants: #17-29-06016_ofi_m (to O.L.P, M.V.Z., M.S.B.-K., V.Y.D., E.A.M., N.A.B., A.A.B., I.V.M), #18-34-00166_mol-a (to M.V.Z., V.Y.D., E.A.M.), and #18-05-600035_Arctika, #18-015-00212_A, #20-015-00328_A (to N.A.B.).

Acknowledgments: The authors are sincerely grateful to all participants of the study. We also wish to acknowledge Vladimir Babenko for his help in the data analysis.

Conflicts of Interest: The authors declare no conflict of interest.

References

1. Del Castillo, F.J.; del Castillo, I. DFNB1 non-syndromic hearing impairment: Diversity of mutations and associated phenotypes. *Front. Mol. Neurosci.* **2017**, *10*, 428. [CrossRef]
2. Stenson, P.D.; Mort, M.; Ball, E.V.; Evans, K.; Hayden, M.; Heywood, S.; Hussain, M.; Phillips, A.D.; Cooper, D.N. The human gene mutation database: Towards a comprehensive repository of inherited mutation data for medical research, genetic diagnosis and next-generation sequencing studies. *Qual. Life Res.* **2017**, *136*, 665–677. [CrossRef]
3. Mahdieh, N.; Rabbani, B. Statistical study of 35delG mutation of *GJB2* gene: A meta-analysis of carrier frequency. *Int. J. Audiol.* **2009**, *48*, 363–370. [CrossRef]
4. Yao, J.; Lu, Y.; Wei, Q.; Cao, X.; Xing, G. A systematic review and meta-analysis of 235delC mutation of GJB2 gene. *J. Transl. Med.* **2012**, *10*, 136. [CrossRef]
5. Chan, D.K.; Chang, K.W. *GJB2*-associated hearing loss: Systematic review of worldwide prevalence, genotype, and auditory phenotype: Systematic review of Cx-26-associated hearing loss. *Laryngoscope* **2014**, *124*, E34–E53. [CrossRef]
6. Gasparini, P.; Rabionet, R.; Barbujani, G.; Melchionda, S.; Petersen, M.; Brøndum-Nielsen, K.; Metspalu, A.; Oitmaa, E.; Pisano, M.; Fortina, M.; et al. High carrier frequency of the 35delG deafness mutation in European populations. *Eur. J. Hum. Genet.* **2000**, *8*, 19–23. [CrossRef] [PubMed]
7. Park, H.-J.; Hahn, S.H.; Chun, Y.-M.; Park, K.; Kim, H.-N. Connexin26 mutations associated with nonsyndromic hearing loss. *Laryngoscope* **2000**, *110*, 1535–1538. [CrossRef] [PubMed]

8. Liu, X.; Xia, X.; Ke, X.; Ouyang, X.; Du, L.; Liu, Y.; Angeli, S.; Telischi, F.F.; Nance, W.E.; Balkany, T.; et al. The prevalence of connexin 26 (*GJB2*) mutations in the Chinese population. *Qual. Life Res.* **2002**, *111*, 394–397. [CrossRef] [PubMed]
9. Ohtsuka, A.; Yuge, I.; Kimura, S.; Namba, A.; Abe, S.; Van Laer, L.; Van Camp, G.; Usami, S. GJB2 deafness gene shows a specific spectrum of mutations in Japan, including a frequent founder mutation. *Qual. Life Res.* **2003**, *112*, 329–333. [CrossRef] [PubMed]
10. Posukh, O.L.; Pallares-Ruiz, N.; Tadinova, V.; Osipova, L.P.; Claustres, M.; Roux, A.-F. First molecular screening of deafness in the Altai Republic population. *BMC Med. Genet.* **2005**, *6*, 12. [CrossRef]
11. Dai, P.; Yu, F.; Han, M.; Liu, X.Z.; Wang, G.; Li, Q.; Yuan, Y.; Liu, X.; Huang, D.; Kang, D.; et al. GJB2 mutation spectrum in 2063 Chinese patients with nonsyndromic hearing impairment. *J. Transl. Med.* **2009**, *7*, 26. [CrossRef]
12. Kim, S.Y.; Kim, A.R.; Han, K.H.; Kim, M.Y.; Jeon, E.-H.; Koo, J.-W.; Oh, S.H.; Choi, B.Y. Residual hearing in dfnb1 deafness and its clinical implication in a Korean population. *PLoS ONE* **2015**, *10*, e0125416. [CrossRef] [PubMed]
13. Tsukada, K.; Nishio, S.Y.; Hattori, M.; Usami, S. Ethnic-specific spectrum of *GJB2* and *SLC26A4* mutations: Their origin and a literature review. *Ann. Otol. Rhinol. Laryngol.* **2015**, *124* (Suppl. 1), 61S–76S. [CrossRef]
14. Erdenechuluun, J.; Lin, Y.-H.; Ganbat, K.; Bataakhuu, D.; Makhbal, Z.; Tsai, C.-Y.; Lin, Y.-H.; Chan, Y.-H.; Hsu, C.-J.; Hsu, W.-C.; et al. Unique spectra of deafness-associated mutations in Mongolians provide insights into the genetic relationships among Eurasian populations. *PLoS ONE* **2018**, *13*, e0209797. [CrossRef]
15. Morell, R.; Kim, H.J.; Hood, L.J.; Goforth, L.; Friderici, K.; Fisher, R.; Van Camp, G.; Berlin, C.I.; Oddoux, C.; Ostrer, H.; et al. Mutations in the connexin 26 Gene (*GJB2*) among Ashkenazi Jews with nonsyndromic recessive deafness. *New. Engl. J. Med.* **1998**, *339*, 1500–1505. [CrossRef] [PubMed]
16. Sobe, T.; Erlich, P.; Berry, A.; Korostichevsky, M.; Vreugde, S.; Avraham, K.B.; Bonné-Tamir, B.; Shohat, M. High frequency of the deafness-associated 167delT mutation in the connexin 26 (*GJB2*) gene in Israeli Ashkenazim. *Am. J. Med. Genet.* **1999**, *86*, 499–500. [CrossRef]
17. Hamelmann, C.; Amedofu, G.K.; Albrecht, K.; Muntau, B.; Gelhaus, A.; Brobby, G.W.; Horstmann, R.D. Pattern of connexin 26 (*GJB2*) mutations causing sensorineural hearing impairment in Ghana. *Hum. Mutat.* **2001**, *18*, 84–85. [CrossRef] [PubMed]
18. Figueroa-Ildefonso, E.; Bademci, G.; Rajabli, F.; Cornejo-Olivas, M.; Villanueva, R.D.C.; Badillo-Carrillo, R.; Inca-Martinez, M.; Neyra, K.M.; Sineni, C.; Tekin, M.; et al. Identification of main genetic causes responsible for non-syndromic hearing loss in a Peruvian population. *Genes* **2019**, *10*, 581. [CrossRef] [PubMed]
19. Minárik, G.; Ferák, V.; Feráková, E.; Ficek, A.; Poláková, H.; Kadasi, L. High frequency of *GJB2* mutation W24X among Slovak Romany (Gypsy) patients with non-syndromic hearing loss (NSHL). *Gen. Physiol. Biophys.* **2003**, *22*, 549–556.
20. Ramshankar, M.; Girirajan, S.; Dagan, O.; Ravi, S.; Jalvi, R.; Rangasayee, R.; Avraham, K.B.; Anand, A. Contribution of connexin26 (*GJB2*) mutations and founder effect to non-syndromic hearing loss in India. *J. Med. Genet.* **2003**, *40*, e68. [CrossRef]
21. Álvarez, A.; Del Castillo, I.; Villamar, M.; Aguirre, L.A.; Gonzalez-Neira, A.; López-Nevot, A.; Moreno-Pelayo, M.A.; Moreno, F. High prevalence of theW24X mutation in the gene encoding connexin-26 (*GJB2*) in Spanish Romani (gypsies) with autosomal recessive non-syndromic hearing loss. *Am. J. Med. Genet. Part. A* **2005**, *137*, 255–258. [CrossRef] [PubMed]
22. Barashkov, N.A.; Dzhemilev, U.M.; Fedorova, S.A.; Teryutin, F.M.; Posukh, O.L.; Fedotova, E.E.; Lobov, S.; Khusnutdinova, E. Autosomal recessive deafness 1A (*DFNB1A*) in Yakut population isolate in Eastern Siberia: Extensive accumulation of the splice site mutation IVS1+1G>A in *GJB2* gene as a result of founder effect. *J. Hum. Genet.* **2011**, *56*, 631–639. [CrossRef] [PubMed]
23. Carranza, C.; Menendez, I.; Herrera, M.; Castellanos, P.; Amado, C.; Maldonado, F.; Rosales, L.; Escobar, N.; Guerra, M.; Alvarez, D.; et al. A Mayan founder mutation is a common cause of deafness in Guatemala. *Clin. Genet.* **2015**, *89*, 461–465. [CrossRef] [PubMed]
24. Van Laer, L.; Coucke, P.; Mueller, R.F.; Caethoven, G.; Flothmann, K.; Prasad, S.D.; Chamberlin, G.P.; Houseman, M.; Taylor, G.R.; van De Heyning, C.; et al. A common founder for the 35delG *GJB2* gene mutation in connexin 26 hearing impairment. *J. Med. Genet.* **2001**, *38*, 515–518. [CrossRef]

25. Tekin, M.; Akar, N.; Cin, Ş.; Blanton, S.; Xia, X.; Liu, X.; Nance, W.; Pandya, A. Connexin 26 (*GJB2*) mutations in the Turkish population: Implications for the origin and high frequency of the 35delG mutation in Caucasians. *Qual. Life Res.* **2001**, *108*, 385–389. [CrossRef]
26. Shahin, H.; Walsh, T.; Sobe, T.; Lynch, E.; King, M.-C.; Avraham, K.B.; Kanaan, M. Genetics of congenital deafness in the Palestinian population: Multiple connexin 26 alleles with shared origins in the Middle East. *Qual. Life Res.* **2002**, *110*, 284–289. [CrossRef]
27. Rothrock, C.R.; Murgia, A.; Sartorato, E.L.; Leonardi, E.; Wei, S.; Lebeis, S.L.; Yu, L.E.; Elfenbein, J.L.; Fisher, R.A.; Friderici, K.H. Connexin 26 35delG does not represent a mutational hotspot. *Qual. Life Res.* **2003**, *113*, 18–23. [CrossRef]
28. Balci, B.; Gerçeker, F.O.; Aksoy, S.; Sennaroğlu, G.; Kalay, E.; Sennaroğlu, L.; Dinçer, P. Identification of an ancestral haplotype of the 35delG mutation in the *GJB2* (connexin 26) gene responsible for autosomal recessive non-syndromic hearing loss in families from the Eastern Black Sea Region in Turkey. *Turk. J. Pediatr.* **2005**, *47*, 213–221.
29. Belguith, H.; Hajji, S.; Salem, N.; Charfeddine, I.; Lahmar, I.; Amor, M.B.; Ouldim, K.; Chouery, E.; Driss, N.; Drira, M.; et al. Analysis of *GJB2* mutation: Evidence for a Mediterranean ancestor for the 35delG mutation. *Clin. Genet.* **2005**, *68*, 188–189. [CrossRef]
30. Tekin, M.; Boğoçlu, G.; Arican, S.; Orman, M.; Tastan, H.; Elsayed, S.; Akar, N. Evidence for single origins of 35delG and delE120 mutations in the *GJB2* gene in Anatolia. *Clin. Genet.* **2004**, *67*, 31–37. [CrossRef]
31. Abidi, O.; Boulouiz, R.; Nahili, H.; Imken, L.; Rouba, H.; Chafik, A.; Barakat, A. The analysis of three markers flanking *GJB2* gene suggests a single origin of the most common 35delG mutation in the Moroccan population. *Biochem. Biophys. Res. Commun.* **2008**, *377*, 971–974. [CrossRef]
32. Kokotas, H.; Van Laer, L.; Grigoriadou, M.; Iliadou, V.; Economides, J.; Pomoni, S.; Pampanos, A.; Eleftheriades, N.; Ferekidou, E.; Korres, S.; et al. Strong linkage disequilibrium for the frequent *GJB2* 35delG mutation in the Greek population. *Am. J. Med. Genet. Part A* **2008**, *146*, 2879–2884. [CrossRef] [PubMed]
33. Kokotas, H.; Grigoriadou, M.; Villamar, M.; Giannoulia-Karantana, A.; Del Castillo, I.; Petersen, M.B. Hypothesizing an ancient greek origin of the *GJB2* 35delG Mutation: Can science meet history? *Genet. Test. Mol. Biomark.* **2010**, *14*, 183–187. [CrossRef] [PubMed]
34. Dzhemileva, L.U.; Posukh, O.L.; Barashkov, N.A.; Fedorova, S.A.; Teryutin, F.M.; Akhmetova, V.L.; Khidiyatova, I.M.; Khusainova, R.I.; Lobov, S.L.; Khusnutdinova, E.K. Haplotype diversity and reconstruction of ancestral haplotype associated with the c.35delG Mutation in the *GJB2* (Cx26) gene among the Volgo-Ural populations of Russia. *Acta Naturae* **2011**, *3*, 52–63. [CrossRef]
35. Norouzi, V.; Azizi, H.; Fattahi, Z.; Esteghamat, F.; Bazazzadegan, N.; Nishimura, C.; Nikzat, N.; Jalalvand, K.; Kahrizi, K.; Smith, R.J.H.; et al. Did the *GJB2* 35delG mutation originate in Iran? *Am. J. Med. Genet. Part A* **2011**, *155*, 2453–2458. [CrossRef] [PubMed]
36. Zytsar, M.V.; Barashkov, N.A.; Bady-Khoo, M.S.; Shubina-Olejnik, O.A.; Danilenko, N.G.; Bondar, A.A.; Morozov, I.V.; Solovyev, A.; Danilchenko, V.Y.; Maximov, V.N.; et al. Updated carrier rates for c.35delG (*GJB2*) associated with hearing loss in Russia and common c.35delG haplotypes in Siberia. *BMC Med. Genet.* **2018**, *19*, 138. [CrossRef]
37. Kudo, T.; Ikeda, K.; Kure, S.; Matsubara, Y.; Oshima, T.; Watanabe, K.-I.; Kawase, T.; Narisawa, K.; Takasaka, T. Novel mutations in the connexin 26 gene (*GJB2*) responsible for childhood deafness in the Japanese population. *Am. J. Med. Genet.* **2000**, *90*, 141–145. [CrossRef]
38. Yan, D.; Park, H.-J.; Ouyang, X.M.; Pandya, A.; Doi, K.; Erdenetungalag, R.; Du, L.L.; Matsushiro, N.; Nance, W.E.; Griffith, A.J.; et al. Evidence of a founder effect for the 235delC mutation of *GJB2* (connexin 26) in east Asians. *Qual. Life Res.* **2003**, *114*, 44–50. [CrossRef]
39. Shinagawa, J.; Moteki, H.; Nishio, S.-Y.; Noguchi, Y.; Usami, S.-I. Haplotype analysis of *GJB2* mutations: Founder effect or mutational hot spot? *Genes* **2020**, *11*, 250. [CrossRef]
40. Gallant, E.; Francey, L.J.; Tsai, E.A.; Berman, M.; Zhao, Y.; Fetting, H.; Kaur, M.; Deardorff, M.A.; Wilkens, A.; Clark, D.; et al. Homozygosity for the V37I *GJB2* mutation in fifteen probands with mild to moderate sensorineural hearing impairment: Further confirmation of pathogenicity and haplotype analysis in asian populations. *Am. J. Med. Genet. Part A* **2013**, *161*, 2148–2157. [CrossRef]

41. Posukh, O.L.; Zytsar, M.V.; Bady-Khoo, M.S.; Danilchenko, V.Y.; Maslova, E.A.; Barashkov, N.A.; Bondar, A.A.; Morozov, I.V.; Maximov, V.N.; Voevoda, M.I. Unique mutational spectrum of the *GJB2* Gene and its pathogenic contribution to deafness in Tuvinians (Southern Siberia, Russia): A high prevalence of rare variant c.516G>C (p.Trp172Cys). *Genes* **2019**, *10*, 429. [CrossRef] [PubMed]
42. Posukh, O.L.; Institute of Cytology and Genetics, Novosibirsk, Russia. Personal communication, 2019.
43. Excoffier, L.; Lischer, H.E.L. Arlequin suite ver 3.5: A new series of programs to perform population genetics analyses under Linux and Windows. *Mol. Ecol. Resour.* **2010**, *10*, 564–567. [CrossRef] [PubMed]
44. Bengtsson, B.O.; Thomson, G. Measuring the strength of associations between HLA antigens and diseases. *Tissue Antigens* **1981**, *18*, 356–363. [CrossRef]
45. Reeve, J.P.; Rannala, B. DMLE+: Bayesian linkage disequilibrium gene mapping. *Bioinform* **2002**, *18*, 894–895. [CrossRef]
46. Risch, N.; De Leon, D.; Ozelius, L.; Kramer, P.; Almasy, L.; Singer, B.; Fahn, S.; Breakefield, X.; Bressman, S. Genetic analysis of idiopathic torsion dystonia in Ashkenazi Jews and their recent descent from a small founder population. *Nat. Genet.* **1995**, *9*, 152–159. [CrossRef]
47. Labuda, M.; Labuda, D.; Korab-Laskowska, M.; Cole, D.E.; Zietkiewicz, E.; Weissenbach, J.; Popowska, E.; Pronicka, E.; Root, A.W.; Glorieux, F.H. Linkage disequilibrium analysis in young populations: Pseudo-vitamin D-deficiency rickets and the founder effect in French Canadians. *Am. J. Hum. Genet.* **1996**, *59*, 633–643. [PubMed]
48. Labuda, D.; Zietkiewicz, E.; Labuda, M. The genetic clock and the age of the founder effect in growing populations: A lesson from French Canadians and Ashkenazim. *Am. J. Hum. Genet.* **1997**, *61*, 768–771. [CrossRef]
49. Colombo, R. Age estimate of the N370S mutation causing gaucher disease in Ashkenazi Jews and European populations: A reappraisal of haplotype data. *Am. J. Hum. Genet.* **2000**, *66*, 692–697. [CrossRef] [PubMed]
50. Weiner, O. Faculty opinions recommendation of mutations of bacteria from virus sensitivity to virus resistance. *Fac. Opin.* **2010**, *28*, 491–511. [CrossRef]
51. Slatkin, M.; Rannala, B. Estimating allele age. *Annu. Rev. Genom. Hum. Genet.* **2000**, *1*, 225–249. [CrossRef]
52. Mongush, M.V. Tuvans of Mongolia and China. *Int. J. Cent. Asian Stud.* **1996**, *1*, 225–243.
53. Chen, Z.; Zhang, Y.; Fan, A.; Zhang, Y.; Wu, Y.; Zhao, Q.; Zhou, Y.; Zhou, C.; Bawudong, M.; Mao, X.; et al. Brief communication: Y-chromosome haplogroup analysis indicates that Chinese Tuvans share distinctive affinity with Siberian Tuvans. *Am. J. Phys. Anthr.* **2011**, *144*, 492–497. [CrossRef]
54. Vainshtein, S.I.; Mannay-Ool, M.H. *History of Tyva*, 2nd ed.; Science: Novosibirsk, Russia, 2001. (In Russian)
55. Mannai-ool, M.K.; Tuvan People. *The Origin and Formation of the Ethnos*; Nauka Publ: Novosibirsk, Russia, 2004; pp. 99–166. (In Russian)
56. Potapov, L.P. *Ethnical structure and origin of Altaians*; Nauka: Leningrad, Soviet Union, 1969.
57. Richards, S.; Aziz, N.; Bale, S.; Bick, D.; Das, S.; Gastier-Foster, J.; Grody, W.W.; Hegde, M.; Lyon, E.; Spector, E.; et al. Standards and guidelines for the interpretation of sequence variants: A joint consensus recommendation of the american college of medical genetics and genomics and the association for molecular pathology. *Genet. Med.* **2015**, *17*, 405–423. [CrossRef]
58. Distefano, M.T.; Hemphill, S.E.; Oza, A.M.; Siegert, R.K.; Grant, A.R.; Hughes, M.Y.; Cushman, B.J.; Azaiez, H.; Booth, K.T.; Chapin, A.; et al. ClinGen expert clinical validity curation of 164 hearing loss gene–disease pairs. *Genet. Med.* **2019**, *21*, 2239–2247. [CrossRef] [PubMed]
59. Tekin, M.; Xia, X.-J.; Erdenetungalag, R.; Cengiz, F.B.; White, T.W.; Radnaabazar, J.; Dangaasuren, B.; Tastan, H.; Nance, W.E.; Pandya, A. *GJB2* mutations in Mongolia: Complex alleles, low frequency, and reduced fitness of the deaf. *Ann. Hum. Genet.* **2010**, *74*, 155–164. [CrossRef] [PubMed]
60. Liu, Y.; Ao, L.; Ding, H.; Zhang, D. Genetic frequencies related to severe or profound sensorineural hearing loss in inner Mongolia autonomous region. *Genet. Mol. Boil.* **2016**, *39*, 567–572. [CrossRef]
61. Yang, X.-L.; Bai-Cheng, X.; Chen, X.-J.; Pan-Pan, B.; Jian-Li, M.; Xiao-Wen, L.; Zhang, Z.-W.; Wan, D.; Zhu, Y.-M.; Guo, Y.-F. Common molecular etiology of patients with nonsyndromic hearing loss in Tibetan, Tu nationality, and Mongolian patients in the northwest of China. *Acta Oto Laryngol.* **2013**, *133*, 930–934. [CrossRef]
62. Tsukada, K.; Nishio, S.-Y.; Usami, S.; The Deafness Gene Study Consortium. A large cohort study of *GJB2* mutations in Japanese hearing loss patients. *Clin. Genet.* **2010**, *78*, 464–470. [CrossRef]

63. Sirmaci, A.; Akcayoz-Duman, D.; Tekin, M. The c.IVS1+1G>A mutation in the *GJB2* gene is prevalent and large deletions involving the *GJB6* gene are not present in the Turkish population. *J. Genet.* **2006**, *85*, 213–216. [CrossRef]
64. Seeman, P.; Sakmaryová, I. High prevalence of the IVS 1+1 G to A/*GJB2* mutation among Czech hearing impaired patients with monoallelic mutation in the coding region of *GJB2*: IVS 1 + 1 G to A *GJB2* mutation in Czech. *Clin. Genet.* **2006**, *69*, 410–413. [CrossRef]
65. Yuan, Y.; Yu, F.; Wang, G.; Huang, S.; Yu, R.; Zhang, X.; Huang, D.-L.; Han, D.-Y.; Dai, P. Prevalence of the *GJB2* IVS1+1G >A mutation in Chinese hearing loss patients with monoallelic pathogenic mutation in the coding region of GJB. *J. Transl. Med.* **2010**, *8*, 127. [CrossRef] [PubMed]
66. Bazazzadegan, N.; Nikzat, N.; Fattahi, Z.; Nishimura, C.; Meyer, N.; Sahraian, S.; Jamali, P.; Babanejad, M.; Kashef, A.; Yazdan, H.; et al. The spectrum of *GJB2* mutations in the Iranian population with non-syndromic hearing loss—A twelve year study. *Int. J. Pediatr. Otorhinolaryngol.* **2012**, *76*, 1164–1174. [CrossRef] [PubMed]
67. Barashkov, N.A.; Pshennikova, V.G.; Posukh, O.L.; Teryutin, F.M.; Solovyev, A.V.; Klarov, L.A.; Romanov, G.P.; Gotovtsev, N.; Kozhevnikov, A.A.; Kirillina, E.V.; et al. Spectrum and frequency of the *GJB2* gene pathogenic variants in a large cohort of patients with hearing impairment living in a subarctic region of Russia (the Sakha Republic). *PLoS ONE* **2016**, *11*, e0156300. [CrossRef]
68. Solovyev, A.; Barashkov, N.A.; Teryutin, F.M.; Pshennikova, V.G.; Romanov, G.P.; Rafailov, A.M.; Sazonov, N.N.; Dzhemilev, U.M.; Tomsky, M.I.; Posukh, O.L.; et al. Selective Heterozygous advantage of carriers of c.-23+1G>A mutation in *GJB2* gene causing autosomal recessive deafness 1A. *Bull. Exp. Boil. Med.* **2019**, *167*, 380–383. [CrossRef] [PubMed]
69. Solovyev, A.V.; Barashkov, N.A.; Bady-Khoo, M.S.; Zytsar, M.V.; Posukh, O.L.; Romanov, G.P.; Rafailov, A.M.; Sazonov, N.N.; Alexeev, A.N.; Dzhemilev, U.M.; et al. Reconstruction of SNP haplotypes with mutation c.-23+1G>A in human gene *GJB2* (Chromosome 13) in some populations of Eurasia. *Russ. J. Genet.* **2017**, *53*, 936–941. [CrossRef]
70. Fedorova, S.A.; Reidla, M.; Metspalu, E.; Metspalu, M.; Rootsi, S.; Tambets, K.; Trofimova, N.; Zhadanov, S.I.; Kashani, B.H.; Olivieri, A.; et al. Autosomal and uniparental portraits of the native populations of Sakha (Yakutia): Implications for the peopling of Northeast Eurasia. *BMC Evol. Boil.* **2013**, *13*, 1–18. [CrossRef]
71. Grillo, A.P.; De Oliveira, F.M.; De Carvalho, G.Q.; Medrano, R.F.V.; Da Silva-Costa, S.M.; Sartorato, E.L.; De Oliveira, C.A. Single nucleotide polymorphisms of the *GJB2* and *GJB6* genes are associated with autosomal recessive nonsyndromic hearing loss. *BioMed Res. Int.* **2015**, *2015*, 1–8. [CrossRef]
72. Parzefall, T.; Lucas, T.; Koenighofer, M.; Ramsebner, R.; Frohne, A.; Czeiger, S.; Baumgartner, W.-D.; Schoefer, C.; Gstoettner, W.; Frei, K. The role of alternative *GJB2* transcription in screening for neonatal sensorineural deafness in Austria. *Acta Oto Laryngol.* **2016**, *137*, 356–360. [CrossRef]

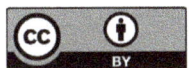

© 2020 by the authors. Licensee MDPI, Basel, Switzerland. This article is an open access article distributed under the terms and conditions of the Creative Commons Attribution (CC BY) license (http://creativecommons.org/licenses/by/4.0/).

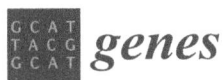

Article

Lights and Shadows in the Genetics of Syndromic and Non-Syndromic Hearing Loss in the Italian Population

Anna Morgan [1,*], Stefania Lenarduzzi [1], Beatrice Spedicati [1,2], Elisabetta Cattaruzzi [1], Flora Maria Murru [1], Giulia Pelliccione [1], Daniela Mazzà [1], Marcella Zollino [3,4], Claudio Graziano [5], Umberto Ambrosetti [6], Marco Seri [5], Flavio Faletra [1] and Giorgia Girotto [1,2]

1. Institute for Maternal and Child Health–IRCCS "Burlo Garofolo", 34137 Trieste, Italy; stefania.lenarduzzi@burlo.trieste.it (S.L.); beatrice.spedicati@burlo.trieste.it (B.S.); elisabetta.cattaruzzi@burlo.trieste.it (E.C.); floramaria.murru@burlo.trieste.it (F.M.M.); giulia.pelliccione@burlo.trieste.it (G.P.); daniela.mazza@burlo.trieste.it (D.M.); flavio.faletra@burlo.trieste.it (F.F.); giorgia.girotto@burlo.trieste.it (G.G.)
2. Department of Medicine, Surgery and Health Sciences, University of Trieste, 34125 Trieste, Italy
3. Fondazione Policlinico Universitario A. Gemelli, IRCCS, UOC Genetica, 00168 Rome, Italy; Marcella.Zollino@Unicatt.it
4. Istituto di Medicina Genomica, Università Cattolica Sacro Cuore, 00168 Rome, Italy
5. Unit of Medical Genetics, S. Orsola-Malpighi Hospital, 40138 Bologna, Italy; claudio.graziano@unibo.it (C.G.); marco.seri@unibo.it (M.S.)
6. Audiology and audiophonology, University of Milano/Fondazione IRCCS Cà Granda Ospedale Maggiore Policlinico, 20122 Milano, Italy; umberto.ambrosetti@unimi.it
* Correspondence: anna.morgan@burlo.trieste.it

Received: 1 October 2020; Accepted: 20 October 2020; Published: 22 October 2020

Abstract: Hearing loss (HL), both syndromic (SHL) and non-syndromic (NSHL), is the most common sensory disorder, affecting ~460 million people worldwide. More than 50% of the congenital/childhood cases are attributable to genetic causes, highlighting the importance of genetic testing in this class of disorders. Here we applied a multi-step strategy for the molecular diagnosis of HL in 125 patients, which included: (1) an accurate clinical evaluation, (2) the analysis of *GJB2, GJB6,* and *MT-RNR1* genes, (3) the evaluation *STRC-CATSPER2* and *OTOA* deletions via Multiplex Ligation Probe Amplification (MLPA), (4) Whole Exome Sequencing (WES) in patients negative to steps 2 and 3. Our approach led to the characterization of 50% of the NSHL cases, confirming both the relevant role of the *GJB2* (20% of cases) and *STRC* deletions (6% of cases), and the high genetic heterogeneity of NSHL. Moreover, due to the genetic findings, 4% of apparent NSHL patients have been re-diagnosed as SHL. Finally, WES characterized 86% of SHL patients, supporting the role of already know disease-genes. Overall, our approach proved to be efficient in identifying the molecular cause of HL, providing essential information for the patients' future management.

Keywords: hereditary hearing loss; MLPA; whole exome sequencing; molecular diagnosis

1. Introduction

Hereditary Hearing Loss (HHL) is the most common sensory disorder in childhood and adulthood, affecting approximately 1–3 out of 1000 newborns [1].

Genetic factors account for more than 50% of all the cases, where the majority exhibit an autosomal recessive (AR) pattern of inheritance (75–80%) followed by 20–25% of autosomal dominant (AD) cases and 1–1.5% of X-linked or mitochondrial ones [2].

More than 200 genes (i.e., ~1% of all the coding genes) are involved in the hearing process [3]; therefore, it is not surprising that HHL displays substantial genetic heterogeneity. The many genetic forms of hearing loss can be further categorized into syndromic and non-syndromic conditions, which, respectively, constitute 30% and 70% of the genetic causes of congenital HHL, with syndromic HHL likely underestimated [4,5]. To date, about 170 loci and 117 genes (36 autosomal dominant (AD), 65 autosomal recessives (AR), 11 AD/AR, and 5 X-linked genes) have been reported as causative of Non-Syndromic Hearing Loss (NSHL) (Hereditary Hearing Loss Homepage; http://hereditaryhearingloss.org/), and more than 400 syndromes associated with hearing loss and other symptoms (Syndromic Hearing Loss—SHL) have been described [6]. In particular, among the syndromes identified so far, some of them appear more frequently than the others (e.g., Usher syndrome compared to Waardenburg syndrome) [7,8]), although, in some cases, the full spectrum of clinical features might be subtle, or even not present until later in life [9].

The implementation of next-generation sequencing technologies (NGS), together with molecular karyotyping (e.g., Single Nucleotide Polymorphism (SNP) array or Comparative Genomic Hybridization (CGH) array) and other validating assays (e.g., Multiplex Ligation Probe Amplification—MLPA), has dramatically increased the diagnostic rate of HHL, leading to the identification of several mutations and Copy Number Variations (CNVs) in known deafness genes, as well as to the discovery of new disease genes [10–13]. The possibility to simultaneously screen large number of genes is essential to address with the genetic heterogeneity of HHL. This aspect is fundamental for NSHL, where, apart from the relevant contribution of the *GJB2* gene and, in some populations of *GJB6* gene, both responsible for ~50% of all AR cases [14–16], and of *STRC* deletions (accounting for 1% to 5% of HL cases [17]), no other worldwide primary players have been identified.

In the present work, we applied a multi-step strategy to identify the genetic cause of HHL in a subset of 125 individuals recruited in the last two years. The protocol included: (1) an accurate clinical evaluation of all the patients and their relatives to exclude all the cases in which HL was due to non-genetic causes (i.e., middle ear anomalies, infections, ototoxic drugs, etc.) and to distinguish between NSHL and SHL; (2) the analysis of *GJB2*, *GJB6* and *MT-RNR1* genes in patients affected by NSHL; (3) the evaluation of *STRC-CATSPER2* and *OTOA* deletions in case of negativity to step (2); (4) Whole Exome Sequencing (WES) analysis in case of negativity to steps (2) and (3) and for patients affected by SHL (Figure 1).

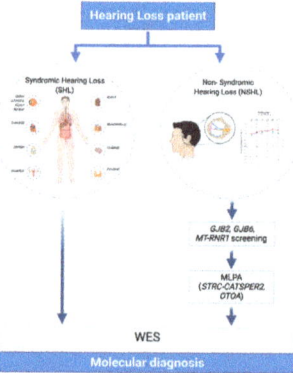

Figure 1. Schematic representation of the multi-step strategy applied for the study of Hereditary Hearing Loss (HHL). All of the patients enrolled in the present study underwent a careful clinical examination to distinguish between Syndromic Hearing Loss (SHL) and Non-Syndromic Hearing Loss (NSHL). Afterwards, NSHL patients were screened for mutation in *GJB2*, *GJB6*, and *MT-RNR1* genes, and for deletions in *STRC-CATSPER2* and *OTOA* genes. All of the NSHL patients negative to the first-level screening, together with SHL patients, have been then analyzed through Whole Exome Sequencing (WES).

The present work results illustrate the genetic heterogeneity of HHL and the importance of a detailed clinical characterization combined with high-throughput technologies for the diagnosis of both NSHL and SHL.

2. Materials and Methods

2.1. Ethical Statement

All patients signed written informed consent forms for both genetic counseling and molecular genetic testing. In the case of minors, informed consent was obtained from the next of kin. The study was approved by the Institutional Review Board (IRB) of the Institute for Maternal and Child Health (IRCCS) Burlo Garofolo, Trieste, Italy. All research was conducted according to the ethical standards as defined by the Helsinki Declaration.

2.2. Clinical Evaluation and Sample Collection

A total of 125 HHL patients have been recruited in the following centers (Otorhinolaryngology or Medical Genetics): Trieste (IRCCS Burlo Garofolo), Milano (IRCCS Cà Granda—Ospedale Maggiore Policlinico), Rome (Policlinico Universitario "A. Gemelli"), and Bologna (Policlinico S. Orsola-Malpighi).

All participants underwent pure tone audiometric testing (PTA) or auditory brainstem response (ABR) in order to characterize the severity of HL according to the international guidelines described by Clark (1981) [18]. Moreover, neurological and ophthalmological examinations, electrocardiogram, kidney ultrasonography, Magnetic Resonance Imaging (MRI) and Computerized Tomography (CT) scan, and thyroid function were carried out on routine basis in all probands.

Based on the clinical findings, 118 patients were classified as NSHL and seven as SHL. Furthermore, depending on the pedigree structure, the cases were divided into sporadic ($n = 90$) and familial ($n = 35$), the latter being classified as likely autosomal recessive (AR) ($n = 9$), and likely autosomal dominant (AD) ($n = 26$).

2.3. GJB2, GJB6, and mtDNA Analysis

For all the patients, the entire coding region of *GJB2* was analyzed by Sanger sequencing (primers available upon request). According to the manufacturer's instructions, DNA was sequenced on a 3500 Dx Genetic Analyzer (Life-Technologies, Carlsbad, CA, USA), using ABI PRISM 3.1 Big Dye terminator chemistry (Life Technologies, Carlsbad, CA, USA). Moreover, *GJB6* deletions (D13S1830-D13S1854) were screened by multiplex PCR using the method described by del Castillo et al. 2002 [19], while The A1555G mtDNA mutation was tested by Restriction Fragment Length Polymorphism (PCR-RFLP) analysis using BsmAI as restriction enzyme, followed by visualization on an agarose gel stained with ethidium bromide.

2.4. Multiplex Ligation Probe Amplification (MLPA)

MLPA analysis for identification of deletion/duplication in *STRC-CATSPER2* and *OTOA* genes was conducted using SALSA® MLPA® probe mixes P461-A1 DIS (MRC-Holland, Amsterdam, the Netherlands) according to the manufacturer's instructions. In brief, 50–100 ng DNA was denatured and hybridized overnight at 60 °C with the SALSA® probe mix. Samples were then treated with DNA ligase for 15 min at 54 °C. The reaction was stopped by incubation at 98 °C for 5 min. Finally, PCR amplification was carried out with specific fluorescent-labeled PCR primers. After amplification, the amplified products' fragment analysis was performed on ABI 3500dx Genetic Analyzer (Life-Technologies, Carlsbad, CA, USA).

Coffalyser.Net software was employed for data analysis in combination with the lot-specific MLPA Coffalyser sheet. The dosage quotient (DQ) of the reference probes in the patient samples was between 0.80 and 1.20. The following cutoff values for the DQ of the probes were used to interpret MLPA results; $0.80 < DQ < 1.20$ (no deletion/duplication), $DQ = 0$ (deletion), and $1.75 < DQ < 2.15$ (duplication).

2.5. Whole Exome Sequencing (WES)

WES was completed on an Illumina NextSeq 550 instrument (Illumina, San Diego, CA, USA) with NextEra Flex for enrichment–Exome panel reagents, according to the manufacturer's protocol.

Secondary analysis has been carried out using Isis Software (v.2.5.42.5-Illumina, Illumina, San Diego, CA, USA), i.e., reads alignment with Burrows-Wheeler Aligner (BWA) 0.7.7-isis-1.0.2 and variant calling with Isaac Variant Caller v. 2.1.4.2.

Single Nucleotides Variations (SNVs) and small Insertions and Deletions (INDELs) were collected into a standardized Variant Call Format (VCF) version 4.1 [20]. SNVs and INDELS were then annotated with ANNOVAR [21] using human genome build 19 (hg19) as the reference.

SNVs leading to synonymous amino acids substitutions not predicted as damaging, not affecting splicing or highly conserved residues were excluded, as well as SNVs/INDELs with quality score (QUAL) < 20 and called in off-target regions.

A comparison between the identified genetic variants and data reported in NCBI dbSNP build153 (http://www.ncbi.nlm.nih.gov/SNP/) as well as in gnomAD (http://gnomad.broadinstitute.org/), and National Heart, Lung and Blood Institute (NHLBI) Exome Sequencing Project (ESP) Exome Variant Server (Exome Variant Server, NHLBI GO Exome Sequencing Project (ESP), Seattle, WA) led to the exclusion of those variants previously reported as polymorphism. In particular, a Minor Allele Frequency (MAF) cutoff of 0.005 for recessive forms and 0.001 for the dominant ones was used.

The pathogenicity of known genetic variants was evaluated using ClinVar (http://www.ncbi.nlm.nih.gov/clinvar/), Deafness Variation Database (http://deafnessvariationdatabase.org/), and The Human Gene Mutation Database (http://www.hgmd.cf.ac.uk/ac/index.php).

Several in silico tools, such as PolyPhen-2 [22], Sorting Intolerant from Toleran (SIFT) [23], MutationTaster [24], Likelihood Ratio Test (LRT) [25], and Combined Annotation Dependent Depletion (CADD) score [26] were used to evaluate the pathogenicity of novel variants. Moreover, the evolutionary conservation of residues across species was evaluated by phyloP [27] and Genomic Evolutionary Rate Profiling (GERP) [28] scores.

Human Splicing Finder (HSF) version 2.4.1 [29] and Splice Site Prediction by Neural Network (NNSPLICE) version 9 (www.fruitfly.org) were adopted to predict the effect of the splice site mutations.

Finally, on a patient by patient basis, variants were discussed in the context of phenotypic data at interdisciplinary meetings and the most likely disease-causing SNVs/INDELs were analyzed by direct Sanger sequencing.

Sanger sequencing was also employed to perform the segregation analysis within the Family.

3. Results

During the last two years, 125 patients have been tested for *GJB2*, *GJB6,* and the A1555G mitochondrial mutation. Twenty percent of them were positive for mutations in the *GJB2* gene (i.e., 25 patients) with the c.35delG being the most frequent mutation (i.e., 44% of patients c.35delG homozygotes and 48% c.35delG carriers, together with other *in-trans* mutations, such as the p.(Glu120del), p.(Trp24 *) and p.(Glu47 *)) (Table 1). None of them carried deletions in *GJB6* or the A1555G mutation in the mitochondrial gene *MT-RNR1*.

Ninety-three NSHL individuals negative to this first-level screening were analyzed through MLPA to search for *STRC-CATSPER2* and *OTOA* deletions. Overall 8% of cases carried a homozygous deletion in *STRC* (*n* = 6) or *OTOA* (*n* = 1) genes (Table 2). The remaining 86 patients, together with their relatives, were then analyzed using WES. Sequencing data analysis led to the molecular diagnosis in 26 additional patients (Table 2) reaching an overall detection rate (i.e., *GJB2/GJB6*/mtDNA screening, MLPA, WES) of 50% (Figure 2A,B).

Table 1. List of patients positive for *GJB2* gene with indication of the identified mutations.

Patient ID	Gene	Variant 1	Variant 2	Status
Patient 1		c.35delG, p.(Gly12Valfs*2)	c.-27C > T	compound heterozygous
Patient 2		c.35delG, p.(Gly12Valfs*2)	c.229T > C, p.(Trp77Arg)	compound heterozygous
Patient 3		c.35delG, p.(Gly12Valfs*2)	c.35delG, p.(Gly12Valfs*2)	homozygous
Patient 4		c.35delG, p.(Gly12Valfs*2)	c.139G > T p.(Glu47*)	compound heterozygous
Patient 5		c.35delG, p.(Gly12Valfs*2)	c.358_360delGAG, p.(Glu120del)	compound heterozygous
Patient 6		c.35delG, p.(Gly12Valfs*2)	c.-23 + 1G > A	compound heterozygous
Patient 7		c.35delG, p.(Gly12Valfs*2)	c.71G > A, p.(Glu24*)	compound heterozygous
Patient 8		c.35delG, p.(Gly12Valfs*2)	c.71G > A, p.(Glu24*)	compound heterozygous
Patient 9		c.35delG, p.(Gly12Valfs*2)	c.35delG, p.(Gly12Valfs*2)	homozygous
Patient 10		c.35delG, p.(Gly12Valfs*2)	c.35delG, p.(Gly12Valfs*2)	homozygous
Patient 11		c.35delG, p.(Gly12Valfs*2)	c.314_327del14, p.(Lys105Argfs*5)	compound heterozygous
Patient 12		c.35delG, p.(Gly12Valfs*2)	c.35delG, p.(Gly12Valfs*2)	homozygous
Patient 13	*GJB2*	c.35delG, p.(Gly12Valfs*2)	c.95G > A, p.(Arg32His)	compound heterozygous
Patient 14		c.35delG, p.(Gly12Valfs*2)	c.35delG, p.(Gly12Valfs*2)	homozygous
Patient 15		c.59T > C, p.(Ile20Thr)	c.314_327del14, p.(Lys105Argfs*5)	compound heterozygous
Patient 16		c.35delG, p.(Gly12Valfs*2)	c.71G > A, p.(Glu24*)	compound heterozygous
Patient 17		c.35delG, p.(Gly12Valfs*2)	c.35delG, p.(Gly12Valfs*2)	homozygous
Patient 18		c.35delG, p.(Gly12Valfs*2)	c.139G > T p.(Glu47*)	compound heterozygous
Patient 19		c.35delG, p.(Gly12Valfs*2)	c.35delG, p.(Gly12Valfs*2)	homozygous
Patient 20		c.35delG, p.(Gly12Valfs*2)	c.35delG, p.(Gly12Valfs*2)	homozygous
Patient 21		c.101T > C, p.(Met34Thr)	c.358_360delGAG, p.(Glu120del)	compound heterozygous
Patient 22		c.35delG, p.(Gly12Valfs*2)	c.35delG, p.(Gly12Valfs*2)	homozygous
Patient 23		c.35delG, p.(Gly12Valfs*2)	c.35delG, p.(Gly12Valfs*2)	homozygous
Patient 24		c.35delG, p.(Gly12Valfs*2)	c.358_360delGAG, p.(Glu120del)	compound heterozygous
Patient 25		c.35delG, p.(Gly12Valfs*2)	c.35delG, p.(Gly12Valfs*2)	homozygous

Table 2. List of likely causative variants identified by WES and Multiplex Ligation Probe Amplification (MLPA). All variants have been classified based on their frequency reported in Genome Aggregation Database (gnomAD, http://gnomad.broadinstitute.org/) and their pathogenicity. In particular, the following tools have been used: CADD PHRED (Pathogenicity score: > 10 predicted to be deleterious), GERP++_RS (higher number is more conserved), and Polyphen-2 (D: Probably damaging, P: possibly damaging; B: benign), SIFT (D: deleterious; T: tolerated), MutationTaster (A (disease_causing_automatic); D (disease_causing); N (polymorphism); P (polymorphism automatic)). NA = not available; hom = homozygous; het = heterozygous.

Family ID	Gene	cDNA Change	Protein Change	dbSNP	gnomAD ALL	CADD PHRED	GERP ++ RS	Polyphen-2	SIFT	Mutatic Taster	References
Family 3	OTOA (NM_144672.3)	entire gene deletion (hom)	NA	NA	NA	NA	NA	NA	NA	NA	Shearer et al., (2014) Genome Med [30]
Family 4	COL11A2 (NM_080680.2)	c.3100C > T (het)	p.(Arg1034Cys)	rs121912947	NA	32	2.95	D	D	D	McGuirt et al., (1999) Nat Genet [31]
Patient 41	MYO7A (NM_000260.3)	c.6236G > A (hom)	p.(Arg2079Gln)	rs765083332	0.00004188	25.5	4.24	P	T	D	NA
Patient 42	ADGRV1 (NM_032119.3)	c.10084C > T (het)	p.(Gln3362 *)	NA	NA	42	3.02	NA	NA	A	NA
		c.13655dupT (het)	p.(Asn4553Glufs *18)	rs765376986	NA	NA	NA	NA	NA	NA	NA
Patient 44	STRC (NM_153700.2)	entire gene deletion (hom)	NA	NA	NA	NA	NA	NA	NA	NA	Vona et al.,(2015) Clin Genet [32]
Patient 45	GJB1 (NM_000166.5)	c.790C > T (het)	p.(Arg264Cys)	rs587777879	0.00005714	25.8	4.9	D	D	D	Numakura et al., (2002) Hum Mutat [33]
Patient 51	CLDN14 (NM_144492.2)	c.301G > A (hom)	p.(Gly101Arg)	rs74315438	0.00004302	26.5	5.42	D	D	D	Wattenhofer et al.,(2005) Hum Mutat [34]
Family 6	SMPX (NM_014332.2)	c.45+1G > A (hemizygous)	NA	NA	NA	24.4	4.9	NA	NA	D	NA
Family 7	SIX1 (NM_005982.3)	c.397_399delGAG (het)	p.(Glu133del)	rs80356460	NA	NA	NA	NA	NA	NA	Ruf et al., (2004) Proc Natl Acad Sci U S A [35]
Family 8	KARS (NM_001130089.1)	c.1423C > T (het)	p.(Leu475Phe)	NA	NA	28.2	5.91	P	T	D	NA
		c.1570T > C (het)	p.(Cys524Arg)	NA	NA	26.9	5.81	D	D	D	NA
Patient 57	OTOG (NM_001277269.1)	c.2500C > T (hom)	p.(Gln834 *)	rs554847663	0.0004274	37	2.01	NA	NA	D	Sheppard et al.,(2018) Genet Med [36]
Family 10	PAX3 (NM_181457.3)	c.220C > T (het)	p.(Arg74Cys)	NA	NA	35	5.24	D	D	D	Lenarduzzi et al, (2019) Hear Res [37]

Table 2. Cont.

Family ID	Gene	cDNA Change	Protein Change	dbSNP	gnomAD_ALL	CADD PHRED	GERP++_RS	Polyphen-2	SIFT	Mutation Taster	References
Patient 62	STRC (NM_153700.2)	entire gene deletion (hom)	NA	NA	NA	NA	NA	NA	NA	NA	Vona et al.,(2015) Clin Genet [32]
Family 13	ESPN (NM_031475.2)	entire gene deletion (hom)	NA	NA	NA	NA	NA	NA	NA	NA	NA
Family 14	MYO6 (NM_004999.3)	c.1525delG (het)	p.(Val509Trpfs *7)	NA	NA	NA	NA	NA	NA	D	NA
Family 15	OTOF (NM_194248.2)	c.2891C > A (hom)	p.(Ala964Glu)	rs201329629	NA	32	5.41	D	D	D	Rodriguez-Ballesteros et al. (2008) Hum Mutat [38] Magliulo et al.,(2017) Otolaryngol Head Neck Surg [39]
Patient 65	ADGRV1 (NM_032119.3)	c.4378G>A (het)	p.(Gly1460Ser)	rs1303930496	0.00001248	32	5.53	D	D	D	NA
		c.13655dupT (het)	p.(Asn4553Glufs *18)	rs765376986	NA	NA	NA	NA	NA	NA	
Family 18	DIAPH1 (NM_005219.4)	c.3556delC (het)	p.(Leu1186Serfs *2)	NA	NA	NA	NA	NA	NA	D	NA
Family 70	GATA3 (NM_002051.2)	c.925-1G > T (het, de novo)	NA	NA	NA	25.9	5.3	NA	NA	NA	NA
Family 20	TECTA (NM_005422.2)	c.3841T > C (het)	p.(Cys1281Arg)	NA	NA	17.03	5.76	T	D	D	NA
Family 21	STRC (NM_153700.2)	entire gene deletion (hom)	NA	NA	NA	NA	NA	NA	NA	NA	Vona et al.,(2015) Clin Genet [32]
Family 23	USH2A (NM_206933.2)	c.2276G > T (het)	p.(Cys759Phe)	rs80338902	0.000947	33	5.79	D	D	D	Rivolta et al.,(2000) Am J Hum Genet [40]
		c.11864G > A (het)	p.(Trp3955 *)	rs111033364	0.000119	51	5.53	NA	NA	D	van Wijk et al., (2004) Am J Hum Genet [41]
	EYA4 (NM_004100.4)	c.714C > A (het)	p.(Tyr238 *)	rs1264401894	0.000004	37	4.77	NA	NA	D	NA
Family 24	WFS1 (NM_006005.3)	c.2567C > A (het)	p.(Pro856His)	NA	NA	23.7	4.82	D	D	D	NA
Family 26	MYO6 (NM_004999.3)	c.613C > T (het)	p.(Arg205 *)	rs557441143	0.00000398	37	3.31	NA	NA	A	Choi ET AL.,(2013) PLoS One 8 [42]
Family 27	COL2A1 (NM_001844.5)	c.4201G > C (het)	p.(Asp1401His)	NA	NA	19.9	5.06	D	D	D	NA
Family 28	ATP2B2 (NM_001001331.4)	c.962C > G (het)	p.(Ser321 *)	NA	NA	42	5.34	NA	T	A	NA

Table 2. Cont.

Family ID	Gene	cDNA Change	Protein Change	dbSNP	gnomAD_ALL	CADD PHRED	GERP ++_RS	Polyphen-2	SIF	Mutatic Taster	References
Patient 79	LARS2	4 Kb gene deletion (hom)	NA	NA	NA	NA	NA	NA	NA	NA	NA
Family 29	PDZD7 (NM_024895.4)	c.166dupC (het)	p.(Arg56Profs * 24)	rs587776894	NA	NA	NA	NA	NA	NA	Ebermann et al.,(2010) J Clin Invest [43]
		c.305G > A (het)	p.(Arg102His)	rs760825921	0.00001061	34	5.07	D	D	D	NA
Family 30	STRC (NM_153700.2)	entire gene deletion (hom)	NA	NA	NA	NA	NA	NA	NA	NA	Vona et al.,(2015) Clin Genet [32]
Family 31	STRC (NM_153700.2)	entire gene deletion (hom)	NA	NA	NA	NA	NA	NA	NA	NA	Vona et al.,(2015) Clin Genet [32]
Family 32	HOMER2 (NM_199330.2)	c.592_597delACCACA (het)	p.(Thr198_Thr199del)	NA	NA	NA	NA	NA	NA	P	NA
Patient 84	STRC (NM_153700.2)	entire gene deletion (hom)	NA	NA	NA	NA	NA	NA	NA	NA	Vona et al.,(2015) Clin Genet [32]
Family 34	STRC (NM_153700.2)	c.4057C > T (hom)	p.(Gln1353 *)	rs774312182	0.00006374	37	4.16	NA	NA	D	Shearer et al., (2010) Proc Natl Acad Sci U S A [44]
Patient 86	TCOF1 (NM_001135243.1)	c.4362_4366del (het)	p.(Lys1457Glufs * 11)	NA	NA	NA	NA	NA	NA	NA	NA
Family 35	COL4A3 (NM_000091.4)	c.3943C > T (het)	p.(Pro1315Ser)	rs760703010	0.00002793	25	5.57	D	D	D	NA
Patient 87	USH2A (NM_206933.2)	c.11864G > A (hom)	p.(Trp3955 *)	rs111033364	0.000119	51	5.53	NA	D	A	van Wijk et al., (2004) Am J Hum Genet [41]
Patient 88	USH2A (NM_206933.2)	c.4933G > T (hom)	p.(Gly1645 *)	NA	NA	38	3.86	NA	NA	A	Sloan-Heggen et al.,(2016) Hum Genet [45]
Patient 89	USH2A (NM_206933.2)	c.2035G > T (het)	p.(Gly679 *)	NA	NA	38	5.26	NA	NA	A	NA
		c.11864G > A (het)	p.(Trp3955 *)	rs111033364	0.000119	51	5.53	NA	D	A	van Wijk et al., (2004) Am J Hum Genet [41]
Patient 90	MYO7A (NM_000260.3)	c.735G > A (het)	(p.Gln245Gln)	NA	NA	NA	NA	NA	NA	A	Atik et al.,(2015) PLoS One 10 [46]
		c.1834_1836delAGC (het)	p.(Ser612del)	NA	NA	NA	NA	NA	NA	D	NA

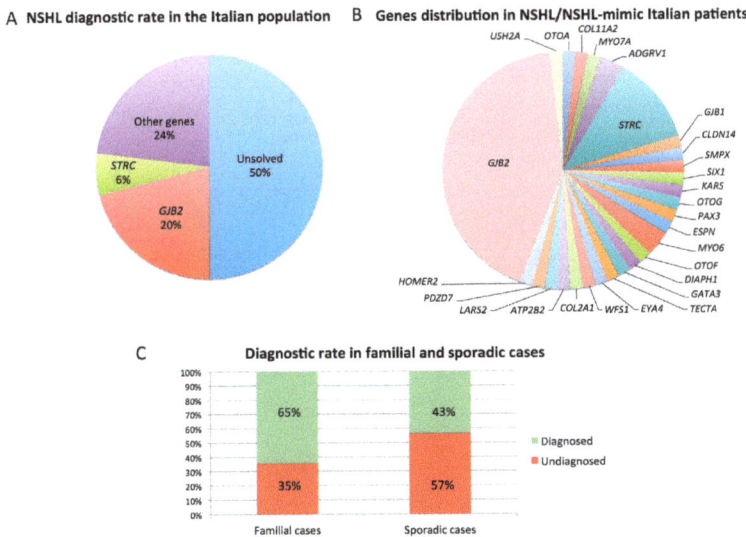

Figure 2. Diagnostic rate and genes distribution in NSHL patients. (**A**) Overall diagnostic rate for NSHL. Moreover, 50% of patients received a conclusive molecular diagnosis, with *GJB2* being the most frequently mutated gene (i.e., 20%), followed by *STRC* (i.e., 6%). (**B**) Genes distribution among all the NSHL and NSHL-mimic patients investigated. (**C**) Diagnostic rate comparison between familial and sporadic cases showing a higher percentage of solved cases among patients presenting with a familial history of HL.

In particular, 65% of familial cases (i.e., 22/34) were genetically characterized, while for sporadic cases, the molecular cause was identified in 43% of patients (i.e., 36/84) (Figure 2C).

WES data allowed unveiling some peculiar scenarios, which reflect the complexity of NSHL.

In particular, WES allowed: (1) to detect syndromes in patients displaying only subtle phenotypic features; (2) to early diagnose diseases with a late-onset clinical manifestations; (3) to identify mutations in more than one gene involved in the same phenotype; (4) to molecularly characterize multiple genetic conditions in the same patient; and (5) to clarify the role of recently discovered genes.

An example of 1) is Family 10, who came to genetic counseling with a clinical diagnosis of NSHL in the proband and in the mother. WES revealed the presence of a novel heterozygous variant in *PAX3* (NM_181457.3) (c.220C > T p.(Arg74Cys)), which occurred as de novo in the mother and was inherited from the proband. *PAX3* is a gene known for being causative of Waardenburg syndrome type 1 and 2 [47], a disease characterized by HL, pigmentation abnormalities and, in some cases, dystopia canthorum or other additional features [8]. A clinical re-evaluation of the patients revealed the presence of mild pigmentary disturbances of the iris, hair, and skin, confirming the molecular diagnosis.

Regarding point 2), three patients who only displayed sensorineural hearing loss have been molecularly classified as Usher patients. In particular, two of them carried pathogenic mutations in the *GPR98* gene (NM_032119.3) while one carried two compound heterozygous mutations in *USH2A* (NM_206933.2) gene (Table 2).

As for point number 3), we were able to identify the simultaneous presence of mutations in both *USH2A* and *EYA4* genes in Family 23, an Italian family apparently affected by autosomal dominant NSHL. WES revealed the presence of two compound heterozygous mutations in *USH2A* (NM_206933.2) in the proband (i.e., c.11864G > A, p.(Trp3955 *) and c.2276G > T, p.(Cys759Phe)) in addition to a stop gain variant in *EYA4* (NM_004100.4), i.e., c.714C > A, p.(Tyr238 *), segregating in the other affected family members (i.e., the proband's mother, the maternal uncle and the maternal grandfather).

Subsequently, the proband's hearing thresholds appeared worse than those of her relatives, possibly due to the simultaneous presence of mutations in both *USH2A* and *EYA4A*.

In other cases, WES revealed the presence of 4) multiple independent genetic conditions that were initially misinterpreted as a single syndrome. An example is Patient 84, who presented with sensorineural hearing loss and periventricular nodular heterotopia (Figure 3).

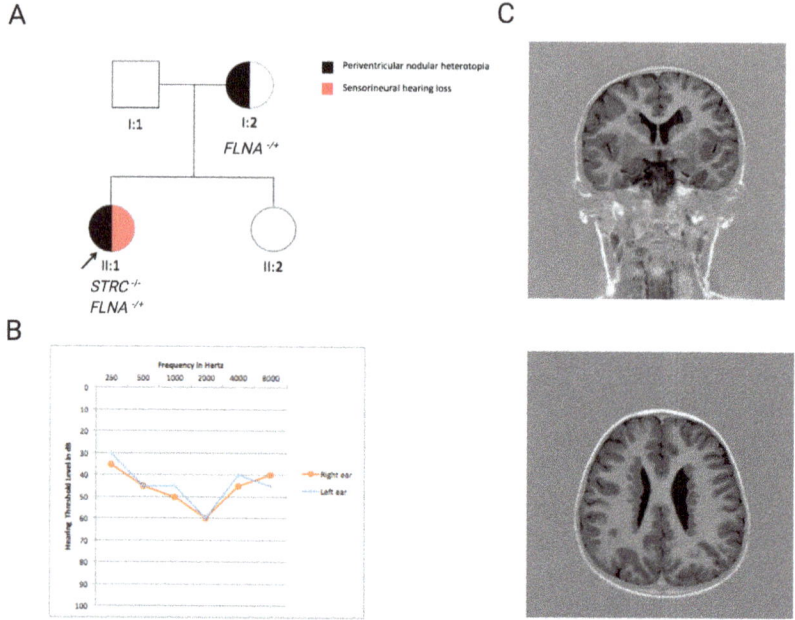

Figure 3. Pedigree, clinical and genetic features of Patient 84. (**A**) Pedigree of Patient 84, affected by both sensorineural hearing loss and periventricular nodular heterotopia. (**B**) Audiometric features of the affected individual, displayed as audiograms (air conduction). The thresholds of the right and left ears are shown. (**C**) Axial (coronal) scan IR T1-weighted. Bilateral periventricular nodules of grey matter are seen immediately deep to the ependymal layer of the bodies of both lateral ventricles.

MLPA detected a homozygous deletion in the *STRC* gene explaining the HL phenotype but not the neurological one. The application of WES allowed to identify a heterozygous nonsense variant in the *FLNA* gene ((NM_001456.3), c.1159C > T p.(Gln387 *)), a gene known for being causative of periventricular nodular heterotopia in an X-linked dominant fashion [48]. The variant was inherited from the mother, whose MRI revealed foci of periventricular nodular heterotopia, confirming the identified allele's pathogenic effect.

WES also allowed 5) to detect novel variants in genes recently described as causative of NSHL, supporting their pathogenic role. An example is the case of Family 28, an Italian family presenting with a likely autosomal dominant NSHL (Figure 4A), where a novel nonsense variant in *ATP2B2* ((NM_001001331.4) c.962C > G, p.(Ser321 *) has been identified.

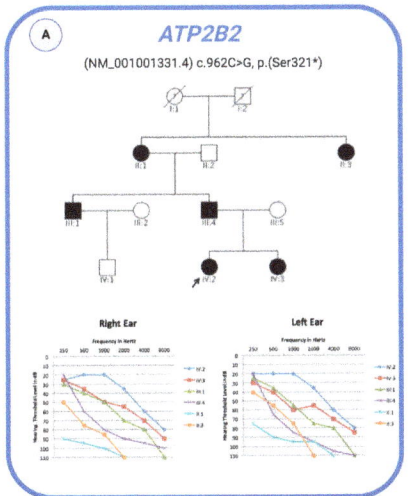
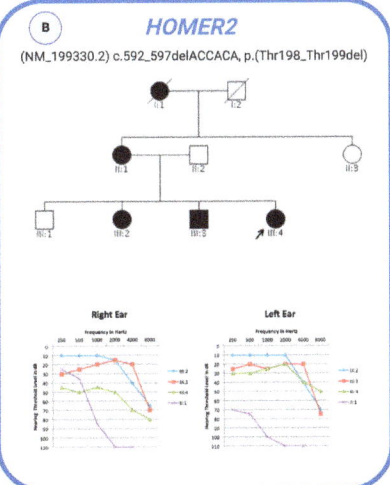

Figure 4. Pedigree and audiometric features of the families with novel variants in *ATP2B2* and *HOMER2* genes. (**A**) Pedigree of the family carrying a novel nonsense variant in the *ATP2B2* gene and audiometric features of the affected individuals. (**B**) Pedigree of the family carrying a novel deletion in the *HOMER2* gene and audiometric features of the affected individuals. Filled symbols represent affected individuals. Probands are indicated with an arrow. Individuals with Roman numeric labels were analyzed in this study. Audiometric features of the subjects are displayed as audiograms (air conduction). The thresholds of the right and left ears are shown.

For many years *ATP2B2* has been described as a modifier of *CDH23* [49], and it has only recently been hypothesized that loss of function mutations in this gene cause autosomal dominant NSHL [50]. The identification of an additional ADNSHL family carrying a nonsense variant strengthens previous findings, confirming the pathogenic role of the ATP2B2 gene.

Another example is Family 32, an Italian family affected by NSHL (Figure 4B). WES revealed the presence of a novel heterozygous deletion in the *HOMER2* gene (NM_199330.2) (i.e., c.592_597delACCACA, p.(Thr198_Thr199del)) segregating within the family in an autosomal dominant fashion. To our knowledge, this represents the third independent NSHL family carrying a variant in this gene [12,51], definitely confirming its relevant role in the etiopathogenesis of hearing loss.

Finally, WES proved to be extremely efficient for the molecular diagnosis of clinically evident SHL. In particular, all the Usher patients (i.e., patients displaying HL and retinitis pigmentosa) were molecularly characterized, identifying homozygous or compound heterozygous mutations in *USH2A* and *MYO7A* genes (Table 2). Among the two suspected Alport patients enrolled in the study, one was a carrier of a variant in *COL4A3* ((NM_000091.5) c.3943C > T, p.(Pro1315Ser)) inherited from the affected father, while the second individual did not display any pathogenic mutation in all the genes known to be causative of such syndrome. Finally, a patient clinically diagnosed with Treacher–Collins syndrome carried a frameshift deletion in *TCOF1* ((NM_000356) c.4131_4135del, p.(K1380Efs * 11)) (Table 2).

4. Discussion

The definition of the molecular basis of HHL has always being a challenge for clinicians and geneticists. The development and application of a multi-step integrated strategy based on (1) an accurate clinical evaluation; (2) *GJB2/GJB6/MT-RNR1* screening; (3) MLPA; and (4) WES has proved to be a powerful approach for the molecular diagnosis of HHL patients.

Regarding NSHL, our data confirmed the relevant role of the *GJB2* gene responsible for 20% of cases, and identified *STRC* as the second major player in the Italian population, being causative of 6%

of all NSHL patients. In this light, the application of MLPA, or other techniques able to identify CNVs, is becoming a crucial test for NSHL patients. Interestingly, in agreement with literature data [17], *STRC* deletions have been identified in patients revealing mild-to-moderate hearing loss (Figure 5), thus, supporting a possible genotype–phenotype correlation between these audiometric features and *STRC* loss.

Audiograms of *STRC* patients

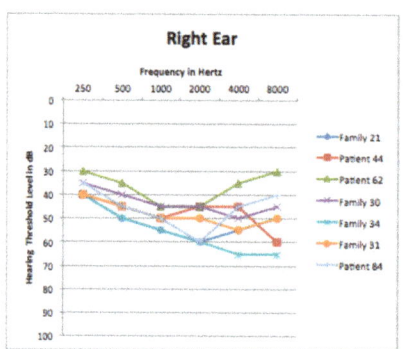 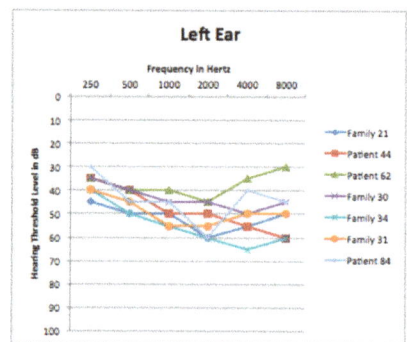

Figure 5. Audiometric features of the patients with *STRC* deletion/mutation. Audiograms of the patients with loss of function mutations or deletions of *STRC* gene display mild-to-moderate hearing loss. The thresholds of the right and left ears are shown.

On the other hand, no deletions in *GJB6* have been detected, and the A1555G mitochondrial mutation. These results, combined with the outcomes of the previous works [10,52] suggest that *GJB6* and *MT-RNR1* are not a common cause of NSHL in the Italian population, despite their relevant role in other areas of the world.

WES allowed the identification of the genetic cause of HHL in 86% of the SHL patients and 23% of the NSHL subjects, revealing some unexpected findings in the latter case. Indeed, 4% of patients received a molecular diagnosis of syndromic HL, despite the first clinical evaluation in favor of NSHL, and multiple genetic causes of the clinical phenotype were identified in two families, hampering the interpretation of the sequencing data.

These findings emphasize the usefulness of WES compared to other approaches, such as the use of comprehensive gene panels. In fact, WES allowed at once (a) an early diagnosis of the syndromic cases that do not already show all the clinical signs or symptoms, (b) the possibility of unveiling unrelated co-existing genetic conditions, (c) the identification of new deafness candidate genes not previously described or only detected as private mutation/gene of a single family worldwide, thus resulting in a cost and time-saving approach.

The results of the present study highlight the complexity of HL and, more importantly, have obvious clinical outcomes. A correct molecular diagnosis provides patients with significant prognostic value and relevant heritability information and influences their management, leading to tailored medical surveillance and different therapeutic options. Moreover, in the case of HHL, it has been demonstrated that knowing the gene involved in the disease can help predict the response to cochlear implantation. As an example, patients carrying mutations in the *GJB2* gene show an excellent response to cochlear implants. In contrast, those with mutations involving genes that affect the cochlear nerve itself gave worse post-implant performance [53]. Knowing this issue before implantation can help define expectations about post-implant auditory function.

Overall, all the examples discussed above point out the complexity of HHL (both syndromic and non-syndromic). When dealing with this phenotype, it is essential to be aware of the difficulties encountered in choosing the most effective approach to arrive at a correct molecular diagnosis. With this in mind, the collaboration between geneticists, clinicians, and otolaryngologists, who have an in-depth knowledge of the clinical features of hearing loss and the genes involved, is fundamental to achieve the ultimate goal of unraveling the genetic bases of HHL and improving the lives of patients.

Author Contributions: Conceptualization, A.M. and G.G.; methodology, A.M., S.L., and G.P.; software, A.M., S.L., and G.G.; validation, S.L., and G.P.; formal analysis, A.M., F.F., and G.G.; investigation, B.S. and F.F.; resources, E.C., F.M.M., D.M., M.Z., C.G., U.A., and M.S.; data curation, A.M., and G.G.; writing—original draft preparation, A.M.; writing—review and editing, G.G.; visualization, A.M., S.L., and G.G.; supervision, F.F. and G.G.; project administration, A.M. and G.G.; funding acquisition: G.G. All authors have read and agreed to the published version of the manuscript.

Funding: This research was supported by D70-RESRICGIROTTO to GG, BENEFICENTIA Stiftung to G.G., and SG-2018-12367867 to A.M. The funders had no role in study design, data collection, and analysis, decision to publish, or preparation of the manuscript.

Acknowledgments: We gratefully acknowledge Martina Bradaschia for the English revision of the manuscript.

Conflicts of Interest: The authors declare no conflict of interest.

References

1. Allen, S.B.; Goldman, J. *Hearing, Inner Ear, Syndromic Sensorineural Loss*; StatPearls Publishing: Tampa, FL, USA, 2019.
2. Likar, T.; Hasanhodžić, M.; Teran, N.; Maver, A.; Peterlin, B.; Writzl, K. Diagnostic outcomes of exome sequencing in patients with syndromic or non-syndromic hearing loss. *PLoS ONE* **2018**, *13*. [CrossRef] [PubMed]
3. Pandey, S.; Pandey, M. Advances in Genetic Diagnosis and Treatment of Hearing Loss—A Thirst for Revolution. In *Update On Hearing Loss*; InTech: London, UK, 2015.
4. Smith, R.J.; Bale, J.F.; White, K.R. Sensorineural hearing loss in children. *Lancet* **2005**, *365*, 879–890. [CrossRef]
5. Korver, A.M.H.; Smith, R.J.H.; Van Camp, G.; Schleiss, M.R.; Bitner-Glindzicz, M.A.K.; Lustig, L.R.; Usami, S.I.; Boudewyns, A.N. Congenital hearing loss. *Nat. Rev. Dis. Prim.* **2017**, *3*, 16094. [CrossRef] [PubMed]
6. Ideura, M.; Nishio, S.Y.; Moteki, H.; Takumi, Y.; Miyagawa, M.; Sato, T.; Kobayashi, Y.; Ohyama, K.; Oda, K.; Matsui, T.; et al. Comprehensive analysis of syndromic hearing loss patients in Japan. *Sci. Rep.* **2019**, *9*. [CrossRef]
7. Wolfrum, U.; Nagel-Wolfrum, K. The Usher Syndrome, a Human Ciliopathy. *Klin. Monbl. Augenheilkd.* **2018**, *235*, 273–280. [CrossRef]
8. Ahmed, J.D.N.; Mui, R.K.; Masood, S. Waardenburg Syndrome. *J. Med Genet.* **2020**, *34*, 656–665.
9. Bademci, G.; Cengiz, F.B.; Foster, J.; Duman, D.; Sennaroglu, L.; Diaz-Horta, O.; Atik, T.; Kirazli, T.; Olgun, L.; Alper, H.; et al. Variations in Multiple Syndromic Deafness Genes Mimic Non-syndromic Hearing Loss. *Sci. Rep.* **2016**, *6*. [CrossRef]
10. Morgan, A.; Lenarduzzi, S.; Cappellani, S.; Pecile, V.; Morgutti, M.; Orzan, E.; Ghiselli, S.; Ambrosetti, U.; Brumat, M.; Gajendrarao, P.; et al. Genomic Studies in a Large Cohort of Hearing Impaired Italian Patients Revealed Several New Alleles, a Rare Case of Uniparental Disomy (UPD) and the Importance to Search for Copy Number Variations. *Front. Genet.* **2018**, *9*, 681. [CrossRef]
11. Cabanillas, R.; Diñeiro, M.; Cifuentes, G.A.; Castillo, D.; Pruneda, P.C.; Álvarez, R.; Sánchez-Durán, N.; Capín, R.; Plasencia, A.; Viejo-Díaz, M.; et al. Comprehensive genomic diagnosis of non-syndromic and syndromic hereditary hearing loss in Spanish patients. *BMC Med. Genom.* **2018**, *11*. [CrossRef]
12. Azaiez, H.; Decker, A.R.; Booth, K.T.; Simpson, A.C.; Shearer, A.E.; Huygen, P.L.M.; Bu, F.; Hildebrand, M.S.; Ranum, P.T.; Shibata, S.B.; et al. HOMER2, a stereociliary scaffolding protein, is essential for normal hearing in humans and mice. *PLoS Genet.* **2015**, *11*, e1005137. [CrossRef]
13. Morgan, A.; Koboldt, D.C.; Barrie, E.S.; Crist, E.R.; García García, G.; Mezzavilla, M.; Faletra, F.; Mihalic Mosher, T.; Wilson, R.K.; Blanchet, C.; et al. Mutations in PLS1, encoding fimbrin, cause autosomal dominant nonsyndromic hearing loss. *Hum. Mutat.* **2019**. [CrossRef] [PubMed]

14. Del Castillo, I.; Moreno-Pelayo, M.A.; Del Castillo, F.J.; Brownstein, Z.; Marlin, S.; Adina, Q.; Cockburn, D.J.; Pandya, A.; Siemering, K.R.; Chamberlin, G.P.; et al. Prevalence and Evolutionary Origins of the del(GJB6-D13S1830) Mutation in the DFNB1 Locus in Hearing-Impaired Subjects: A Multicenter Study. *Am. J. Hum. Genet.* **2003**, *73*, 1452–1458. [CrossRef]
15. Cama, E.; Melchionda, S.; Palladino, T.; Carella, M.; Santarelli, R.; Genovese, E.; Benettazzo, F.; Zelante, L.; Arslan, E. Hearing loss features in GJB2 biallelic mutations and GJB2/GJB6 digenic inheritance in a large Italian cohort. *Int. J. Audiol.* **2009**, *48*, 12–17. [CrossRef] [PubMed]
16. Morton, C.C.; Nance, W.E. Newborn Hearing Screening—A Silent Revolution. *N. Engl. J. Med.* **2006**, *354*, 2151–2164. [CrossRef]
17. Yokota, Y.; Moteki, H.; Nishio, S.Y.; Yamaguchi, T.; Wakui, K.; Kobayashi, Y.; Ohyama, K.; Miyazaki, H.; Matsuoka, R.; Abe, S.; et al. Frequency and clinical features of hearing loss caused by STRC deletions. *Sci. Rep.* **2019**, *9*. [CrossRef]
18. Clark, J.G. Uses and abuses of hearing loss classification. *ASHA* **1981**, *23*, 493–500.
19. Del Castillo, I.; Villamar, M.; Moreno-Pelayo, M.A.; del Castillo, F.J.; Alvarez, A.; Tellería, D.; Menéndez, I.; Moreno, F. A deletion involving the connexin 30 gene in nonsyndromic hearing impairment. *N. Engl. J. Med.* **2002**, *346*, 243–249. [CrossRef]
20. Danecek, P.; Auton, A.; Abecasis, G.; Albers, C.A.; Banks, E.; DePristo, M.A.; Handsaker, R.E.; Lunter, G.; Marth, G.T.; Sherry, S.T.; et al. The variant call format and VCFtools. *Bioinformatics* **2011**, *27*, 2156–2158. [CrossRef]
21. Wang, K.; Li, M.; Hakonarson, H. ANNOVAR: Functional annotation of genetic variants from high-throughput sequencing data. *Nucleic Acids Res.* **2010**, *38*, e164. [CrossRef]
22. Adzhubei, I.; Jordan, D.M.; Sunyaev, S.R. Predicting functional effect of human missense mutations using PolyPhen-2. *Curr. Protoc. Hum. Genet.* **2013**, *7*. [CrossRef]
23. Ng, P.C.; Henikoff, S. SIFT: Predicting amino acid changes that affect protein function. *Nucleic Acids Res.* **2003**, *31*, 3812–3814. [CrossRef] [PubMed]
24. Schwarz, J.M.; Rödelsperger, C.; Schuelke, M.; Seelow, D. MutationTaster evaluates disease-causing potential of sequence alterations. *Nat. Methods* **2010**, *7*, 575–576. [CrossRef] [PubMed]
25. Chun, S.; Fay, J.C. Identification of deleterious mutations within three human genomes. *Genome Res.* **2009**, *19*, 1553–1561. [CrossRef] [PubMed]
26. Kircher, M.; Witten, D.M.; Jain, P.; O'Roak, B.J.; Cooper, G.M.; Shendure, J. A general framework for estimating the relative pathogenicity of human genetic variants. *Nat. Genet.* **2014**, *46*, 310–315. [CrossRef] [PubMed]
27. Pollard, K.S.; Hubisz, M.J.; Rosenbloom, K.R.; Siepel, A. Detection of nonneutral substitution rates on mammalian phylogenies. *Genome Res.* **2010**, *20*, 110–121. [CrossRef] [PubMed]
28. Cooper, G.M.; Stone, E.A.; Asimenos, G.; NISC Comparative Sequencing Program; Green, E.D.; Batzoglou, S.; Sidow, A. Distribution and intensity of constraint in mammalian genomic sequence. *Genome Res.* **2005**, *15*, 901–913. [CrossRef] [PubMed]
29. Desmet, F.-O.; Hamroun, D.; Lalande, M.; Collod-Béroud, G.; Claustres, M.; Béroud, C. Human Splicing Finder: An online bioinformatics tool to predict splicing signals. *Nucleic Acids Res.* **2009**, *37*, e67. [CrossRef]
30. Shearer, A.E.; Kolbe, D.L.; Azaiez, H.; Sloan, C.M.; Frees, K.L.; Weaver, A.E.; Clark, E.T.; Nishimura, C.J.; Black-Ziegelbein, E.A.; Smith, R.J.H. Copy number variants are a common cause of non-syndromic hearing loss. *Genome Med.* **2014**, *6*, 37. [CrossRef]
31. McGuirt, W.T.; Prasad, S.D.; Griffith, A.J.; Kunst, H.P.M.; Green, G.E.; Shpargel, K.B.; Runge, C.; Huybrechts, C.; Mueller, R.F.; Lynch, E.; et al. Mutations in COL11A2 cause non-syndromic hearing loss (DFNA13). *Nat. Genet.* **1999**, *23*, 413–419. [CrossRef]
32. Vona, B.; Hofrichter, M.A.H.; Neuner, C.; Schröder, J.; Gehrig, A.; Hennermann, J.B.; Kraus, F.; Shehata-Dieler, W.; Klopocki, E.; Nanda, I.; et al. DFNB16 is a frequent cause of congenital hearing impairment: Implementation of STRC mutation analysis in routine diagnostics. *Clin. Genet.* **2015**, *87*, 49–55. [CrossRef]
33. Numakura, C.; Lin, C.; Ikegami, T.; Guldberg, P.; Hayasaka, K. Molecular analysis in Japanese patients with Charcot-Marie-Tooth disease: DGGE analysis for PMP22, MPZ, and Cx32/GJB1 mutations. *Hum. Mutat.* **2002**, *20*, 392–398. [CrossRef] [PubMed]

34. Wattenhofer, M.; Reymond, A.; Falciola, V.; Charollais, A.; Caille, D.; Borel, C.; Lyle, R.; Estivill, X.; Petersen, M.B.; Meda, P.; et al. Different mechanisms preclude mutant CLDN14 proteins from forming tight junctions in vitro. *Hum. Mutat.* **2005**, *25*, 543–549. [CrossRef] [PubMed]
35. Ruf, R.G.; Xu, P.X.; Silvius, D.; Otto, E.A.; Beekmann, F.; Muerb, U.T.; Kumar, S.; Neuhaus, T.J.; Kemper, M.J.; Raymond, R.M.; et al. SIX1 mutations cause branchio-oto-renal syndrome by disruption of EYA1-SIX1-DNA complexes. *Proc. Natl. Acad. Sci. USA* **2004**, *101*, 8090–8095. [CrossRef] [PubMed]
36. Sheppard, S.; Biswas, S.; Li, M.H.; Jayaraman, V.; Slack, I.; Romasko, E.J.; Sasson, A.; Brunton, J.; Rajagopalan, R.; Sarmady, M.; et al. Utility and limitations of exome sequencing as a genetic diagnostic tool for children with hearing loss. *Genet. Med.* **2018**, *20*, 1663–1676. [CrossRef]
37. Lenarduzzi, S.; Morgan, A.; Faletra, F.; Cappellani, S.; Morgutti, M.; Mezzavilla, M.; Peruzzi, A.; Ghiselli, S.; Ambrosetti, U.; Graziano, C.; et al. Next generation sequencing study in a cohort of Italian patients with syndromic hearing loss. *Hear. Res.* **2019**, *381*. [CrossRef]
38. Rodríguez-Ballesteros, M.; Reynoso, R.; Olarte, M.; Villamar, M.; Morera, C.; Santarelli, R.; Arslan, E.; Medá, C.; Curet, C.; Völter, C.; et al. A multicenter study on the prevalence and spectrum of mutations in the otoferlin gene (*OTOF*) in subjects with nonsyndromic hearing impairment and auditory neuropathy. *Hum. Mutat.* **2008**, *29*, 823–831. [CrossRef]
39. Magliulo, G.; Iannella, G.; Gagliardi, S.; Iozzo, N.; Plateroti, R.; Mariottini, A.; Torricelli, F. Usher's Syndrome Type II: A Comparative Study of Genetic Mutations and Vestibular System Evaluation. *Otolaryngol. Head Neck Surg.* **2017**, *157*, 853–860. [CrossRef]
40. Rivolta, C.; Sweklo, E.A.; Berson, E.L.; Dryja, T.P. Missense mutation in the USH2A gene: Association with recessive retinitis pigmentosa without hearing loss. *Am. J. Hum. Genet.* **2000**, *66*, 1975–1978. [CrossRef]
41. Van Wijk, E.; Pennings, R.J.E.; Te Brinke, H.; Claassen, A.; Yntema, H.G.; Hoefsloot, L.H.; Cremers, F.P.M.; Cremers, W.R.J.; Kremer, H. Identification of 51 Novel Exons of the Usher Syndrome Type 2A (USH2A) Gene That Encode Multiple Conserved Functional Domains and That Are Mutated in Patients with Usher Syndrome Type II. *Am. J. Hum. Genet.* **2004**, *74*, 738–744. [CrossRef]
42. Choi, B.Y.; Park, G.; Gim, J.; Kim, A.R.; Kim, B.J.; Kim, H.S.; Park, J.H.; Park, T.; Oh, S.H.; Han, K.H.; et al. Diagnostic Application of Targeted Resequencing for Familial Nonsyndromic Hearing Loss. *PLoS ONE* **2013**, *8*. [CrossRef]
43. Ebermann, I.; Phillips, J.B.; Liebau, M.C.; Koenekoop, R.K.; Schermer, B.; Lopez, I.; Schäfer, E.; Roux, A.F.; Dafinger, C.; Bernd, A.; et al. PDZD7 is a modifier of retinal disease and a contributor to digenic Usher syndrome. *J. Clin. Invest.* **2010**, *120*, 1812–1823. [CrossRef]
44. Shearer, A.E.; DeLuca, A.P.; Hildebrand, M.S.; Taylor, K.R.; Gurrola, J.; Scherer, S.; Scheetz, T.E.; Smith, R.J.H. Comprehensive genetic testing for hereditary hearing loss using massively parallel sequencing. *Proc. Natl. Acad. Sci. USA* **2010**, *107*, 21104–21109. [CrossRef]
45. Sloan-Heggen, C.M.; Bierer, A.O.; Shearer, A.E.; Kolbe, D.L.; Nishimura, C.J.; Frees, K.L.; Ephraim, S.S.; Shibata, S.B.; Booth, K.T.; Campbell, C.A.; et al. Comprehensive genetic testing in the clinical evaluation of 1119 patients with hearing loss. *Hum. Genet.* **2016**, *135*, 441–450. [CrossRef] [PubMed]
46. Atik, T.; Onay, H.; Aykut, A.; Bademci, G.; Kirazli, T.; Tekin, M.; Ozkinay, F. Comprehensive analysis of deafness genes in families with autosomal recessive nonsyndromic hearing loss. *PLoS ONE* **2015**, *10*. [CrossRef]
47. Tassabehji, M.; Read, A.P.; Newton, V.E.; Patton, M.; Gruss, P.; Harris, R.; Strachan, T. Mutations in the PAX3 gene causing Waardenburg syndrome type 1 and type 2. *Nat. Genet.* **1993**, *3*, 26–30. [CrossRef] [PubMed]
48. Chen, M.H.; Walsh, C.A. *FLNA-Related Periventricular Nodular Heterotopia*; University of Washington: Seattle, WA, USA, 1993.
49. Schultz, J.M.; Yang, Y.; Caride, A.J.; Filoteo, A.G.; Penheiter, A.R.; Lagziel, A.; Morell, R.J.; Mohiddin, S.A.; Fananapazir, L.; Madeo, A.C.; et al. Modification of human hearing loss by plasma-membrane calcium pump PMCA2. *N. Engl. J. Med.* **2005**, *352*, 1557–1564. [CrossRef] [PubMed]
50. Smits, J.J.; Oostrik, J.; Beynon, A.J.; Kant, S.G.; de Koning Gans, P.A.M.; Rotteveel, L.J.C.; Klein Wassink-Ruiter, J.S.; Free, R.H.; Maas, S.M.; van de Kamp, J.; et al. De novo and inherited loss-of-function variants of ATP2B2 are associated with rapidly progressive hearing impairment. *Hum. Genet.* **2019**, *138*, 61–72. [CrossRef] [PubMed]

51. Lu, X.; Wang, Q.; Gu, H.; Zhang, X.; Qi, Y.; Liu, Y. Whole exome sequencing identified a second pathogenic variant in HOMER2 for autosomal dominant non-syndromic deafness. *Clin. Genet.* **2018**, *94*, 419–428. [CrossRef]
52. Vozzi, D.; Morgan, A.; Vuckovic, D.; D'Eustacchio, A.; Abdulhadi, K.; Rubinato, E.; Badii, R.; Gasparini, P.; Girotto, G. Hereditary hearing loss: A 96 gene targeted sequencing protocol reveals novel alleles in a series of Italian and Qatari patients. *Gene* **2014**, *542*, 209–216. [CrossRef]
53. Shearer, A.E.; Eppsteiner, R.W.; Frees, K.; Tejani, V.; Sloan-Heggen, C.M.; Brown, C.; Abbas, P.; Dunn, C.; Hansen, M.R.; Gantz, B.J.; et al. Genetic variants in the peripheral auditory system significantly affect adult cochlear implant performance. *Hear. Res.* **2017**, *348*, 138–142. [CrossRef]

Publisher's Note: MDPI stays neutral with regard to jurisdictional claims in published maps and institutional affiliations.

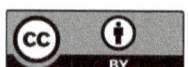

© 2020 by the authors. Licensee MDPI, Basel, Switzerland. This article is an open access article distributed under the terms and conditions of the Creative Commons Attribution (CC BY) license (http://creativecommons.org/licenses/by/4.0/).

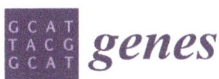

Article

Improving the Management of Patients with Hearing Loss by the Implementation of an NGS Panel in Clinical Practice

Gema García-García [1,2,*], Alba Berzal-Serrano [1], Piedad García-Díaz [3], Rebeca Villanova-Aparisi [1], Sara Juárez-Rodríguez [1], Carlos de Paula-Vernetta [3,4], Laura Cavallé-Garrido [1,3,4], Teresa Jaijo [1,2,5], Miguel Armengot-Carceller [1,3,4,6], José M Millán [1,2] and Elena Aller [1,2,5]

1. Group of Molecular, Cellular and Genomic Biomedicine, IIS-La Fe, 46026 Valencia, Spain; berzalserrano@gmail.com (A.B.-S.); rebeca.va95@gmail.com (R.V.-A.); sarajuarezrodriguez@gmail.com (S.J.-R.); cavalle_lau@gva.es (L.C.-G.); jaijo_ter@gva.es (T.J.); miguel.armengot@uv.es (M.A.-C.); millan_jos@gva.es (J.M.M.); aller_ele@gva.es (E.A.)
2. CIBER of Rare Diseases (CIBERER), 28029 Madrid, Spain
3. ENT Department, Polytechnic and University Hospital La Fe, 46026 Valencia, Spain; piedadgardiaz@gmail.com (P.G.-D.); depaula_car@gva.es (C.d.P.-V.)
4. Surgery Department, University of Valencia, 46026 Valencia, Spain
5. Units of Genetics, Polytechnic and University Hospital La Fe, 46026 Valencia, Spain
6. CIBER of Respiratory Diseases (CIBERES), 28029 Madrid, Spain
* Correspondence: gegarcia@ciberer.es; Tel.: +34-961246678

Received: 3 November 2020; Accepted: 3 December 2020; Published: 7 December 2020

Abstract: A cohort of 128 patients from 118 families diagnosed with non-syndromic or syndromic hearing loss (HL) underwent an exhaustive clinical evaluation. Molecular analysis was performed using targeted next-generation sequencing (NGS) with a custom panel that included 59 genes associated with non-syndromic HL or syndromic HL. Variants were prioritized according to the minimum allele frequency and classified according to the American College of Medical Genetics and Genomics guidelines. Variant(s) responsible for the disease were detected in a 40% of families including autosomal recessive (AR), autosomal dominant (AD) and X-linked patterns of inheritance. We identified pathogenic or likely pathogenic variants in 26 different genes, 15 with AR inheritance pattern, 9 with AD and 2 that are X-linked. Fourteen of the found variants are novel. This study highlights the clinical utility of targeted NGS for sensorineural hearing loss. The optimal panel for HL must be designed according to the spectrum of the most represented genes in a given population and the laboratory capabilities considering the pressure on healthcare.

Keywords: hearing loss; next-generation sequencing; genetics; molecular analysis; clinical evaluation

1. Introduction

Hearing loss (HL) is the most common sensory deficit in humans [1]. According to data from the World Health Organization, it is estimated that more than 5% of the world's population suffers from this disease, that is, around 360 million people.

HL can be classified as conductive, sensorineural or mixed (a combination of both); acquired or hereditary; prelingual or postlingual; and non-syndromic (NSHL) or syndromic, as a part of a more complex phenotype, that account up to 30% of HL cases [2].

HL is one of the most common birth defects, with an incidence of 1–2 per 1000 newborns and growing as age increases, reaching more than 300 per 1000 in those over 75 years of age. This high incidence is due to both environmental and genetic factors. The genetic contribution to newborn HL has been reported to be 50–60% depending of the study and the population [3,4].

As the rate of acquired hearing loss secondary to environmental causes decreases, the significance of genetic factors that lead to deafness increases [5]. To date, over 120 genes have been associated with NSHL (Hereditary Hearing Loss Homepage: https://hereditaryhearingloss.org/), and over 400 syndromes have been associated with hearing impairment [6]. These genes encode proteins of a very diverse nature and are involved in different pathways, such as mechanotransduction, ear structures, ion homeostasis, etc.

Genetic confirmation of hearing loss is essential to the provision of genetic counseling, to ascertain the risk of recurrence and, in some cases, to determine the prognosis and select the best rehabilitation options. Furthermore, although the utility of molecular diagnosis is still limited for therapeutic approaches, a growing number of gene-based strategies to treat HL have been carried out in recent years at preclinical stages [7].

In the last decade, next generation sequencing (NGS), including custom targeted panels and whole exome sequencing, has revolutionized the genetic screening of disorders with high genetic and allelic heterogeneity, such as hearing loss, allowing hundreds of genes in several patients to be screened simultaneously in a short time and in a cost-effective manner.

In this study, we assess the efficacy of a home-designed panel for hearing loss in the Genetics Department of a tertiary university hospital.

2. Materials and Methods

2.1. Patients and Samples

A total of 128 patients from 118 families diagnosed with non-syndromic or syndromic HL were included in our study. Most patients were of Spanish origin, except for three patients that came from Eastern Europe, two patients that were from Maghreb, two patients that were of sub-Saharan origin and one patient that was from East Asia. Patients were recruited from September 2017 to December 2019. Most patients presented with non-syndromic hearing loss, but we also received for screening four patients with Usher syndrome (USH), two with Waardenburg syndrome (WS) and two patients with branchio-oto-renal syndrome (BOR). Patients were enrolled through the Department of Otolaryngology of the University Hospital La Fe, according to standard assistance procedures. Comprehensive clinical evaluations, imaging examination, pure-tone audiograms, auditory brainstem response and other relevant medical information were collected for the probands to characterize the type and severity of HL. All recruited patients presented sensorineural or mixed HL. Hearing loss severity was established as mild (between >25 and ≤40 dB), moderate (between >40 and ≤70 dB) or severe/profound (>70 dB).

Written informed consent was obtained from all participants or their legal guardians. This study was approved by the Hospital La Fe Ethics Committee in agreement with the Declaration of Helsinki (REV03/5/2014).

Genomic DNA (gDNA) from the patients and relatives was obtained and purified using the automated DNA extractor QIAsymphony (QIAGEN, Hombrechtikon, Switzerland). The concentration of the resulting DNA samples was determined with Nanodrop and Qubit fluorometer (Thermo Fisher Scientific, Waltham, MA, USA)

2.2. Panel Design

We designed an NGS panel for the analysis of hereditary hearing loss using the SureDesign tool (Agilent Technologies, Santa Clara, CA, USA). The genes that were included in this panel were selected according to the prevalence reported in different studies [1,8–10] choosing those with the highest prevalence. Finally, the panel included the coding regions and flanking intronic regions (+/−25 bp) of 59 genes, 35 of them associated with non-syndromic HL, and 24 genes associated with syndromic HL (Table 1). The panel also included five deep intronic regions of the *USH2A* gene [11–13].

Table 1. The Table Indicates the Genes Included in this Study and the Associated Phenotype.

Gene	Phenotype	Gene	Phenotype
ACTG1	NSHL	TRIOBP	NSHL
CEP250	NSHL	CDH23	USH/NSHL
CHD7	CHARGE	CIB2	USH/NSHL
CISD2	NSHL	DFNB31	USH/NSHL
CLDN14	NSHL	MYO7A	USH/NSHL
COCH	NSHL	PCDH15	USH/NSHL
DFNA5	NSHL	USH1C	USH/NSHL
DFNB59	NSHL	USH1G	USH/NSHL
ESPN	NSHL	EDN3	WS
EYA4	NSHL	EDNRB	WS
GJB2	NSHL	MITF	WS
GJB6	NSHL	PAX3	WS
KCNQ4	NSHL	SNAI2	WS
LHFPL5	NSHL	SOX10	WS
LOXHD1	NSHL	EYA1	BOR
LRTOMT	NSHL	SIX1	BOR
MYH9	NSHL	SIX5	BOR
MYH14	NSHL	ADGRV1	USH
MYO6	NSHL	CLRN1	USH
MYO15A	NSHL	USH2A	USH
OTOA	NSHL	KCNE1	JLNS
OTOF	NSHL	KCNQ1	JLNS
OTOG	NSHL	COL11A2	Stickler/NSHL
OTOGL	NSHL	SEMA3E	CHARGE
POU3F4	NSHL	SLC26A4	Pendred/NSHL
PTPRQ	NSHL	WFS1	WF/NSHL
SMPX	NSHL	chr1:215827262-215827362	USH
STRC	NSHL	chr1:215967733-215967833	USH
TECTA	NSHL	chr1:216039671-216039771	USH
TIMM8A	NSHL	chr1:216064520-216064560	USH
TMC1	NSHL	chr1:216247426-216247526	USH
TMPRSS3	NSHL		
TPRN	NSHL		

NSHL: Non-syndromic hearing loss, USH: Usher syndrome, WS: Waardenburg syndrome, BOR: BOR syndrome, JLNS: Jervell and Lange-Nielsen syndrome, Stickler: Stickler syndrome, CHARGE: Charge syndrome, Pendred: Pendred syndrome, WF: Wolfram syndrome.

We tried to include some extra probes for the regions of *ESPN*, *OTOA* and *STRC* genes showing high homology with their pseudogenes, in addition to the default probes generated by the *SureDesign* software (Agilent Technologies, Santa Clara, CA, USA). Three extra probes were designed and included for *ESPN* (chr1:6500314-6500500, chr1:6500686-6500868, chr1:6505724-6505995) and seven for *OTOA* (chr16:21742158-21742251, chr16:21752042-21752229, chr16:21756202-21756357, chr16:21763256-21763398, chr16:21763690-21763826, chr16:21768403-21768598, chr16:21771791-21772050). However, bioinformatic tools failed to design extra probes for *STRC*, due to the fact that *STRC* is 99.6% identical to its pseudogene (*pSTRC*).

2.3. Library Preparation and Sequencing

The library preparation was carried out according to the Bravo NGS SureSelectQXT Automated Target Enrichment protocol (Agilent Technologies, Santa Clara, CA, USA) for Illumina Multiplexed Sequencing. Sequencing analysis was performed sequentially in batches of 16 patients. The libraries were sequenced on a MiSeq instrument with a MiSeq v2 300 cycle reagent kit (Illumina, San Diego, CA, USA).

2.4. Data Analysis

The resulting sequencing data were analyzed with the Alissa software tool (Agilent Technologies, Santa Clara, CA, USA) in regard to the human assembly GRCh37/hg19. This software performs the alignment, variant calling and annotation of the variants. The annotated variants were filtered according to a minor allele frequency (MAF) value ≤ 0.02 (the frequency of the variants was explored in the Exome Aggregation Consortium (ExAC) database, genomeAD (https://gnomad.broadinstitute.org/) and 1000 genomes (https://www.internationalgenome.org/). To classify the variants, we also took into account their annotation in the dbSNP (www.ncbi.nlm.nih.gov/SNP/), their description in ClinVar (https://www.ncbi.nlm.nih.gov/clinvar/), Varsome (https://Varsome.com/), HGMD (http://www.hgmd.cf.ac.uk/), LOVD (https://www.lovd.nl/) and Deafness Variation Database (http://deafnessvariationdatabase.org/) and the variant type. Novel missense variants were evaluated with the predictors included in the Varsome website and Alissa software: *BayesDel_addAF, DANN, DEOGEN2, EIGEN, FATHMM-MKL, M-CAP, MVP, MutationAssessor, MutationTaster, REVEL* and *SIFT*.

To predict the potential effect of the variants on the splicing, we used the bioinformatic tools *MaxEnt* and *Splice AI*.

Sanger sequencing (BigDye Terminator kit v1.1, Applied Biosystems, Carlsbad, CA, USA) was carried out to validate the pathogenic and likely pathogenic point variants and to perform segregation analysis when patients' relatives were available.

To detect copy number variations (CNVs), we carried out an analysis using the DECoN v1.0.2 program [14], which is a tool that detects variants in copy number from aligned sequences based on the number of reads for each position. The CNVs obtained by this program were checked using the multiplex ligation-dependent probe amplification technique (MLPA): *OTOA + STRC* (P461 salsa) (MRC-Holland, Amsterdam, The Netherlands). Deletions previously described to affect the DFNB1 locus were confirmed by multiplex PCR [15]. These MLPA reagents were also performed in patients with only one pathogenic variant detected in a gene with (autosomal recessive) AR inheritance.

3. Results

We aimed to obtain a median read depth greater than 100×. Coverages obtained were around 150×–200×, and 98% of analyzable target regions were covered by at least 20 reads. However, some regions of 3 genes with homologous pseudogenes (*ESPN, OTOA* and especially *STRC*) were not well covered. These regions are detailed in Table S1.

We detected the variant(s) responsible for the disease in 47 out of 118 families (40%), 27 with an AR inheritance pattern, 18 with AD and 2 with an X-linked pattern (Table 2). Detailed clinical data from the diagnosed patients are shown in Table 2.

We identified candidate variants in 26 different genes, 15 with AR inheritance pattern, 9 with AD and 2 with an X-linked pattern (Figure 1). Among the 54 different candidate variants detected, 24 were missense, 7 frameshift, 11 nonsense, 2 inframe ins/del, 3 CNVs and 7 affected to the splice-site. Fourteen out of 54 variants were novel (Tables 2 and 3).

Table 2. Disease Causing Variants Detected and Clinical Data of the Diagnosed Patients.

(A) Patients Diagnosed with Autosomal Recessive Deafness

Family	Patient	Sex	Age	Diagnosis	Gene	Allele 1	Allele 2	Phenotype
1	33311	M	1	NSHL	GJB2 NM_004004.5	c.35del/p.(Gly12Valfs *2) [16]	c.35del/p.(Gly12Valfs *2) [16]	SNHL, bilateral, symmetrical, prelingual, severe, stable
2	35961	F	2	NSHL	GJB2 NM_004004.5	c.35del/p.(Gly12Valfs *2) [16]	c.35del/p.(Gly12Valfs *2) [16]	SNHL, bilateral, symmetrical, prelingual, moderate, stable
3	39026	F	0	NSHL	GJB2 NM_004004.5	c.35del/p.(Gly12Valfs *2) [16]	c.35del/p.(Gly12Valfs *2) [16]	SNHL, bilateral, symmetrical, prelingual, severe-profound, stable
4	39611	F	5	NSHL	GJB2 NM_004004.5	c.596C > T/p.(Ser199Phe) [17]	c.35del/p.(Gly12Valfs *2) [16]	SNHL, bilateral, symmetrical, postlingual, severe, stable
5	40372	M	5	NSHL	GJB2 NM_004004.5	c.617A > G/p.(Asn206Ser) [18]	c.269dup/p.(Val91Serfs *11) [19]	SNHL, bilateral, symmetrical, postlingual, mild-moderate, stable
6	42105	M	0	NSHL	GJB2 NM_004004.5	c.101T > C/p.(Met34Thr) [20]	c.427C > T/p.(Arg143Trp) [21]	SNHL, bilateral, symmetrical, prelingual, moderate, stable
7	28981	M	0	NSHL	GJB2 NM_004004.5 / GJB6 NM_001110219.2	c.35del/p.(Gly12Valfs *2) [16]	del(GJB6-D13S1830) [22]	SNHL, bilateral, symmetrical, prelingual, profound, stable
8	34307	M	0	NSHL	GJB2 NM_004004.5 / GJB6 NM_001110219.2	c.269dup/p.(Val91Serfs *11) [19]	del(GJB6-D13S1830) [22]	SNHL, bilateral, symmetrical, prelingual, profound, stable
9	37468	M	1	NSHL	GJB2 NM_004004.5 / GJB6 NM_001110219.2	c.617A > G/p.(Asn206Ser) [18]	del(GJB6-D13S1830) [22]	SNHL, bilateral, symmetrical, prelingual, profound, stable

Table 2. Cont.

#	ID	Sex	Age	Type	Gene	Variant 1	Variant 2	Phenotype
10	37439	F	5	NSHL	STRC NM_153700.2	Whole gene deletion (15q15) [23]	Whole gene deletion (15q15) [23]	SNHL, bilateral, symmetrical, postlingual, moderate, stable
					GJB2 NM_004004.5	c.101T > C/p.(Met34Thr) [20]	—	
11	33416	F	7	NSHL	STRC NM_153700.2	Whole gene deletion (15q15) [23]	Whole gene deletion (15q15) [23]	SNHL, bilateral, symmetrical, postlingual, moderate, stable
12	37112	M	4	NSHL	STRC NM_153700.2	Whole gene deletion (15q15) [23]	Whole gene deletion (15q15) [23]	SNHL, bilateral, symmetrical, postlingual, moderate, stable
13	31410	M	5	NSHL	OTOF NM_194248.2	c.4275G > A/p.(Trp1425 *) [24]	c.2485C > T/p.(Gln829 *) [25]	SNHL, bilateral, symmetrical, prelingual, profound, stable
14	40184	F	0	NSHL	OTOF NM_194248.2	c.2485C > T/p.(Gln829 *) [25]	c.2485C > T/p.(Gln829 *) [25]	SNHL, bilateral, symmetrical, prelingual, profound, stable
14	41793	F	0	NSHL	OTOF NM_194248.2	c.2485C > T/p.(Gln829 *) [25]	c.2485C > T/p.(Gln829 *) [25]	SNHL, bilateral, symmetrical, prelingual, profound, stable
15	34197	F	54	NSHL	LOXHD1 NM_144612.6	c.3419dup/p.(Leu1140Phefs *5)	c.3419dup/p.(Leu1140Phefs *5)	SNHL, bilateral, symmetrical, postlingual, moderate–severe, stable
16	34865	M	7	NSHL	LOXHD1 NM_144612.6	c.4480C > T/p.(Arg1494 *) [26]	c.4480C > T/p.(Arg1494 *) [26]	SNHL, bilateral, symmetrical, postlingual, moderate, stable
17	29440	M	33	NSHL	OTOA NM_144672.3	c.877C > T/p.(Gln293 *)	Whole gene deletion (16q12.2 region) [27]	SNHL, bilateral, postlingual, moderate, stable
18	37140	M	4	NSHL	OTOA NM_144672.3	Whole gene deletion (16q12.2 region) [27]	Whole gene deletion (16q12.2 region) [27]	SNHL, bilateral, symmetrical, postlingual, moderate, stable

Table 2. Cont.

	ID	Sex	Age	Type	Gene	Variant 1	Variant 2	Phenotype
19	29865	F	46	NSHL	TMPRSS3 NM_024022.2	c.1276G > A/p.(Ala426Thr) [28]	c.1159G > A/p.(Ala387Thr) [29]	SNHL, bilateral, symmetrical, postlingual, mild–moderate, progressive
19	38198	F	40	NSHL	TMPRSS3 NM_024022.2	c.1276G > A/p.(Ala426Thr) [28]	**c.235T > C/p.(Cys79Arg)**	SNHL, bilateral, symmetrical, postlingual, profound, progressive
20	42108	F	1	NSHL	MYO15A NM_016239.3	c.8968-1G > T [30]	c.8968-1G > T [30]	SNHL, bilateral, symmetrical, prelingual, severe, stable
21	37513	M	4	NSHL/EVA	SLC26A4 NM_000441.1	c.1540C > A/p.(Gln514Lys) [31]	c.1540C > A/p.(Gln514Lys) [31]	SNHL, bilateral, asymmetrical, postlingual, Right: profound Left: moderate, stable, EVA
22	36777	F	1	NSHL	OTOG NM_001277269.1	**c.2140dup/p.(Ser714Lysfs *22)**	**c.2140dup/p.(Ser714Lysfs *22)**	SNHL, bilateral, symmetrical, prelingual, moderate, stable
23	39949	F	18	NSHL	TECTA NM_005422.2	c.4055G > A/p.(Cys1352Tyr) [32]	c.4055G > A/p.(Cys1352Tyr) [32]	SNHL, bilateral, moderate
					MYO7A NM_000260.3	c.5648G > A/p.(Arg1883Gln) [33]		
24	40453	F	40	NSHL	MYO7A NM_000260.3	c.1232T > C/p.(Val411Ala) [34]	c.6025del/p.(Ala2009Profs *32) [35]	SNHL, bilateral, symmetrical, postlingual, mild, stable
25	27862	M	30	USH	ADGRV1 NM_032119.3	c.12528-1G > T [36]	c.17933A > G/p.(His5978Arg) [37]	SNHL, congenital, moderate, retinitis pigmentosa
26	30816	F	1	USH	CDH23 NM_022124.5	**c.310G > T/p.(Glu104*)**	c.2289 + 1G > A [38]	SNHL, bilateral, symmetrical, prelingual, profound, stable, bilateral, vestibular areflexia, retinitis pigmentosa

Table 2. Cont.

Family	Patient	Sex	Age	Diagnosis	Gene	Allele 1	Allele 2	Phenotype
27	27734	F	49	USH	USH2A NM_206933.2	c.9799T > C/p.(Cys3267Arg) [39]	c.9676C > T/p.(Arg3226 *) [40]	SNHL, bilateral, symmetrical, postlingual, moderate, stable, retinitis pigmentosa
(B) Patients Diagnosed with Autosomal Dominant Deafness								
Family	Patient	Sex	Age	Diagnosis	Gene	Allele 1	Allele 2	Phenotype
28	32954	M	46	NSHL	MYO6 NM_004999.3	c.2545C > T/p.(Arg849 *) [41]		SNHL, bilateral, symmetrical, postlingual, moderate, stable
28	32955	F	15	NSHL	MYO6 NM_004999.3	c.2545C > T/p.(Arg849 *) [41]		SNHL, bilateral, symmetrical, moderate, stable
29	35197	F	37	NSHL	MYO6 NM_004999.3	c.1666C > T/p.(Arg556 *)		SNHL, bilateral, symmetrical, postlingual, moderate, stable
30	40488	F	30	NSHL	MYO6 NM_004999.3	c.1224-9del		SNHL, bilateral, asymmetrical, postlingual, severe-profound, progressive
31	31110	M	42	NSHL	MYO6 NM_004999.3	c.1674 + 1G > A		SNHL, bilateral, symmetrical, postlingual, moderate, stable
31	36163	M	32	NSHL	ESPN NM_031475.2	c.1674 + 1G > A	c.2467C > T/p.(Gln823 *)	SNHL, bilateral, symmetrical, postlingual, moderate, stable
32	29272	M	46	NSHL	MYO6 NM_004999.3	c.2751dup/p.(Gln918Thrfs *24) [42]		SNHL, postlingual
32					ESPN NM_031475.2	c.2230G > A/p.(Asp744Asn) [43]		

Table 2. Cont.

32	41950	F 61	NSHL	MYO6 NM_004999.3	c.2751dup/p.(Gln918Thrfs *24) [42]	SNHL, postlingual
33	41268	M 18	NSHL	ESPN NM_031475.2 MYO6 NM_004999.3	c.2230G > A/p.(Asp744Asn) [43] **c.494T > G/p.(Leu165Arg)**	SNHL, bilateral, symmetrical, postlingual, profound, progressive, tinnitus
34	33945	M 3	NSHL	MYO7A NM_000260.3 TECTA NM_005422.2	c.1997G > A/p.(Arg666Gln) [44] c.3527G > A/p.(Ser1176Asn) [8]	SNHL, bilateral, asymmetrical, prelingual, stable
35	35453	M 2	NSHL	TECTA NM_005422.2	c.5668C > T/p.(Arg1890Cys) [45]	SNHL, bilateral, symmetrical, prelingual, moderate, stable
36	38971	F 0	NSHL	TECTA NM_005422.2	c.5383 + 5_5383 + 8del [46]	SNHL, bilateral, symmetrical, prelingual, moderate, stable
36	39927	F 0	NSHL	TECTA NM_005422.2	c.5509T > G/p.(Cys1837Gly) [47] c.5509T > G/p.(Cys1837Gly) [47]	SNHL, unilateral, asymmetrical, prelingual, moderate-severe, progressive
37	4293	M 6	NSHL	COL11A2 NM_080680.2	**c.1748G > A/p.(Gly583Asp)**	SNHL, bilateral, symmetrical, postlingual, stable
37	31449	M 35	NSHL	COL11A2 NM_080680.2	**c.1748G > A/p.(Gly583Asp)**	SNHL, bilateral, asymmetrical, postlingual, Right: mild–moderate; Left: moderate-severe, stable

Table 2. Cont.

					Gene	Variant	Phenotype
38	35238	M	6	NSHL/Stickler	COL11A2 NM_080680.2	c.4392 + 1G > A [48]	SNHL, bilateral, symmetrical, postlingual, moderate, stable, flattened facial profile, sunken nasal root, short nose with anteverted nostrils, osteorticular problems
38	42783	F	37	NSHL/Stickler	COL11A2 NM_080680.2	c.4392 + 1G > A [48]	SNHL, flattened facial profile, osteorticular problems and maxillofacial alterations
39	40431	M	5	NSHL	WFS1 NM_006005.3	c.1463_1474dup/ p.(Val491_Pro492insLeuIleThrVal)	SNHL, bilateral, asymmetrical, postlingual, Right: profound Left: severe, progressive
40	42125	F	5	NSHL	WFS1 NM_006005.3	c.2108G > A/p.(Arg703His) [49]	SNHL, bilateral, symmetrical, postlingual, severe-profound, progressive
41	36655	M	7	NSHL	KCNQ4 NM_004700.3	c.857A > G/p.(Tyr286Cys) [50]	SNHL, bilateral, symmetrical, postlingual, moderate, stable
41	44138	M	46	NSHL	KCNQ4 NM_004700.3	c.857A > G/p.(Tyr286Cys) [50]	
42	39490	F	45	NSHL	ACTG1 NM_001199954.1	c.895C > G/p.(Leu299Val) [29]	SNHL, bilateral, asymmetrical, postlingual, right: moderate left: severe, progressive
43	40519	M	40	NSHL	EYA4 NM_004100.4	c.988C > T/p.(Gln330 *) [51]	SNHL, bilateral, asymmetrical, postlingual, right: profound left: severe, progressive, tinnitus, decrease in size of both cochlear nerves

Table 2. Cont.

Family	Patient	Sex	Age	Diagnosis	Gene	Allele 1	Allele 2	Phenotype
44	12227	M	34	WS	MITF NM_198159.2	c.943C > T/p.(Arg315 *) [52]		HL, prelingual, White forelock, Heterochromia iridis
					GJB6 NM_001110219.2	del(GJB6-D13S1830) [22]		
45	37350	M	2	BOR	EYA1 NM_000503.5	c.1540_1542del/p.(Leu514del) [53]		Mixed HL, bilateral, symmetrical, prelingual, severe, stable, 2nd branchial arch fistula, facial dysmorphia

(C) Patients Diagnosed with X-Linked Deafness

Family	Patient	Sex	Age	Diagnosis	Gene	Allele 1	Allele 2	Phenotype
46	34796	M	1	NSHL	POU3F4 (XLR) NM_000307.4	c.977T > C/p.(Phe326Ser)		Mixed HL, bilateral symmetrical, prelingual, moderate, stable, bilateral corkscrew cochlea, incomplete splitting of turns, absence of meatus and stapes fixation
47	14285	M	3	NSHL	SMPX (XLD) NM_014332.2	c.20del/p.(Pro7Glnfs *74)		SNHL, bilateral, symmetrical, postlingual, moderate, stable
47	41863	F	30	NSHL	SMPX (XLD) NM_014332.2	c.20del/p.(Pro7Glnfs *74)		SNHL, bilateral, symmetrical, postlingual, moderate, stable

The table indicates the patient and family code, sex, age (indicated in years), diagnosis, mutated gene, variants and phenotype. The variants described in the table are pathogenic or probably pathogenic, and novel variants are marked in bold. M: male, F: female, NSHL: non-syndromic hearing loss, HL: hearing loss, EVA: enlarged vestibular aqueduct, USH: Usher syndrome, WS: Waardenburg syndrome, BOR: branchio–oto–renal, XLR: recessive X-linked, XLD: dominant X-linked.

Table 3. Classification of Novel Variants Identified in this Study.

Gene	Variant		Classification	Frequency			Pathogenicity Scores		
	Nucleotide	Protein		GnomAD Exomes	GnomAD Genomes	Deafness Variation Database	Missense Pathogenicity Scores	Conservation Score (GERP)	MaxEnt
LOXHD1 NM_144612.6	c.3419dup	p.(Leu1140Phefs *5)	Pathogenic	0.0000267	NF	NF	NA	5.05	-
OTOA NM_144672.3	c.877C > T	p.(Gln293 *)	Pathogenic	NF	NF	NF	NA	5.41	-
TMPRSS3 NM_024022.2	c.235T > C	p.(Cys79Arg)	Likely Pathogenic	NF	NF	NF	11/13	5.23	-
OTOG NM_001277269.1	c.2140dup	p.(Ser714Lysfs *22)	Pathogenic	NF	NF	NF	NA	4.9	-
CDH23 NM_022124.5	c.310G > T	p.(Glu104 *)	Pathogenic	NF	NF	NF	NA	5.43	-
MYO6 NM_004999.3	c.1666C > T	p.(Arg556 *)	Pathogenic	0.0000119	NF	Unknown significance–Impact High	NA	5.77	-
MYO6 NM_004999.3	c.1224-9del	-	VUS	NF	NF	NF	NA	5.23	AS broken (from 7.08 to −4.37)
MYO6 NM_004999.3	c.1674 + 1G > A	-	Pathogenic	0.00000736	NF	Unknown significance–Impact High	NA	5.77	DS broken (from 7.94 to −0.24)
ESPN NM_031475.2	c.2467C > T	p.(Gln823 *)	Pathogenic	NF	NF	NF	NA	4.28	-
MYO6 NM_004999.3	c.494T > G	p.(Leu165Arg)	VUS	NF	NF	NF	13/13	5.45	-
COL11A2 NM_080680.2	c.1748G > A	p.(Gly583Asp)	Likely Pathogenic	NF	NF	NF	11/11	3.89	-
WFS1 NM_006005.3	c.1463_1474dup	p.(Val491_Pro492insLeuIleThrVal)	VUS	NF	NF	NF	NA	4.25	-
POU3F4 NM_000307.4	c.977T > C	p.(Phe326Ser)	Likely Pathogenic	NF	NF	NF	10/10	5.07	-
SMPX NM_014332.2	c.20del	p.(Pro7Glnfs *74)	Pathogenic	NF	NF	NF	NA	5.78	-

NF: not found; NA: not available; AS: acceptor splice-site; DS: donor splice-site. "Classification": Variants are classified according to the guidelines of the ACMG [54]. "Pathogenicity Scores" refer to the number of in silico tools that classify the variant as pathogenic/likely pathogenic versus the total of predictors used. The scores were obtained from https://Varsome.com/ (accessed November 2020) and included the followings predictors: BayesDel_addAF, DANN, DEOGEN2, EIGEN,FATHMM-MKL, LIST-S2, M-CAP, MVP, MutationAssessor, MutationTaster, PrimateAI, REVEL and SIFT. Not all predictors were available for all analyzed variants. GERP is a conservation score. The values range from −12.3 to 6.17, with 6.17 being the most conserved.

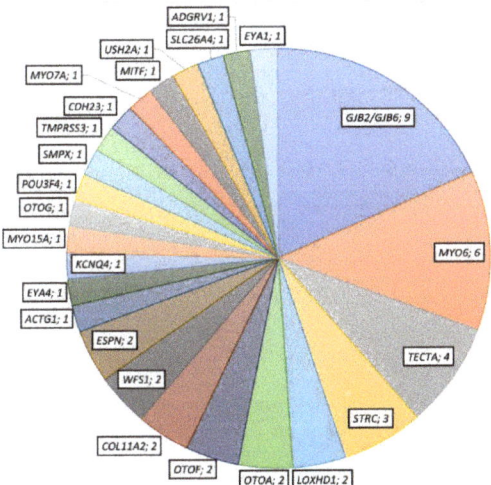

Figure 1. Number of diagnosed patients with putative disease-responsible variants in each represented gene.

3.1. Autosomal Recessive HL

Twenty-nine cases belonging to 27 families carried biallelic pathogenic or likely pathogenic variants associated with an autosomal recessive pattern of inheritance (Table 2A).

Twenty-six cases presented with NSHL. These were linked to *GJB2/GJB6* (DFNB1) (nine cases), *STRC* (three cases), *OTOF* (three cases belonging to two families), *LOXHD1* (two cases), *OTOA* (two cases), *TMPRSS3* (two cases belonging to one family) and one case in the *MYO15A*, *SLC26A4*, *OTOG*, *TECTA* and *MYO7A* genes (Figure 1). Family trees for families with more than one affected patient are displayed in Figure 2. The remaining three solved cases suffered from Usher syndrome due to putative pathogenic variants in *ADGRV1*, *CDH23* and *USH2A*, one family for each gene.

The most prevalent variants found were c.35del (*GJB2*) and del (*GJB6*-D13S1830), both affecting DFNB1 locus, followed by the complete deletion of the *STRC* gene. In all cases, the deletion of *STRC* was associated with mild to moderate postlingual hearing loss.

Five of the detected pathogenic variants were novel. Four of them produced a premature stop codon: three frameshift variants (c.3419dup/p.(Leu1140Phefs *5) in *LOXHD1*, c.877C > T/p.(Gln293 *) in *OTOA* and c.2140dup/p.(Ser714Lysfs *22) in *OTOG*) and one nonsense variant (c.310G > T/p.(Glu104 *) in *CDH23*). The only novel missense variant detected was c.235T > C/p.(Cys79Arg) in *TMPRSS3*.

3.2. Autosomal Dominant HL

We identified variants responsible for the disease associated with an autosomal dominant pattern of inheritance in 25 patients belonging to 18 families (Table 2B).

Twenty-four of these patients had been referred as non-syndromic HL. Nine patients belonging to six families presented variants in *MYO6*, four patients from three families in *TECTA*, four patients from two families in *COL11A2*, two patients from two families in *WFS1* and two patients from the same family in *KCNQ4*; pathogenic variants in *ACTG1* and *EYA4* were detected in one patient each (Table 2B and Figure 2).

One of the families linked to *COL11A2* (family 38) was found to present the pathogenic variant c.4392 + 1G > A, previously described by Brunner et al. (1994) [48] as associated with Stickler syndrome without eye affectation. This family was clinically re-evaluated and re-classified as Stickler syndrome.

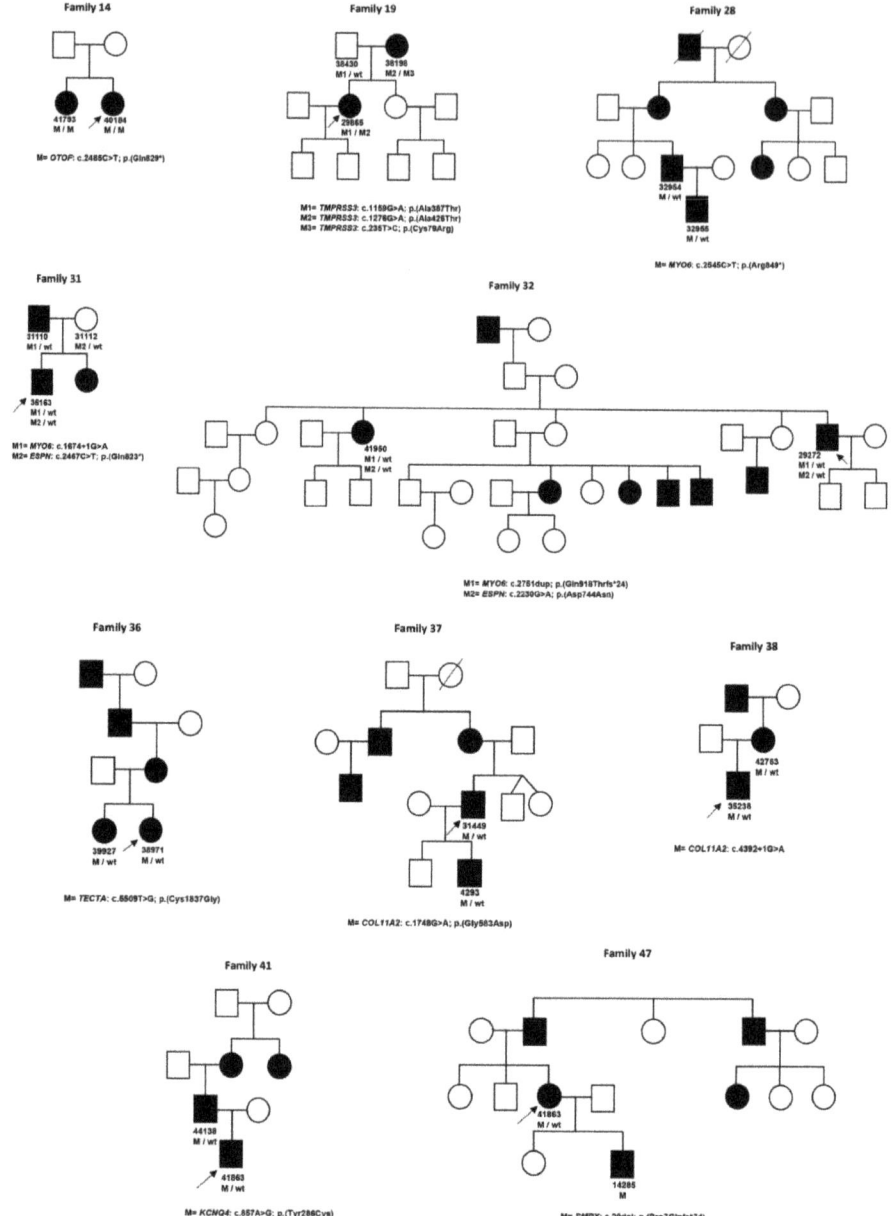

Figure 2. Pedigrees of the families and segregation analysis of the detected pathogenic or likely pathogenic variants. Arrows indicate the proband case, M indicates the pathogenic or likely pathogenic variant and wt indicates wild type sequence.

Additionally, we also detected pathogenic variants in two families with syndromic hearing loss. We found the variants responsible for the disease in one patient diagnosed with Waardenburg syndrome, presenting the variant responsible for the disease in *MITF*, and one patient diagnosed with BOR syndrome was found to present with the pathogenic variant in *EYA1*.

No prevalent pathogenic variants associated with an autosomal dominant (AD) pattern of inheritance was detected. Seven of the AD pathogenic variants identified in the present study were novel. One novel stop codon (c.1666C > T/p.(Arg556 *)) was detected in *MYO6*. Two splicing variants, none previously described, were detected; one of them was located at a canonical site (c.1674 + 1G > A in *MYO6*), and the other was located at c.1224-9del in *MYO6*. Furthermore, an in-frame novel duplication was found in *WFS1*, c.1463_1474dup/p.(Val491_Pro492insLeuIleThrVal) and two missenses variants in *COL11A2* (c.1748G > A/p.(Gly583Asp)) and *MYO6* (c.494T > G/p.(Leu165Arg)) (Table 3).

The audiogram of patient 40431, harboring the c.1463_1474dup/p.(Val491_Pro492insLeuIleThrVal) variant, showed a characteristic profile with severe threshold increases for low-frequency tones (Figure 3).

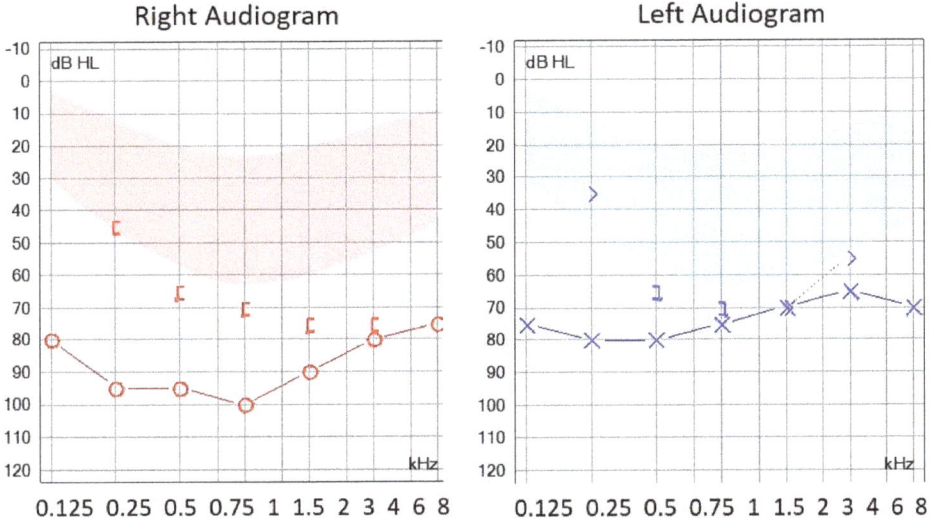

Figure 3. Audiogram performed in patient 40431 harboring the c.1463_1474dup/p.(Val491_Pro492insLeuIleThrVal) variant in the *WFS1* gene.

3.3. X-Linked HL

Variants responsible for the disease associated with an X-linked pattern of inheritance were found in three cases belonging to two families (Table 2C). One case presented a novel missense variant in *POU3F4* (recessive X-linked) and the other two cases were a boy and his mother, both carrying a novel frameshift variant in *SMPX* (dominant X-linked) (Figure 2 and Table 3).

3.4. Partially Diagnosed Patients

In 11 patients we detected one or several pathogenic variants in the heterozygous state in genes with an AR inheritance pattern. In seven cases we identified a pathogenic variant in only one gene: *USH2A* (2), *GJB2* (2), *STRC* (1), *OTOF* (1) and *CDH23* (1). In four patients we detected pathogenic variants in several different genes (Table 4)

Table 4. Patients with only One Heterozygous Pathogenic or Likely Pathogenic Variant in Genes Associated with an Autosomal Recessive Inheritance Pattern.

Patient	Diagnosis	Gene	Allele 1
40056	NSHL	USH2A NM_206933.2	c.4325T > C/p.(Phe1442Ser) [55]
31443	USH	USH2A NM_206933.2	c.2431_2432del/p.(Lys811Aspfs*11) [35]
28523	NSHL	USH2A NM_206933.2	c.2135del/p.(Ser712*) [56]
		MYO7A NM_000260.3	c.5581C > T/p.(Arg1861*) [57]
37248	NSHL	USH2A NM_206933.2	c.9244A > G/p.(Ile3082Val) [58]
		GJB2 NM_004004.5	c.109G > A/p.(Val37Ile) [59]
37986	NSHL	GJB2 NM_004004.5	c.269T > C/(p.Leu90Pro) [19]
39353	NSHL	GJB2 NM_004004.5	c.445G > A/p.(Ala149Thr) [60]
12228	NSHL	STRC NM_153700.2	**Complex rearrangement**
28358	NSHL	OTOF NM_194248.2	c.2485C > T/p.(Gln829*) [25]
35862	NSHL	OTOF NM_194248.2	c.2485C > T/p.(Gln829*) [25]
		CDH23 NM_022124.5	c.4762C > T/p.(Arg1588Trp) [61]
33335	USH	CDH23 NM_022124.5	c.2289 + 1G > A [38]
34978	NSHL	TMC1 NM_138691.2	c.1763 + 3A > G [62]
		TMPRSS3 NM_024022.2	c.280G > A/p.(Gly94Arg) [29]

NSHL: non-syndromic hearing loss, USH: Usher syndrome. Novel variants are marked in bold.

4. Discussion

The genetic diagnosis of hereditary hearing loss is highly difficult due to its enormous underlying genetic heterogeneity (more than 120 genes described up to date), which is a reflection of the high complexity of the ear structure and organization.

In the last 10 years (from 2006 to 2016), the genetic analysis of patients with hearing loss in our tertiary hospital was restricted to detect the most frequent pathogenic variants responsible for hereditary sensorineural hearing loss in Spain, specifically the complete coding sequence of the GJB2 gene, the deletions D13S1830 and delD13S1854 in the GJB6 gene and the OTOF p.Q829X variants. The implementation of our custom NGS panel containing 59 HL genes improved the management of our patients, as it has allowed us to detect putative pathogenic variants in 26 different genes. Furthermore, we have been able to genetically diagnose syndromic cases suffering from Deafness Infertility syndrome, Usher syndrome, Stickler syndrome, Waardenburg syndrome and BOR syndrome.

However, pathogenic variants in a few genes still explain a great number of hearing loss cases. The main example is GJB2, encoding connexin 26. Pathogenic variants in this gene are the most common cause of hereditary hearing loss in many populations [63]. In the present work, biallelic variants in GJB2, together with GJB6 (DFNB1 locus), were responsible for the disease in nine families with AR inheritance, followed by pathogenic variants in STRC (three AR families). Regarding AD inheritance families, heterozygous pathogenic variants in MYO6 were found in six families, followed by pathogenic variants in *TECTA* (four AD families). An additional patient presented a homozygous AR pathogenic variant in *TECTA*. All inheritance patterns have been described for HL: recessive, dominant, X-linked and mitochondrial. In some genes (like *MYO6*, *TECTA* or *ESPN*), a group of variants follow a dominant inheritance pattern, whereas others follow a recessive inheritance pattern, complicating the interpretation of genetic analysis [64]. Another feature that complicates the genetic studies of HL is the existence of some pseudogenes with high homology to some prevalent genes (like *STRC*, *OTOA* or *ESPN*). In the panel design, we tried to include some extra probes for the regions of these genes showing high homology with their pseudogenes, in addition to the default probes generated by SureDesign. However, low coverage was still obtained, and those point variants suspected to be pathogenic had to be confirmed by Sanger sequencing using primers specifically designed to hybridize only with the gene, not the pseudogene [65,66].

When a CNV affecting *STRC* or *OTOA* was suspected after DECoN v1.0.2 analysis, its presence was confirmed by MLPA using SALSA P461 (MRC Holland).

Several pathogenic variants identified in this study are reported in a large number of studies, suggesting a high prevalence. The pathogenic variant in *OTOF* c.2485C > T/p.(Gln829 *) is the third most frequent in the Spanish population that causes prelingual hearing loss [67], and *STRC* deletions are the second most frequent cause of mild-to-moderate hearing loss after the DFNB1 locus [68]. The variant c.1540C > A/p.(Gln514Lys) is the most frequent variant in *SLC26A4* in the Spanish population, described in more than 36 Spanish families to date [69]. Furthermore, the pathogenic change c.9799T > C/p.(Cys3267Arg) in *USH2A* is one of the most frequent variants in the Spanish population, specifically the third most common cause of Usher syndrome [70,71]. Finally, the pathogenic variant c.5668C T/p.(Arg1890Cys) that affects the *TECTA* gene has been described in some families from Spain, America and The Netherlands. In the most unrelated families, patients present the same haplotype, which suggests that the variant is derived from a common ancestor (founder effect) [46].

Nowadays, all known HL genes can be simultaneously analyzed thanks to the technological development of NGS. Even so, the rate of genetic diagnosis using NGS in patients with hearing loss varies around 40–60% [8,29,64,72–76] depending on many factors: the degree of HL (profound, severe, moderate), age of HL onset, the existence of family history, the ethnic origin or the number of genes contained in the NGS panel. The highest rates have usually been obtained for patients with a positive family history or when the HL was congenital and symmetric [8]. In the present work, the global diagnostic yield was 40%. This is a satisfactory yield, since our custom NGS panel included a limited number of genes (59), and the exclusion criteria for the genetic testing was very lax. Thus, the analyzed patient sample was very heterogeneous, including all types of sensorineural/mixed hearing loss (congenital, prelingual and postlingual; mild, moderate, severe and profound; and stable and progressive) with ages ranging from 0 to 61 years.

4.1. Novel VUS/Likely Pathogenic Variants

The development of NGS has revolutionized the field of genetic diagnosis, especially in extremely genetically heterogeneous diseases, such as hereditary HL. However, an elevated number of genetic variants of uncertain clinical significance (VUS) has been detected using this technology [77]. Variants predicted to generate direct stop codons or changes in the reading frame of the proteins and variants located at canonical splice sites (+/−1 and +/−2 positions of introns) are usually classified as pathological for proteins for which loss of function is reported as cause of the disease. However, the interpretation of missense, isocoding and intronic variants located out of canonical splice sites is more complex, and many times these variants remain classified as VUS. In these cases, bioinformatics predictions, segregation analyses or functional studies are required to infer the pathological character of these variants. In our study, a lot of a priori VUS variants were detected, and only seven of them were classified as likely pathogenic based upon bioinformatics predictions and/or segregation analyses: four missense, one intronic variant and one in-frame duplication.

Missense variants: The c.235T > C/p.(Cys79Arg) change in *TMPRSS3* was not found in gnomAD exomes/genomes, and 11 computational programs predicted it as pathogenic in Varsome. Furthermore, it was found in *trans* with other previously described pathogenic variants in the *TMPRSS3* (see Table 2 and Figure 2). The *MYO6* (c.494T > G/p.(Leu165Arg)) variant was found in patient 41268. He was referred to as AD non-syndromic hearing loss, being her mother, her sister and her sister's son were also affected. Although this variant was classified as VUS following the ACMG guidelines, we should not rule it out since it was not found in healthy control databases, had a high conservation score and showed a pathogenic computational verdict based on 13 pathogenic predictions. The *COL11A2* (c.1748G > A/p.(Gly583Asp)) change was found in a patient and his affected father (family 37). This variant was not present in healthy population databases, and it showed pathogenic predictions in the Alissa Interpret program based on *MutationTaster*, *MutationAssessor*, *LRT*, *PolyPhen2* and *PROVEAN*. Finally, the c.977T > C/p.(Phe326Ser) (*POU3F4*) variant was found in a boy with mixed hearing loss and cochlear malformations (bilateral corkscrew cochlea, incomplete splitting of turns, absence of meatus and stapes fixation); clinical characteristics of hearing loss are linked to this gene. Furthermore, this change was absent in healthy controls databases, and it showed a pathogenic computational verdict based on 10 pathogenic predictions in Varsome.

Intronic variant: The c.1224-9del variant in *MYO6* was found in a patient with an AD pattern of inheritance in her family, given that her mother was also affected. Unfortunately, the patient's mother refused to collaborate in the genetic study. This variant was not found in healthy control population databases, and the *MaxEnt* bioinformatic tool predicted the loss of the wild-type acceptor site. This variant was classified as VUS following the AMCG, but we consider that *MYO6* c.1224-9del could be a good candidate, and functional studies at the RNA level would be necessary to definitively confirm or discard the pathologic effect of this novel variant.

In frame duplication: The *WFS1* in-frame duplication (c.1463_1474dup/p.(Val491_Pro492insLeuIleThrVal)) was detected in a patient presenting HL also in a cousin and her son, but they did not collaborate in the study. This change was classified as VUS according to the ACMG. However, we consider that it is necessary to take this variant into account since it is not described in the population databases, has an acceptable value of conservation and, following the criteria of the ACMG, if it had been possible to show that the variant segregates correctly within the family, the WFS1 c.1463_1474dup/p.(Val491_Pro492insLeuIleThrVal) variant would be directly classified as likely pathogenic. Additionally, the clinical phenotype of this patient is similar to other patients with pathogenic variants in *WFS1*, showing a characteristic audiogram with low frequencies more affected (Figure 3).

4.2. Patients with Pathogenic Variants in Two Different Genes

NGS panels allow the simultaneous analysis of a great number of genes, and, sometimes, pathogenic variants in different genes are found in the same patient.

In the present work, the 37439 patient presented the AR c.101T > C/p.(Met34Thr) variant in *GJB2* in addition to the homozygous *STRC* whole gene deletion. Patient 39949 presented the AR c.5648G > A/p.(Arg1883Gln) variant in *MYO7A* in addition to the homozygous c.4055G > A/p.(Cys1352Tyr) AR variant in *TECTA*. These findings have important implications for reproductive genetic counseling.

The 36163 patient was found to carry two different heterozygous novel pathogenic variants in two different genes: c.1674 + 1G > A in *MYO6* and c.2467C > T/p.(Gln823 *) in *ESPN*. Segregation analysis in this family showed that the affected father also carried the variant in *MYO6*, whereas the healthy mother carried the variant in *ESPN*. From these results it can be deduced that the variant in *MYO6* is responsible for AD hearing loss, whereas the *ESPN* variant presents an AR inheritance pattern (Figure 2).

The 29272 and the 41950 patients from the same family carried two different previously described AD pathogenic variants in two different genes: c.2751dup/p.(Gln918Thrfs *24) in *MYO6* and c.2230G > A/p.(Asp744Asn) in *ESPN*. These two patients belong to a large family with more affected members, but these were geographically dispersed, and it was not possible to segregate these two variants with all family members in order to definitely elucidate the genetic basis and the inheritance pattern of HL in this case (Figure 2).

Finally, the likely pathogenic novel *MYO6* (c.494T > G/p.(Leu165Arg)) variant was found in patient 41268, referred to as AD non-syndromic hearing loss. Furthermore, two previously described AR pathogenic variants in *MYO7A* (c.1997G > A/p.(Arg666Gln) and c.3527G > A/p.(Ser1176Asn)) were found in this patient. Segregation analysis would be necessary to definitely elucidate the genetic basis and the inheritance pattern of HL in this family and to offer accurate genetic reproductive genetic counseling.

4.3. Syndromic Cases

Most patients included in this study suffered from non-syndromic hearing loss, but eight cases were referred as syndromic: four patients with Usher syndrome (USH), two Waardenburg syndrome (WS) patients and two branchio-oto-renal syndrome (BOR) patients. We could find the variants responsible for the disease in five of them (Table 2A,B).

The patient 35238 and his mother (42783) were referred as NSHL, but they were found to carry a pathogenic variant in *COL11A2*: c.4392 + 1G > A. This variant had been previously reported by Brunner et al. (1994) [48] associated with Stickler syndrome without eye affectation. These patients were clinically re-evaluated, and both presented with osteoarticular problems and flattened facial profiles (Table 2B). Thus, this family was re-classified as Stickler syndrome.

Three unrelated cases with bilateral, symmetrical, postlingual, moderate and stable HL (33416, 37112 and 37439) presented biallelic contiguous-gene deletions at chromosome 15q15.3 that included both *CATSPER2* and *STRC*. This deletion causes deafness–infertility syndrome (DIS) in males due to *CATSPER* haploinsufficiency results in sperm abnormalities [78]. The patient 37112 was a male of 4 years old. Thus, the patient´s parents were informed that their son will be infertile in adulthood.

In another case (12228), a complex rearrangement involving *STRC* and *CATSPER2* was detected (Table 3 and Figure 4). *DECoN* analysis using NGS data showed a partial deletion involving exons 1–15 of *STRC*. However, based on coverage data from NGS, we could not differentiate between *STRC* and *pSTRC*. Thus, an MLPA analysis was performed using P-461 SALSA (MRC Holland). This SALSA includes specific probes only for exons 19, 24–25 of *STRC* and also some specific probes for some exons of *CATSPER2*. MLPA results showed a partial deletion affecting exons 23, 24 and 25 of *STRC* (chr15:41680256-41682666), whereas *STRC* exon 19 showed a normal dosage (chr15:41684606-41684940). However, chromosome coordinates chr15:41711482-41728076 corresponding to *CATSPER2* showed again a ratio of 0.5. Segregation analysis would be helpful in this case to find out if this complex rearrangement is carried in the same chromosome or if there are two different deletions affecting the 15q15.3 locus, located in different alleles.

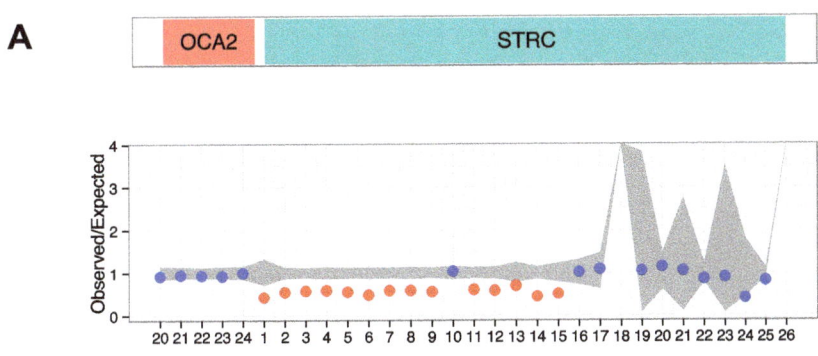

Figure 4. *Cont.*

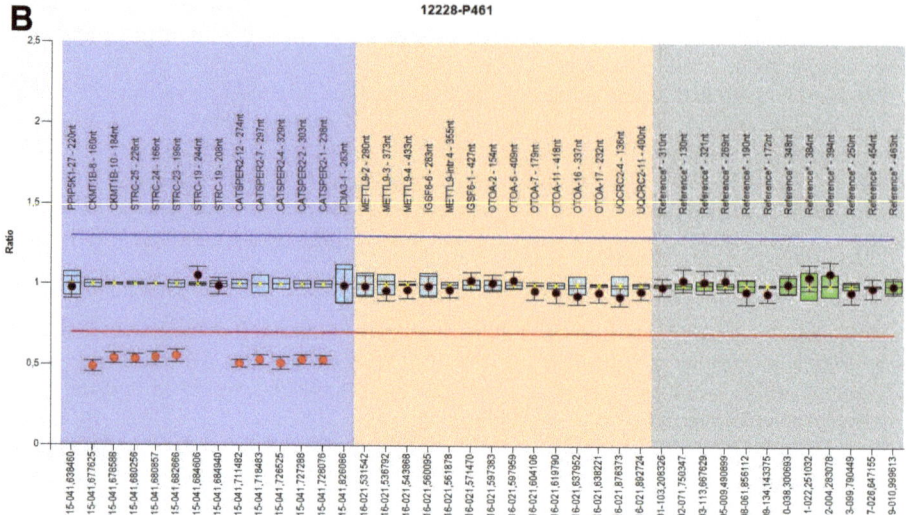

Figure 4. Complex rearrangement identified in patient 12228 in the *STRC* gene. (**A**) Result obtained from *Decon* software. The x-axis represents the exon number. Blue points reflect a normal value. Red points reflect a possible deletion for the exon. (**B**) MLPA representation of patient 12228 with the P461 salsa using the Coffalyzer.Net program (MRC Holland). Normal range: 0.7–1.3 (indicated with red and blue line, respectively).

5. Conclusions

A large number of genes has been associated with HL, but still many cases remain unexplained. Novel HL genes are expected to be discovered and also genetic variants affecting regulatory regions of the genome, which are currently not screened in diagnosis genetic testing. Furthermore, the possibility of multigenic inheritance patterns must be explored in the near future [79].

Nowadays, a huge number of DNA variants are being detected in countless genetic diagnostic laboratories around the world, and a non-negligible number of them are possibly being misinterpreted. It is necessary to share this information with the scientific community and to establish close collaborations to interpret the functional implications of DNA variability. Working altogether, we will be able to decipher the secrets that we still ignore about the human genome.

Supplementary Materials: The following are available online at http://www.mdpi.com/2073-4425/11/12/1467/s1, Table S1: Regions of the panel design with a poor coverage.

Author Contributions: Conceptualization, M.A.-C., J.M.M. and E.A.; Formal analysis, A.B.-S., P.G.-D., R.V.-A., S.J.-R. and C.d.P.-V.; Funding acquisition, J.M.M.; Investigation, G.G.-G., A.B.-S., M.A.-C., R.V.-A., S.J.-R. and T.J.; Methodology, G.G.-G., T.J. and E.A.; Project administration, L.C.-G., M.A.-C., J.M.M. and E.A.; Validation, A.B.-S., R.V.-A. and S.J.-R.; Writing—original draft, G.G.-G. and E.A.; Writing—review and editing, C.d.P.-V., L.C.-G., T.J., M.A.-C. and J.M.M. All authors have read and agreed to the published version of the manuscript.

Funding: This work was financially supported by grants from the Institute of Health Carlos III (ISCIII), including the Center for Biomedical Research Network on Rare Diseases (CIBERER), FIS (PI19/00303). GGG is a recipient of a senior postdoctoral contract from CIBERER.

Conflicts of Interest: The authors declare no conflict of interest.

References

1. Shearer, A.E.; Smith, R.J.H. Massively Parallel Sequencing for Genetic Diagnosis of Hearing Loss: The New Standard of Care. *Otolaryngol. Head Neck Surg.* **2015**, *153*, 175–182. [CrossRef] [PubMed]
2. Hoefsloot, L.H.; Feenstra, I.; Kunst, H.P.M.; Kremer, H. Genotype phenotype correlations for hearing impairment: Approaches to management. *Clin. Genet.* **2014**, *85*, 514–523. [CrossRef] [PubMed]
3. Morton, C.C.; Nance, W.E. Newborn hearing screening—A silent revolution. *N. Engl. J. Med.* **2006**, *354*, 2151–2164. [CrossRef]
4. Smith, R.J.H.; Bale, J.F.; White, K.R. Sensorineural hearing loss in children. *Lancet* **2005**, *365*, 879–890. [CrossRef]
5. Kochhar, A.; Hildebrand, M.S.; Smith, R.J.H. Clinical aspects of hereditary hearing loss. *Genet. Med.* **2007**, *9*, 393–408. [CrossRef] [PubMed]
6. Alford, R.L.; Arnos, K.S.; Fox, M.; Lin, J.W.; Palmer, C.G.; Pandya, A.; Rehm, H.L.; Robin, N.H.; Scott, D.A.; Yoshinaga-Itano, C.; et al. American College of Medical Genetics and Genomics guideline for the clinical evaluation and etiologic diagnosis of hearing loss. *Genet. Med. Off. J. Am. Coll. Med. Genet.* **2014**, *16*, 347–355. [CrossRef]
7. Delmaghani, S.; El-Amraoui, A. Inner Ear Gene Therapies Take Off: Current Promises and Future Challenges. *J. Clin. Med.* **2020**, *9*, 2309. [CrossRef]
8. Sloan-Heggen, C.M.; Bierer, A.O.; Shearer, A.E.; Kolbe, D.L.; Nishimura, C.J.; Frees, K.L.; Ephraim, S.S.; Shibata, S.B.; Booth, K.T.; Campbell, C.A.; et al. Comprehensive genetic testing in the clinical evaluation of 1119 patients with hearing loss. *Hum. Genet.* **2016**, *135*, 441–450. [CrossRef]
9. Yan, D.; Xiang, G.; Chai, X.; Qing, J.; Shang, H.; Zou, B.; Mittal, R.; Shen, J.; Smith, R.J.H.; Fan, Y.-S.; et al. Screening of deafness-causing DNA variants that are common in patients of European ancestry using a microarray-based approach. *PLoS ONE* **2017**, *12*, e0169219. [CrossRef]
10. Domínguez-Ruíz, M. *Estudio Molecular de Genes Implicados en Hipoacusia No Sindrómica Autosómica Recesiva Mediante Secuenciación Sanger y de Nueva Generación*; UAM: Madrid, Spain, 2015.
11. Baux, D.; Vaché, C.; Blanchet, C.; Willems, M.; Baudoin, C.; Moclyn, M.; Faugère, V.; Touraine, R.; Isidor, B.; Dupin-Deguine, D.; et al. Combined genetic approaches yield a 48% diagnostic rate in a large cohort of French hearing-impaired patients. *Sci. Rep.* **2017**, *7*, 16783. [CrossRef]
12. Liquori, A.; Vaché, C.; Baux, D.; Blanchet, C.; Hamel, C.; Malcolm, S.; Koenig, M.; Claustres, M.; Roux, A.-F. Whole USH2A Gene Sequencing Identifies Several New Deep Intronic Mutations. *Hum. Mutat.* **2016**, *37*, 184–193. [CrossRef] [PubMed]
13. Vaché, C.; Besnard, T.; Le Berre, P.; García-García, G.; Baux, D.; Larrieu, L.; Abadie, C.; Blanchet, C.; Bolz, H.J.; Millan, J.; et al. Usher syndrome type 2 caused by activation of an USH2A pseudoexon: Implications for diagnosis and therapy. *Hum. Mutat.* **2012**, *33*, 104–108. [CrossRef] [PubMed]
14. Fowler, A.; Mahamdallie, S.; Ruark, E.; Seal, S.; Ramsay, E.; Clarke, M.; Uddin, I.; Wylie, H.; Strydom, A.; Lunter, G.; et al. Accurate clinical detection of exon copy number variants in a targeted NGS panel using DECoN. *Wellcome Open Res.* **2016**, *1*, 20. [CrossRef] [PubMed]
15. del Castillo, F.J.; Rodríguez-Ballesteros, M.; Alvarez, A.; Hutchin, T.; Leonardi, E.; de Oliveira, C.A.; Azaiez, H.; Brownstein, Z.; Avenarius, M.R.; Marlin, S.; et al. A novel deletion involving the connexin-30 gene, del(GJB6-d13s1854), found in trans with mutations in the GJB2 gene (connexin-26) in subjects with DFNB1 non-syndromic hearing impairment. *J. Med. Genet.* **2005**, *42*, 588–594. [CrossRef]
16. Zelante, L.; Gasparini, P.; Estivill, X.; Melchionda, S.; D'Agruma, L.; Govea, N.; Milá, M.; Monica, M.D.; Lutfi, J.; Shohat, M.; et al. Connexin26 mutations associated with the most common form of non-syndromic neurosensory autosomal recessive deafness (DFNB1) in Mediterraneans. *Hum. Mol. Genet.* **1997**, *6*, 1605–1609. [CrossRef]
17. Green, G.E.; Scott, D.A.; McDonald, J.M.; Woodworth, G.G.; Sheffield, V.C.; Smith, R.J. Carrier rates in the midwestern United States for GJB2 mutations causing inherited deafness. *JAMA* **1999**, *281*, 2211–2216. [CrossRef]
18. Marlin, S.; Garabédian, E.N.; Roger, G.; Moatti, L.; Matha, N.; Lewin, P.; Petit, C.; Denoyelle, F. Connexin 26 gene mutations in congenitally deaf children: Pitfalls for genetic counseling. *Arch. Otolaryngol. Head Neck Surg.* **2001**, *127*, 927–933. [CrossRef]

19. Denoyelle, F.; Marlin, S.; Weil, D.; Moatti, L.; Chauvin, P.; Garabédian, E.N.; Petit, C. Clinical features of the prevalent form of childhood deafness, DFNB1, due to a connexin-26 gene defect: Implications for genetic counselling. *Lancet* **1999**, *353*, 1298–1303. [CrossRef]
20. Kelsell, D.P.; Dunlop, J.; Stevens, H.P.; Lench, N.J.; Liang, J.N.; Parry, G.; Mueller, R.F.; Leigh, I.M. Connexin 26 mutations in hereditary non-syndromic sensorineural deafness. *Nature* **1997**, *387*, 80–83. [CrossRef]
21. Brobby, G.W.; Müller-Myhsok, B.; Horstmann, R.D. Connexin 26 R143W mutation associated with recessive nonsyndromic sensorineural deafness in Africa. *N. Engl. J. Med.* **1998**, *338*, 548–550. [CrossRef]
22. del Castillo, I.; Villamar, M.; Moreno-Pelayo, M.A.; del Castillo, F.J.; Alvarez, A.; Tellería, D.; Menéndez, I.; Moreno, F. A deletion involving the connexin 30 gene in nonsyndromic hearing impairment. *N. Engl. J. Med.* **2002**, *346*, 243–249. [CrossRef]
23. Zhang, Y.; Malekpour, M.; Al-Madani, N.; Kahrizi, K.; Zanganeh, M.; Lohr, N.J.; Mohseni, M.; Mojahedi, F.; Daneshi, A.; Najmabadi, H.; et al. Sensorineural deafness and male infertility: A contiguous gene deletion syndrome. *J. Med. Genet.* **2007**, *44*, 233–240. [CrossRef] [PubMed]
24. Rodríguez-Ballesteros, M.; del Castillo, F.J.; Martín, Y.; Moreno-Pelayo, M.A.; Morera, C.; Prieto, F.; Marco, J.; Morant, A.; Gallo-Terán, J.; Morales-Angulo, C.; et al. Auditory neuropathy in patients carrying mutations in the otoferlin gene (OTOF). *Hum. Mutat.* **2003**, *22*, 451–456. [CrossRef] [PubMed]
25. Migliosi, V.; Modamio-Høybjør, S.; Moreno-Pelayo, M.A.; Rodríguez-Ballesteros, M.; Villamar, M.; Tellería, D.; Menéndez, I.; Moreno, F.; Del Castillo, I. Q829X, a novel mutation in the gene encoding otoferlin (OTOF), is frequently found in Spanish patients with prelingual non-syndromic hearing loss. *J. Med. Genet.* **2002**, *39*, 502–506. [CrossRef] [PubMed]
26. Eppsteiner, R.W.; Shearer, A.E.; Hildebrand, M.S.; Deluca, A.P.; Ji, H.; Dunn, C.C.; Black-Ziegelbein, E.A.; Casavant, T.L.; Braun, T.A.; Scheetz, T.E.; et al. Prediction of cochlear implant performance by genetic mutation: The spiral ganglion hypothesis. *Hear. Res.* **2012**, *292*, 51–58. [CrossRef] [PubMed]
27. Shahin, H.; Walsh, T.; Rayyan, A.A.; Lee, M.K.; Higgins, J.; Dickel, D.; Lewis, K.; Thompson, J.; Baker, C.; Nord, A.S.; et al. Five novel loci for inherited hearing loss mapped by SNP-based homozygosity profiles in Palestinian families. *Eur. J. Hum. Genet. EJHG* **2010**, *18*, 407–413. [CrossRef] [PubMed]
28. Wattenhofer, M.; Di Iorio, M.V.; Rabionet, R.; Dougherty, L.; Pampanos, A.; Schwede, T.; Montserrat-Sentis, B.; Arbones, M.L.; Iliades, T.; Pasquadibisceglie, A.; et al. Mutations in the TMPRSS3 gene are a rare cause of childhood nonsyndromic deafness in Caucasian patients. *J. Mol. Med. Berl. Ger.* **2002**, *80*, 124–131. [CrossRef]
29. Miyagawa, M.; Nishio, S.; Ikeda, T.; Fukushima, K.; Usami, S. Massively parallel DNA sequencing successfully identifies new causative mutations in deafness genes in patients with cochlear implantation and EAS. *PLoS ONE* **2013**, *8*, e75793. [CrossRef]
30. Kalay, E.; Uzumcu, A.; Krieger, E.; Caylan, R.; Uyguner, O.; Ulubil-Emiroglu, M.; Erdol, H.; Kayserili, H.; Hafiz, G.; Başerer, N.; et al. MYO15A (DFNB3) mutations in Turkish hearing loss families and functional modeling of a novel motor domain mutation. *Am. J. Med. Genet. Part A* **2007**, *143*, 2382–2389. [CrossRef]
31. Pera, A.; Villamar, M.; Viñuela, A.; Gandía, M.; Medà, C.; Moreno, F.; Hernández-Chico, C. A mutational analysis of the SLC26A4 gene in Spanish hearing-impaired families provides new insights into the genetic causes of Pendred syndrome and DFNB4 hearing loss. *Eur. J. Hum. Genet. EJHG* **2008**, *16*, 888–896. [CrossRef]
32. Hutchin, T.; Coy, N.N.; Conlon, H.; Telford, E.; Bromelow, K.; Blaydon, D.; Taylor, G.; Coghill, E.; Brown, S.; Trembath, R.; et al. Assessment of the genetic causes of recessive childhood non-syndromic deafness in the UK—Implications for genetic testing. *Clin. Genet.* **2005**, *68*, 506–512. [CrossRef] [PubMed]
33. Ouyang, X.M.; Yan, D.; Du, L.L.; Hejtmancik, J.F.; Jacobson, S.G.; Nance, W.E.; Li, A.R.; Angeli, S.; Kaiser, M.; Newton, V.; et al. Characterization of Usher syndrome type I gene mutations in an Usher syndrome patient population. *Hum. Genet.* **2005**, *116*, 292–299. [CrossRef]
34. Kothiyal, P.; Cox, S.; Ebert, J.; Husami, A.; Kenna, M.A.; Greinwald, J.H.; Aronow, B.J.; Rehm, H.L. High-throughput detection of mutations responsible for childhood hearing loss using resequencing microarrays. *BMC Biotechnol.* **2010**, *10*, 10. [CrossRef] [PubMed]
35. Nájera, C.; Beneyto, M.; Blanca, J.; Aller, E.; Fontcuberta, A.; Millán, J.M.; Ayuso, C. Mutations in myosin VIIA (MYO7A) and usherin (USH2A) in Spanish patients with Usher syndrome types I and II, respectively. *Hum. Mutat.* **2002**, *20*, 76–77. [CrossRef]
36. García-García, G.; Besnard, T.; Baux, D.; Vaché, C.; Aller, E.; Malcolm, S.; Claustres, M.; Millan, J.M.; Roux, A.-F. The contribution of GPR98 and DFNB31 genes to a Spanish Usher syndrome type 2 cohort. *Mol. Vis.* **2013**, *19*, 367–373. [PubMed]

37. Besnard, T.; Vaché, C.; Baux, D.; Larrieu, L.; Abadie, C.; Blanchet, C.; Odent, S.; Blanchet, P.; Calvas, P.; Hamel, C.; et al. Non-USH2A mutations in USH2 patients. *Hum. Mutat.* **2012**, *33*, 504–510. [CrossRef] [PubMed]
38. Astuto, L.M.; Bork, J.M.; Weston, M.D.; Askew, J.W.; Fields, R.R.; Orten, D.J.; Ohliger, S.J.; Riazuddin, S.; Morell, R.J.; Khan, S.; et al. CDH23 mutation and phenotype heterogeneity: A profile of 107 diverse families with Usher syndrome and nonsyndromic deafness. *Am. J. Hum. Genet.* **2002**, *71*, 262–275. [CrossRef]
39. Aller, E.; Jaijo, T.; Beneyto, M.; Nájera, C.; Oltra, S.; Ayuso, C.; Baiget, M.; Carballo, M.; Antiñolo, G.; Valverde, D.; et al. Identification of 14 novel mutations in the long isoform of USH2A in Spanish patients with Usher syndrome type II. *J. Med. Genet.* **2006**, *43*, e55. [CrossRef]
40. Neuhaus, C.; Eisenberger, T.; Decker, C.; Nagl, S.; Blank, C.; Pfister, M.; Kennerknecht, I.; Müller-Hofstede, C.; Charbel Issa, P.; Heller, R.; et al. Next-generation sequencing reveals the mutational landscape of clinically diagnosed Usher syndrome: Copy number variations, phenocopies, a predominant target for translational read-through, and PEX26 mutated in Heimler syndrome. *Mol. Genet. Genomic Med.* **2017**, *5*, 531–552. [CrossRef]
41. Sanggaard, K.M.; Kjaer, K.W.; Eiberg, H.; Nürnberg, G.; Nürnberg, P.; Hoffman, K.; Jensen, H.; Sørum, C.; Rendtorff, N.D.; Tranebjaerg, L. A novel nonsense mutation in MYO6 is associated with progressive nonsyndromic hearing loss in a Danish DFNA22 family. *Am. J. Med. Genet. Part A* **2008**, *146*, 1017–1025. [CrossRef]
42. Kwon, T.-J.; Oh, S.-K.; Park, H.-J.; Sato, O.; Venselaar, H.; Choi, S.Y.; Kim, S.; Lee, K.-Y.; Bok, J.; Lee, S.-H.; et al. The effect of novel mutations on the structure and enzymatic activity of unconventional myosins associated with autosomal dominant non-syndromic hearing loss. *Open Biol.* **2014**, *4*. [CrossRef] [PubMed]
43. Donaudy, F.; Zheng, L.; Ficarella, R.; Ballana, E.; Carella, M.; Melchionda, S.; Estivill, X.; Bartles, J.R.; Gasparini, P. Espin gene (ESPN) mutations associated with autosomal dominant hearing loss cause defects in microvillar elongation or organisation. *J. Med. Genet.* **2006**, *43*, 157–161. [CrossRef] [PubMed]
44. Bonnet, C.; Riahi, Z.; Chantot-Bastaraud, S.; Smagghe, L.; Letexier, M.; Marcaillou, C.; Lefèvre, G.M.; Hardelin, J.-P.; El-Amraoui, A.; Singh-Estivalet, A.; et al. An innovative strategy for the molecular diagnosis of Usher syndrome identifies causal biallelic mutations in 93% of European patients. *Eur. J. Hum. Genet. EJHG* **2016**, *24*, 1730–1738. [CrossRef]
45. Plantinga, R.F.; de Brouwer, A.P.M.; Huygen, P.L.M.; Kunst, H.P.M.; Kremer, H.; Cremers, C.W.R.J. A novel TECTA mutation in a Dutch DFNA8/12 family confirms genotype-phenotype correlation. *J. Assoc. Res. Otolaryngol. JARO* **2006**, *7*, 173–181. [CrossRef] [PubMed]
46. Hildebrand, M.S.; Morín, M.; Meyer, N.C.; Mayo, F.; Modamio-Hoybjor, S.; Mencía, A.; Olavarrieta, L.; Morales-Angulo, C.; Nishimura, C.J.; Workman, H.; et al. DFNA8/12 caused by TECTA mutations is the most identified subtype of nonsyndromic autosomal dominant hearing loss. *Hum. Mutat.* **2011**, *32*, 825–834. [CrossRef] [PubMed]
47. Moreno-Pelayo, M.A.; del Castillo, I.; Villamar, M.; Romero, L.; Hernández-Calvín, F.J.; Herraiz, C.; Barberá, R.; Navas, C.; Moreno, F. A cysteine substitution in the zona pellucida domain of alpha-tectorin results in autosomal dominant, postlingual, progressive, mid frequency hearing loss in a Spanish family. *J. Med. Genet.* **2001**, *38*, E13. [CrossRef] [PubMed]
48. Brunner, H.G.; van Beersum, S.E.; Warman, M.L.; Olsen, B.R.; Ropers, H.H.; Mariman, E.C. A Stickler syndrome gene is linked to chromosome 6 near the COL11A2 gene. *Hum. Mol. Genet.* **1994**, *3*, 1561–1564. [CrossRef]
49. Sun, Y.; Cheng, J.; Lu, Y.; Li, J.; Lu, Y.; Jin, Z.; Dai, P.; Wang, R.; Yuan, H. Identification of two novel missense WFS1 mutations, H696Y and R703H, in patients with non-syndromic low-frequency sensorineural hearing loss. *J. Genet. Genom. Yi Chuan Xue Bao* **2011**, *38*, 71–76. [CrossRef]
50. Escribano, L.B. *Epidemiología Genética en Pacientes Españoles con Hipoacusia de Herencia Autosómica Dominante, Sindrómica y No Sindrómica, Utilizando Herramientas de Nueva Generación: Array-CGH y Secuenciación Masiva*; UAM: Madrid, Spain, 2016.
51. Shinagawa, J.; Moteki, H.; Nishio, S.-Y.; Ohyama, K.; Otsuki, K.; Iwasaki, S.; Masuda, S.; Oshikawa, C.; Ohta, Y.; Arai, Y.; et al. Prevalence and clinical features of hearing loss caused by EYA4 variants. *Sci. Rep.* **2020**, *10*, 3662. [CrossRef] [PubMed]

52. Nobukuni, Y.; Watanabe, A.; Takeda, K.; Skarka, H.; Tachibana, M. Analyses of loss-of-function mutations of the MITF gene suggest that haploinsufficiency is a cause of Waardenburg syndrome type 2A. *Am. J. Hum. Genet.* **1996**, *59*, 76–83.
53. Wu, C.-C.; Tsai, C.-Y.; Lin, Y.-H.; Chen, P.-Y.; Lin, P.-H.; Cheng, Y.-F.; Wu, C.-M.; Lin, Y.-H.; Lee, C.-Y.; Erdenechuluun, J.; et al. Genetic Epidemiology and Clinical Features of Hereditary Hearing Impairment in the Taiwanese Population. *Genes* **2019**, *10*, 772. [CrossRef] [PubMed]
54. Richards, S.; Aziz, N.; Bale, S.; Bick, D.; Das, S.; Gastier-Foster, J.; Grody, W.W.; Hegde, M.; Lyon, E.; Spector, E.; et al. Standards and Guidelines for the Interpretation of Sequence Variants: A Joint Consensus Recommendation of the American College of Medical Genetics and Genomics and the Association for Molecular Pathology. *Genet. Med.* **2015**, *17*, 405–424. [CrossRef] [PubMed]
55. Méndez-Vidal, C.; González-Del Pozo, M.; Vela-Boza, A.; Santoyo-López, J.; López-Domingo, F.J.; Vázquez-Marouschek, C.; Dopazo, J.; Borrego, S.; Antiñolo, G. Whole-exome sequencing identifies novel compound heterozygous mutations in USH2A in Spanish patients with autosomal recessive retinitis pigmentosa. *Mol. Vis.* **2013**, *19*, 2187–2195. [PubMed]
56. Bernal, S.; Medà, C.; Solans, T.; Ayuso, C.; Garcia-Sandoval, B.; Valverde, D.; Del Rio, E.; Baiget, M. Clinical and genetic studies in Spanish patients with Usher syndrome type II: Description of new mutations and evidence for a lack of genotype—Phenotype correlation. *Clin. Genet.* **2005**, *68*, 204–214. [CrossRef]
57. Adato, A.; Weil, D.; Kalinski, H.; Pel-Or, Y.; Ayadi, H.; Petit, C.; Korostishevsky, M.; Bonne-Tamir, B. Mutation profile of all 49 exons of the human myosin VIIA gene, and haplotype analysis, in Usher 1B families from diverse origins. *Am. J. Hum. Genet.* **1997**, *61*, 813–821. [CrossRef]
58. Xu, Y.; Guan, L.; Shen, T.; Zhang, J.; Xiao, X.; Jiang, H.; Li, S.; Yang, J.; Jia, X.; Yin, Y.; et al. Mutations of 60 known causative genes in 157 families with retinitis pigmentosa based on exome sequencing. *Hum. Genet.* **2014**, *133*, 1255–1271. [CrossRef]
59. Abe, S.; Usami, S.; Shinkawa, H.; Kelley, P.M.; Kimberling, W.J. Prevalent connexin 26 gene (GJB2) mutations in Japanese. *J. Med. Genet.* **2000**, *37*, 41–43. [CrossRef]
60. Rabionet, R.; Zelante, L.; López-Bigas, N.; D'Agruma, L.; Melchionda, S.; Restagno, G.; Arbonés, M.L.; Gasparini, P.; Estivill, X. Molecular basis of childhood deafness resulting from mutations in the GJB2 (connexin 26) gene. *Hum. Genet.* **2000**, *106*, 40–44. [CrossRef]
61. Wagatsuma, M.; Kitoh, R.; Suzuki, H.; Fukuoka, H.; Takumi, Y.; Usami, S. Distribution and frequencies of CDH23 mutations in Japanese patients with non-syndromic hearing loss. *Clin. Genet.* **2007**, *72*, 339–344. [CrossRef]
62. de Heer, A.-M.R.; Collin, R.W.J.; Huygen, P.L.M.; Schraders, M.; Oostrik, J.; Rouwette, M.; Kunst, H.P.M.; Kremer, H.; Cremers, C.W.R.J. Progressive sensorineural hearing loss and normal vestibular function in a Dutch DFNB7/11 family with a novel mutation in TMC1. *Audiol. Neurootol.* **2011**, *16*, 93–105. [CrossRef]
63. Duman, D.; Tekin, M. Autosomal recessive nonsyndromic deafness genes: A review. *Front. Biosci.* **2012**, *17*, 2213–2236. [CrossRef] [PubMed]
64. Shearer, A.E.; Hildebrand, M.S.; Smith, R.J. Hereditary Hearing Loss and Deafness Overview. In *GeneReviews*; Adam, M.P.; Ardinger, H.H.; Pagon, R.A.; Wallace, S.E.; Bean, L.J.; Stephens, K.; Amemiya, A., Eds.; University of Washington: Seattle, WA, USA, 1993.
65. Mandelker, D.; Amr, S.S.; Pugh, T.; Gowrisankar, S.; Shakhbatyan, R.; Duffy, E.; Bowser, M.; Harrison, B.; Lafferty, K.; Mahanta, L.; et al. Comprehensive diagnostic testing for stereocilin: An approach for analyzing medically important genes with high homology. *J. Mol. Diagn.* **2014**, *16*, 639–647. [CrossRef] [PubMed]
66. Zwaenepoel, I.; Mustapha, M.; Leibovici, M.; Verpy, E.; Goodyear, R.; Liu, X.Z.; Nouaille, S.; Nance, W.E.; Kanaan, M.; Avraham, K.B.; et al. Otoancorin, an inner ear protein restricted to the interface between the apical surface of sensory epithelia and their overlying acellular gels, is defective in autosomal recessive deafness DFNB22. *Proc. Natl. Acad. Sci. USA* **2002**, *99*, 6240–6245. [CrossRef] [PubMed]
67. Carvalho, G.M.D.; Ramos, P.Z.; Castilho, A.M.; Guimarães, A.C.; Sartorato, E.L. Molecular study of patients with auditory neuropathy. *Mol. Med. Rep.* **2016**, *14*, 481–490. [CrossRef] [PubMed]
68. Yokota, Y.; Moteki, H.; Nishio, S.; Yamaguchi, T.; Wakui, K.; Kobayashi, Y.; Ohyama, K.; Miyazaki, H.; Matsuoka, R.; Abe, S.; et al. Frequency and clinical features of hearing loss caused by STRC deletions. *Sci. Rep.* **2019**, *9*. [CrossRef] [PubMed]

69. Yazdanpanahi, N.; Tabatabaiefar, M.A.; Bagheri, N.; Azadegan Dehkordi, F.; Farrokhi, E.; Hashemzadeh Chaleshtori, M. The role and spectrum of SLC26A4 mutations in Iranian patients with autosomal recessive hereditary deafness. *Int. J. Audiol.* **2015**, *54*, 124–130. [CrossRef]
70. Jaijo, T.; Aller, E.; García-García, G.; Aparisi, M.J.; Bernal, S.; Avila-Fernández, A.; Barragán, I.; Baiget, M.; Ayuso, C.; Antiñolo, G.; et al. Microarray-based mutation analysis of 183 Spanish families with Usher syndrome. *Invest. Ophthalmol. Vis. Sci.* **2010**, *51*, 1311–1317. [CrossRef]
71. Blanco-Kelly, F.; Jaijo, T.; Aller, E.; Avila-Fernandez, A.; López-Molina, M.I.; Giménez, A.; García-Sandoval, B.; Millán, J.M.; Ayuso, C. Clinical aspects of Usher syndrome and the USH2A gene in a cohort of 433 patients. *JAMA Ophthalmol.* **2015**, *133*, 157–164. [CrossRef]
72. Butz, M.; McDonald, A.; Lundquist, P.A.; Meyer, M.; Harrington, S.; Kester, S.; Stein, M.I.; Mistry, N.A.; Zimmerman Zuckerman, E.; Niu, Z.; et al. Development and Validation of a Next-Generation Sequencing Panel for Syndromic and Nonsyndromic Hearing Loss. *J. Appl. Lab. Med.* **2020**, *5*, 467–479. [CrossRef]
73. Cabanillas, R.; Diñeiro, M.; Cifuentes, G.A.; Castillo, D.; Pruneda, P.C.; Álvarez, R.; Sánchez-Durán, N.; Capín, R.; Plasencia, A.; Viejo-Díaz, M.; et al. Comprehensive genomic diagnosis of non-syndromic and syndromic hereditary hearing loss in Spanish patients. *BMC Med. Genom.* **2018**, *11*, 58. [CrossRef]
74. Diaz-Horta, O.; Duman, D.; Foster, J.; Sırmacı, A.; Gonzalez, M.; Mahdieh, N.; Fotouhi, N.; Bonyadi, M.; Cengiz, F.B.; Menendez, I.; et al. Whole-exome sequencing efficiently detects rare mutations in autosomal recessive nonsyndromic hearing loss. *PLoS ONE* **2012**, *7*, e50628. [CrossRef] [PubMed]
75. Tekin, D.; Yan, D.; Bademci, G.; Feng, Y.; Guo, S.; Foster, J.; Blanton, S.; Tekin, M.; Liu, X. A next-generation sequencing gene panel (MiamiOtoGenes) for comprehensive analysis of deafness genes. *Hear. Res.* **2016**, *333*, 179–184. [CrossRef] [PubMed]
76. Zou, S.; Mei, X.; Yang, W.; Zhu, R.; Yang, T.; Hu, H. Whole-exome sequencing identifies rare pathogenic and candidate variants in sporadic Chinese Han deaf patients. *Clin. Genet.* **2020**, *97*, 352–356. [CrossRef] [PubMed]
77. Vears, D.F.; Sénécal, K.; Borry, P. Reporting practices for variants of uncertain significance from next generation sequencing technologies. *Eur. J. Med. Genet.* **2017**, *60*, 553–558. [CrossRef] [PubMed]
78. Hoppman, N.; Aypar, U.; Brodersen, P.; Brown, N.; Wilson, J.; Babovic-Vuksanovic, D. Genetic testing for hearing loss in the United States should include deletion/duplication analysis for the deafness/infertility locus at 15q15.3. *Mol. Cytogenet.* **2013**, *6*, 19. [CrossRef] [PubMed]
79. Kremer, H. Hereditary hearing loss; about the known and the unknown. *Hear. Res.* **2019**, *376*, 58–68. [CrossRef] [PubMed]

Publisher's Note: MDPI stays neutral with regard to jurisdictional claims in published maps and institutional affiliations.

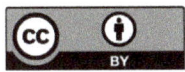

© 2020 by the authors. Licensee MDPI, Basel, Switzerland. This article is an open access article distributed under the terms and conditions of the Creative Commons Attribution (CC BY) license (http://creativecommons.org/licenses/by/4.0/).

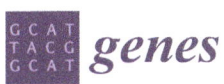

Article

Genetic Spectrum of Syndromic and Non-Syndromic Hearing Loss in Pakistani Families

Julia Doll [1], Barbara Vona [1,2,*], Linda Schnapp [1], Franz Rüschendorf [3], Imran Khan [4], Saadullah Khan [5], Noor Muhammad [5], Sher Alam Khan [5], Hamed Nawaz [5], Ajmal Khan [6], Naseer Ahmad [7], Susanne M. Kolb [1], Laura Kühlewein [8], Jonathan D. J. Labonne [9], Lawrence C. Layman [9,10], Michaela A. H. Hofrichter [1], Tabea Röder [1], Marcus Dittrich [1,11], Tobias Müller [11], Tyler D. Graves [9], Il-Keun Kong [12], Indrajit Nanda [1], Hyung-Goo Kim [13,*] and Thomas Haaf [1]

[1] Institute of Human Genetics, Julius Maximilians University Würzburg, 97074 Würzburg, Germany; julia.doll@uni-wuerzburg.de (J.D.); schnapp-linda@web.de (L.S.); susi_kolb@yahoo.com (S.M.K.); michaela.hofrichter@uni-wuerzburg.de (M.A.H.H.); tabea.roeder@uni-wuerzburg.de (T.R.); marcus.dittrich@biozentrum.uni-wuerzburg.de (M.D.); nanda@biozentrum.uni-wuerzburg.de (I.N.); thomas.haaf@uni-wuerzburg.de (T.H.)
[2] Tübingen Hearing Research Centre, Department of Otolaryngology-Head and Neck Surgery, Eberhard Karls University, 72076 Tübingen, Germany
[3] Max Delbrück Center for Molecular Medicine in the Helmholtz Association, 13125 Berlin, Germany; fruesch@mdc-berlin.de
[4] Department of Chemistry, Bacha Khan University Charsadda, Khyber Pakhtunkhwa 24420, Pakistan; imrangnu@gmail.com
[5] Department of Biotechnology and Genetic Engineering, Kohat University of Science and Technology, Kohat, Khyber Pakhtunkhwa 24420, Pakistan; saadkhanwazir@gmail.com (S.K.); noormwazir@yahoo.com (N.M.); sakmarwat79@gmail.com (S.A.K.); hamedwazir@gmail.com (H.N.)
[6] Department of Biotechnology, Bacha Khan University Charsadda, Khyber Pakhtunkhwa 24420, Pakistan; ajmalkhanbbt@gmail.com
[7] District Eye Specialist, Police and Services Hospital Peshawar, Khyber Pakhtunkkhwa 24420, Pakistan; na_safi1982@yahoo.com
[8] Department of Ophthalmology, Eberhard Karls University, 72076 Tübingen, Germany; laura.kuehlewein@med.uni-tuebingen.de
[9] Section of Reproductive Endocrinology, Infertility & Genetics, Department of Obstetrics and Gynecology, Medical College of Georgia, Augusta University, Augusta, GA 30912, USA; molgenetics_and_epigenetics@hotmail.com (J.D.J.L.); lalayman@augusta.edu (L.C.L.); tylergraves14@hotmail.com (T.D.G.)
[10] Department of Neuroscience and Regenerative Medicine, Medical College of Georgia, Augusta University, Augusta, GA 30912, USA
[11] Department of Bioinformatics, Julius Maximilians University Würzburg, 97074 Würzburg, Germany; tobias.mueller@biozentrum.uni-wuerzburg.de
[12] Department of Animal Sciences, Division of Applied Life Science (BK21 Four), Gyeongsang National University, Jinju 52828, Korea; ikong7900@gmail.com
[13] Neurological Disorders Research Center, Qatar Biomedical Research Institute, Hamad Bin Khalifa University, 34110 Doha, Qatar
* Correspondence: barbara.vona@uni-tuebingen.de (B.V.); hkim@hbku.edu.qa (H.-G.K.); Tel.: +49-7071-298-8154 (B.V.); +974-4454-5856 (H.-G.K.)

Received: 14 September 2020; Accepted: 9 November 2020; Published: 11 November 2020

Abstract: The current molecular genetic diagnostic rates for hereditary hearing loss (HL) vary considerably according to the population background. Pakistan and other countries with high rates of consanguineous marriages have served as a unique resource for studying rare and novel forms of recessive HL. A combined exome sequencing, bioinformatics analysis, and gene mapping approach for 21 consanguineous Pakistani families revealed 13 pathogenic or likely pathogenic variants in the genes *GJB2, MYO7A, FGF3, CDC14A, SLITRK6, CDH23,* and *MYO15A,* with an overall resolve rate of 61.9%. *GJB2* and *MYO7A* were the most frequently involved genes in this cohort. All the identified variants were either homozygous or compound heterozygous, with two of them not previously described in the literature (15.4%). Overall, seven missense variants (53.8%), three nonsense variants (23.1%), two frameshift variants (15.4%), and one splice-site variant (7.7%) were observed. Syndromic HL was identified in five (23.8%) of the 21 families studied. This study reflects the extreme genetic heterogeneity observed in HL and expands the spectrum of variants in deafness-associated genes.

Keywords: genetic diagnosis; consanguinity; genome-wide linkage analysis; hearing loss; Pakistan; exome sequencing

1. Introduction

In parts of the world where consanguinity is prevalent, it is not uncommon to see a high prevalence of genetic diseases. The consanguineous marriage rates in Pakistan are among the highest worldwide [1]. Approximately 60% of marriages in Pakistan are consanguineous, with roughly 80% of these marriages being between first cousins [2]. The prevalence of autosomal recessive diseases associated with a monogenic background, such as profound hearing loss (HL), is high in countries where consanguineous marriages are common [3].

Hereditary HL is one of the most prevalent sensory disorders that affects 1 to 2 per 1000 live births worldwide. Genetic factors are responsible for over half of all HL [4]. Studies describing genetic variants in Pakistani families with HL show evidence of the extreme clinical and genetic heterogeneity of this sensory disease and support the importance of investigating and characterizing families from this region of the world [5–7]. Over 120 genes have been identified as causing non-syndromic hearing loss (NSHL), which comprises approximately 70% of all forms of hereditary HL (http://hereditaryhearingloss.org). Autosomal recessive HL (ARHL) is the most commonly observed inheritance pattern. There are presently over 600 syndromic forms of deafness [8], which appear in approximately 30% of patients with genetic HL. Many of these deafness syndromes mimic non-syndromic deafness at onset [9]. Hearing impairment profoundly complicates speech and language development in prelingual children and can negatively impact education and employment prospects [10].

Exome sequencing (ES) allows for the parallel sequencing of all coding regions of the human genome and has accelerated the process of identifying causally associated variants in patients with HL [11]. In 13 consanguineous families with diverse forms of HL, we identified 13 variants in 7 HL-associated genes using ES and gene mapping approaches in 21 Pakistani families. Two of the 13 variants were not previously described in the literature. The present study underscores the importance of genetically characterizing consanguineous families with HL to expand the spectrum of clinically relevant variants in genetically diverse populations, thus improving our understanding of the alleles involved in ARHL and enhancing genetic counseling.

2. Materials and Methods

2.1. Clinical Evaluation

This study was approved by the Ethics Committees of Augusta University (624456-4), Kohat University of Science and Technology (16–25), and the University of Würzburg (46/15). Fully informed written consent was obtained prior to initiating our study. Informed written consent from minors was provided from parent(s) or legal guardians. We recruited 21 consanguineous Pakistani families with congenital, bilateral, and severe-to-profound HL. The affected individuals in family 6 and 7 were audiologically tested by pure-tone audiometry, conforming with the established guidelines described by Mazzoli et al. [12]. Hearing thresholds were measured at 0.25, 0.5, 1, 2, 4, 6, and 8 kHz. HL was self-reported in all other families but clearly noted as severe-to-profound. Ophthalmic examinations of families 4, 5, 6, 7, and 8 were performed.

2.2. Autozygosity Mapping and Linkage Analysis

2.2.1. Genotyping and Quality Control

The Illumina Infinium HumanCore-24 v1.0 Bead Chip array (Illumina, Inc., San Diego, CA, USA) was used for genotyping. From the 306,670 markers on the array, we filtered out indels, MT- and Y-chromosomal SNPs, and variations without physical positions, resulting in 259,460 biallelic SNPs for quality control (QC) and linkage analysis. Data conversion to linkage format files and QC was managed with ALOHOMORA software [13]. The sex of individuals was estimated by counting heterozygous genotypes on the X-chromosome and compared to the upraised pedigree data. The relationships between family members were verified with the program GRR [14]. PedCheck [15] was used to detect Mendelian errors (ME) and SNPs with ME were removed from the data set. Unlikely genotypes—e.g., double recombinants—were identified with Merlin [16] and deleted in the individuals.

2.2.2. Linkage Analysis

Linkage analysis was performed with Merlin using an autosomal recessive mode of inheritance and complete penetrance. We assumed 0.001 as the mutant allele frequency. We executed Merlin twice, once with a full marker set of around 258,000 SNPs after QC. This calculation was used to obtain the best positions for recombination events. The second analysis was conducted with a reduced marker set (~119,000 SNPs), where a minimal distance of 10,000 bases between markers was used. This calculation, where the linkage disequilibrium (LD) between markers is reduced, identifies linkage peaks which were inflated by markers in LD. We removed the linkage regions where the LOD score broke down more than 0.3 in the LD-reduced analysis. In summary, we selected regions where the LOD score reached the maximal LOD score of a family and where the LOD score was stable in the less dense, LD-reduced marker set. Under the given inheritance model (recessive) and the pedigree structure with a consanguinity loop, this linkage analysis is called autozygosity mapping.

2.3. Exome Sequencing

Genomic DNA (gDNA) was extracted from peripheral blood lymphocytes using a standard phenol/chloroform [17] and ethanol precipitation [18]. A total of 50 ng of gDNA from the proband from each family was subjected to ES with the Nextera Rapid Capture Exome or the TruSeq Exome Enrichment kits (Illumina, Inc., San Diego, CA, USA) according to the manufacturer's protocol. An additional family member (IV.1) of family 5 was exome sequenced due to the presence of two distinct phenotypes in the family—namely, HL and a suspected bone disorder. A 2×76 bp paired-end read sequencing was performed using a v2 high-output reagent kit with the NextSeq500 sequencer (Illumina, Inc., San Diego, CA, USA). Raw bcl sequencing files were converted with the bcl2fastq software (Illumina, Inc., San Diego, CA, USA) and the data were aligned to the human reference genome GRCh37 [19] (hg19).

2.4. Variant Analysis and Prioritization

Single-nucleotide variants (SNVs) and small indels (<15 bp) were analyzed with the GensearchNGS software (PhenoSystems SA, Wallonia, Belgium). Analysis was supported using an established in-house bioinformatics pipeline based on the GATK toolkit including Burrows-Wheeler (BWA)-based read alignment, base quality score recalibration, indel realignment, duplicate removal, and SNP and indel discovery, with subsequent score recalibration according to the GATK Best Practice recommendations [19–21]. Variant filtering and prioritization were performed using a conservative minor allele frequency <0.01 based on population databases and an alternate allele frequency present at >20% referring to reads. Additional variants not removed by minor allele frequency filtering were subjected to an in-house allele count filter ($n = 300$) that removed variants appearing >2%, as these are too common in our exome dataset to enter manual analysis. Variant prioritization included the tools PolyPhen-2 (PP) [22], SIFT [23], MutationTaster (MT) [24], fathmm [25], LRT [26], and GERP [27]. The Deafness Variation Database [28] was also integrated into our pipeline to permit the quick assessment of variants in known deafness genes. Frequency-based filtering was performed according to a population-specific manner that includes The Greater Middle East Variome Project [29] and gnomAD [30] to account for varying allele frequencies across ethnicities. CNV analysis was performed for 19 out of 21 families using the eXome Hidden MarkovModel (XHMM, version 1.0) approach [31].

2.5. Variant Validation and Segregation Testing

The candidate variants remaining after filtering were amplified by PCR using primers designed from the Primer3 software [32]. The primer sequences are shown in Table S1. PCR products were bidirectionally sequenced with an ABI 3130xl 16-capillary sequencer (Life Technologies, Carlsbad, CA, USA). Sequence reactions were completed with 5× sequencing buffer and big dye terminator (Applied Biosystems, Waltham, MA, USA). DNA sequence analysis was performed using the Gensearch software (Phenosystems SA, Wallonia, Belgium).

3. Results

3.1. Summary of Affected Genes and Genetic Context

Using ES and bioinformatics analysis, 13 different variants in seven HL-associated genes were identified, including two that have not been previously described in the literature (15.4%). In aggregate, these variants are likely causally associated in 13 out of 21 (61.9%) consanguineous Pakistani families. Pathogenic and likely pathogenic variants were identified in the genes *GJB2*, *MYO7A*, *FGF3*, *CDC14A*, *SLITRK6*, *CDH23*, and *MYO15A* (Table 1). *GJB2* and *MYO7A* were implicated in the genetic diagnosis of almost half of all cases (46.2%). Among the different variant types observed, seven were missense (53.8%), three were nonsense (23.1%), two were frameshift (15.4%), and one was a splice-site variant (7.7%). All the variants were either homozygous or compound heterozygous, showed an autosomal recessive inheritance pattern, and were validated by segregation testing (Figure 1, Figure S1).

Table 1. Likely causal variants identified in Pakistani families with hearing loss (HL).

ID	Gene	DFN locus	Transcript	Nucleotide	Protein	Zygosity	MT	PP	SIFT	GERP	LRT	DVD
Family 1	FGF3	–	NM_005247.2	c.166C>T	p.(Leu56Phe)	1/1	DC	PrD	D	C	U	U
Family 2	FGF3	–	NM_005247.2	c.166C>T	p.(Leu56Phe)	1/1	DC	PrD	D	C	U	U
Family 3	GJB2	DFNB1	NM_004004.5	c.231G>A	p.(Trp77*)	1/1	DC	–	–	C	D	P [33]
Family 4	MYO7A	DFNB2	NM_000260.3	c.470G>A	p.(Ser157Asn)	1/1	DC	PrD	D	C	D	P [34]
Family 5	MYO7A	DFNB2	NM_000260.3	c.3502C>T	p.(Arg1168Trp)	1/1	DC	PrD	D	C	D	LP [35]
Family 6	CDC14A	DFNB32	NM_033312.2	c.1041dup [36]	p.(Ser348Glnfs*2) [36]	1/1	–	–	–	–	–	–
Family 7	**SLITRK6**	–	NM_032229.2	**c.120_121insT**	**p.(Asp41*)**	1/1	–	–	–	–	–	–
Family 8	MYO7A	DFNB2	NM_000260.3	c.1258A>T c.1849T>C c.4505A>G	p.(Lys420*) p.(Ser617Pro) p.(Asp1502Gly)	0/1 0/1 0/1	DC DC DC	– PrD PrD	– D D	C C C	D D D	P [37] U [38] U [6]
Family 9	CDH23	DFNB12	NM_022124.5	c.2968G>A	p.(Asp990Asn)	1/1	DC	PrD	D	C	D	P [39]
Family 10	GJB2	DFNB1	NM_004004.5	c.35delG	p.(Gly12Valfs*2)	1/1	–	–	–	–	–	P [40]
Family 11	GJB2	DFNB1	NM_004004.5	c.35delG	p.(Gly12Valfs*2)	1/1	–	–	–	–	–	P [40]
Family 12	MYO15A	DFNB3	NM_016239.3	c.9518-2A>G		1/1	DC	–	–	C	–	U [5]
Family 13	CDH23	DFNB12	NM_022124.5	c.4688T>C	p.(Leu1563Pro)	1/1	DC	PrD	D	C	D	P [41]

1/1 homozygous; 0/1 heterozygous. Previously undescribed variants are marked in bold. Abbreviations: LRT, Likelihood Ratio Test; MT, MutationTaster; PP, PolyPhen-2; SIFT, Sorting Intolerant from Tolerant; GERP, Genomic Evolutionary Rate Profiling; DVD, Deafness Variation Database; C, conserved; D, deleterious; DC, disease causing; P, pathogenic; LP, likely pathogenic; PrD, probably damaging; U, unknown significance.

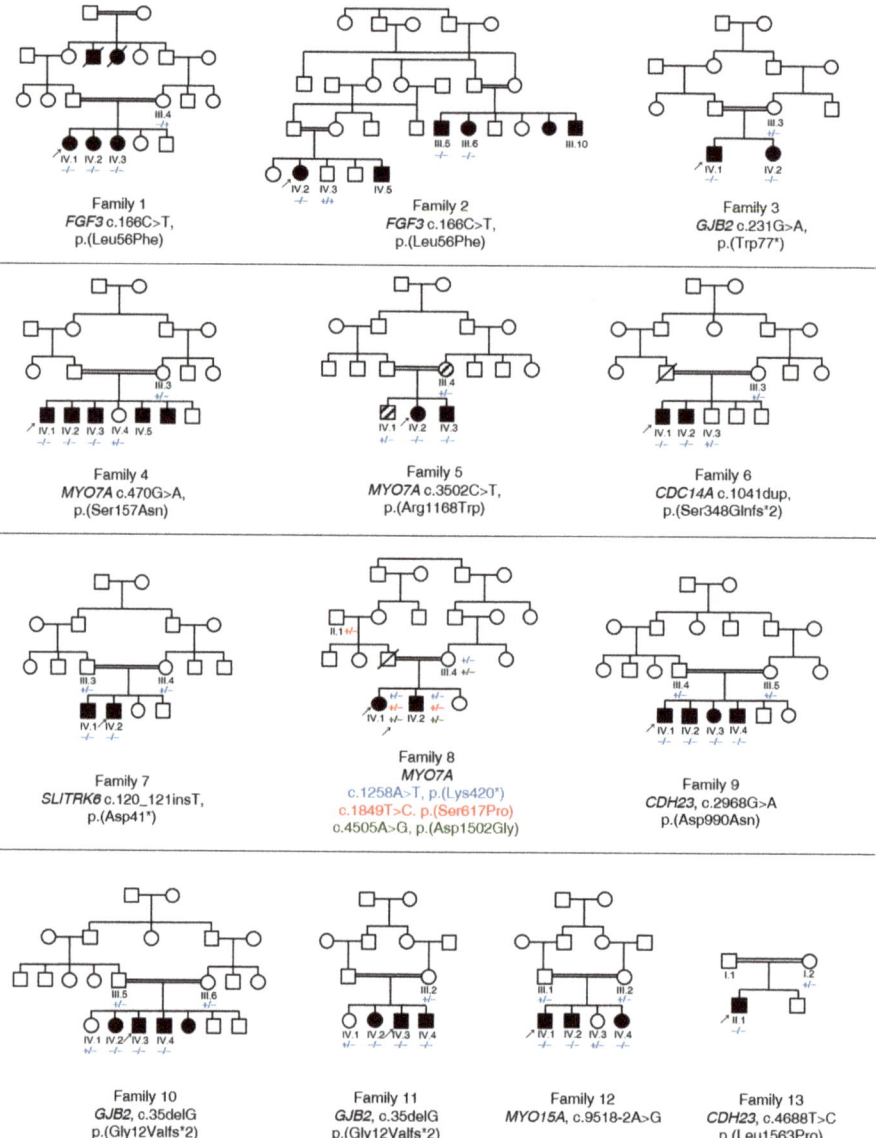

Figure 1. Pedigree and segregation analysis of known and previously undescribed variants in 13 Pakistani families with HL. All the families have a consanguineous background, marked with double lines. Affected individuals are shown in black symbols, and unaffected parents and siblings are shown in unfilled symbols. Individuals with a bone disorder, but without HL, are shown in striped symbols. Probands who were exome sequenced are marked with an arrow. Deceased individuals are marked with a diagonal line. The mutated and wild type alleles are illustrated with "−" (mutated) and "+" (wild type) symbols, respectively.

3.2. Clinical Features and Genetic Spectrum of Patients with Syndromic HL

FGF3, MYO7A and SLITRK6

All the affected individuals were clinically diagnosed with congenital, bilateral HL and have a consanguineous background. Five of 21 families (23.8%) revealed a syndromic form of HL. Two of the 21 families were clinically diagnosed with Usher syndrome, one of the most common forms of syndromic HL [8].

The affected individuals who were available for testing in families 1 and 2 reported severe HL and cupped ears (Figure 2A, Table 2) (IV.1, IV.2, IV.3, family 1; III.5, III.6, III.10, IV.2, IV.5, family 2). A homozygous missense c.166C>T, p.(Leu56Phe) variant was identified in *FGF3* (NM_005247.2; Figure S2) in families 1 and 2 that co-segregated with HL in both families (Figure 1). The variant is predicted to be disease causing (MT, PP, SIFT), involves the substitution of a conserved amino acid (aa), and was not previously published in the literature. The variant is classified as likely pathogenic according to the ClinGen HL working group expert specification [41]. Homozygous variants in *FGF3* have been associated with deafness, accompanied by inner ear agenesis, microtia, and microdontia [42].

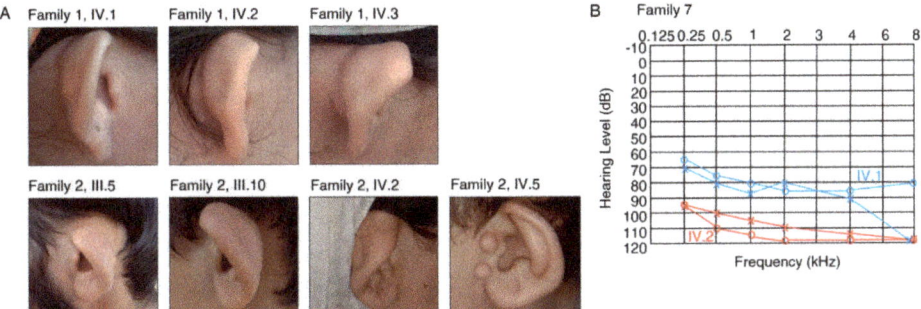

Figure 2. Clinical aspects of patients with previously unreported variants. (**A**) Affected individuals in family 1 (IV.1, IV.2, IV.3) and family 2 (only III.5, III.10, IV.2, IV.5 were available for photographs) show cupped ears and report severe HL. (**B**) Pure-tone audiogram for affected family members IV.1 (blue) and IV.2 (red) in family 7. Left-ear measurements are represented as "x" and right-ear measurements are shown with "o".

The proband (IV.1) in family 4 and his affected siblings (IV.2, IV.3, IV.5) were diagnosed with Usher syndrome and revealed a homozygous pathogenic missense c.470G>A, p.(Ser157Asn) variant [34] in *MYO7A*. Ophthalmological examination of the proband IV.3 revealed high myopia, cataract, and retinitis pigmentosa in both eyes. Visual acuity was reduced to 5/60 (Snellen equivalent, 20/250), with corrective lenses of −12.00/0/0° in both eyes. Ophthalmological examination of the proband IV.5 revealed high myopia, cataract, and retinitis pigmentosa in both eyes. Visual acuity was reduced to light perception in the right eye, and 1/60 (Snellen equivalent, worse than 20/1000) in the left eye. Thus, the patient was legally blind. Cataract was more pronounced in the right eye. Ultrasonographic findings of the right eye were within normal limits. The aa substitution weakens the 5′ donor splice-site predicted by several in silico prediction tools. A previously published minigene assay that was conducted using nasal epithelial cells proved the skipping of exon 5 in the mutant transcript, which likely results in a truncated protein [43] (Figure 1). Two individuals in family 5 (III.4, IV.1) suffer from a bone disorder but have normal hearing in contrast to the affected family members (IV.2, IV.3), who show a distinct Usher syndrome phenotype (Table 2). The ophthalmological examination of proband IV.2 revealed hyperopia in both eyes (+9/0/0° in the right eye, and +11/0/0° in the left eye) and lenticular opacity (cataract) in both eyes. Retinitis pigmentosa was confirmed with indirect ophthalmoscopy with a 20 Diopter power lens. We identified a homozygous pathogenic missense c.3502C>T, p.(Arg1168Trp) variant [35] in the gene *MYO7A* in affected individuals (IV.2, IV.3) that segregated in family 5. An ES analysis of III.3 and IV.1 did not uncover any variants in genes associated with bone disorders or neuropathies. Both variants that have been identified in family 4 and family 5 are known to cause Usher syndrome type 1 [34,35].

The affected individuals in family 7 (IV.1, IV.2) reported severe-to-profound HL (Table 2, Figure 2B). Ophthalmological examination in IV.1 revealed compound myopic astigmatism and grossly cupped discs diagnosed as glaucoma in both eyes. The macula appeared normal in both eyes. Visual acuity was reduced to 0.5 logMAR in both eyes (Snellen equivalent: 20/63), with corrective lenses of −5.50/−2.50/90° in the right eye and −6.50/−1.00/60° in the left eye. Intraocular pressure was 17 mmHg in both eyes. Additionally, Duane retraction syndrome (a congenital neuromuscular dysfunction of the eye movement caused by a failure of the sixth cranial nerve) was diagnosed in the left eye. Other data (e.g., axial length, status of lens, macula/retina, visual field, treatment of glaucoma) were not available. Ophthalmological examination in IV.2 revealed compound myopic astigmatism and myopic alterations with macular degeneration in both eyes. Visual acuity was reduced to count fingers with corrective lenses of −5.00/−2.50/90° in the right eye and −4.00/−3.00/90° in the left eye. Intraocular pressure was 15 mmHg in both eyes. Thus, the patient was legally blind. Other data (e.g., axial length, status of lens, macula/retina, visual field, treatment of glaucoma) were not available. Family 7 revealed a segregating novel homozygous nonsense variant c.120_121insT, p.(Asp41*) in the gene *SLITRK6* (NM_032229.2; Figure S2) that was present in both affected family members (IV.1, IV.2) (Figure 1) and was absent in population databases. The variant is classified as likely pathogenic according to the ClinGen HL working group expert specification [41]. Homozygous variants in this gene are known to cause sensorineural deafness and high myopia in humans [44].

Both previously unreported variants have been submitted to the Leiden Open Variation Database (LOVD) v3.0 under the accession IDs 00307903 (*FGF3* c.166C>T, p.(Leu56Phe)) and 00307904 (*SLITRK6* c.120_121insT, p.(Asp41*)).

3.3. Identification of Causative Variants in Patients with NSHL

3.3.1. GJB2

Variants in the gene *GJB2* (NM_004004.5; DFNB1A, DFNA3A) were identified in three families (3, 10, 11). The proband (IV.1) and his affected sibling (IV.2) in family 3 revealed a common homozygous pathogenic nonsense variant c.231G>A, p.(Trp77*) [33] that was consistent with the familial segregation analysis (Figure 1). The probands in families 10 (IV.3) and 11 (IV.3) revealed a prevalent homozygous pathogenic frameshift variant c.35delG, p.(Gly12Valfs*2) [40] thatsegregated in both families (Figure 1). In this study, variants in *GJB2* accounted for 23.1% of the 13 resolved families and comprised 14.3% (3 out of 21) of the total diagnostic yield.

3.3.2. MYO7A

Family 8 revealed three different heterozygous *MYO7A* variants: c.1258A>T, p.(Lys420*) [37], c.1849T>C, p.(Ser617Pro) [38], and c.4505A>G, p.(Asp1502Gly) [6]. All three heterozygous variants were identified exclusively in the affected individuals (IV.1, IV.2). The unaffected mother (III.4) revealed only two of the variants (c.1258A>T, p.(Lys420*); c.4505A>G, p.(Asp1502Gly)) and the unaffected paternal grandfather (II.1) was confirmed with the third variant c.1849T>C, p.(Ser617Pro), confirming a compound heterozygosity of p.(Lys420*) and p.(Ser617Pro) (Figure 1). Vision was normal in all the affected individuals, and Usher syndrome was not confirmed. Ophthalmological examination in proband IV.1 revealed no significant ocular problems in either eye. Visual acuity was 6/6 (Snellen equivalent, 20/20) in both eyes. Photographs of the central retina showed the optic disc, macula, and vessels within normal limits in both eyes.

In aggregate, *MYO7A* (NM_000260.3; DFNA11, DFNB2, USH1B) was affected in three families, accounting for 23.1% of the overall diagnostic yield.

Table 2. Clinical information for Pakistani families.

ID	Phenotype	Affected Family Members	Unaffected Family Members
Family 1	HL, cupped ears	IV.1, IV.2, IV.3	III.4
Family 2	HL, cupped ears	III.5, III.6, III.10 [1], IV.2, IV.5 [1]	IV.3
Family 3	HL	IV.1 (25 y/o), IV.2 (10 y/o)	III.3
Family 4	Usher syndrome	IV.1 (35 y/o), IV.2 (33 y/o), IV.3 (32 y/o), IV.5 (33 y/o) [1]	III.3, IV.4
Family 5	Usher syndrome [2], bone disorder [2]	IV.2 (30 y/o), IV.3 (18 y/o); Usher syndrome	III.4, IV.1; bone disorder
Family 6	severe-to-profound HL, compound myopic astigmatism	IV.1 (30 y/o), IV.2 (28 y/o)	III.3, IV.3
Family 7	severe-to-profound HL, compound myopic astigmatism, glaucoma	IV.1 (26 y/o), IV.2 (23 y/o)	III.3, III.4
Family 8	HL	IV.1 (13 y/o), IV.2 (12 y/o)	II.1, III.4
Family 9	HL	IV.1 (33 y/o), IV.2 (32 y/o), IV.3 (20 y/o), IV.4 (18 y/o)	III.4, III.5
Family 10	HL	IV.2 (14 y/o), IV.3 (13 y/o), IV.4 (12 y/o)	III.5, III.6, IV.1
Family 11	HL	IV.2 (16 y/o), IV.3 (14 y/o), IV.4 (12 y/o)	III.2, IV.1
Family 12	HL	IV.1 (15 y/o), IV.2 (15 y/o), IV.4 (10 y/o)	III.1, III.2, IV.3
Family 13	HL	II.1 (11 y/o)	I.2

Abbreviations: HL, hearing loss; y/o, years old available ages for affected individuals; [1] no DNA available for testing, only clinical photographs (Figure 2A) or ophthalmological examination; [2] two distinct phenotypes within the family.

3.3.3. CDC14A, CDH23 and MYO15A

Family 6 reported severe-to-profound HL and suffers from compound myopic astigmatism (IV.1, IV.2). A frameshift variant (c.1041dup, p.(Ser348Glnfs*2)) was identified in the deafness gene *CDC14A* (NM_033312.2, DFNB32) in affected family members of family 6 (IV.1, IV.2) and co-segregated with HL in this family (Figure 1). Both affected individuals are unmarried and have no children. This variant was described as disease causing supported by functional RT-qPCR validation [36].

We identified two families with variants in the gene *CDH23*. The proband of family 9 (IV.1) revealed a homozygous pathogenic *CDH23* (NM_022124.5, DFNB12) missense variant c.2968G>A, p.(Asp990Asn) [39] that was validated via Sanger sequencing and was also present in three affected siblings (IV.2, IV.3, IV.4) (Figure 1). The affected proband in family 13 showed a segregating homozygous pathogenic missense variant c.4688T>C, p.(Leu1563Pro) [45] in the gene *CDH23* (Figure 1).

Furthermore, we identified a homozygous splice-site variant c.9518-2A>G in *MYO15A* (NM_016239.3, DFNB3) in the proband (IV.1) and affected siblings (IV.2, IV.4) in family 12 (Figure 1). This variant likely mediates the loss of the canonical splice acceptor site predicted by several in silico prediction tools and was previously reported in another Pakistani family with NSHL [5].

3.4. Autosomal Recessive HL Loci

Genome-wide genotyping and autozygosity mapping that were performed for 13 Pakistani families revealed loci for autosomal recessive HL (hg19) (Table 3).

The homozygous c.166C>T, p.(Leu56Phe) variant in *FGF3* was identified and supported by linkage intervals spanning 33.5 Mb and 6.1 Mb for families 1 and 2 (Table 3), respectively. The 19.4 Mb interval in family 4 (Table 3) included the homozygous c.470G>A, p.(Ser157Asn) variant in *MYO7A*. Family 5 revealed a 3.7 Mb interval that contained the c.3502C>T, p.(Arg1168Trp) variant in *MYO7A*. The longest interval (13.6 Mb) of the mapping data in family 6 (Table 3) was concordant with the homozygous c.1041dup, p.(Ser348Glnfs*2) variant in *CDC14A* detected by exome analysis. Family 7 revealed a 15.9 Mb interval (Table 3) on chromosome 13, encompassing *SLITRK6* and its homozygous c.120_121insT, p.(Asp41*) variant. The longest interval in family 9 (13.9 Mb, Table 3) included the homozygous *CDH23* c.2968G>A, p.(Asp990Asn) variant. Both intervals in families 10 (3.3 Mb, Table 3) and 11 (4.4 Mb, Table 3) included *GJB2*. Family 12 revealed a 7.7 Mb interval (Table 3) that was consistent with the exome data and includes *MYO15A*. The longest interval in family 13 (29.0 Mb) contained the homozygous *CDH23* c.4688T>C, p.(Leu1563Pro) variant (Table 3).

The most significant linkage intervals in families 3 and 8 did not include the affected genes *GJB2* and *MYO7A*. However, the longest interval in family 3 is located slightly outside of the *GJB2* gene coordinates.

Table 3. Loci for autosomal recessive HL in 13 Pakistani families.

Family ID	Chromosomal Band	Region of Autozygosity Identified by Linkage Analysis (hg19)	Length (Mb)	LOD	Causal Gene in Locus	Gene Coordinates (hg19)
Family 1	11p12-q13.4	39,536,493–73,025,971	33.5	2.529	FGF3	chr11:69,624,736–69,634,192
Family 2	11q13.1-q13.3	63,870,810–69,964,525	6.1	3.73	FGF3	chr11:69,624,736–69,634,192
Family 3 *	13q12.11-q14.11	22,661,666–41,063,028	18.4	1.927		
Family 4	11q13.3-q14.3	69,063,393–88,489,081	19.4	2.529	MYO7A	chr11:76,839,310–76,926,284
Family 5	11q13.5-q14.1	76,792,431–80,457,784	3.7	1.927	MYO7A	chr11:76,839,310–76,926,284
Family 6	1p22.2-p21.2	88,430,037–102,069,696	13.6	1.927	CDC14A	chr1:100,810,598–100,985,833
Family 7	13q22.1-q31.3	74,995,660–90,925,494	15.9	1.2	SLITRK6	chr13:86,366,925–86,373,554
Family 8	No interval close to MYO7A					
Family 9	10q21.2-q22.3	64,059,261–78,005,230	13.9	3.006	CDH23	chr10:73,156,691–73,575,702
Family 10	13q11-q12.11	19,121,950–22,395,049	3.3	2.529	GJB2	chr13:20,761,609–20,767,037
Family 11	13q11-q12.12	19,121,950–23,534,670	4.4	2.529	GJB2	chr13:20,761,609–20,767,037
Family 12	17p12-p11.2	13,801,016–21,539,613	7.7	2.529	MYO15A	chr17:18,012,020–18,083,116
Family 13	10q21.2-q23.31	61,998,060–91,002,927	29.0	1.2	CDH23	chr10:73,156,691–73,575,702

Abbreviations: LOD, logarithm of the odds. * Family 3 revealed a homozygous interval outside but near the GJB2 gene locus.

4. Discussion

Geographically or culturally isolated populations that have high rates of consanguinity, such as the Pakistani families included in this study, have proven valuable for novel HL gene identification studies and for contributing to a greater understanding of the alleles implicated in HL [46–48]. Although our patient cohort was relatively small, the overall resolve rate in this study of 61.9% is nonetheless comparable to other studies with consanguineous families that have showed a resolve rate of 67% [49]. As expected, most of the families revealed variants that were homozygous (92.3%) and compound heterozygous (7.7%) and were primarily found in ARHL-associated genes.

We identified causative variants in seven HL-associated genes. Many of these variants were missense (53.8%, Figure 3B), which is consistent with the mutational characteristics of deafness genes [50]. Unlike previous studies investigating the genetic spectrum of hearing-impaired Pakistani patients that have described SLC26A4 as a frequent cause of HL in this population, causal variants in this gene were not present in our cohort. This is likely explained due to the restricted geographical region from which our families were recruited and the existence of prevalent founder variants in this gene, especially in the Pakistani population, that were absent in our relatively small cohort [51].

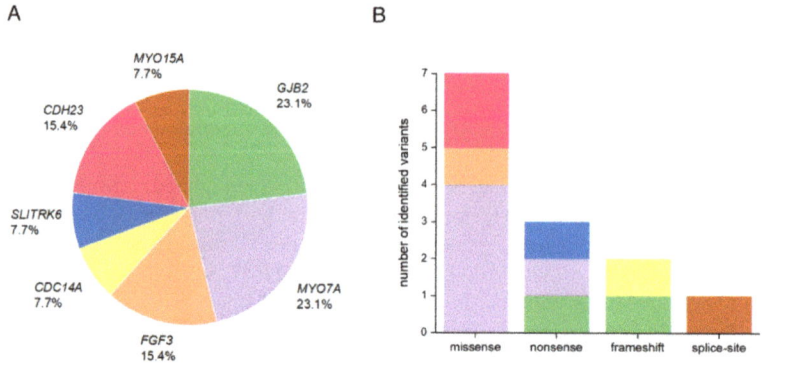

Figure 3. Overview of the affected genes and the distribution of different variant types in Pakistani families with HL. (**A**) Overall percentage of each affected gene in 13 Pakistani families. (**B**) Number of identified variants by type (missense, nonsense, frameshift, splice-site). The color code refers to the genes that are marked in (**A**).

Genes that are most frequently implicated in autosomal recessive NSHL (ARNSHL) in consanguineous families from Pakistan are GJB2 (MIM *121011), SLC26A4 (MIM *605646), MYO15A (MIM *602666), OTOF (MIM *603681), CDH23 (MIM *605516), TMC1 (MIM *606706), MYO7A (MIM *276903), and HGF (MIM *142409) [6,52,53]. Variants in the genes MYO7A and GJB2 accounted for a combined 46.2% of all diagnoses in the present study which is consistent with previously published rates from Pakistani cohort studies (Figure 3A) [5–7]. We also identified the c.231G>A, p.(Trp77*) variant in one family that has been reported as one of the most common *GJB2* alleles in Pakistani HL patients [54].

Interestingly, disease-causing variants in Pakistani patients with NSHL often involved genes that were also associated with syndromic HL, such as *MYO7A* [55] or *CDH23* [39]. For example, patients with a diagnosis of Usher syndrome type 1B (MIM *276900) show profound congenital hearing impairment, retinitis pigmentosa, vestibular dysfunction, and biallelic causal variants in *MYO7A* [56]. In this study, pathogenic variants of *MYO7A* were identified in three families (4, 5, 8). Affected individuals in family 4 and family 5 were confirmed with Usher syndrome, which is characterized by severe auditory and ophthalmic symptoms. Both of the homozygous variants that have been identified in family 4 (c.470G>A, p.(Ser157Asn)) and 5 (c.3502C>T, p.(Arg1168Trp)) are known to cause Usher syndrome type 1 [34,35].

Family 8 revealed three different heterozygous variants in *MYO7A*, with all three of them exclusively present in both affected siblings (IV.1, IV.2), in whom Usher syndrome was excluded. Interestingly, two of the three identified variants (c.1258A>T, c.4505A>G) were previously described in a Pakistani family reporting ARNSHL [6]. Richard et al. [6] also described a third heterozygous variant (c.3502C>T) that differs from the third variant in the present study (c.1849T>C). In family 8, the two c.1258A>T and c.4505A>G variants were inherited from the maternal allele (III.4), and the c.1849T>C variant was an inferred paternally inherited allele, thus confirming compound heterozygosity in both affected patients (IV.1, IV.2) of c.1258A>T, p.(Lys420*) and c.1849T>C, p.(Ser617Pro) (Figure 1). The absent homozygous interval in a region that contains *MYO7A* supports a suspected compound heterozygosity for the variants in this family. It remains to be determined if the double mutated maternal allele is either a broadly segregating allele in the Pakistani population or if the two families are possibly distantly related.

The homozygous c.2968G>A, p.(Asp990Asn) missense variant in *CDH23* segregating in family 9 was identified as a recurrent variant in South Indian families with HL [57] and is known to cause ARNSHL [39]. The second pathogenic homozygous missense variant in *CDH23* (c.4688T>C, p.(Leu1563Pro)), which is known to cause non-syndromic deafness, has been identified in family 13 [45].

We identified two unrelated families (1, 2) with the same c.166C>T, p.(Leu56Phe) variant in the gene *FGF3*. Recessive variants in *FGF3* have been described in patients diagnosed with LAMM syndrome, which is characterized by congenital deafness with labyrinthine aplasia (LA), microtia (M) and microdontia (M) (MIM *610706) [42]. The phenotypic characteristics in patients can vary from fully penetrant LAMM syndrome to milder forms with less severe syndromic features [58]. Probands from families 1 and 2 show HL and cupped ears (Figure 2A), which overlap with milder phenotypic characteristics such as minor dental and external ear phenotypes that were previously described in the literature. We cannot exclude an inner ear malformation in the affected individuals due to absent temporal bone CTs.

Three nonsense variants were found in the genes *GJB2*, *SLITRK6*, and *MYO7A* (Figure 3). While the c.231G>A, p.(Trp77*) variant in *GJB2* and the c.1258A>T, p.(Lys420*) variant in *MYO7A* were previously described as pathogenic, the nonsense variant c.120_121insT, p.(Asp41*) in *SLITRK6*, segregating in family 7, was novel. The effect of the induced stop-codon at amino acid position 41 out of 841 amino acids encoding SLITRK6 would truncate 95% of the protein and likely be targeted by nonsense-mediated mRNA decay (NMD) [59]. To date, only five variants are known to cause the associated autosomal recessive deafness and myopia syndrome [44,60,61] that is consistent with the phenotype in family 7. Myopia in deafness and myopia syndrome has been reported to range between −6 and −11 diopters [44,62]. Findings in both siblings (IV.1, IV.2) in family 7 and affected individuals (IV.3, IV.5) in family 4, who had undergone ophthalmological examination were consistent with high myopia. Additionally, IV.3 and IV.5 in family 4, and IV.2 in family 5 showed findings typical for retinitis pigmentosa. Interestingly, all the previously identified variants are also either nonsense or frameshift variants, suggesting loss-of-function as an underlying mechanism. Consistently, *Slitrk6* knock-out mice showed distinct reduction in cochlear innervation and a defective auditory brainstem response [44].

Family 12 revealed a homozygous splice-site variant c.9518-2A>G in intron 57 of *MYO15A* [5]. This variant likely mediates the complete loss of the 3′ acceptor site according to several in silico prediction tools, and possibly results in the skipping of exon 58. Variants that occur in important consensus sequences at the exon-intron boundaries, thus disrupting the actual splicing process, are known to be the cause of a variety of human diseases [63].

5. Conclusions

The present study of 21 Pakistani families identified two novel alleles causing HL and emphasizes the importance of investigating different populations and their heterogeneous genetic background. The fact that 38.1% of the 21 examined families are still considered unresolved highlights a possible area in which the further application of advanced sequencing and analysis methods could uncover currently unrecognized genetic changes due to technical limitations. Candidate genes have been identified in four families that are presently undergoing functional analysis. In families without candidate genes identified, genome sequencing would support uniform copy number variation analysis and the analysis of deep intronic or regulatory variants that are difficult to ascertain by ES. Some of the limitations of the study include potentially insufficient coverage of homopolymeric or GC-rich regions and the existence of mapping difficulties for regions containing pseudogenes or larger deletions, insertions, or structural rearrangements, as listed in previous ES studies, and may diagnose some of the unresolved families [64]. Nevertheless, an ES approach is still the method of choice for elucidating genetic variants in a large portion of heritable human disorders, including HL.

Supplementary Materials: The following are available online at http://www.mdpi.com/2073-4425/11/11/1329/s1: Figure S1: Sanger-sequencing chromatograms of 13 Pakistani families with HL. Figure S2: Overview of previously undescribed and known HL-related variants in *FGF3* and *SLITRK6*. Table S1: Primer sequences for identified variants in 13 Pakistani families with HL.

Author Contributions: Conceptualization, T.H., H.-G.K., B.V.; Manuscript drafting, J.D., B.V.; Ascertained families and obtained clinical data, S.K., N.M., S.A.K., H.N., A.K., N.A., L.C.L., I.K., I.-K.K., H.-G.K.; Supervision, T.H., I.N., B.V.; Exome sequencing and segregation analysis, J.D., L.S., S.M.K., M.A.H.H., T.R., T.D.G., J.D.J.L., B.V.; Autozygosity mapping and linkage analysis, F.R.; Interpretation of ophthalmological data, L.K.; Bioinformatics support, T.M., M.D. All the authors participated in final review and editing of the manuscript. All authors have read and agreed to the published version of the manuscript.

Funding: This research received no external funding.

Acknowledgments: The authors would like to express their sincere gratitude to the families for their participation in this study.

Conflicts of Interest: The authors declare no conflict of interest.

References

1. Hamamy, H. Consanguineous marriages: Preconception consultation in primary health care settings. *J. Community Genet.* **2012**, *3*, 185–192. [CrossRef] [PubMed]
2. Hussain, R.; Bittles, A.H. The prevalence and demographic characteristics of consanguineous marriages in Pakistan. *J. Biosoc. Sci.* **1998**, *30*, 261–275. [CrossRef] [PubMed]
3. Zakzouk, S. Consanguinity and hearing impairment in developing countries: A custom to be discouraged. *J. Laryngol. Otol.* **2002**, *116*, 811–816. [CrossRef] [PubMed]
4. Morton, C.C.; Nance, W.E. Newborn hearing screening–a silent revolution. *N. Engl. J. Med.* **2006**, *354*, 2151–2164. [CrossRef] [PubMed]
5. Khan, A.; Han, S.; Wang, R.; Ansar, M.; Ahmad, W.; Zhang, X. Sequence variants in genes causing nonsyndromic hearing loss in a Pakistani cohort. *Mol. Genet. Genom. Med.* **2019**, *7*, e917. [CrossRef] [PubMed]

6. Richard, E.M.; Santos-Cortez, R.L.P.; Faridi, R.; Rehman, A.U.; Lee, K.; Shahzad, M.; Acharya, A.; Khan, A.A.; Imtiaz, A.; Chakchouk, I.; et al. Global genetic insight contributed by consanguineous Pakistani families segregating hearing loss. *Hum. Mutat.* **2019**, *40*, 53–72. [CrossRef]
7. Shafique, S.; Siddiqi, S.; Schraders, M.; Oostrik, J.; Ayub, H.; Bilal, A.; Ajmal, M.; Seco, C.Z.; Strom, T.M.; Mansoor, A.; et al. Genetic spectrum of autosomal recessive non-syndromic hearing loss in Pakistani families. *PLoS ONE* **2014**, *9*, e100146. [CrossRef]
8. Parker, M.; Bitner-Glindzicz, M. Genetic investigations in childhood deafness. *Arch. Dis. Child.* **2015**, *100*, 271–278. [CrossRef]
9. Bademci, G.; Cengiz, F.B.; Foster Ii, J.; Duman, D.; Sennaroglu, L.; Diaz-Horta, O.; Atik, T.; Kirazli, T.; Olgun, L.; Alper, H.; et al. Variations in Multiple Syndromic Deafness Genes Mimic Non-syndromic Hearing Loss. *Sci. Rep.* **2016**, *6*, 31622. [CrossRef]
10. Sajjad, M.; Khattak, A.A.; Bunn, J.E.; Mackenzie, I. Causes of childhood deafness in Pukhtoonkhwa Province of Pakistan and the role of consanguinity. *J. Laryngol. Otol.* **2008**, *122*, 1057–1063. [CrossRef]
11. Vona, B.; Nanda, I.; Hofrichter, M.A.; Shehata-Dieler, W.; Haaf, T. Non-syndromic hearing loss gene identification: A brief history and glimpse into the future. *Mol. Cell Probes* **2015**, *29*, 260–270. [CrossRef] [PubMed]
12. Mazzoli, M.; Van Camp, G.; Newton, V.; Giarbini, N.; Declau, F.; Parving, A. Recommendations for the description of genetic and audiological data for families with nonsyndromic hereditary hearing impairment. *Audiol. Med.* **2003**, *1*, 148–150.
13. Ruschendorf, F.; Nurnberg, P. ALOHOMORA: A tool for linkage analysis using 10K SNP array data. *Bioinformatics* **2005**, *21*, 2123–2125. [CrossRef] [PubMed]
14. Abecasis, G.R.; Cherny, S.S.; Cookson, W.O.; Cardon, L.R. GRR: Graphical representation of relationship errors. *Bioinformatics* **2001**, *17*, 742–743. [CrossRef] [PubMed]
15. O'Connell, J.R.; Weeks, D.E. PedCheck: A program for identification of genotype incompatibilities in linkage analysis. *Am. J. Hum. Genet.* **1998**, *63*, 259–266. [CrossRef] [PubMed]
16. Abecasis, G.R.; Cherny, S.S.; Cookson, W.O.; Cardon, L.R. Merlin-rapid analysis of dense genetic maps using sparse gene flow trees. *Nat. Genet.* **2002**, *30*, 97–101. [CrossRef]
17. Sambrook, J.; Russell, D.W. Purification of nucleic acids by extraction with phenol: Chloroform. *CSH Protoc.* **2006**, *2006*. [CrossRef]
18. Green, M.R.; Sambrook, J. Precipitation of DNA with Ethanol. *Cold Spring Harb. Protoc.* **2016**, *2016*. [CrossRef]
19. Li, H.; Durbin, R. Fast and accurate long-read alignment with Burrows-Wheeler transform. *Bioinformatics* **2010**, *26*, 589–595. [CrossRef]
20. DePristo, M.A.; Banks, E.; Poplin, R.; Garimella, K.V.; Maguire, J.R.; Hartl, C.; Philippakis, A.A.; del Angel, G.; Rivas, M.A.; Hanna, M.; et al. A framework for variation discovery and genotyping using next-generation DNA sequencing data. *Nat. Genet.* **2011**, *43*, 491–498. [CrossRef]
21. McKenna, A.; Hanna, M.; Banks, E.; Sivachenko, A.; Cibulskis, K.; Kernytsky, A.; Garimella, K.; Altshuler, D.; Gabriel, S.; Daly, M.; et al. The Genome Analysis Toolkit: A MapReduce framework for analyzing next-generation DNA sequencing data. *Genome Res.* **2010**, *20*, 1297–1303. [CrossRef] [PubMed]
22. Adzhubei, I.A.; Schmidt, S.; Peshkin, L.; Ramensky, V.E.; Gerasimova, A.; Bork, P.; Kondrashov, A.S.; Sunyaev, S.R. A method and server for predicting damaging missense mutations. *Nat. Methods* **2010**, *7*, 248–249. [CrossRef] [PubMed]
23. Ng, P.C.; Henikoff, S. Predicting the effects of amino acid substitutions on protein function. *Annu. Rev. Genom. Hum. Genet.* **2006**, *7*, 61–80. [CrossRef] [PubMed]
24. Schwarz, J.M.; Cooper, D.N.; Schuelke, M.; Seelow, D. MutationTaster2: Mutation prediction for the deep-sequencing age. *Nat. Methods* **2014**, *11*, 361–362. [CrossRef] [PubMed]
25. Shihab, H.A.; Gough, J.; Cooper, D.N.; Stenson, P.D.; Barker, G.L.; Edwards, K.J.; Day, I.N.; Gaunt, T.R. Predicting the functional, molecular, and phenotypic consequences of amino acid substitutions using hidden Markov models. *Hum. Mutat.* **2013**, *34*, 57–65. [CrossRef]
26. Chun, S.; Fay, J.C. Identification of deleterious mutations within three human genomes. *Genome Res.* **2009**, *19*, 1553–1561. [CrossRef]
27. Cooper, G.M.; Stone, E.A.; Asimenos, G.; Green, E.D.; Batzoglou, S.; Sidow, A. Distribution and intensity of constraint in mammalian genomic sequence. *Genome Res.* **2005**, *15*, 901–913. [CrossRef]

28. Shearer, A.E.; Eppsteiner, R.W.; Booth, K.T.; Ephraim, S.S.; Gurrola, J., II; Simpson, A.; Black-Ziegelbein, E.A.; Joshi, S.; Ravi, H.; Giuffre, A.C.; et al. Utilizing ethnic-specific differences in minor allele frequency to recategorize reported pathogenic deafness variants. *Am. J. Hum. Genet.* **2014**, *95*, 445–453. [CrossRef]
29. Scott, E.M.; Halees, A.; Itan, Y.; Spencer, E.G.; He, Y.; Azab, M.A.; Gabriel, S.B.; Belkadi, A.; Boisson, B.; Abel, L.; et al. Characterization of Greater Middle Eastern genetic variation for enhanced disease gene discovery. *Nat. Genet.* **2016**, *48*, 1071–1076. [CrossRef]
30. Karczewski, K.J.; Francioli, L.C.; Tiao, G.; Cummings, B.B.; Alföldi, J.; Wang, Q.; Collins, R.L.; Laricchia, K.M.; Ganna, A.; Birnbaum, D.P.; et al. Variation across 141,456 human exomes and genomes reveals the spectrum of loss-of-function intolerance across human protein-coding genes. *bioRXiv* **2019**. [CrossRef]
31. Fromer, M.; Purcell, S.M. Using XHMM Software to Detect Copy Number Variation in Whole-Exome Sequencing Data. *Curr. Protoc. Hum. Genet.* **2014**, *81*, 7–23. [CrossRef] [PubMed]
32. Untergasser, A.; Cutcutache, I.; Koressaar, T.; Ye, J.; Faircloth, B.C.; Remm, M.; Rozen, S.G. Primer3-new capabilities and interfaces. *Nucleic Acids Res.* **2012**, *40*, e115. [CrossRef] [PubMed]
33. Kelsell, D.P.; Dunlop, J.; Stevens, H.P.; Lench, N.J.; Liang, J.N.; Parry, G.; Mueller, R.F.; Leigh, I.M. Connexin 26 mutations in hereditary non-syndromic sensorineural deafness. *Nature* **1997**, *387*, 80–83. [CrossRef] [PubMed]
34. Jaijo, T.; Aller, E.; Oltra, S.; Beneyto, M.; Najera, C.; Ayuso, C.; Baiget, M.; Carballo, M.; Antinolo, G.; Valverde, D.; et al. Mutation profile of the MYO7A gene in Spanish patients with Usher syndrome type I. *Hum. Mutat.* **2006**, *27*, 290–291. [CrossRef] [PubMed]
35. Le Guedard-Mereuze, S.; Vache, C.; Baux, D.; Faugere, V.; Larrieu, L.; Abadie, C.; Janecke, A.; Claustres, M.; Roux, A.F.; Tuffery-Giraud, S. Ex vivo splicing assays of mutations at noncanonical positions of splice sites in USHER genes. *Hum. Mutat.* **2010**, *31*, 347–355. [CrossRef] [PubMed]
36. Doll, J.; Kolb, S.; Schnapp, L.; Rad, A.; Ruschendorf, F.; Khan, I.; Adli, A.; Hasanzadeh, A.; Liedtke, D.; Knaup, S.; et al. Novel Loss-of-Function Variants in CDC14A are Associated with Recessive Sensorineural Hearing Loss in Iranian and Pakistani Patients. *Int. J. Mol. Sci.* **2020**, *21*, 311. [CrossRef]
37. Cremers, F.P.; Kimberling, W.J.; Kulm, M.; de Brouwer, A.P.; van Wijk, E.; te Brinke, H.; Cremers, C.W.; Hoefsloot, L.H.; Banfi, S.; Simonelli, F.; et al. Development of a genotyping microarray for Usher syndrome. *J. Med. Genet.* **2007**, *44*, 153–160. [CrossRef]
38. Carss, K.J.; Arno, G.; Erwood, M.; Stephens, J.; Sanchis-Juan, A.; Hull, S.; Megy, K.; Grozeva, D.; Dewhurst, E.; Malka, S.; et al. Comprehensive Rare Variant Analysis via Whole-Genome Sequencing to Determine the Molecular Pathology of Inherited Retinal Disease. *Am. J. Hum. Genet.* **2017**, *100*, 75–90. [CrossRef]
39. Bork, J.M.; Peters, L.M.; Riazuddin, S.; Bernstein, S.L.; Ahmed, Z.M.; Ness, S.L.; Polomeno, R.; Ramesh, A.; Schloss, M.; Srisailpathy, C.R.; et al. Usher syndrome 1D and nonsyndromic autosomal recessive deafness DFNB12 are caused by allelic mutations of the novel cadherin-like gene CDH23. *Am. J. Hum. Genet.* **2001**, *68*, 26–37. [CrossRef]
40. Zelante, L.; Gasparini, P.; Estivill, X.; Melchionda, S.; D'Agruma, L.; Govea, N.; Mila, M.; Monica, M.D.; Lutfi, J.; Shohat, M.; et al. Connexin26 mutations associated with the most common form of non-syndromic neurosensory autosomal recessive deafness (DFNB1) in Mediterraneans. *Hum. Mol. Genet.* **1997**, *6*, 1605–1609. [CrossRef]
41. Schultz, J.M.; Bhatti, R.; Madeo, A.C.; Turriff, A.; Muskett, J.A.; Zalewski, C.K.; King, K.A.; Ahmed, Z.M.; Riazuddin, S.; Ahmad, N.; et al. Allelic hierarchy of CDH23 mutations causing non-syndromic deafness DFNB12 or Usher syndrome USH1D in compound heterozygotes. *J. Med. Genet.* **2011**, *48*, 767–775. [CrossRef] [PubMed]
42. Oza, A.M.; DiStefano, M.T.; Hemphill, S.E.; Cushman, B.J.; Grant, A.R.; Siegert, R.K.; Shen, J.; Chapin, A.; Boczek, N.J.; Schimmenti, L.A.; et al. Expert specification of the ACMG/AMP variant interpretation guidelines for genetic hearing loss. *Hum. Mutat.* **2018**, *39*, 1593–1613. [CrossRef] [PubMed]
43. Tekin, M.; Hismi, B.O.; Fitoz, S.; Ozdag, H.; Cengiz, F.B.; Sirmaci, A.; Aslan, I.; Inceoglu, B.; Yuksel-Konuk, E.B.; Yilmaz, S.T.; et al. Homozygous mutations in fibroblast growth factor 3 are associated with a new form of syndromic deafness characterized by inner ear agenesis, microtia, and microdontia. *Am. J. Hum. Genet.* **2007**, *80*, 338–344. [CrossRef] [PubMed]
44. Aparisi, M.J.; Garcia-Garcia, G.; Aller, E.; Sequedo, M.D.; de la Camara, C.M.-F.; Rodrigo, R.; Armengot, M.; Cortijo, J.; Milara, J.; Diaz, L.M.; et al. Study of USH1 splicing variants through minigenes and transcript analysis from nasal epithelial cells. *PLoS ONE* **2013**, *8*, e57506. [CrossRef] [PubMed]

45. Tekin, M.; Chioza, B.A.; Matsumoto, Y.; Diaz-Horta, O.; Cross, H.E.; Duman, D.; Kokotas, H.; Moore-Barton, H.L.; Sakoori, K.; Ota, M.; et al. SLITRK6 mutations cause myopia and deafness in humans and mice. *J. Clin. Investig.* **2013**, *123*, 2094–2102. [CrossRef]
46. Yan, D.; Kannan-Sundhari, A.; Vishwanath, S.; Qing, J.; Mittal, R.; Kameswaran, M.; Liu, X.Z. The Genetic Basis of Nonsyndromic Hearing Loss in Indian and Pakistani Populations. *Genet. Test. Mol. Biomark.* **2015**, *19*, 512–527. [CrossRef]
47. Heutink, P.; Oostra, B.A. Gene finding in genetically isolated populations. *Hum. Mol. Genet.* **2002**, *11*, 2507–2515. [CrossRef]
48. Friedman, T.B.; Griffith, A.J. Human nonsyndromic sensorineural deafness. *Annu. Rev. Genom. Hum. Genet.* **2003**, *4*, 341–402. [CrossRef]
49. Sloan-Heggen, C.M.; Babanejad, M.; Beheshtian, M.; Simpson, A.C.; Booth, K.T.; Ardalani, F.; Frees, K.L.; Mohseni, M.; Mozafari, R.; Mehrjoo, Z.; et al. Characterising the spectrum of autosomal recessive hereditary hearing loss in Iran. *J. Med. Genet.* **2015**, *52*, 823–829. [CrossRef]
50. Azaiez, H.; Booth, K.T.; Ephraim, S.S.; Crone, B.; Black-Ziegelbein, E.A.; Marini, R.J.; Shearer, A.E.; Sloan-Heggen, C.M.; Kolbe, D.; Casavant, T.; et al. Genomic Landscape and Mutational Signatures of Deafness-Associated Genes. *Am. J. Hum. Genet.* **2018**, *103*, 484–497. [CrossRef]
51. Anwar, S.; Riazuddin, S.; Ahmed, Z.M.; Tasneem, S.; Ateequl, J.; Khan, S.Y.; Griffith, A.J.; Friedman, T.B.; Riazuddin, S. SLC26A4 mutation spectrum associated with DFNB4 deafness and Pendred's syndrome in Pakistanis. *J. Hum. Genet.* **2009**, *54*, 266–270. [CrossRef] [PubMed]
52. Hilgert, N.; Smith, R.J.; Van Camp, G. Forty-six genes causing nonsyndromic hearing impairment: Which ones should be analyzed in DNA diagnostics? *Mutat. Res.* **2009**, *681*, 189–196. [CrossRef] [PubMed]
53. Schultz, J.M.; Khan, S.N.; Ahmed, Z.M.; Riazuddin, S.; Waryah, A.M.; Chhatre, D.; Starost, M.F.; Ploplis, B.; Buckley, S.; Velasquez, D.; et al. Noncoding mutations of HGF are associated with nonsyndromic hearing loss, DFNB39. *Am. J. Hum. Genet.* **2009**, *85*, 25–39. [CrossRef] [PubMed]
54. Anjum, S.; Azhar, A.; Tariq, M.; Baig, S.M.; Bolz, H.J.; Qayyum, M.; Naqvi, S.M.S.; Raja, G.K. GJB2 Gene Mutations Causing Hearing Loss in Pakistani Families. *Pak. J. Life Soc. Sci.* **2014**, *12*, 126–131.
55. Liu, X.Z.; Walsh, J.; Mburu, P.; Kendrick-Jones, J.; Cope, M.J.; Steel, K.P.; Brown, S.D. Mutations in the myosin VIIA gene cause non-syndromic recessive deafness. *Nat. Genet.* **1997**, *16*, 188–190. [CrossRef] [PubMed]
56. Weil, D.; Blanchard, S.; Kaplan, J.; Guilford, P.; Gibson, F.; Walsh, J.; Mburu, P.; Varela, A.; Levilliers, J.; Weston, M.D.; et al. Defective myosin VIIA gene responsible for Usher syndrome type 1B. *Nature* **1995**, *374*, 60–61. [CrossRef]
57. Vanniya, S.P.; Chandru, J.; Pavithra, A.; Jeffrey, J.M.; Kalaimathi, M.; Ramakrishnan, R.; Karthikeyen, N.P.; Srikumari, C.R.S. Recurrence of reported CDH23 mutations causing DFNB12 in a special cohort of South Indian hearing impaired assortative mating families—An evaluation. *Ann. Hum. Genet.* **2018**, *82*, 119–126. [CrossRef]
58. Riazuddin, S.; Ahmed, Z.M.; Hegde, R.S.; Khan, S.N.; Nasir, I.; Shaukat, U.; Riazuddin, S.; Butman, J.A.; Griffith, A.J.; Friedman, T.B.; et al. Variable expressivity of FGF3 mutations associated with deafness and LAMM syndrome. *BMC Med. Genet.* **2011**, *12*, 21. [CrossRef]
59. Maquat, L.E. Nonsense-mediated mRNA decay: Splicing, translation and mRNP dynamics. *Nat. Rev. Mol. Cell Biol.* **2004**, *5*, 89–99. [CrossRef]
60. Salime, S.; Riahi, Z.; Elrharchi, S.; Elkhattabi, L.; Charoute, H.; Nahili, H.; Rouba, H.; Kabine, M.; Bonnet, C.; Petit, C.; et al. A novel mutation in SLITRK6 causes deafness and myopia in a Moroccan family. *Gene* **2018**, *659*, 89–92. [CrossRef]
61. Van Beeck Calkoen, E.A.; Engel, M.S.D.; van de Kamp, J.M.; Yntema, H.G.; Goverts, S.T.; Mulder, M.F.; Merkus, P.; Hensen, E.F. The etiological evaluation of sensorineural hearing loss in children. *Eur. J. Pediatr.* **2019**, *178*, 1195–1205. [CrossRef] [PubMed]
62. Ordonez, J.L.; Tekin, M. Deafness and Myopia Syndrome. In *GeneReviews((R))*; Adam, M.P., Ardinger, H.H., Pagon, R.A., Wallace, S.E., Bean, L.J.H., Stephens, K., Amemiya, A., Eds.; University of Washington: Seattle, WA, USA, 1993.
63. Anna, A.; Monika, G. Splicing mutations in human genetic disorders: Examples, detection, and confirmation. *J. Appl. Genet.* **2018**, *59*, 253–268. [CrossRef] [PubMed]

64. Sheppard, S.; Biswas, S.; Li, M.H.; Jayaraman, V.; Slack, I.; Romasko, E.J.; Sasson, A.; Brunton, J.; Rajagopalan, R.; Sarmady, M.; et al. Utility and limitations of exome sequencing as a genetic diagnostic tool for children with hearing loss. *Genet. Med.* **2018**, *20*, 1663–1676. [CrossRef] [PubMed]

Publisher's Note: MDPI stays neutral with regard to jurisdictional claims in published maps and institutional affiliations.

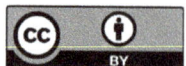

© 2020 by the authors. Licensee MDPI, Basel, Switzerland. This article is an open access article distributed under the terms and conditions of the Creative Commons Attribution (CC BY) license (http://creativecommons.org/licenses/by/4.0/).

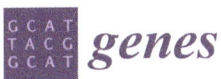

Review

Systematic Review of Sequencing Studies and Gene Expression Profiling in Familial Meniere Disease

Alba Escalera-Balsera [1], Pablo Roman-Naranjo [1] and Jose Antonio Lopez-Escamez [1,2,3,*]

[1] Otology & Neurotology Group CTS 495, Department of Genomic Medicine, Centro Pfizer-Universidad de Granada-Junta de Andalucía de Genómica e Investigación Oncológica, 18016 Granada, Spain; alba.escalera@genyo.es (A.E.-B.); pablo.roman@genyo.es (P.R.-N.)

[2] Department of Otolaryngology, Instituto de Investigación Biosanitaria, ibs.GRANADA, Hospital Universitario Virgen de las Nieves, 18014 Granada, Spain

[3] Department of Surgery, Division of Otolaryngology, Universidad de Granada, 18016 Granada, Spain

* Correspondence: antonio.lopezescamez@genyo.es; Tel.: +34-958-715-500 (ext. 160)

Received: 1 October 2020; Accepted: 25 November 2020; Published: 27 November 2020

Abstract: Familial Meniere Disease (FMD) is a rare inner ear disorder characterized by episodic vertigo associated with sensorineural hearing loss, tinnitus and/or aural fullness. We conducted a systematic review to find sequencing studies segregating rare variants in FMD to obtain evidence to support candidate genes for MD. After evaluating the quality of the retrieved records, eight studies were selected to carry out a quantitative synthesis. These articles described 20 single nucleotide variants (SNVs) in 11 genes (*FAM136A*, *DTNA*, *PRKCB*, *COCH*, *DPT*, *SEMA3D*, *STRC*, *HMX2*, *TMEM55B*, *OTOG* and *LSAMP*), most of them in singular families—the exception being the *OTOG* gene. Furthermore, we analyzed the pathogenicity of each SNV and compared its allelic frequency with reference datasets to evaluate its role in the pathogenesis of FMD. By retrieving gene expression data in these genes from different databases, we could classify them according to their gene expression in neural or inner ear tissues. Finally, we evaluated the pattern of inheritance to conclude which genes show an autosomal dominant (AD) or autosomal recessive (AR) inheritance in FMD.

Keywords: Meniere's disease; exome sequencing; sensorineural hearing loss; vestibular disorders; familial segregation; single nucleotide variant; rare variant; Mendelian disorders; inheritance pattern

1. Introduction

The human inner ear is formed by six sensory organs: the spiral organ of Corti, located in the anterior part of the temporal bone, and the vestibular organs that consist of the utricle, the saccule, and the three semicircular canals that form the posterior labyrinth. These organs share a highly specialized tissue, the neurosensory epithelium, which contains the auditory and vestibular hair cells (HCs). The displacement of HC stereocilia opens the mechanotransduction channels at the hair bundle that mediates the conversion of mechanical signals to neural impulses at the afferent synapses to drive acoustic or acceleration information to the cochlear or vestibular nuclei in the brainstem [1,2].

Meniere Disease (MD) is an inner ear disorder that is characterized by episodic vertigo and associated with sensorineural hearing loss (SNHL), tinnitus and/or aural fullness. It is a multifactorial disorder where the combined effect of genetics and environmental factors probably determine the onset of the condition. The criteria to diagnose MD are based on the clinical symptoms occurring during the attacks of vertigo and the documentation of SNHL by a pure tone audiogram before, during or after the episode of vertigo [3]. Notably, MD and vestibular migraine, whose clinical features could overlap, are the most common causes of spontaneous recurrent vertigo [4].

Histopathological and MRI studies have demonstrated an enlargement of the endolymphatic space in patients with MD, with an accumulation of endolymph in the saccule and the cochlea—termed as endolymphatic hydrops [5].

The prevalence of MD in a population changes according to the geographical region and the ethnic background. Epidemiology records report a prevalence of MD that varies from 17 to 200 cases/100,000. In general, MD is more common in European descendants [6], and the age of onset ranges from 30 to 70 years. Moreover, MD is associated with several comorbid conditions such as autoimmune arthritis, psoriasis, irritable bowel syndrome and migraine [7].

Hierarchical clustering methods have identified five clinical subgroups of patients with MD, one of them being familial MD (FMD) [8,9]. FMD is a rare disease that is defined if at least another family member in the first or second degree, in addition to the proband, fulfills all the clinical criteria of definite or probable MD [3].

In populations of European descent, the FMD represents 8–9% of cases [10,11]. The pattern of inheritance is autosomal dominant (AD) in most families; however, genetic heterogeneity is found and recessive inheritance has also been reported [10]. A family history where several members have SNHL, migraine or recurrent vertigo, justifies the investigation of the proband and their relatives to verify if any of them accomplish the diagnostic criteria for MD [3].

Early studies in multiplex families with FMD using microsatellite markers and segregation analysis pointed to different loci [12–14], but no causal gene was identified. However, the development of exome sequencing has facilitated the identification of few novel candidate genes in singular families [15–17].

The aim of this systematic review is to critically analyze the evidence to support causal genes in FMD and to describe the potential role of these genes in the pathogenesis of MD by retrieving information from gene expression databases.

2. Materials and Methods

2.1. Study Design

This is a systematic review of sequencing studies in FMD, which follows Preferred Reporting Items for Systematic Reviews (PRISMA) guidelines (Supplementary Table S1) [18]. We also conducted an additional search in general and tissue specific databases to retrieve gene expression profiles of candidate genes for FMD.

2.2. Research Question and Selection Criteria

This systematic review aims to describe genes reported in FMD in sequencing studies and to find which cell types and extracellular structures are potentially involved. Therefore, we formulated the question "which genes have been found to be associated with FMD?". In concordance with the methodology for systematic reviews, this question was answered following the PICOS strategy:

- Population: Patients diagnosed with FMD.
- Intervention: Sequencing studies (Sanger or exome/genome sequencing) in FMD searching for rare variants to target candidate genes.
- Comparison: Allelic frequency (AF) was compared with population specific reference datasets (gnomAD: Genome Aggregation Database, CSVS: Collaborative Spanish Variant Server, SweGen and ExAC: Exome Aggregation Consortium) [19–22], for candidate variants in selected genes.
- Outcome: Genetic findings and pathogenicity scores reported (rare variants, candidate genes).
- Study design: Familial segregation studies.

2.3. Search Strategies

The literature search was carried out on 11th August 2020 using the PubMed database with the following keywords: (familial [Title/Abstract] OR family [Title/Abstract] OR gene [Title/Abstract] OR genes [Title/Abstract] OR inheritance [Title/Abstract] OR variation [Title/Abstract] OR mutation [Title/Abstract]) AND (Meniere Disease [Title/Abstract] OR Meniere's Disease [Title/Abstract]). The search was filtered by the last 20 years (2000–2020) and written in English, by configuring an advanced search on PubMed.

Gene expression profiles for the candidate genes retrieved from the different studies were analyzed using the following datasets:

- Gene transcripts identified in the Neuropil and Somata layers of CA1 region in the Hippocampus in *Rattus norvegicus* by Cajigas et al. [23].
- Human synaptic genes in SynaptomeDB [24].
- Transcriptome catalogue of adult human inner ear, and the list of preferentially expressed mRNA genes in the inner ear when compared to 32 other tissues [25].

Additionally, the following datasets were obtained from the gEAR portal (https://umgear.org/):

- RNA-Seq in embryonic day 16.5 (E16.5) and postnatal day 0 (P0) from cochlear and vestibular sensory epithelium in mouse [26].
- RNA-Seq in P0 from cochlea and vestibule in mouse, where HCs were compared with epithelial non-HCs [27].
- RNA-Seq in P0 from cochlea in mouse to contrast HC with the rest of cochlear duct [28].
- RNA-Seq in adult mice from organ of Corti, comparing inner HCs (IHC), outer HC (OHCs), Deiters' cells and pillar cells [29].
- Single cell RNA-Seq in postnatal day 1 (P1) and 7 (P7) from organ of Corti in mouse [30].

Furthermore, the SHIELD database [31] was used to retrieve the following datasets:

- RNA expression by microarray from adult mice from cochlea to analyze IHC and OHC [32].
- RNA expression by microarray from developmental stages of mice from spiral ganglion (SG) and vestibular ganglion (VG) [2].

2.4. Exclusion Criteria

Articles that accomplish the following characteristics were excluded from the systematic review:

- Animal studies were excluded from the first analysis.
- Studies not published in English.

2.5. Quality Assessment of Selected Studies

After screening titles and abstracts of the selected records, reviews, meta-analysis, and irrelevant records (non-genetic studies, pharmacogenomics or clinical studies) were removed. Articles that did not meet the eligibility criteria were discarded. The criteria were composed by three main questions:

- Is the study performed with two or more members of a family diagnosed with MD or with patients from different families but all of them diagnosed with FMD?
- Has the study reported a gene or a position in the genome statistically significant when it was compared to genome reference datasets?
- Has the study used an accurate methodology and is it described with enough details to validate its findings?

If all these questions were answered with "yes", the record was selected for synthesis. Next, each reported variant was assessed and classified as benign/likely benign/unknown significance/likely pathogenic or pathogenic according to the American College of Medical Genetics and Genomics (ACMG) criteria [33,34] and a Combined Annotation Dependent Depletion (CADD) score [35,36].

2.6. Data Extraction and Synthesis

From each article selected, the following information was extracted to perform the synthesis: first author's last name, publication year, study design, population, number of patients in the study, sex of the patients, diagnostic criteria used for MD, sequencing method and genetic findings, gene and genomic position of the variant type (single nucleotide or structural variant). Moreover, the Reference Single Nucleotide Polymorphism (rs), the AF in gnomAD, CSVS, SweGen and ExAC, the pathogenicity score according to the ACMG criteria, the CADD score and the inheritance pattern were obtained or calculated. In this systematic review, the list of retrieved candidate genes and the classification of these genes according to their inheritance pattern were the main outcomes. Furthermore, the gene expression profile in neural or inner ear tissues was used to define the cell types involved with each gene.

3. Results

3.1. Selection and Characteristics of FMD Studies

With the objective of knowing which of the rare variants or genes related to FMD, we obtained 191 articles from PubMed. Afterwards, reviews, meta-analysis and irrelevant records were removed. Finally, we evaluated if the 64 remaining articles met the eligibility criteria and eight of them were selected for qualitative synthesis (Figure 1).

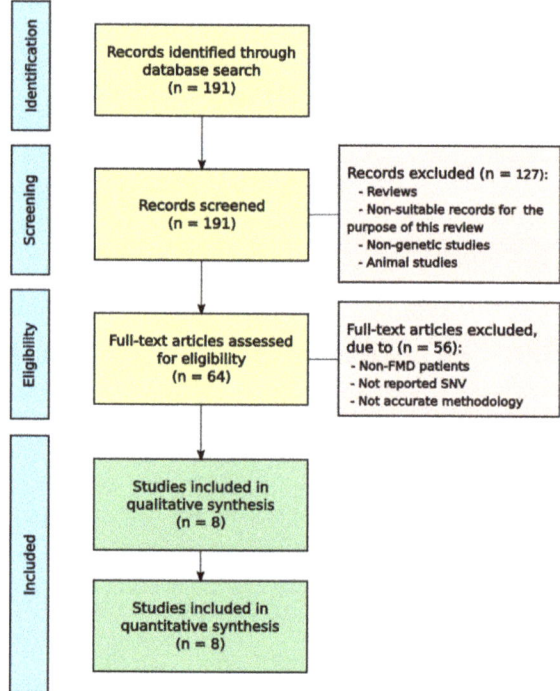

Figure 1. Flowchart to select Familial Meniere Disease (FMD) studies.

One of the questions to accomplish the eligibility criteria was if all reported patients in each family were diagnosed as FMD, preferably they should be diagnosed following the diagnostic criteria described by the International Classification Committee for Vestibular Disorders of the Barany Society in 2015 [3]; however, only three of eight studies used these criteria; another three studies used the diagnostic criteria of the Committee on Hearing and Equilibrium of the American Academy of

Otolaryngology–Head and Neck Surgery (AAO-HNS) published in 1995 [37], and two studies did not clarify the diagnostic criteria. One of them included three individuals in the same family with SNHL and episodic vertigo, and the other reported definite MD in two sisters without stating if they used the AAO-HNS or the Barany criteria to define MD. The diagnostic criteria of the Barany Society and the AAO-HNS are described in the Supplementary Table S2.

Among the eight selected studies, three articles reported candidate variants in two genes, one of them, *FAM136A* and *DTNA* in the same Spanish family, another record reported *DPT* and *SEMA3D* in two unrelated Spanish families and the other *HMX2* and *TMEM55B* in the same Finnish family. Five studies confirmed only one gene (*PRKCB*, *COCH*, *STRC*, *OTOG* and *LSAMP*) in families from Iran, South Korea, Spain and Sweden.

All studies used Whole Exome Sequencing (WES), and seven of them also performed Sanger sequencing to validate the variants. Moreover, all of them have data about the population ancestry, the sex and the number of individuals affected. A summary of these studies is shown in Table 1.

Table 1. Summary of studies which describe single nucleotide variants (SNVs) selected for quantitative synthesis.

Ref.	Population	Patients	Sex	Diagnosis	Genetic Findings	
					Gene	SNV
[15]	Spanish	3	F	AAO-HNS	FAM136A	2:70527974G>A
					DTNA	18:32462094G>T
[16]	Spanish	2	M	AAO-HNS	PRKCB	16:23999898G>T
[38]	Korean	3	F, M	Barany Society	COCH	14:31349796G>A
[17]	Spanish	3	F	Barany Society	DPT	1:168665849G>A
		3	F, M		SEMA3D	7:84642128G>A
[39]	Swedish–Norwegian	3	M	SNHL and episodic vertigo	STRC	15:43896948G>A
[40]	Finnish	2	M	AAO-HNS	HMX2	10:124909634T>A
					TMEM55B	14:20927370G>A
[41]	Spanish	73	F, M	Barany Society	OTOG	11:17574758G>A
						11:17578774G>A
						11:17594747C>A
						11:17621218C>T
						11:17627548G>A
						11:17631453C>T
						11:17632921C>T
						11:17656672G>A
						11:17663747G>A
						11:17667139G>C
[42]	Iranian	2	F, M	Definite MD	LSAMP	3:115561402T>C *

F: female; M: male; AAO-HNS: American Academy of Otolaryngology–Head and Neck Surgery; SNHL: sensorineural hearing loss; MD: Meniere Disease; *: this SNV was not validated by Sanger sequencing.

3.2. Inheritance of SNVs Associated with FMD

Requena et al. [15] studied a family with three affected women in consecutive generations with definite MD. All cases segregated two heterozygous rare variants in *FAM136A* and *DTNA* genes, which suggests an AD pattern of inheritance. The variant chr2:70527974G>A in *FAM136A* (NM_032822.3) was a nonsense novel variant leading to a stop codon; the ultrarare heterozygous variant chr18:32462094G>T reported in the *DTNA* gene (NM_001390.4) produces an amino acid change from valine to phenylalanine and generates a novel splice-site sequence predicted as a constitutive acceptor. Both variants were classified as pathogenic (Table 2).

The novel missense variant in the *PRKCB* gene (NM_002738.7) [16] was found in a family with two cases of complete MD phenotype and the father of the proband with SNHL (incomplete phenotype), and the pattern of inheritance was considered AD with incomplete penetrance. The chr16:23999898G>T variant causes an amino acid change from glycine to valine and it was considered likely pathogenic.

The chr14:31349796G>A variant in the *COCH* gene was reported in a Korean family with DFNA9 phenotype [38]; of note, two siblings and her mother presented episodic vertigo and SNHL fulfilling criteria for definite MD and another two siblings had an incomplete phenotype. This SNV showed an AD inheritance pattern with incomplete phenotype and this family should be considered as FMD. This SNV is not described in gnomAD or ClinVar and it was classified as likely pathogenic.

The SNV in the *SEMA3D* gene (NM_152754.2) [17] was found in a family with three individuals affected by MD in the same generation, all of them segregated the novel missense variant; in addition, there were another three individuals with incomplete phenotype in different generations. This variant, in chr7:84642128G>A, causes an amino acid change from proline to serine and it was classified as pathogenic. In the same article, Martín-Sierra et al. found a missense variant in the *DPT* gene (NM_001937.4) in a family with three sisters affected by MD, and one of the probands had anti-ribonucleoprotein antibodies, suggesting a comorbid immune disorder without all criteria for systemic lupus erythematosus.

Furthermore, in the family, seven relatives had incomplete phenotype (SNHL or episodic vertigo). The three patients with MD and two individuals presenting progressive bilateral SNHL and sudden SNHL, segregated the variant. The chr1:168665849G>A produces an amino acid change from arginine to cysteine and it was classified as likely pathogenic. Both SNVs had an AD inheritance pattern with an incomplete penetrance.

Frykholm et al. [39] described a family with two brothers and a first cousin with moderate, non-progressive SNHL and episodic vertigo. The two brothers shared a nonsense homozygous variant, which is chr15:43896948G>A, in the *STRC* gene (NM_153700.2), and the cousin had the same variant in heterozygosis inherited from the mother and a deletion of approximately 97 kb spanning the *STRC* gene, inherited from the father. None of the parents had symptoms of the disease, which suggests that it had an AR inheritance pattern.

Skarp et al. [40] found two heterozygous variants in *HMX2* and *TMEM55B*, which were present in an individual and his grandfather, both affected with MD. The father of the first individual did not report any symptoms of MD, and he would be an obligate carrier of these variants, but it was not possible to validate them because he did not donate a DNA sample for the study. Since these SNVs do not lead to MD with full penetrance, additional heterozygous variants in these genes should be considered to confirm recessive inheritance in this family. Both missense variants, chr10:124909634T>A in the *HMX2* gene (NM_005519.1) lead to an amino acid change from tyrosine to asparagine and chr14:20927370G>A in the *TMEM55B* gene (NM_001100814.2) from leucine to phenylalanine and were classified as likely pathogenic and with uncertain significance, respectively.

Roman-Naranjo et al. [41] reported several missense variants in the *OTOG* gene (NM_001277269.2) in multiplex Spanish families with FMD. Moreover, this study used a group of sporadic cases with MD, and AFs were compared with the non-Finnish European and Spanish (gnomAD) reference population datasets (CSVS). A heterozygous variant (chr11:17574758G>A), classified as pathogenic, was observed in two cases from two unrelated families; both families also shared the rare variant chr11:17663747G>A and one of them also had a third variant, chr11:17627548G>A. Moreover, two heterozygous variants, chr11:17578774G>A and chr11:17632921C>T, were found in four additional patients from four different unrelated families. In both sets of families, heterozygous compound recessive inheritance pattern was suggested. The rest of the variants were reported in three, two or one unrelated patients with FMD.

Table 2. Genetic findings for each SNV (single nucleotide variant), pathogenicity and inheritance pattern.

Gene	Chr	Position	ID	cDNA	Protein	Variant Effect	Allelic Frequency [1] gnomAD	Allelic Frequency [1] Other	ACMG Classification	CADD Score	Inheritance Pattern
FAM136A	2	70527974	rs690016537	c.226C>T	p.Gln76*	Nonsense	Novel		Pathogenic (PS3, PS4, PM2, PM4, PP3)	41.00	AD
DTNA	18	32462094	rs533568822	c.2143G>T	p.Val715Phe	Missense	8.79×10^{-6}	NF (CSVS)	Pathogenic (PS3, PS4, BP1)	24.90	AD
PRKCB	16	23999898	rs1131692056	c.275G>T	p.Gly92Val	Missense	Novel		Likely Pathogenic (PS4, PM2, PP3, PP5)	28.20	AD [2]
COCH	14	31349796	-	-	-	-	Novel		Likely Pathogenic (PS4, PM2, PP2, PP3, PP5)	28.10	AD [2]
DPT	1	168665849	rs748718975	c.544C>T	p.Arg182Cys	Missense	1.72×10^{-5}	NF (CSVS)	Likely Pathogenic (PS4, PM1, PP3, PP5, BP1)	32.00	AD [2]
SEMA3D	7	84642128	rs1057519374	c.1738C>T	p.Pro580Ser	Missense	Novel		Pathogenic (PS4, PM1, PM2, PP3, PP5)	25.00	AD [2]
STRC	15	43896948	rs144948296	c.4027C>T	p.Gln1343*	Nonsense	3.62×10^{-4}	0.001 (SweGen)	Pathogenic (PSV1, PS4, PM2, PP3, PP5)	40.00	AR
HMX2	10	124909634	rs1274867386	c.817T>A	p.Tyr273Asn	Missense	Novel		Likely Pathogenic (PS4, PM2, PP3)	31.00	AR [3]
TMEM55B	14	20927370	rs201529818	c.706C>T	p.Leu229Phe	Missense	9.56×10^{-4}	8.2×10^{-5} (ExAC)	Uncertain Significance (PS4, PP3, BS1)	25.80	AR [3]

Table 2. Cont.

Gene	Chr	Position	ID	cDNA	Protein	Variant Effect	Allelic Frequency [1]		ACMG Classification	CADD Score	Inheritance Pattern
							gnomAD	Other CSVS			
OTOG	11	17574758	rs552304627	c.421G>A	p.Val141Met	Missense	0.001288	0.004	Pathogenic (PVS1, PS4, PM2, PP3, BP1)	33.00	AR [3]
	11	17578774	rs61978648	c.805G>A	p.Val269Ile	Missense	0.004439	0.014	Likely Benign (PS4, BP1, BP4, BP6)	19.12	AR [3]
	11	17594747	-	-	p.Pro747Thr	Missense	Novel		Uncertain Significance (PS4, PM2, BP1, BP4)	21.90	-
	11	17621218	rs117005078	c.3719C>T	p.Pro1240Leu	Missense	0.005740	0.004	Likely Pathogenic (PS4, PM2, PP3, BP1)	33.00	-
	11	17627548	rs145689709	c.4058G>A	p.Arg1353Gln	Missense	0.004040	0.006	Uncertain Significance (PS4, PM2, BP1, BP4, BP6)	22.00	AR [3]
	11	17631453	rs117380920	c.4642C>T	p.Leu1548Phe	Missense	0.012350	0.013	Benign (PS4, BS1, BS2, BP1, BP4, BP6)	12.42	-
	11	17632921	rs61736002	c.6110C>T	p.Ala2037Val	Missense	0.001207	0.004	Uncertain Significance (PS4, PM2, BP1, BP4)	7.61	AR [3]
	11	17656672	rs76461792	c.7667G>A	p.Arg2556Gln	Missense	0.004671	0.004	Benign (PS4, BS1, BS2, BP1, BP4, BP6)	23.50	-
	11	17663747	rs117315845	c.8405G>A	p.Arg2802His	Missense	0.002725	0.006	Uncertain Significance (PS4, PM2, BP1, BP4, BP6)	16.79	AR [3]
	11	17667139	rs61997203	c.8526G>C	p.Lys2842Asn	Missense	0.023350	0.019	Benign (PS4, BS1, BS2, BP1, BP6)	24.20	-
LSAMP	3	115561402	-	c.673A>G	p.Lys225Glu	Missense	Novel		Likely Pathogenic (PS4, PM2)	25.90	AR

ID: reference Single Nucleotide Polymorphism identifier; *: stop codon; NF: not found; [1]: allelic frequencies reported in the original reports have been updated according to the available information in the last version of the reference database; gnomAD: Genome Aggregation Database; CSVS: Collaborative Spanish Variant Server; ExAC: Exome Aggregation Consortium; ACMG: American College of Medical Genetics and Genomics; CADD: Combined Annotation Dependent Depletion; AD: autosomal dominant inheritance pattern; AR: autosomal recessive inheritance pattern; [2]: incomplete penetrance; [3]: multiple inheritance.

Recently, Mehrjoo et al. [42] studied a family with consanguineous parents with four descendants, two of them with definite MD and two unaffected siblings with an AR inheritance pattern. Both affected patients had poor senses of smell, which suggests that the phenotype could be MD-like phenotype. A novel homozygous variant chr3:115561402T>C in the LSAMP gene (NM_001318915) was reported in the two affected siblings with MD and it was classified as likely pathogenic. This SNV is not described in gnomAD or ClinVar.

3.3. Classification of Genes

Genes were classified according to the gene expression profile in neural or the inner ear databases (Figures 2 and 3).

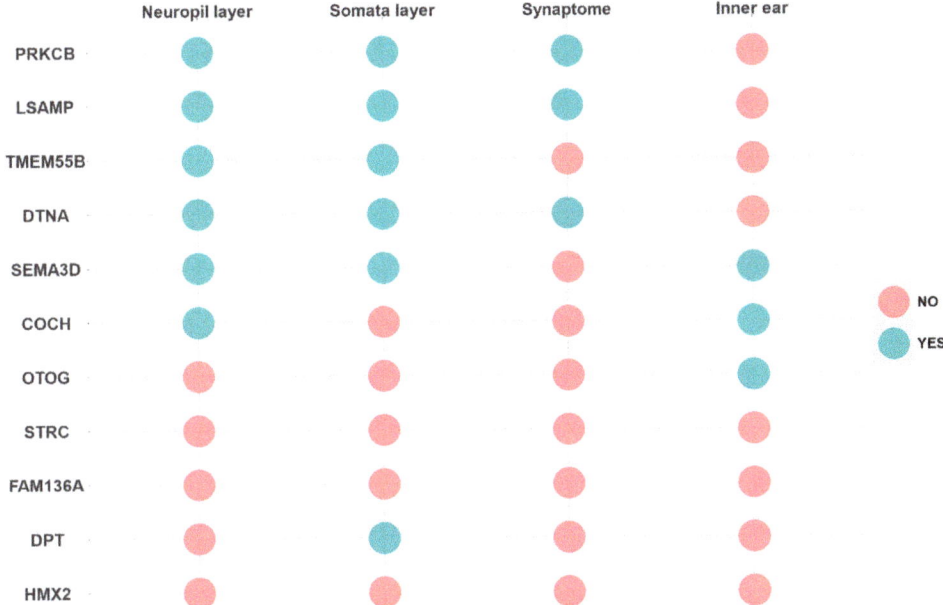

Figure 2. Summary of candidate FMD genes expressed in neural tissues and human inner ear databases, and in cyan genes that appear in the databases and in red genes that do not appear. Genes were identified in Neuropil layer and Somata layer of CAI Hippocampus in *R. norvegicus* (columns 1 and 2); genes that encode proteins of human synapsis (column 3) and preferentially expressed genes in the human inner ear compared to 32 other tissues (column 4).

First, *PRKCB* and *LSAMP* genes have gene expression in the three neural tissues and they are highly expressed in SG and VG, and they show a rather low expression in HCs. Remarkably, *PRKCB*, which encodes the β subunit of protein kinase C, shows a tonotopic distribution in tectal cells and inner border cells in the organ of Corti [16].

The *TMEM55B* gene is reported in neural tissues, the exception being the Synaptome database, and it is also highly expressed in both SG and VG. According to these data, the genes *PRKCB*, *LSAMP* and *TMEMB55B* will have a gene expression profile related to supporting cells in the neurosensory epithelia, sensory neurons or neural tissues.

However, *COCH* and *OTOG* encode the extracellular proteins cochlin and otogelin, and they are differentially expressed in the human inner ear. Moreover, gene expression datasets show that both are expressed in cochlea and vestibule; particularly, *OTOG* is expressed in non-HC of vestibular epithelia and cochlear HC in the organ of Corti, and *COCH* in the lateral wall of the cochlea, close to the organ of Corti. For these reasons, *COCH* and *OTOG* genes are predominantly expressed in inner ear tissues, although *COCH* was also reported in neuropil layer.

The *STRC* gene is not differentially expressed in the human inner ear, but it has a specific high expression in HCs, particularly in OHC, highlighting a key role in the OHC stereocilia in the organ of Corti.

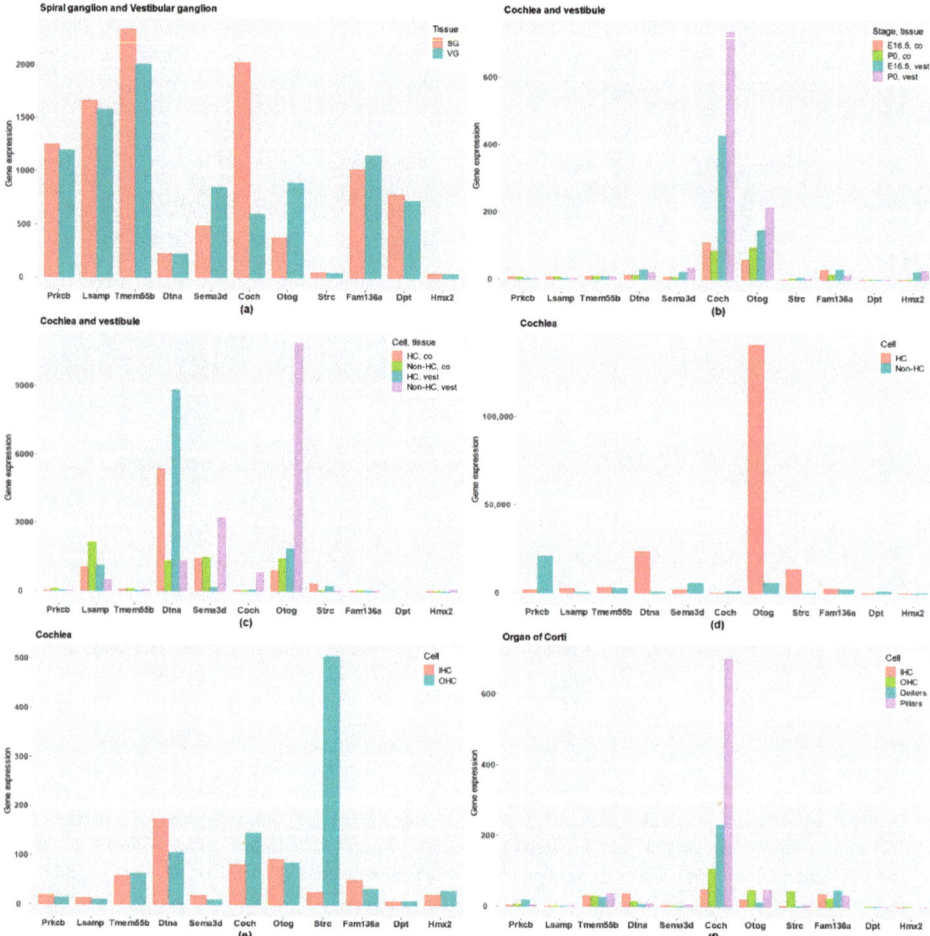

Figure 3. Gene expression profile in candidate genes for FMD in different tissues: (**a**) RNA expression data across inner ear developmental stages in mice comparing SG and VG; (**b**) RNA-Seq data comparing embryonic day 16.5 (E16.5) and postnatal day (P0) between cochlea (co) and vestibule (vest); (**c**) RNA-Seq data at postnatal day (P0) in mice comparing hair cells (HCs) with epithelial non-HCs in both cochlea (co) and vestibule (vest); (**d**) RNA-Seq data from postnatal day (P0) in mice comparing HCs with the rest of cochlear duct in cochlea; (**e**) RNA expression data from adult mice cochlea comparing inner HCs (IHCs) and outer HCs (OHCs); (**f**) RNA-Seq data from adult mice in the organ of Corti, comparing IHCs, OHCs, Deiters' cells and pillar cells.

DTNA presents a preferential gene expression in the three neural tissues and not in human inner ear, although the gene is expressed in both auditory and vestibular HCs in mouse, showing a low expression in non-HC. *SEMA3D* encodes the axonal guidance signaling protein semaphoring 3D, and it has an important role in neural tissues and in inner ear tissues. It is expressed in the human inner ear, but also in the Neuropil and Somata layers in neural tissues. In addition, it is higher expressed in non-HC than in HC, and is expressed in both SG and VG.

Finally, no conclusive gene expression data were found for *FAM136A*, *DPT* and *HMX2* genes, which have a low expression in inner ear tissues or neural tissues. However, the *DPT* gene seems to have a higher expression in the Somata layer.

FMD genes show a different expression profile during development in the mouse organ of Corti. By retrieving single cell gene expression data from P1 and P7, we could establish which cell types reveal a relatively high expression from early stages to adult inner ear (Figure 4). *COCH* is highly expressed in the organ of Corti, particularly in the outer sulcus cells. There are genes that show a high expression in P1, but their expression decreases at P7, such as *PRKCB*, *SEMA3D* or *LSAMP*, suggesting a relevant role during the maturation of the organ of Corti.

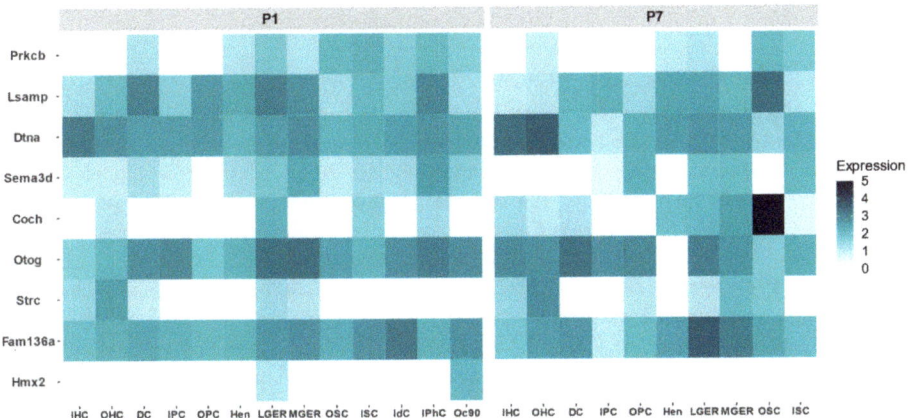

Figure 4. Relative gene expression of candidate genes for FMD in the mouse organ of Corti in postnatal days 1 (P1) and 7 (P7) comparing different cell types: inner hair cells (IHC), outer hair cells (OHC), Deiters' cells (DC), inner pillar cells (IPC), outer pillar cells (OPC), Hensen cells (Hen), lateral greater epithelial ridge cells (LGER), medial greater epithelial ridge cells (MGER), outer sulcus cells (OSC), inner sulcus cells (ISC), interdental cells (IdC), inner phalangeal cells (IPhC), cells expressing Oc90 (Oc90).

4. Discussion

4.1. Main Findings in FMD Candidate Genes

FMD is not a monogenic disorder. In this systematic review, we have found 11 candidate genes related with FMD, which supports the genetic heterogeneity of the condition. Although further evidence from cellular and animal models is needed, the finding of rare missense variants in the *OTOG* gene in multiplex unrelated families strongly support their role in the pathogenesis of FMD. Some SNVs in *OTOG* (chr11:17574758G>A, chr11:17578774G>A, chr11:17621218C>T, chr11:17632921C>T, chr11:17663747G>A and chr11:17667139G>C) [41] were reported in multiplex families with different unrelated individuals with FMD. Whereas SNVs in *PRKCB* [16], *DPT*, *SEMA3D* [17], *COCH* [38], *STRC* [39], *HMX2*, *TMEM55B* [40] and *LSAMP* [42] were only described in simplex families. Hence, it would be necessary to find new additional cases or families with these variations to support their involvement in FMD.

The heterogeneity observed in the genetics of FMD suggests that different causes could lead to the same syndrome, consisting of episodic vertigo associated SNHL and tinnitus during the attacks. This complex phenotype is the result of genetic and environmental factors and several genes will play a role in specific cell types in the inner ear, and other genes will encode essential neural signals to support the innervation of the sensorineural epithelia, such as *SEMA3D*. Therefore, one of the objectives of this systematic review is to classify the genes related to FMD in these two groups, according to their predominant gene expression profile.

4.2. Inheritance Pattern in FMD

In this systematic review, we have found evidence to support that the inheritance pattern in FMD could be AD or AR. As it was previously reported, some of these AD families have a partial syndrome (SNHL or vertigo). The SNVs in *FAM136A*, *DTNA*, *PRKCB*, *COCH*, *DPT* and *SEMA3D* have and AD inheritance pattern; specifically, there are variants in *PRKCB*, *COCH*, *DPT* and *SEMA3D* segregates with an incomplete penetrance because in the families reported, there were some relatives that presented an incomplete phenotype of MD.

On the other hand, SNVs in *STRC* and *LSAMP* had an AR inheritance pattern. Moreover, SNVs in *HMX2* and *TMEM55B* and five SNVs of *OTOG* also have an AR inheritance.

4.3. Classification of Genes

Familial MD genes with a predominant gene expression profile in neural tissues are *PRKCB*, *TMEM55* and *LSAMP*. It is possible that rare missense SNVs in these genes could contribute to the MD phenotype by affecting protein function and thus hindering neural development, maintenance or function, for example, by reducing the trophic support to hair cells at the nerve endings. An enrichment of rare missense variants in genes involved in axonal guidance signaling has been reported in MD [43].

In the first place, *PRKCB* gene encodes Protein kinase C (PKC), which is a serine- and threonine-specific protein kinases that can be activated by calcium and the second messenger diacylglycerol [44]. Martin-Sierra et al. [16] described that the protein encoded by *PRKCB* gene was highly expressed in the tectal cells of rat cochlea, and it showed a tonotopic expression gradient from the apical turn, where it demonstrated a strong labeling to the middle and basal turn of the cochlea. These results confirmed previous gene expression datasets generated from the mouse cochlea with higher expression in the apical and middle turns in mice [45], which matches with the low-frequency SNHL in the studied family.

TMEM55 (transmembrane protein 55B) interacts with various proteins [46] and participates in the lysosomal dynamics [47]. Furthermore, it is part of a family of transmembrane proteins to which *TMEM132E* gene belongs, where mutations that cause DFNB99 nonsyndromic hearing loss were also described [48].

LSAMP (limbic-system-associated membrane protein) is a neuronal surface glycoprotein distributed in cortical and subcortical regions of the limbic system [49]; it is involved in neurite formation and outgrowth [50], and it was previously related to schizophrenia and bipolar disorder [51]. Its role in the innervation of the organ of Corti or vestibular organs has not been established.

However, *COCH*, *OTOG* and *STRC* have a higher expression in the inner ear, which suggests that changes in their protein products could cause structural modifications in the inner ear, leading to a fragile structure. *COCH* gene produces cochlin protein, which is the most abundant protein in human and mouse cochlea, and in vestibular organs of mice the second most frequent protein. Cochlin is present in the spiral ligament and spiral limbus, in the lateral wall close to the organ of Corti [52]. It is an essential structural protein to maintain the complex architecture of the lateral wall of the cochlea.

The *OTOG* gene, which encodes otogelin, is mainly expressed in acellular structures that cover the sensory inner ear epithelia: the tectorial membrane, the otoconial membranes and the cupula over the cristae ampullaris of the semicircular canals [25]. Otogelin also contributes to the horizontal top connectors and tectorial membrane-attachment crowns of OHC stereocilia, where they interact, directly or indirectly, with stereocilin [53]. The tectorial membrane is in close connection to HC stereocilia, which explains the high expression of *OTOG* in cochlear HC in the inner ear. Moreover, in the vestibular non-HC *OTOG* also had a very high expression, suggesting that these cell types could synthetize otogelin.

The *STRC* gene encodes the Stereocilin protein in cochlea and vestibule; it is associated with the gelatinous membrane overlaying the vestibular kinocilia, which suggests a role of the protein in sensing balance and spatial orientation [39]. Verpy et al. [54] reported the functional association between Stereocilin and OHC; moreover, they conclude that it is essential to the formation of horizontal top connectors, which maintain the cohesiveness of the mature OHC hair bundle, and are required for the tip-link turn over.

DTNA and *SEMA3D* have a relevant gene expression in neural tissues and within the inner ear. *DTNA* encodes α-dystrobrevin, which is a structural protein of the dystrophin-associated protein complex whose absence in the mouse model causes abnormalities of the blood–brain barrier and progressive edema [55]. Furthermore, Requena et al. [15] confirmed the expression of α-dystrobrevin in supporting cells by immunohistochemistry in a rat model. This also suggested that changes in this protein in the intermediate filament network can affect the motility of HC, as is reported in gene expression databases showing a high expression of *DTNA* in both cochlear and vestibular HCs.

SEMA3D encodes Semaphorin-3D, which belongs to the axon guidance pathway and inhibits the neural growth [56]. Gallego-Martinez et al. [43] reported an enrichment of rare missense variants in axonal guidance signaling in sporadic MD. The genes in the axon guidance pathway regulate the neurite attraction and repulsion; consequently, they patterned the auditory projections, allowing the tonotopy established by the auditory HC [57]. *SEMA3D* may be relevant to the formation or maintenance of inner ear tissues [17]; Requena et al. [58] reported that the most significant pathway in cochlear supporting cells was axonal guidance signaling, and also it was one of the most significant pathways in vestibular supporting cells, according to the differentially expressed genes in mice HC and non-HCs.

Finally, three FMD genes (*FAM136A*, *DPT* and *HMX2*) do not have a predominant gene expression in neural or inner ear tissue databases and they could not be classified in a group.

4.4. Limitations of Systematic Review in FMD Studies

The main weakness in FMD is that most of the SNVs and candidate genes reported were only found in single families. Additional families with pathogenic or likely pathogenic variants in the same gene segregating the phenotype would support the association between candidate genes and FMD.

A second limitation observed is that all studies that found SNVs in FMD were performed with Whole Exome Sequencing or genotyping and there are no datasets using Whole Genome Sequencing. Intronic or intergenic regions could harbor SNV, or structural variants in FMD, which are missing.

Additionally, a large set of families is necessary to perform case-control studies with a larger sample size and with patients from different families, to compare AF of the rare variants in FMD with sporadic cases as was performed in the *OTOG* study [41].

Finally, an important limitation in this systematic review was the comparison of gene expression among different databases during development and across different species. Moreover, there are few expression datasets for the vestibular organs, which did not allow us to compare between cochlear and vestibular datasets.

5. Conclusions

- The inheritance pattern in FMD can be AD or AR.
- Although 11 candidate genes have been reported in FMD, these genes need replication in new families and imaging studies to define which cell types are involved; they could be classified according to the gene expression profile in neural or inner ear tissues genes.

Supplementary Materials: The following are available online at http://www.mdpi.com/2073-4425/11/12/1414/s1, Table S1: Preferred Reporting Items for Systematic Reviews and Meta-Analyses (PRISMA); Table S2: Barany Society and AAO-HNS criterion to define MD.

Author Contributions: J.A.L.-E. conceived the study design and developed the scientific arguments. J.A.L.-E. and A.E.-B. performed literature search, quality assessment of the studies, interpretation of data, drafting the manuscript and revised the final version. P.R.-N. also helped in the interpretation of the data, developing the scientific arguments and revised the final draft. All authors have read and agreed to the published version of the manuscript.

Funding: This work was supported by PE-0356-2018 from Consejeria de Salud y Familias.

Acknowledgments: We would like to thank Marisa Flook for the revision of the English grammar style and Sana Amanat and Alvaro Gallego-Martinez for their advice in the interpretation of the data.

Conflicts of Interest: The authors declare no conflict of interest.

References

1. Kwan, K.Y.; Shen, J.; Corey, D.P. C-MYC Transcriptionally Amplifies SOX2 Target Genes to Regulate Self-Renewal in Multipotent Otic Progenitor Cells. *Stem Cell Rep.* **2015**, *4*, 47–60. [CrossRef]
2. Lu, C.C.; Appler, J.M.; Houseman, E.A.; Goodrich, L.V. Developmental profiling of spiral ganglion neurons reveals insights into auditory circuit assembly. *J. Neurosci.* **2011**, *31*, 10903–10918. [CrossRef]
3. Lopez-Escamez, J.A.; Carey, J.; Chung, W.-H.; Goebel, J.A.; Magnusson, M.; Mandalà, M.; Newman-Toker, D.E.; Strupp, M.; Suzuki, M.; Trabalzini, F.; et al. Diagnostic criteria for Menière's disease. *J. Vestib. Res.* **2015**, *25*, 1–7. [CrossRef]
4. Lopez-Escamez, J.A.; Dlugaiczyk, J.; Jacobs, J.; Lempert, T.; Teggi, R.; von Brevern, M.; Bisdorff, A. Accompanying symptoms overlap during attacks in menière's disease and vestibular migraine. *Front. Neurol.* **2014**, *5*. [CrossRef]
5. Hallpike, C.S.; Cairns, H. Observations on the pathology of ménière's syndrome. *J. Laryngol. Otol.* **1938**, *53*, 625–655. [CrossRef]
6. Alexander, T.H.; Harris, J.P. Current epidemiology of meniere's syndrome. *Otolaryngol. Clin. N. Am.* **2010**, *43*, 965–970. [CrossRef]
7. Tyrrell, J.S.; Whinney, D.J.D.; Ukoumunne, O.C.; Fleming, L.E.; Osborne, N.J. Prevalence, Associated Factors, and Comorbid Conditions for Ménière's Disease. *Ear Hear.* **2014**, *35*, e162. [CrossRef] [PubMed]
8. Frejo, L.; Martin-Sanz, E.; Teggi, R.; Trinidad, G.; Soto-Varela, A.; Santos-Perez, S.; Manrique, R.; Perez, N.; Aran, I.; Almeida-Branco, M.S.; et al. Extended phenotype and clinical subgroups in unilateral Meniere disease: A cross-sectional study with cluster analysis. *Clin. Otolaryngol.* **2017**, *42*, 1172–1180. [CrossRef] [PubMed]
9. Frejo, L.; Soto-Varela, A.; Santos-Perez, S.; Aran, I.; Batuecas-Caletrio, A.; Perez-Guillen, V.; Perez-Garrigues, H.; Fraile, J.; Martin-Sanz, E.; Tapia, M.C.; et al. Clinical Subgroups in Bilateral Meniere Disease. *Front. Neurol.* **2016**, *7*. [CrossRef] [PubMed]
10. Requena, T.; Espinosa-Sanchez, J.M.; Cabrera, S.; Trinidad, G.; Soto-Varela, A.; Santos-Perez, S.; Teggi, R.; Perez, P.; Batuecas-Caletrio, A.; Fraile, J.; et al. Familial clustering and genetic heterogeneity in Meniere's disease. *Clin. Genet.* **2014**, *85*, 245–252. [CrossRef] [PubMed]
11. Hietikko, E.; Kotimäki, J.; Sorri, M.; Männikkö, M. High incidence of Meniere-like symptoms in relatives of Meniere patients in the areas of Oulu University Hospital and Kainuu Central Hospital in Finland. *Eur. J. Med. Genet.* **2013**, *56*, 279–285. [CrossRef] [PubMed]
12. Klar, J.; Frykholm, C.; Friberg, U.; Dahl, N. A Meniere's disease gene linked to chromosome 12p12.3. *Am. J. Med. Genet. Part. B Neuropsychiatr. Genet.* **2006**, *141B*, 463–467. [CrossRef] [PubMed]
13. Gabriková, D.; Frykholm, C.; Friberg, U.; Lahsaee, S.; Entesarian, M.; Dahl, N.; Klar, J. Familiar Meniere's disease restricted to 1.48 Mb on chromosome 12p12.3 by allelic and haplotype association. *J. Hum. Genet.* **2010**, *55*, 834–837. [CrossRef] [PubMed]
14. Hietikko, E.; Kotimäki, J.; Kentala, E.; Klockars, T.; Sorri, M.; Männikkö, M. Finnish familial Meniere disease is not linked to chromosome 12p12.3, and anticipation and cosegregation with migraine are not common findings. *Genet. Med.* **2011**, *13*, 415–420. [CrossRef]
15. Requena, T.; Cabrera, S.; Martín-Sierra, C.; Price, S.D.; Lysakowski, A.; Lopez-Escamez, J.A. Identification of two novel mutations in FAM136A and DTNA genes in autosomal-dominant familial Meniere's disease. *Hum. Mol. Genet.* **2015**, *24*, 1119–1126. [CrossRef]

16. Martín-Sierra, C.; Requena, T.; Frejo, L.; Price, S.D.; Gallego-Martinez, A.; Batuecas-Caletrio, A.; Santos-Pérez, S.; Soto-Varela, A.; Lysakowski, A.; Lopez-Escamez, J.A. A novel missense variant in PRKCB segregates low-frequency hearing loss in an autosomal dominant family with Meniere's disease. *Hum. Mol. Genet.* **2016**, *25*, 3407–3415. [CrossRef]
17. Martín-Sierra, C.; Gallego-Martinez, A.; Requena, T.; Frejo, L.; Batuecas-Caletrío, A.; Lopez-Escamez, J.A. Variable expressivity and genetic heterogeneity involving DPT and SEMA3D genes in autosomal dominant familial Meniere's disease. *Eur. J. Hum. Genet.* **2017**, *25*, 200–207. [CrossRef]
18. Moher, D.; Liberati, A.; Tetzlaff, J.; Altman, D.G. Preferred reporting items for systematic reviews and meta-analyses: The PRISMA statement. *J. Clin. Epidemiol.* **2009**, *62*, 1006–1012. [CrossRef]
19. Karczewski, K.J.; Francioli, L.C.; Tiao, G.; Cummings, B.B.; Alföldi, J.; Wang, Q.; Collins, R.L.; Laricchia, K.M.; Ganna, A.; Birnbaum, D.P.; et al. The mutational constraint spectrum quantified from variation in 141,456 humans. *Nature* **2020**, *581*, 434–443. [CrossRef]
20. Peña-Chilet, M.; Roldán, G.; Perez-Florido, J.; Ortuño, F.M.; Carmona, R.; Aquino, V.; Lopez-Lopez, D.; Loucera, C.; Fernandez-Rueda, J.L.; Gallego, A.; et al. CSVS, a crowdsourcing database of the Spanish population genetic variability. *Nucleic Acids Res.* **2020**. [CrossRef]
21. Ameur, A.; Dahlberg, J.; Olason, P.; Vezzi, F.; Karlsson, R.; Martin, M.; Viklund, J.; Kähäri, A.K.; Lundin, P.; Che, H.; et al. SweGen: A whole-genome data resource of genetic variability in a cross-section of the Swedish population. *Eur. J. Hum. Genet.* **2017**, *25*, 1253–1260. [CrossRef] [PubMed]
22. Karczewski, K.J.; Weisburd, B.; Thomas, B.; Solomonson, M.; Ruderfer, D.M.; Kavanagh, D.; Hamamsy, T.; Lek, M.; Samocha, K.E.; Cummings, B.B.; et al. The ExAC browser: Displaying reference data information from over 60,000 exomes. *Nucleic Acids Res.* **2017**, *45*, D840–D845. [CrossRef] [PubMed]
23. Cajigas, I.J.; Tushev, G.; Will, T.J.; tom Dieck, S.; Fuerst, N.; Schuman, E.M. The local transcriptome in the synaptic neuropil revealed by deep sequencing and high-resolution imaging. *Neuron* **2012**, *74*, 453–466. [CrossRef]
24. Pirooznia, M.; Wang, T.; Avramopoulos, D.; Valle, D.; Thomas, G.; Huganir, R.L.; Goes, F.S.; Potash, J.B.; Zandi, P.P. SynaptomeDB: An ontology-based knowledgebase for synaptic genes. *Bioinformatics* **2012**, *28*, 897–899. [CrossRef] [PubMed]
25. Schrauwen, I.; Hasin-Brumshtein, Y.; Corneveaux, J.J.; Ohmen, J.; White, C.; Allen, A.N.; Lusis, A.J.; Van Camp, G.; Huentelman, M.J.; Friedman, R.A. A comprehensive catalogue of the coding and non-coding transcripts of the human inner ear. *Hear. Res.* **2016**, *333*, 266–274. [CrossRef] [PubMed]
26. Rudnicki, A.; Isakov, O.; Ushakov, K.; Shivatzki, S.; Weiss, I.; Friedman, L.M.; Shomron, N.; Avraham, K.B. Next-generation sequencing of small RNAs from inner ear sensory epithelium identifies microRNAs and defines regulatory pathways. *BMC Genom.* **2014**, *15*, 484. [CrossRef] [PubMed]
27. Elkon, R.; Milon, B.; Morrison, L.; Shah, M.; Vijayakumar, S.; Racherla, M.; Leitch, C.C.; Silipino, L.; Hadi, S.; Weiss-Gayet, M.; et al. RFX transcription factors are essential for hearing in mice. *Nat. Commun.* **2015**, *6*, 8549. [CrossRef]
28. Cai, T.; Jen, H.-I.; Kang, H.; Klisch, T.J.; Zoghbi, H.Y.; Groves, A.K. Characterization of the transcriptome of nascent hair cells and identification of direct targets of the Atoh1 transcription factor. *J. Neurosci.* **2015**, *35*, 5870–5883. [CrossRef]
29. Liu, H.; Chen, L.; Giffen, K.P.; Stringham, S.T.; Li, Y.; Judge, P.D.; Beisel, K.W.; He, D.Z.Z. Cell-specific transcriptome analysis shows that adult pillar and deiters' cells express genes encoding machinery for specializations of cochlear hair cells. *Front. Mol. Neurosci.* **2018**, *11*, 356. [CrossRef]
30. Kolla, L.; Kelly, M.C.; Mann, Z.F.; Anaya-Rocha, A.; Ellis, K.; Lemons, A.; Palermo, A.T.; So, K.S.; Mays, J.C.; Orvis, J.; et al. Characterization of the development of the mouse cochlear epithelium at the single cell level. *Nat. Commun.* **2020**, *11*. [CrossRef]
31. Shen, J.; Scheffer, D.I.; Kwan, K.Y.; Corey, D.P. SHIELD: An integrative gene expression database for inner ear research. *Database* **2015**, *2015*. [CrossRef] [PubMed]
32. Liu, H.; Pecka, J.L.; Zhang, Q.; Soukup, G.A.; Beisel, K.W.; He, D.Z.Z. Characterization of transcriptomes of cochlear inner and outer hair cells. *J. Neurosci.* **2014**, *34*, 11085–11095. [CrossRef]
33. Green, R.C.; Berg, J.S.; Grody, W.W.; Kalia, S.S.; Korf, B.R.; Martin, C.L.; McGuire, A.L.; Nussbaum, R.L.; O'Daniel, J.M.; Ormond, K.E.; et al. ACMG recommendations for reporting of incidental findings in clinical exome and genome sequencing. *Genet. Med.* **2013**, *15*, 565–574. [CrossRef]

34. Richards, S.; Aziz, N.; Bale, S.; Bick, D.; Das, S.; Gastier-Foster, J.; Grody, W.W.; Hegde, M.; Lyon, E.; Spector, E.; et al. Standards and guidelines for the interpretation of sequence variants: A joint consensus recommendation of the American College of Medical Genetics and Genomics and the Association for Molecular Pathology. *Genet. Med.* **2015**, *17*, 405–423. [CrossRef]
35. Kircher, M.; Witten, D.M.; Jain, P.; O'Roak, B.J.; Cooper, G.M.; Shendure, J. A general framework for estimating the relative pathogenicity of human genetic variants. *Nat. Genet.* **2014**, *46*, 310–315. [CrossRef]
36. Rentzsch, P.; Witten, D.; Cooper, G.M.; Shendure, J.; Kircher, M. CADD: Predicting the deleteriousness of variants throughout the human genome. *Nucleic Acids Res.* **2019**, *47*, D886–D894. [CrossRef] [PubMed]
37. Committee on Hearing and Equilibrium guidelines for the diagnosis and evaluation of therapy in Menière's disease. *Otolaryngol. Head Neck Surg.* **1995**, *113*, 181–185. [CrossRef]
38. Kim, B.J.; Kim, A.R.; Han, K.-H.; Rah, Y.C.; Hyun, J.; Ra, B.S.; Koo, J.-W.; Choi, B.Y. Distinct vestibular phenotypes in DFNA9 families with COCH variants. *Eur. Arch. Otorhinolaryngol.* **2016**, *273*, 2993–3002. [CrossRef] [PubMed]
39. Frykholm, C.; Klar, J.; Tomanovic, T.; Ameur, A.; Dahl, N. Stereocilin gene variants associated with episodic vertigo: Expansion of the DFNB16 phenotype. *Eur. J. Hum. Genet.* **2018**, *26*, 1871–1874. [CrossRef] [PubMed]
40. Skarp, S.; Kanervo, L.; Kotimäki, J.; Sorri, M.; Männikkö, M.; Hietikko, E. Whole-exome sequencing suggests multiallelic inheritance for childhood-onset Ménière's disease. *Ann. Hum. Genet.* **2019**, *83*, 389–396. [CrossRef] [PubMed]
41. Roman-Naranjo, P.; Gallego-Martinez, A.; Soto-Varela, A.; Aran, I.; Moleon, M.D.C.; Espinosa-Sanchez, J.M.; Amor-Dorado, J.C.; Batuecas-Caletrio, A.; Perez-Vazquez, P.; Lopez-Escamez, J.A. Burden of Rare Variants in the OTOG Gene in Familial Meniere's Disease. *Ear Hear.* **2020**. [CrossRef] [PubMed]
42. Mehrjoo, Z.; Kahrizi, K.; Mohseni, M.; Akbari, M.; Arzhangi, S.; Jalalvand, K.; Najmabadi, H.; Farhadi, M.; Mohseni, M.; Asghari, A.; et al. Limbic system associated membrane protein mutation in an iranian family diagnosed with ménière's disease. *Arch. Iran. Med.* **2020**, *23*, 319–325. [CrossRef] [PubMed]
43. Gallego-Martinez, A.; Requena, T.; Roman-Naranjo, P.; May, P.; Lopez-Escamez, J.A. Enrichment of damaging missense variants in genes related with axonal guidance signalling in sporadic Meniere's disease. *J. Med. Genet.* **2020**, *57*, 82–88. [CrossRef] [PubMed]
44. O'Leary, N.A.; Wright, M.W.; Brister, J.R.; Ciufo, S.; Haddad, D.; McVeigh, R.; Rajput, B.; Robbertse, B.; Smith-White, B.; Ako-Adjei, D.; et al. Reference sequence (RefSeq) database at NCBI: Current status, taxonomic expansion, and functional annotation. *Nucleic Acids Res.* **2016**, *44*, D733–D745. [CrossRef] [PubMed]
45. Yoshimura, H.; Takumi, Y.; Nishio, S.; Suzuki, N.; Iwasa, Y.; Usami, S. Deafness Gene Expression Patterns in the Mouse Cochlea Found by Microarray Analysis. *PLoS ONE* **2014**, *9*. [CrossRef] [PubMed]
46. Hashimoto, Y.; Shirane, M.; Nakayama, K.I. TMEM55B contributes to lysosomal homeostasis and amino acid–induced mTORC1 activation. *Genes Cells* **2018**, *23*, 418–434. [CrossRef] [PubMed]
47. Takemasu, S.; Nigorikawa, K.; Yamada, M.; Tsurumi, G.; Kofuji, S.; Takasuga, S.; Hazeki, K. Phosphorylation of TMEM55B by Erk/MAPK regulates lysosomal positioning. *J. Biochem.* **2019**, *166*, 175–185. [CrossRef]
48. Li, J.; Zhao, X.; Xin, Q.; Shan, S.; Jiang, B.; Jin, Y.; Yuan, H.; Dai, P.; Xiao, R.; Zhang, Q.; et al. Whole-exome sequencing identifies a variant in TMEM132E causing autosomal-recessive nonsyndromic hearing loss DFNB99. *Hum. Mutat.* **2015**, *36*, 98–105. [CrossRef]
49. Pimenta, A.F.; Fischer, I.; Levitt, P. cDNA cloning and structural analysis of the human limbic-system-associated membrane protein (LAMP). *Gene* **1996**, *170*, 189–195. [CrossRef]
50. Philips, M.-A.; Lilleväli, K.; Heinla, I.; Luuk, H.; Hundahl, C.A.; Kongi, K.; Vanaveski, T.; Tekko, T.; Innos, J.; Vasar, E. Lsamp is implicated in the regulation of emotional and social behavior by use of alternative promoters in the brain. *Brain Struct. Funct.* **2015**, *220*, 1381–1393. [CrossRef]
51. Behan, A.T.; Byrne, C.; Dunn, M.J.; Cagney, G.; Cotter, D.R. Proteomic analysis of membrane microdomain-associated proteins in the dorsolateral prefrontal cortex in schizophrenia and bipolar disorder reveals alterations in LAMP, STXBP1 and BASP1 protein expression. *Mol. Psychiatry* **2009**, *14*, 601–613. [CrossRef] [PubMed]
52. Robertson, N.G.; Cremers, C.W.R.J.; Huygen, P.L.M.; Ikezono, T.; Krastins, B.; Kremer, H.; Kuo, S.F.; Liberman, M.C.; Merchant, S.N.; Miller, C.E.; et al. Cochlin immunostaining of inner ear pathologic deposits and proteomic analysis in DFNA9 deafness and vestibular dysfunction. *Hum. Mol. Genet.* **2006**, *15*, 1071–1085. [CrossRef]

53. Avan, P.; Gal, S.L.; Michel, V.; Dupont, T.; Hardelin, J.-P.; Petit, C.; Verpy, E. Otogelin, otogelin-like, and stereocilin form links connecting outer hair cell stereocilia to each other and the tectorial membrane. *Proc. Natl. Acad. Sci. USA* **2019**, *116*, 25948–25957. [CrossRef] [PubMed]
54. Verpy, E.; Leibovici, M.; Michalski, N.; Goodyear, R.J.; Houdon, C.; Weil, D.; Richardson, G.P.; Petit, C. Stereocilin connects outer-hair-cell stereocilia to one another and to the tectorial membrane. *J. Comp. Neurol* **2011**, *519*, 194–210. [CrossRef] [PubMed]
55. Lien, C.F.; Mohanta, S.K.; Frontczak-Baniewicz, M.; Swinny, J.D.; Zablocka, B.; Górecki, D.C. Absence of glial α-Dystrobrevin causes abnormalities of the blood-brain barrier and progressive brain edema. *J. Biol. Chem.* **2012**, *287*, 41374–41385. [CrossRef] [PubMed]
56. Aghajanian, H.; Choi, C.; Ho, V.C.; Gupta, M.; Singh, M.K.; Epstein, J.A. Semaphorin 3d and Semaphorin 3e Direct Endothelial Motility through Distinct Molecular Signaling Pathways. *J. Biol. Chem.* **2014**, *289*, 17971–17979. [CrossRef] [PubMed]
57. Webber, A.; Raz, Y. Axon guidance cues in auditory development. *Anat. Rec. Part A Discov. Mol. Cell. Evol. Biol.* **2006**, *288A*, 390–396. [CrossRef]
58. Requena, T.; Gallego-Martinez, A.; Lopez-Escamez, J.A. Bioinformatic integration of molecular networks and major pathways involved in mice cochlear and vestibular supporting cells. *Front. Mol. Neurosci.* **2018**, *11*. [CrossRef]

Publisher's Note: MDPI stays neutral with regard to jurisdictional claims in published maps and institutional affiliations.

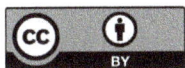

© 2020 by the authors. Licensee MDPI, Basel, Switzerland. This article is an open access article distributed under the terms and conditions of the Creative Commons Attribution (CC BY) license (http://creativecommons.org/licenses/by/4.0/).

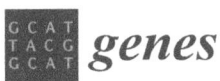

Article

Mouse Models of Human Pathogenic Variants of *TBC1D24* Associated with Non-Syndromic Deafness DFNB86 and DFNA65 and Syndromes Involving Deafness

Risa Tona [1], Ivan A. Lopez [2], Cristina Fenollar-Ferrer [1,3], Rabia Faridi [1], Claudio Anselmi [4,5], Asma A. Khan [6], Mohsin Shahzad [7,8], Robert J. Morell [9], Shoujun Gu [10], Michael Hoa [10], Lijin Dong [11], Akira Ishiyama [2], Inna A. Belyantseva [1], Sheikh Riazuddin [7] and Thomas B. Friedman [1,*]

[1] Laboratory of Molecular Genetics, National Institute on Deafness and Other Communication Disorders, Porter Neuroscience Research Center, National Institutes of Health, Bethesda, MD 20892, USA; risa.tona@nih.gov (R.T.); cristina.fenollarferrer@nih.gov (C.F.-F.); rabia.faridi@nih.gov (R.F.); belyants@nidcd.nih.gov (I.A.B.)
[2] The NIDCD National Temporal Laboratory at UCLA, Department of Head and Neck Surgery, David Geffen School of Medicine at UCLA, Los Angeles, CA 90095, USA; ilopez@ucla.edu (I.A.L.); ishiyama@ucla.edu (A.I.)
[3] Laboratory of Molecular & Cellular Neurobiology, National Institute of Mental Health, National Institutes of Health, Bethesda, MD 20892, USA
[4] Research Center for Genetic Medicine, Children's National Hospital, Washington, DC 20010, USA; canselmi@childrensnational.org
[5] Department of Genomics and Precision Medicine, The George Washington University, Washington, DC 20052, USA
[6] National Centre of Excellence in Molecular Biology, University of the Punjab Lahore, Lahore 53700, Pakistan; asmaalikan@gmail.com
[7] Department of Molecular Biology, Shaheed Zulfiqar Ali Bhutto Medical University, Islamabad 44080, Pakistan; mohsinshahzad@szabmu.edu.pk (M.S.); riazuddin@aimrc.org (S.R.)
[8] Jinnah Burn and Reconstructive Surgery Center, Allama Iqbal Medical Research Center, Jinnah Hospital, University of Health Sciences, Lahore 54550, Pakistan
[9] Genomics and Computational Biology Core, National Institute on Deafness and Other Communication Disorders, NIH, Bethesda, MD 20892, USA; morellr@nidcd.nih.gov
[10] Auditory Development and Restoration Program, National Institute on Deafness and Other Communication Disorders, National Institutes of Health, Bethesda, MD 20892, USA; shoujun.gu@nih.gov (S.G.); michael.hoa@nih.gov (M.H.)
[11] Genetic Engineering Core, National Eye Institute, National Institutes of Health, Bethesda, MD 20892, USA; dongl@nei.nih.gov
* Correspondence: friedman@nidcd.nih.gov; Tel.: +1-301-496-7882

Received: 3 September 2020; Accepted: 21 September 2020; Published: 24 September 2020

Abstract: Human pathogenic variants of *TBC1D24* are associated with clinically heterogeneous phenotypes, including recessive nonsyndromic deafness DFNB86, dominant nonsyndromic deafness DFNA65, seizure accompanied by deafness, a variety of isolated seizure phenotypes and DOORS syndrome, characterized by deafness, onychodystrophy, osteodystrophy, intellectual disability and seizures. Thirty-five pathogenic variants of human *TBC1D24* associated with deafness have been reported. However, functions of TBC1D24 in the inner ear and the pathophysiology of TBC1D24-related deafness are unknown. In this study, a novel splice-site variant of *TBC1D24* c.965 +1G > A in compound heterozygosity with c.641G > A p.(Arg214His) was found to be segregating in a Pakistani family. Affected individuals exhibited, either a deafness-seizure syndrome or nonsyndromic deafness. In human temporal bones, TBC1D24 immunolocalized in hair cells and spiral ganglion neurons, whereas in mouse cochlea, *Tbc1d24* expression was detected only in spiral ganglion neurons. We engineered mouse models of *DFNB86* p.(Asp70Tyr) and *DFNA65* p.(Ser178Leu) nonsyndromic deafness and syndromic forms of deafness p.(His336Glnfs*12) that have the same pathogenic variants that were reported for human *TBC1D24*. Unexpectedly, no auditory dysfunction was detected in *Tbc1d24* mutant mice, although homozygosity for some of the variants caused seizures or lethality. We provide some insightful supporting data to explain the phenotypic differences resulting from equivalent pathogenic variants of mouse *Tbc1d24* and human *TBC1D24*.

Keywords: *Tbc1d24* mouse models; hearing loss; DFNB86; DFNA65; DOORS; syndromic deafness; human temporal bone

1. Introduction

Sensorineural hearing loss is a heterogenous disorder with a great variety of etiologies, including inherited and de novo pathogenic variants, infections, ototoxic drugs, and aging [1,2]. Variants of hundreds of different human genes are associated with deafness affecting approximately 0.2% of newborns [3]. Non-syndromic hearing loss transmitted as an autosomal recessive trait is often congenital, while transmission as an autosomal dominant trait often results in a progressive loss of hearing [4]. Approximately one-third of individuals with an inherited hearing loss have additional impairments in other organs [5], and of the more than 400 reported syndromic forms of hearing loss, many are not yet well-understood at the molecular level [6]. Moreover, different pathogenic variants of a gene may be associated with dominant or recessive modes of inheritance, and the phenotypic outcome may be syndromic or non-syndromic. For example, some variants of *MYO7A* are associated with dominant (*DFNA11*) or recessive (*DFNB2*) inheritance of non-syndromic deafness, while the majority of *MYO7A* pathogenic variants cause Usher syndrome (USH1B) [7–9].

Another example is pathogenic variants of *TBC1D24* that are associated with non-syndromic hearing loss, segregating as a recessive (*DFNB86*) [10] or a dominant trait (*DFNA65*) [11,12]. Variants of *TBC1D24* are also associated with syndromic hearing loss, which includes hearing loss with seizures, or a multisystem disorder named DOORS (Deafness, Onychodystrophy, Osteodystrophy, mental Retardation and Seizures). Following the first report of two recessive variants of human *TBC1D24* associated with *DFNB86* [10], six additional pathogenic variants of *TBC1D24* have been reported to associate with non-syndromic deafness (Figure 1A). Twenty-eight pathogenic variants of *TBC1D24* are associated with syndromic deafness (Figure 1A), including a novel splice-site variant c.965 + 1G > A which is segregating in a Pakistani family reported in this study (Figure 1B). At present, there are 96 variants of *TBC1D24*, including missense, nonsense, splice site, small indels and gross insertion and deletions that are associated with non-syndromic and syndromic forms of deafness as well as seizures.

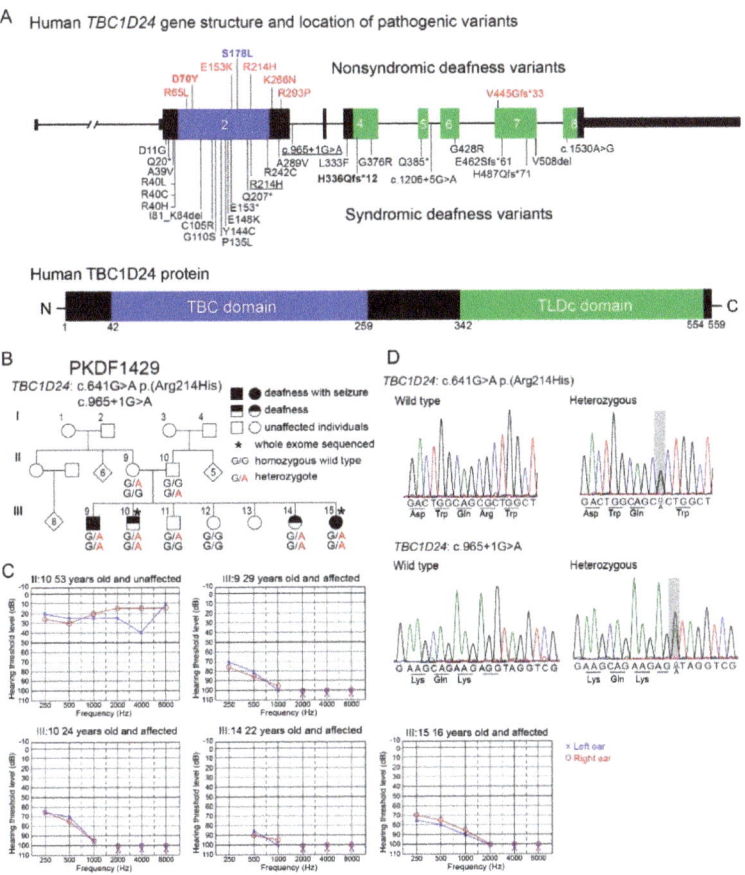

Figure 1. (**A**) A diagram of the human *TBC1D24* gene displaying the approximate locations of pathogenic variants associated with non-syndromic deafness and syndromic forms of deafness. The eight annotated exons of human *TBC1D24* encode a TBC domain (blue) and a TLDc domain (green). Eight reported pathogenic variants associated with non-syndromic deafness are drawn above the gene structure. p.Ser178Leu (blue) is an autosomal dominant variant associated with progressive deafness DFNA65 reported to be segregating in two unrelated families [11,12]. Other non-syndromic variants (red font) are associated with DFNB86 recessively inherited deafness. Twenty-eight pathogenic variants including three splice-site variants are associated with syndromic forms of deafness (deafness and epilepsy or DOORS) and are shown under the schematic of the gene. p.Arg214His and a splice-site variant c.965 + 1G > A (underlined) are segregating in family PKDF1429 in this study. The murine equivalent of the known human pathogenic variants of p.Asp70Tyr, p.Ser178Leu and p.His336Glnfs*12 together with p.S324Tfs*3 are characterized in this study. A, Alanine; C, Cysteine; D, Aspartic acid; E, Glutamic acid; F, Phenylalanine; G, Glycine; H, Histidine; I, Isoleucine; K, Lysine; L, Leucine; N, Asparagine; P, Proline; Q, Glutamine; R, Arginine; S, Serine; T, Threonine; V, Valine; Y, Tyrosine; *, stop codon. (**B**) Pedigree of Pakistani family PKDF1429. A novel likely pathogenic donor splice-site variant c.965 + 1G > A and a previously reported p.Arg214His pathogenic variant are associated in family PKDF1429 with apparent non-syndromic deafness and syndromic deafness, as two deaf individuals in this family were reported to have had seizures. All affected individuals self-reported to be congenitally profoundly deaf. Individual III:9 (29 years old) had simple partial seizures and III:15 (16 years old) had tonic-clonic seizures

in childhood from six months to three years. Individuals III:10 (24 years old) and III:14 (22 years old) have not had seizures that were obvious to their parents. (**C**) Audiograms from member of family PKDF1429. All affected individuals showed bilateral profound deafness. (**D**) Representative chromatograms of genomic DNA sequences of c.641G > A p.(Arg214His) and c.965 + 1G > A with wild type allele. The variants are shaded in gray.

There are several alternative transcripts of human *TBC1D24* including a transcript that skips micro exon 3 [10,13]. The largest *TBC1D24* transcript encodes a TBC domain (Tre-2-Bub2-Cdc16) and a TLDc domain (TBC, LysM, domain catalytic) (Figure 1A). The functions of the TBC and TLDc domains are different and pathogenic variants of TBC1D24 have been reported in both domains (Figure 1A). Some members of the large family of TBC domain-containing proteins have been shown to function as GTPase-activating proteins (GAPs), which are involved in the regulation of membrane-trafficking in partnership with Rab-GTPases [14,15]. However, the TBC domain of TBC1D24 lacks a critical arginine residue in order to function as a Rab-GTPase, an assumption that is yet to be experimentally demonstrated with purified TBC1D24 protein [10,14]. There are five proteins encoded in the human genome that have a TLDc domain and two of them, OXR1 and NCOA7, have been shown to provide an important neuro-protective role against oxidative stress [16]. It is not known whether human *TBC1D24* function in the inner ear or in the hippocampus requires the anti-oxidative function of its TLDc domain [17].

Here, we identified a novel pathogenic splice-site variant of *TBC1D24* in family PKDF1429 from Pakistan. To investigate the localization and possible function of TBC1D24 in the human inner ear, we performed immunostaining using human temporal bones. In addition, using CRISPR/Cas9 editing of *Tbc1d24*, we engineered mice with some of the same pathogenic mutations reported for human *TBC1D24*. We previously reported the first mouse model of human early infantile epileptic encephalopathy 16 (EIEE16) due to *TBC1D24* p.Ser324Thrfs*3 variant. In mouse, this variant recapitulated the seizure phenotype reported in the human family [13,18]. Here, we evaluated the phenotypes of a mouse with p.Asp70Tyr variant of *Tbc1d24* as a model of human *DFNB86* [10] and a mouse with *Tbc1d24* p.Ser178Leu variant as a model of human *DFNA65* [11,12]. We also undertook molecular modeling together with molecular dynamic (MD) simulations to evaluate the effects of a substitution of leucine for the serine-178 residue on human and mouse TBC1D24. A *Tbc1d24* p.His336Glnfs*12 allele was also engineered, which, depending on the second variant in trans-configuration, could lead to a mouse model of human DOORS or early infantile epileptic encephalopathy 16 (EIEE16) with deafness [19,20].

2. Materials and Methods

2.1. Ethic Approval and Clinical Evaluation

Our study was approved by and conducted in accordance with The Office of Human Subjects Research Protection (OH-93-N-016 to TBF) at the National Institutes of Health, Bethesda, Maryland and from the IRB-DF/2020 in Lahore, Pakistan (OH-93-DC-0016 to SR). Written informed consent was obtained from and signed by all individuals in this study. Clinical history, including a pedigree, onset of hearing loss and episodes of seizure were obtained during interviews with family members. Pure tone audiometry for all affected individuals and their parents in family PKDF1429 were obtained in home settings. The existence of morphological features of DOORS were evaluated in all affected individuals and their obligate carrier parents.

2.2. Whole Exome Sequencing (WES) and Bioinformatic Analyses

For family PKDF1429, sequence capture was performed using an Illumina Truseq Rapid Capture Enrichment Kit to create libraries (Illumina, San Diego, CA, USA). Genomic DNA samples of the hearing-impaired siblings III:10 and III:15 (Figure 1) were exome sequenced to an average depth of 56× and 68×, respectively. Sequence reads were mapped against the GRCh38 assembly using BWA (Burrows-Wheeler Alignment) [21] with recalibration performed using the GATK pipeline

(Genome Analysis Toolkit, https://gatk.broadinstitute.org/hc/en-us). Variant calls were annotated with ANNOVAR. Variant Call Format (VCF) files were imported into Ingenuity Variant Analysis (IVA, Qiagen, Germantown, MD, USA) for further downstream analyses. Variants were prioritized based on their allele frequency, pathogenicity, conservation and zygosity. Sanger sequencing validated co-segregation of the variant with the phenotype.

2.3. Mouse Models of Human TBC1D24-Associated Deafness

The analyses of mice in this study were conducted according to the National Institutes of Health Guidelines for the Care and Use of Laboratory Animals. All experimental procedures were approved by the NINDS/NIDCD Animal Care and Use Committee (ACUC) at the National Institutes of Health (protocol 1263-15 to TBF and protocol NEI-626 to LD). We engineered mouse *Tbc1d24* c.208 G > T p.(Asp70Tyr) and c.[533 C > T; 534 T > G] p.(Ser178Leu) which are the equivalent of human *TBC1D24* c.208 G > T p.(Asp70Tyr) (*DFNB86*), and c.533 C > T p.(Ser178Leu) (*DFNA65*) variants, respectively [10–12]. In mouse, we also engineered a *Tbc1d24* c.1008delT p.(His336Glnfs*12) variant, which in human is associated with DOORS or early infantile epileptic encephalopathy 16 (EIEE16) with deafness [19,20]. Since homozygosity for the p.His336Glnfs*12 variant in mouse is an embryonic lethal, mice that are compound heterozygous for two variants p.Ser324Thrfs*3 and p.His336Glnfs*12 were studied as they are viable. *Tbc1d24* missense alleles were created using CRISPR/Cas9-mediated homologous recombination directly in C57BL/6J zygotes with a single-strand DNA oligo as the recombination template (IDT, Integrated DNA Technologies, Coralville, IA, USA) in each allele. Briefly, guide RNAs (gRNA, for SpCas9, PAM = NGG) were selected for each intended allele based on their relative positions to target codons, and ranking by the online gRNA selection tool (www.CRISPRscan.org). gRNAs were synthesized with T7 in vitro transcription as described [22] and further tested for their efficiencies of in vitro cleavage and in-cell culture indel mutagenesis activities. For the in vitro cleavage assay, genomic PCR product, containing the target sites of selected gRNAs was incubated with SpCas9 protein (NEB, New England Biolabs, Ipswich, MA, USA) by following manufacturer's suggested protocol and analyzed on 2% agarose gel stained with ethidium bromide. Guide RNAs were further tested for their efficiencies inducing indels at target sites in an immortalized mouse embryonic fibroblast (MEF) cell line engineered to carry a tet-inducible Cas9 expression cassette. Upon confirmation of efficient target cleavage activity in MEF cells, gRNAs were mixed with SpCas9 protein (PNA Bio, Thousand Oaks, CA, USA) along with a synthetic single-strand donor DNA oligo template as described above. The single-strand donor DNA oligo templates were designed to repair the cleavage gap by the gRNA to restore the open reading frame, while having the desired single amino acid changes introduced based on Richardson et al. [23]. The mixture of gRNAs, Cas9 protein and the donor oligos were microinjected into zygotes of C57BL/6 background as described [24]. gRNAs used to generate *Tbc1d24* mutations p.Asp70Tyr, p.Ser178Leu and p.His336Glnfs*12 were 5′-GGCATAAGGTGTGACTGTG-3′, 5′-GTCATACAGGAAGACTCAA-3′ and 5′-CTGAGTGGAAGTTCTCTGCA-3′, respectively. Donor oligo sequences of p.Asp70Tyr, p.Ser178Leu and p.His336Glnfs*12 were 5′-GAGCCACACCCTGCGCGGGAAAGTGTACCAGCGCCTGATCCGGGACA TCCCCTGCCGCACAGTCACACCTTATGCCAGCGTGTACAGTGACATTG-3′ (96 mer oligo), 5′-GA TGAAGCTGAGTGTTTCGAAAAAGCCTGCCGCATCTTATCCTGCAATGACCCCACCAAGAAGCTCA TTGACCAGAGCTTCCTGGCCTTTGAGTTGTCCTGTATG ACATTTGGGGACCTGGTGAACA -3′ (127 mer oligo) and 5′-ACTGTGGGCTCTGATCCCTCCTCGCTTTTCCCAGGCAGTTTGTGCACTT AGCTGT CCAGCAGAGAACTTCCACTCAGAGATTGTCAGCGTGAAGGA-3′ (96 mer oligo), respectively.

F0 founder mice were screened for their CRISPR/Cas9 edited mutations as described below. Mice carrying each mutation were backcrossed to C57BL/6J mice for more than three generations. The p.Asp70Tyr allele was genotyped by Sanger sequencing; a 403 bp amplified fragment was generated by PCR using primers (5′-CAGCCTAGGACCTGCCTTG-3′, 5′-TGGCAATACACAG GAGGATCT-3′). Mice carrying the p.Ser178Leu variant were genotyped using PCR primers 5′-CGCAAGATCCTCCTGTGTATTG-3′ and 5′-AGAACTTGAGGATGGCCAGA-3′. The resulting

409 bp amplicon was analyzed after a *HinFI* restriction endonuclease digestion (NEB). The wild type amplicon was cut once with restriction endonuclease *HinFI* producing 187 bp and 222 bp restriction fragments. The p.Ser178Leu amplicon was uncut by *HinFI*. p.His336Glnfs*12 mice were genotyped by PCR using primers 5′-GGGACTTCTAGGAATAATTTCACC-3′ and 5′-TGCTGCAGTG ATGAGAAGAG-3′. The resulting 325 bp amplicon was analyzed after a *NlaIIII* restriction endonuclease digestion (NEB). The wild type 325 bp amplicon was digested by *NlaIIII* and produced 115 bp and 210 bp restriction fragments, while the p.His336Glnfs*12 allele generated a 324 bp amplicon and was uncut by *NlaIIII*. The engineering and genotyping of mice carrying the p.Ser324Thrfs*3 allele were described in Tona et al. 2019 [13].

The human *TBC1D24* p.Ser178Leu variant is associated with DFNA65 autosomal dominant nonsyndromic hearing loss with an onset reported in the third decade and initially affecting the high frequencies [11,12]. Since C57BL/6J mice show age-related hearing loss due to the *Cdh23* c.753G > A variant [25,26], mice carrying the *Tbc1d24* p.Ser178Leu allele were backcrossed with *Cdh23* wild type (*Cdh23*^{753G}) mice with a C57BL/6J background (B6.CAST-Cdh23^{Ahl+}, The Jackson Laboratory, Bar Harbor, ME). In this study, all *Tbc1d24* p.Ser178Leu mice were homozygous for *Cdh23*^{753G}, which was genotyped by PCR using primers 5′-CTAGAGAACCCACGCAGGAC-3′ and 5′-TCAGCCCAAGCCTCTACTGT-3′. The resulting 430 bp amplicon was analyzed after *BsrI* restriction endonuclease digestion (NEB). The *Cdh23*^{753G} allele was uncut by *BsrI* while *Cdh23*$^{753G>A}$ allele generated 66 bp and 364 bp restriction fragments.

2.4. ABR and DPOAE Measurements of Hearing Ability

Auditory testing was performed in the NIDCD/NIH Mouse Auditory Testing Core facility as described [27]. Briefly, mice were anesthetized by an intraperitoneal (IP) injection of a combination of 56 mg/kg body weight of ketamine (VetOne, MWI, Boise, ID, USA) and 0.375 mg/kg body weight of dexdomitor (Putney, Portland, ME, USA). Both auditory brainstem responses (ABR) and distortion product otoacoustic emissions (DPOAE) were measured in the right ear using Tucker-Davis Technologies hardware (TDT, Alachua, FL, RZ6 Multi I/O processor, MF-1 speakers) and software (BioSigRz, v. 5.7.2). ABR wave 1 latencies and amplitudes were measured at 80 dB SPL at 8 kHz, 16 kHz, 32 kHz and 40 kHz. To evaluate the hearing status of the *Tbc1d24* p.Asp70Tyr allele, five wild types (1 male, 4 females), 6 heterozygotes p.Asp70Tyr (1 male, 5 females) and 6 homozygotes p.Asp70Tyr (1 male, 5 females) were tested at P30, P60 and P90. For the *Tbc1d24* p.Ser178Leu allele with *Cdh23* c.753G > A variant (*Cdh23*$^{753G>A}$), three wild types (2 males, 1 female), three heterozygotes p.Ser178Leu (2 males, 1 female) and three homozygotes p.Ser178Leu (2 males, 1 female) were tested at P30, P60 and P90. The *Tbc1d24* p.Ser178Leu was homozygous for the wild type *Cdh23* (Cdh23^{753G}) and there were three wild types (2 males, 1 female), four heterozygotes p.Ser178Leu (3 males, 1 female) and six homozygotes p.Ser178Leu (4 males, 2 females), which were tested at P30, P60, P90 and P180. Since *Tbc1d24* compound heterozygous p.Ser324Thrfs*3/p.His336Glnfs*12 mice die by P20, three heterozygous p.Ser324Thrfs*3 (1 male, 2 females) and three compound heterozygous p.Ser324Thrfs*3/p.His336Glnfs*12 (1 male, 2 females) mice were evaluated only at P17.

2.5. Immunofluorescence Staining in Celloidin Sections of Human Cochleae

Human temporal bone specimens were obtained within 12 to 24 h of death from subjects without a hearing loss history [28]. The temporal bones were stored in 10% neutral-buffered formalin at 4 °C for 4 weeks, decalcified with 5% EDTA for 9 to 12 months, dehydrated in a graded ascending ethyl alcohol series and embedded in celloidin over a 3-month period. Temporal bones embedded in celloidin were cut in 20 μm thick serial sections of which every tenth section was mounted and stained with hematoxylin and eosin. The rest of the sections were stored in a glass jar and immersed in 80% ethanol and 20% double distilled water. Celloidin sections containing the cochlea (mid-modiolar area) were removed from the jar and mounted on Superfrost Plus slides (Thermo Fisher Scientific, Waltham, MA, USA) and used for immunofluorescence staining.

To remove the celloidin [28], sections were placed in a glass Petri dish and immersed in ethanol saturated with sodium hydroxide solution (100 g NaOH in 100 mL of ethanol), diluted 1:3 with 100% ethanol for 1 h, followed by 100% ethanol, 50% ethanol, and distilled water for 10 min each. Slides were placed horizontally in a glass Petri dish containing antigen retrieval solution (Vector Antigen Unmasking Solution, Vector Labs, Burlingame, CA, USA diluted 1:250 with distilled water) and heated in the microwave oven using intermittent heating of two 2 min cycles with an interval of 1 min between the heating cycles, Slides were allowed to cool for 15 min, followed by 10 min wash with phosphate buffered saline solution (PBS, 0.1 M, pH 7.4). A drop of trypsin antigen retrieval solution (#ab970, Abcam, Boston, MA, USA 1 drop of concentrated trypsin in 4 drops of PBS for 3 min) was added to each section. Sections were washed with PBS 4 × 15 min.

Sections were blocked in PBS containing 1% bovine serum albumin fraction V (Sigma-Aldrich, St. Louis, MO, USA) and 0.1% Triton X-100 (Sigma-Aldrich, St Louis, MO, USA) for 1 h, and incubated subsequently with the rabbit antibody against TBC1D24 (ab101933, RRID: AB_10712373 or ab234723, Abcam) and mouse monoclonal antibody against acetylated tubulin (T745, Sigma-Aldrich, St Louis, MO, USA) in blocking solution for 72 h at 4 °C in a humid chamber. After 4 washes (15 min) in PBS, a mixture of Alexa-488 conjugated goat anti-rabbit polyclonal IgG and Alexa-564 conjugated horse anti-mouse polyclonal IgG (both from Molecular Probes, Carlsbad, CA, USA) was added at a dilution of 1:500 in blocking solution and incubated at room temperature for 3 h in the dark. Slides were mounted in Vectashield mounting media (Vector Labs) containing DAPI. Background immunofluorescence was removed using the Vector True VIEW kit (Vector Labs).

Negative controls, consisting of secondary antibody only, and unstained human cochlea sections were used to assess for background staining and auto-fluorescence, respectively. Negative controls exhibited minimal staining or auto-fluorescence. As positive controls, mouse cochlea sections were immuno-stained with TBC1D24 antibody as previously reported [10]. The Institutional Review Board (IRB) of UCLA approved this study of human temporal bones (IRB protocol #10-001449, AI) and methods used in this study are in accordance with NIH and IRB guidelines and regulations. Informed consent was obtained from each patient before inclusion in the study of temporal bone sections; temporal bone specimens came from five individuals with normal hearing, of which three were female and two were male, ranging from 55 to 78 years old.

2.6. In Situ Hybridization and Immunohistochemistry Using Mouse Cochleae

In situ hybridizations were performed using RNAscope assays (Advanced Cell Diagnostics (ACD), Newark, CA, USA). Cochleae from C57BL/6J wild type mice at postnatal day three (P3) were fixed overnight at 4 °C in 4% PFA (Electron Microscopy Sciences, Hatfield, PA, USA) in 1 PBS. Fixed cochleae were cryopreserved in 15% sucrose in 1× PBS for overnight at 4 °C and then in 30% sucrose in 1× PBS for overnight at 4 °C. Each cochlea was embedded and frozen in Super Cryoembedding Medium (Section-Lab, Hiroshima, Japan). Frozen cochleae were sectioned (12 μm thick) using a CM3050S cryostat microtome (Leica, Vienna, Austria). RNAscope Multiplex Fluorescent V2 Assays (ACD) were conducted using Probe-Mm-Tbc1d24 (target region: 839 to 1739 nucleotides, NM_001163847.1), Probe-Mm-Tubb3-C4 (target region: 2 to 1636 nucleotides, NM_023279.2) and Probe-Mm-Myo7a-C2 (target region: 1365 to 2453 nucleotides, NM_001256081.1). Images were taken with an LSM880 confocal microscope equipped with 63× and 40× objectives (Carl Zeiss Microscopy, Thornwood, NY, USA).

Immunolocalization of TBC1D24 protein was examined in mouse cochleae at P8. The dissected cochleae were fixed overnight with 4% PFA in 1× PBS at 4 °C. Permeabilization was done with 0.5% Triton X-100 and blocking was performed with 2% BSA and 5% goat serum in 1× PBS. To verify localization of TBC1D24 protein, we used four antibodies (ab101933, RRID: AB_10712373, Abcam; ab234723, Abcam; NBP1-82925, RRID: AB_11061868, Novus Biologicals, Littleton, CO; sc-390237, Santa Cruz Biotechnology, Dallas, TX, USA). Samples were incubated with one of the anti-TBC1D24 antibodies and anti-Tubulin Beta 3 (TUBB3) antibody (801202, RRID: AB_10063408, BioLegend, San Diego, CA, USA) for 2 h, washed with 1× PBS and stained with anti-rabbit and anti-mouse secondary antibodies (Alexa Flour 488 and 568, respectively). Specimen were mounted using ProLong Gold Antifade Mountant with DAPI (Thermo Fisher Scientific, Carlsbad, CA, USA) and observed with the 63× objective using LSM780 (Carl Zeiss Microscopy).

2.7. scRNA-Seq

Single cell RNA-Seq (scRNA-Seq) datasets [29] of the developing cochlear epithelium at E16.5, P1 and P7 were analyzed. Briefly, normalized count tables of E16.5, P1 and P7 cochlear samples were obtained from GSE137299. Genes without canonical names (starting with "Gm-" or ending with "Rik") were removed before further analyses. Modularity-based clustering with Leiden algorithm was implemented in Scanpy (v1.4.5). Briefly, principal component analysis (PCA) was performed on all remaining genes. A KNN graph was constructed based on the Euclidean distance by the function *pp.neighbors* using default settings. Cells were clustered by the function *tl.leiden* with the resolution E16.5 = 10, P1 = 2 and P7 = 0.8. Expression of *Myo6* was used as a general hair cell marker and *Fgf8* expression was used as an inner hair cell (IHC) marker. *Neurod6* was used as an outer hair cell (OHC) marker of E16 and P1 data, and *Slc26a5* was used as a P7 OHC marker. Violin plots for *Myo6*, *Myo15*, *Cldn11* and *Tbc1d24* at E16.5, P1 and P7 were generated by Seaborn (v0.10.1) in Python (v3.8.2).

2.8. Computational Modeling

A three-dimensional (3D) structure of the TBC domain of human TBC1D24 (hTBC1D24) was obtained using template-based modelling. A critical step in molecular modelling is the selection of a template. The implementation of Hidden-Markov profiles in template-search algorithms increases sensitivity, especially in the identification of templates that share very low sequence identity with the query sequence, but still share the same fold. This is the case of the fold-recognition algorithm implemented in HHpred server [30], which led to the identification of the TBC domain of Skywalker (PDB id: 5HJQ and resolution 2.3 Å) [31] as a suitable template of the human TBC domain of TBC1D24 after scanning the hTBC1D24 profile against each of the profiles of the structures deposited in the Protein Data Bank [32]. The initial alignment of hTBC1D24 and 5HJQ amino-acid sequences covers residues 11-311 of hTBC1D24 (NP_001186036.1) and shows 24% amino acid sequence identity, with all the secondary structural elements aligned. This alignment was subsequently refined using an iterative process that places the most conserved residues packing towards the core of the protein and avoids gaps within secondary-structural elements. This refinement was guided by the conservation scores calculated by the Consurf server [33] and by the ProQ2 score calculated for each residue position (local ProQ2 score) [34], which evaluates the compatibility between the TBC1D24 sequence and the structural fold at a given segment. The final alignment of hTBC1D24 (residues 11-314) and 5HJQ (residues 55-338) together with that of mouse and human TBC1D24 obtained with Clustal Omega (https://www.ebi.ac.uk/Tools/msa/clustalo/) was then used to create 2000 models of human TBC (hTBC) and mouse TBC (mTBC) domains using Modeller [35]. The final models were those with the best ProQ2 score and Procheck analysis from each set and covered more sequence than that reported by Finelli et al. [36]. α-Helical restraints were applied during the two production runs to residues 300-314 (NP_001186036.1) to complete the C-terminal helix of the TBC domain, which was missing in the template.

2.9. Molecular Dynamic Simulations

The all-atom models of human and mouse TBC were enclosed in a simulation box of dimensions ~97 × 97 × 120 Å comprising a hydrated bilayer and 150 mM KCl as electrolyte. Each system included ~116,000 atoms. The initial setup for a hydrated bilayer was made of 288 POPC (1-palmitoyl-2-oleoyl-sn-glycero-3-phosphocholine) and one PIP2 lipid molecules and was generated by using the CHARMM-GUI web-based interface [37] and then relaxed for 50 nanoseconds (ns). For each system, first, water molecules were placed within the protein structure with Dowser [38]. The protein was then inserted into the simulation box by superimposing the coordinates of the PIP2 heads into the lipid bilayer associated with the protein model and removing the overlapping water molecules. To optimize the protein-solvent and protein-lipid interfaces in the model, and to thermalize the system, a series of short simulations were carried out with gradually weaker positional restraints applied to the protein, the PIP2 head, the Dowser-added water molecules, and the z-coordinates of the lipid atoms (excluding hydrogen atoms). The whole relaxation process was carried out for 23 ns. In order to run two independent simulations, the relaxation was repeated starting from a different set of velocities. Finally, two fully independent unrestrained simulations were carried out for a total of 400 ns for each system.

The final simulation snapshots were extracted and used to initiate the free-energy perturbation (FEP) calculations. Here, a given side-chain, Ser178, is mutated alchemically to leucine using a step-wise protocol controlled by a parameter λ that reflects the weights of the serine and the leucine in the potential energy function of the system. FEP calculations were carried out with 21 intermediate λ steps. For each λ, the system was simulated for 50 ns. The initial 10 ns of each simulation were considered as an equilibration. The final 40 ns were split into two sets to have two independent estimates of the free-energy. Free energy differences were evaluated by using the BAR algorithm [39]. To evaluate the free-energy of the unfolded state, the FEP protocol was repeated for a tripeptide (Ala-Ser-Ala), capped with acetyl and N-methylamine groups at the N and C termini, embedded in a cubic water box of dimensions ~97 × 97 × 97 Å with KCl 150 mM as electrolyte. In this case, the snapshot after 50 ns of simulation was used to initiate the FEP calculations.

All molecular dynamics simulations were carried out with Gromacs version 2018.3 [40], using an integration time-step of 2 femtoseconds (fs), periodic boundary conditions, and a Nose-Hoover temperature coupling set to 303.15 K. The pressure was maintained at 1 bar using Parrinello-Rahman coupling semi-isotropically in the x, y plane and z direction. Electrostatic interactions were calculated using the Particle-Mesh-Ewald algorithm, with a real-space cut-off of 12 Å. A shifted Lennard-Jones potential, also cut-off at 12 Å, was used to compute van-der-Waals interactions. The CHARMM36 force field for proteins [41] and lipids [42] was used in all calculations.

3. Results

3.1. Novel Splice Variant of Human TBC1D24 Associated with Deafness and Seizures

Clinical histories and phenotypes were obtained from four affected and two unaffected siblings and their unaffected parents of family PKDF1429 (Figure 1B). All affected individuals in family PKDF1429 had congenital pre-lingual profound hearing loss (Figure 1C). Individual III:9 also had simple partial seizures while III:15 had tonic-clonic seizures in childhood from six months to three years of age. Individuals III:10 and III:14 did not show seizures. Physical examinations in this family did not reveal any dysmorphic features of DOORS. These data indicated that deafness segregating in this family appears to be non-syndromic (only hearing loss) for individuals III:10 and III:14, although admittedly subtle seizures in these two individuals may not have been noticed.

To determine the molecular genetic causes for the apparent non-syndromic and syndromic hearing loss segregating in family PKDF1429, whole exome sequencing (WES) was performed using gDNA from individuals III:10 and III:15 (Figure 1B). Compound heterozygous variants of *TBC1D24* (NM_001199107.1): c.641G > A p.(Arg214His) and c.965 + 1G > A were identified in affected individuals III:10 and III:15, which were confirmed by Sanger sequencing (Figure 1D). The donor splice-site pathogenic variant c.965 + 1G > A of intron 2 of *TBC1D24* is novel. The c.965 + 1G > A is absent from gnomAD (v2.1.1) database of 125,748 exome and 45,708 whole genome sequences from unrelated individuals and the G nucleotide is conserved from human to lamprey with a CADD score of 35, indicating deleteriousness of this variant (https://cadd.gs.washington.edu/). The novel variant has been submitted to ClinVar (https://www.ncbi.nlm.nih.gov/clinvar/) under submission ID SUB7952908. The variant of c.641G > A p.(Arg214His) was reported in compound heterozygosity with variants p.Glu153Lys or with p.Val445Glyfs*33 and associated with non-syndromic deafness *DFNB86* [43].

Sanger sequencing confirmed the genotypes of eight members of family PKDF1429. Parents of affected children were heterozygous, confirming the trans-configuration of the two variants, and unaffected members of the family were either heterozygous for p.Arg214His variant or homozygous for the wild type allele (Figure 1B). The clinical heterogeneity of affected members of family PKDF1429 suggests that the *TBC1D24* genotype alone does not unequivocally dictate the phenotype, i.e., either non-syndromic deafness or the combination of deafness and seizures.

3.2. TBC1D24 Protein Localization in Human and Mouse Temporal Bone and Tbc1d24 mRNA Expression in Wild Type Mouse Cochlea

In P3 wild type mouse cochlea, in situ hybridization using RNAscope probes demonstrated that *Tbc1d24* mRNA was expressed in spiral ganglion neurons. However, no *Tbc1d24* mRNA was detected in mouse organ of Corti, including inner and outer hair cells (Figure 2A). Moreover, in RNAseq databases, there were only background levels of *Tbc1d24* mRNA expression present in mouse hair cells at E16.5, P1 and P7. It was similar to the background levels of *Cldn11* mRNA in hair cells, which we used as our negative hair cell expression control (Figure S1). *Cldn11* is abundantly expressed in the basal cells of the stria vascularis, but not in hair cells [44–47]. In addition, we immunolocalized TBC1D24 protein in the cell bodies of mouse spiral ganglion neurons (Figure 2B) corroborating published data [10,13]. However, TBC1D24 has also been reported to be localized in stereocilia at E14.5 and P0 to P3 but not at P7 using an sc-390237 antibody [12], an observation we reproduced with this same commercial antiserum against TBC1D24. Nevertheless, three other antibodies against TBC1D24 that showed immunoreactivity in spiral ganglion neurons, did not detect any immunofluorescence signal in hair cells at various ages of mouse, including adult. Among these three antibodies, the rabbit polyclonal ab101933 antibody was developed against an antigenic sequence of human TBC1D24 (aa 467–515) that is present within the antigenic sequence of human origin of the mouse monoclonal sc-390237 antibody (aa 437–559). The specificity of the second out of these three antibodies, NBP1-82925 antibody, was confirmed previously using *Tbc1d24* p.Val67Serfs*4 (TBC1D24 null) mouse inner ear [14]. By comparison, in temporal bone sections from deceased presumably normal hearing individuals, TBC1D24 protein was immunolocalized in spiral ganglion neurons and outer and inner hair cells using two different TBC1D24 antibodies from Abcam, including ab101933 antibody (Figure 3). Taken together, these data indicate that mouse hair cell TBC1D24 immunoreactivity using mouse monoclonal sc-390237 antibody is likely to be non-specific. In both human and mouse, there is abundant expression of *TBC1D24* mRNA and TBC1D24 protein in spiral ganglion neurons, but in hair cells, TBC1D24 expression is detected only in human, while it was undetectable in mouse hair cells.

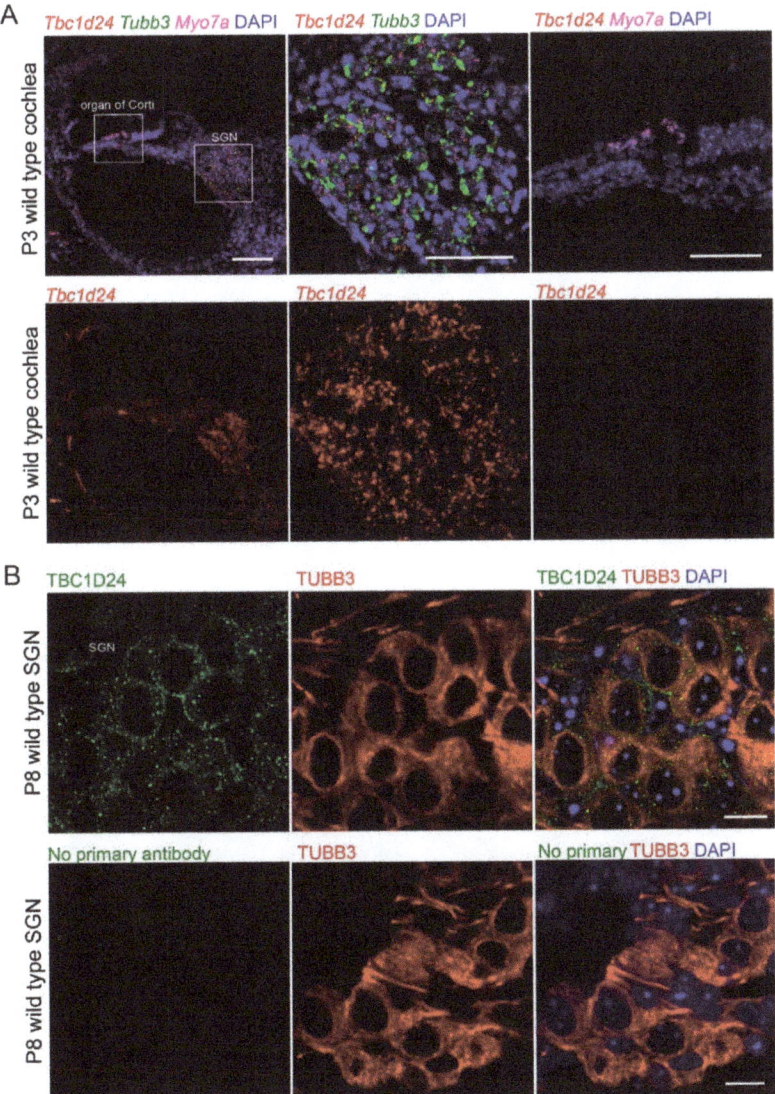

Figure 2. Expressions of mouse *Tbc1d24* mRNA and TBC1D24 protein in spiral ganglion neurons (SGN). (**A**) In situ hybridization using an RNAscope probe in wild type mouse cochlea at P3. *Tbc1d24* mRNA (red, probe-Mm-Tbc1d24) is present in SGN. Expression of *Tbc1d24* mRNA was not detected in the organ of Corti. Hair cells and SGN were labeled using RNAscope probes that recognize *Myo7a* (magenta, Probe-Mm-Myo7a-C2), and *Tubb3* (green, Probe-Mm-Tubb3-C4), respectively. Middle panels are enlarged images of the SGN. Right panels are enlarged images of the organ of Corti. Scale bars are 100 μm (left panel) and 50 μm (middle and right panels). (**B**) Localization of TBC1D24 in wild type mouse SGN. TBC1D24 (green) colocalizes with TUBB3 (red), a marker for the cell body of spiral ganglion neurons, in P8 mouse cochlea. Scale bars are 10 μm.

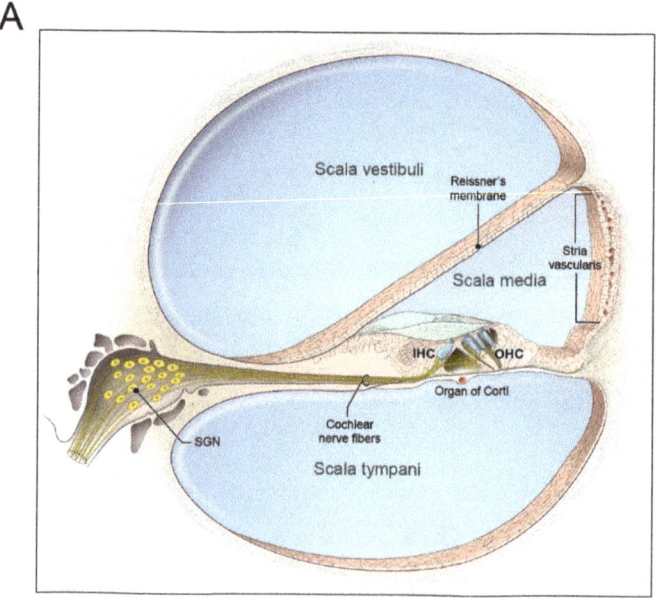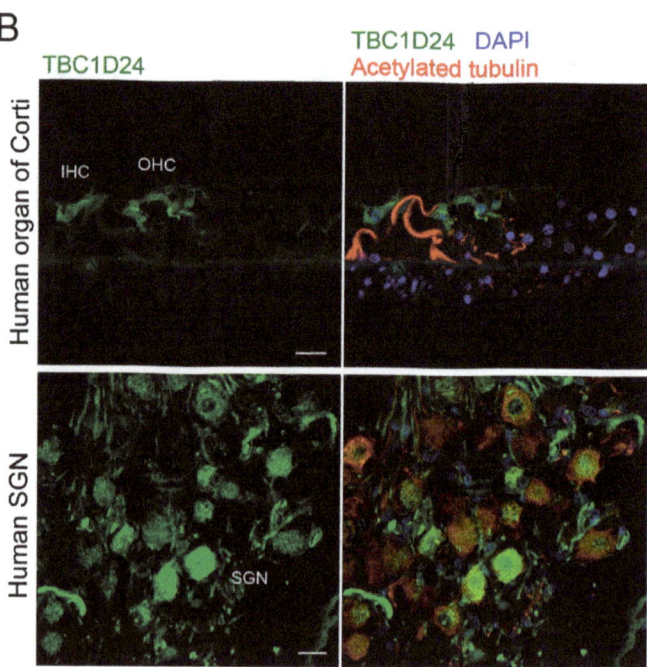

Figure 3. TBC1D24 expression in spiral ganglion neurons (SGN) and organ of Corti from human temporal bones. (**A**) Drawing of a cochlea in cross-section including the organ of Corti and SGN. The organ of Corti contains various supporting cells, one row of inner hair cells (IHC) and three rows of outer hair cells (OHC). (**B**) Representative images of localization of TBC1D24 in human temporal bone cross-sections. TBC1D24 is detected in an IHC and OHC (upper panels) and SGN (lower panels). Scale bars are 20 μm.

3.3. Auditory Function in the Mouse Models of DFNB86 and DFNA65

The hearing status of mouse models of human *DFNB86* and *DFNA65* deafness was quantitatively evaluated using auditory brainstem responses (ABR) and distortion product otoacoustic emissions (DPOAE), which are measures of spiral ganglion neurons and outer hair cell functions, respectively. For the p.Asp70Tyr allele, which is a mouse model of the human DFNB86 p.Asp70Tyr variant [10], ABRs were measured at P30, P60 and P90 in heterozygous and homozygous mutant mice and control homozygous wild type littermates (Figure 4A and Figure S2B). ABR thresholds were within the normal range for all three genotypes. TBC1D24 protein was localized to spiral ganglion neurons in both human and P8 mouse. Therefore, we focused on ABR wave 1 because wave 1 originates from the action potential in the auditory nerve [48]. ABR wave 1 latencies and wave 1 amplitudes were measured at 80 dB SPL at four frequencies (8, 16, 32 and 40 kHz). No significant differences were detected among the three genotypes (Figure 4A), suggesting normal auditory nerve function in *Tbc1d24* homozygous p.Asp70Tyr mutant mice. Homozygous p.Asp70Tyr mice and their littermate controls also have normal distortion product otoacoustic emissions (DPOAE), indicating that outer hair cell amplification of basilar membrane vibrations is indistinguishable from the wild type (Figure 4B).

The human *TBC1D24* c.533C > T p.(Ser178Leu) variant is associated with dominantly inherited loss of hearing DFNA65, segregating in two apparently unrelated families [11,12]. Affected individuals in these two families showed progressive high frequency hearing loss [11,12]. The Ser178 residue is conserved in human and mouse TBC1D24 (Figure S2), although there are other differences in amino acid sequence nearby the Ser178 residue and elsewhere between wild type human and mouse TBC1D24 proteins. We engineered a mouse model of the human *TBC1D24* dominant p.Ser178Leu allele associated with deafness DFNA65. Both homozygous and heterozygous p.Ser178Leu mutant mice with a C57BL/6J genetic background have hearing indistinguishable from their wild type littermates (Figure S2D). Given that mice with a C57BL/6J background show age-related high frequency hearing loss due to *Cdh23* c.753G > A variant [25,26], both wild type littermates and p.Ser178Leu mutant mice showed the expected age-related hearing loss due to this allele of *Cdh23* (Cdh23^{753A}) [25,26]. To exclude association of progressive hearing loss in this *Tbc1d24* p.Ser178Leu mouse with p.Ser178Leu variant, we measured ABR and DPOAE in *Tbc1d24* p.Ser178Leu mouse with the wild type *Cdh23* allele (Cdh23^{753G}). Homozygous and heterozygous p. Ser178Leu mice with the Cdh23^{753G} allele in the background also showed normal ABR thresholds, wave 1 latencies, wave 1 amplitudes and DPOAE (Figure 4C,D and Figure S2C), arguing that the observed age-related hearing loss was exclusively due to *Cdh23* (Cdh23^{753A}) allele.

To evaluate the auditory function of a mouse model of human *TBC1D24* syndromic deafness, we tested hearing by ABR analyses using compound heterozygous p.Ser324Thrfs*3/p.His336Glnfs*12 mice. The human *TBC1D24* p.His336Glnfs*12 variant is associated with syndromic hearing loss. Compound heterozygosity for human p.His336Glnfs*12 and the 1206 + 5G > A exon 5 donor splice site variant of *TBC1D24* is associated with DOORS [19], whereas compound heterozygosity for p.His336Glnfs*12 and perhaps the less disabling p.Asp11Gly single amino acid substitution is associated with early-infantile epileptic encephalopathy 16 (EIEE16) with hearing loss [20]. Using CRISPR/Cas9 editing, we engineered the p.His336Glnfs*12 allele in mouse *Tbc1d24*. However, homozygous p.His336Glnfs*12 mice die during embryonic development. Human p.His336Glnfs*12 homozygotes have not been reported. Consequently, we generated compound heterozygous p.Ser324Thrfs*3/p.His336Glnfs*12 mice. As homozygous p.Ser324Thrfs*3 mice had severe seizures but normal hearing at two weeks of age [13], the p.Ser324Thrfs*3 allele was a logical variant to evaluate the p.His336Glnfs*12 allele in compound heterozygosity. Compound heterozygous p.Ser324Thrfs*3/p.His336Glnfs*12 mice also died around P20 due to seizures; however, their auditory functions at P17 were within the same range as their normal hearing heterozygous p.Ser324Thrfs*3 littermates (Figure S2A). These findings indicate that several different variants of *Tbc1d24* in mouse, unlike the homologous human recessive and dominant variants of *TBC1D24*, are not associated with hearing loss. However, the seizure phenotypes in humans, due to variants of *TBC1D24* are recapitulated in our mouse *Tbc1d24* models [13].

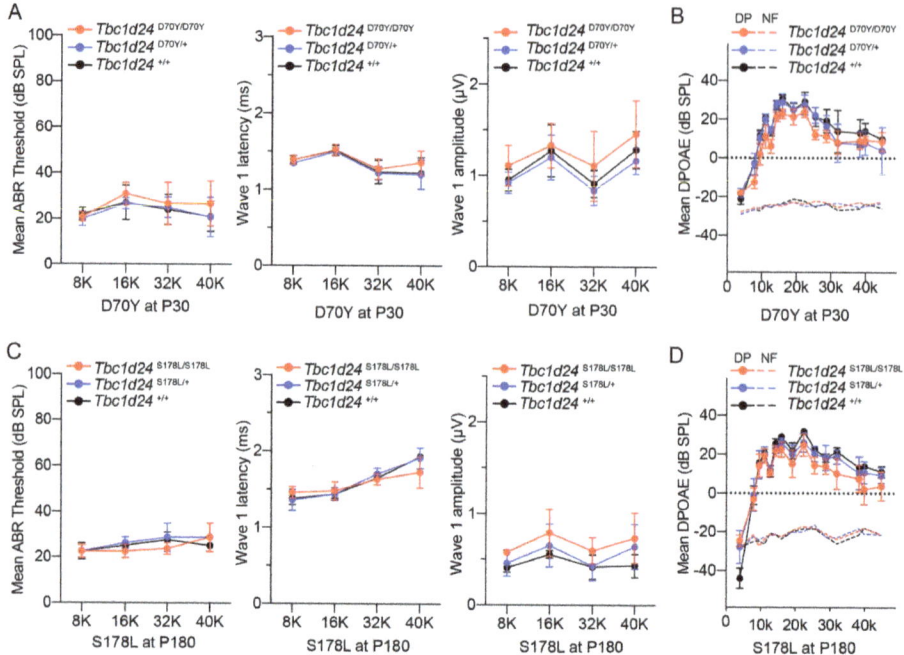

Figure 4. Auditory function measurements of wild type, heterozygous and homozygous *Tbc1d24* mutant mice. (**A**) Mean ABR thresholds, ABR wave 1 latency and ABR wave 1 amplitude of *Tbc1d24* homozygous p.Asp70Tyr (D70Y) ($n = 6$), heterozygous p.Asp70Tyr ($n = 5$) and wild type littermate ($n = 5$) mice at P30. No significant differences were detected between homozygous p.Asp70Tyr, heterozygous p.Asp70Tyr and wild type in threshold, wave 1 latency and wave 1 amplitude. ABR threshold at P60 and P90 are shown in Supplementary Figure S2. (**B**) Mean DPOAE levels for the same *Tbc1d24* p.Asp70Tyr mice tested with ABR. There was no significant difference among the three genotypes. (**C**) Mean ABR thresholds, ABR wave 1 latency and ABR wave 1 amplitude of *Tbc1d24* homozygous p.Ser178Leu ($n = 6$), heterozygous p.Ser178Leu (S178L) ($n = 4$) and wild type littermates ($n = 3$) at P180. As *Tbc1d24* p.Ser178Leu mice and wild type littermate controls had homozygous wild type alleles of *Cdh23* (*Cdh23*^{753G}), they didn't show a high frequency progressive age-related hearing loss. Homozygous p.Ser178Leu mice and heterozygous p.Ser178Leu mice have normal hearing at P30 to P180. ABR threshold of *Tbc1d24* p.Ser178Leu with *Cdh23*^{753G} and *Tbc1d24* p.Ser178Leu with *Cdh23*$^{753G>A}$ at P30 to P90 are shown in Supplementary Figure S2. (**D**) Mean DPOAE levels in mice with the same *Tbc1d24* p.Ser178Leu allele but the wild type *Cdh23*^{753G} were tested by ABR. Dash lines indicate noise floors (NF). No significant differences were detected between homozygous p.Ser178Leu, heterozygous p.Ser178Leu and wild type controls. All data represent mean ± SD.

Human TBC1D24 has an essential function required for normal hearing, since several different human variants of *TBC1D24* are associated with non-syndromic deafness or syndromic deafness (Figure 1A). However, in mouse, TBC1D24 appears not to be required for hearing perhaps because the loss of TBC1D24 function may be compensated by a paralogous protein. However, there might be other explanations as to why particular homozygous or compound heterozygous variants of *TBC1D24* are deafness-causing in humans, while the very same variants in mouse *Tbc1d24* did not affect hearing. Next, we used computational modeling and molecular dynamic simulations to identify additional non-mutually exclusive reasons beyond the cell type-specific differences in the expression of TBC1D24 to explain the different species-specific phenotypic outcome.

3.4. Template-Based Models of Mouse and Human TBC1D24

The final models of human and mouse TBC domain of TBC1D24 show just one residue in disallowed regions from the PROCHECK analyses, indicating that the models have overall good stereochemistry. In order to analyze the compatibility of the TBC1D24 sequence with the fold of the template, 5HJQ, we calculated the ProQ2 score normalized by the number of amino acid residues (global ProQ2 score). Both models have a normalized ProQ2 score of ~0.6, similar to that of the template (0.7). In summary, both analyses highlight the good stereochemical quality of the models and adequate selection of the template. Both models were used to analyze in further details the sites close to residues Asp70 and Ser178 in mouse and human TBC for any structural difference (Figure 5A). In particular, we considered the neighboring residues within 6 Å of Asp70 and Ser178. In both mouse and human, Asp70 is located in a loop and exposed to the solvent with adjacent residues that are strictly conserved (Figure 5A,B and Figure S3), indicating that this residue may be part of a post-translational motif or a partner-protein binding site. This observation suggests that deafness arising from p.Asp70Tyr substitution in human, but normal hearing in p.Asp70Tyr mouse, is not likely due to differences in the identity of the neighboring amino acids. Alternatively, the different phenotypic outcomes are related to an evolutionary divergence in the functional necessity and cell-type specific regulation of expression of human *TBC1D24* compared to mouse *Tbc1d24*.

The Ser178 residue is located in a α-helix (Figure 5A) and is part of a hydrophobic site with neighboring residues that are mostly conserved. However, there is a notable difference between mouse and human at residue 167. In mouse, there is a lysine and in human there is an arginine (Figure 5B and Figure S3). Even though both residues are positively charged, the chemical nature of the arginine provides a more bulky side chain compared to lysine and may indicate why the p.Ser178Leu substitution may result in a different hearing phenotype in mouse compared to human when expressed in the same cell types. Nevertheless, specific details at a structural level of this different phenotype cannot be identified by analyzing mouse and human TBC models (Figure S4). Therefore, we took advantage of Molecular Dynamics (MD).

To gain insight on the effect of p.Ser178Leu substitution, we carried out a series of MD simulations of human hTBC and mouse mTBC, enclosed in a simulation box comprising a hydrated bilayer. One PIP2 molecule anchored the protein to the bilayer (Figure S5). For each system, we first carried out two independent, unrestrained simulations of 200 ns. During these simulations, the protein structures conserved essentially all the structural features of the initial models, with hTBC and mTBC sharing the same tertiary structure except for a remarkable conformational difference (Figure 6A and Table S1). In fact, the C-terminal helix of each domain, which in the initial models laid close to the membrane plane, moved toward Ser178, practically packing the serine side chain in between residues 304 and 308. This conformational change was observed in all simulations and, except in one case, it took place either during the relaxation phase or within the first 2 ns of unrestrained simulations (Figure 7). This finding suggests that the Ser178 residue is critical for packing the C-terminal helix to the protein core, and, as a consequence, stabilizing the folding of the global TBC domain.

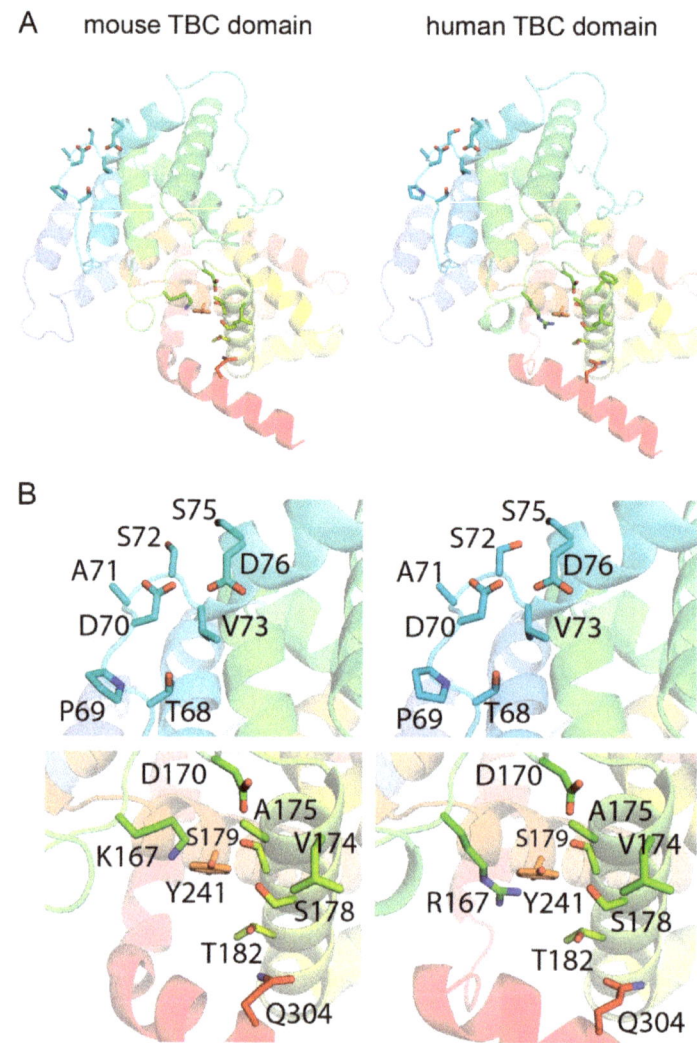

Figure 5. Computational modeling of human TBC1D24 and mouse TBC1D24. (**A**) Models of the TBC domains of mouse (left) and human (right) of TBC1D24 shown as a cartoon. Residues Asp70 and Ser178 as well as those within 6 Å are shown as sticks. (**B**) Enlarged view of the Asp70 (top) and Ser178 (bottom) sites in mouse (left) and human (right) models. Residues within 6 Å of Asp70 or Ser178 are also shown as sticks and indicated with labels. A, Alanine; D, Aspartic acid; K, Lysine; P, Proline; Q, Glutamine; R, Arginine; S, Serine; T, Threonine; V, Valine; Y, Tyrosine.

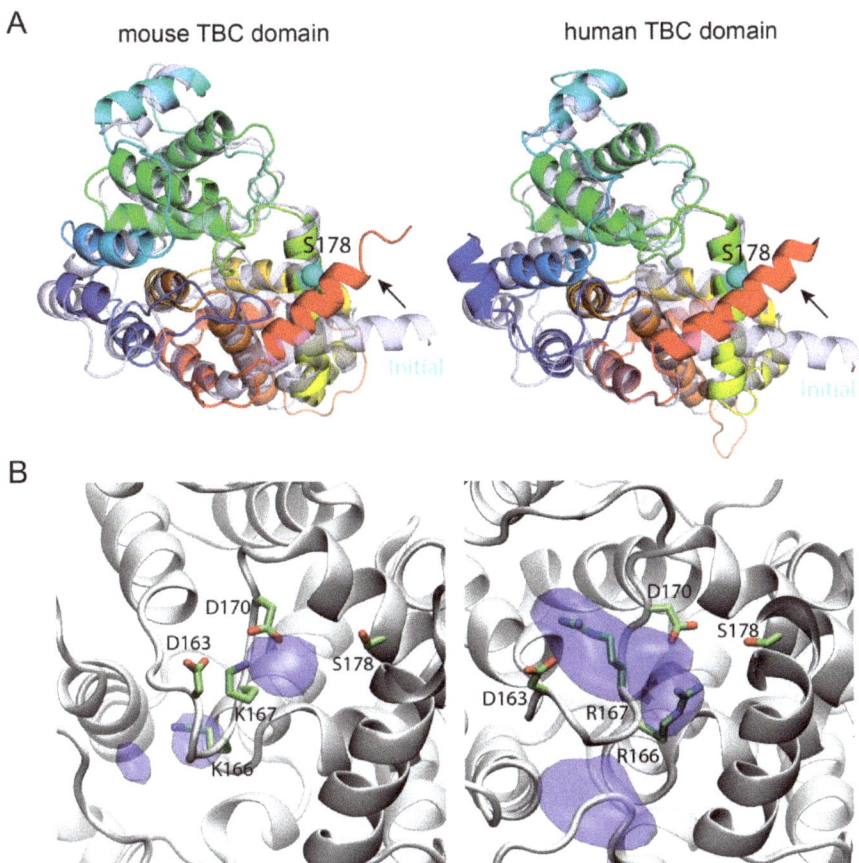

Figure 6. (**A**) Structural superimposition of the initial models of mouse (left) and human (right (light blue colored) with their corresponding final structures after 200-ns molecular dynamics (MD) simulations (rainbow-colored). The reorientation of the C-terminal helix of the TBC domain when comparing the initial model (α-helix colored in light red) and that after Molecular Dynamics simulation was applied (α-helix colored in bright red) is indicated as an arrow. The Cα of Ser178 in both cases is shown as a cyan sphere. (**B**) Side-chain distribution of residues 166 and 167. The isosurfaces of the distribution of the guanidinium moieties of Arg166 and Arg167 (right panel), calculated from the hTBC simulations and that of the ε-amine moieties of Lys166 and Lys167 (left panel), calculated from the mTBC simulations (nitrogens only), are shown in dark blue. In both cases the isosurfaces refer to the density value of 0.05 atomic mass units per Å^3. The protein snapshots correspond to the final snapshots from the respective simulations (sim. 2) where the protein is shown as a gray cartoon and the side-chains of residues Asp163, Lys/Arg166, Lys/Arg167 and Asp170 as gray sticks with the headgroups colored by element: N is blue; O is red. D, Aspartic acid; K, Lysine; R, Arginine; S, Serine.

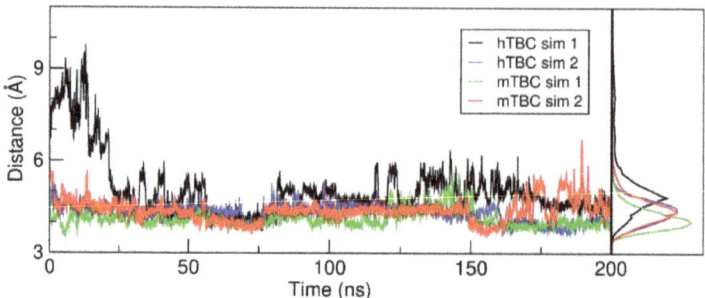

Figure 7. Distance between Ser178 and the C-terminal helix. Left panel: The minimal distance between the Cβ of Ser178 and the Cα of the residues from 304 to 308 is plotted as a function of simulated time, showing how Ser178 is adjacent to the TBC C-terminal helix in most of the snapshots extracted from both human and mouse simulations. Right panel: normalized distributions of the values in the left panel.

To cast light on the role in stabilization of the TBC domain that is played by the Ser178 residue and how the substitution of leucine affects it, we carried out free-energy perturbation (FEP) simulations. Here, Ser178 is mutated, through a number of unphysical (alchemical) intermediates to leucine using a step-wise protocol controlled by a parameter λ that reflects the weights of serine and leucine in the potential energy function of the system. To relate the calculated free-energy values to the folding free-energy differences, we performed similar FEP simulations of a tripeptide in water, which is adopted as representative of the domain unfolded state. The substitution of a leucine-178 for serine-178 showed little effect on the hTBC domain. In fact, the calculated ΔΔG was 0.47 kcal/mol, therefore comparable to the thermal energy fluctuations, in the direction of a slight destabilization of the fold. On the other hand, surprisingly, the same mutation stabilized the folding of mTBC by 3.1 kcal/mol (Table S2). Leucine is significantly more hydrophobic than serine and is found among the most frequent amino acids at α-helical interfaces of soluble proteins, whereas serine is mostly found in non-interfacial regions [49]. Therefore, it is not surprising that the p.Ser178Leu mutation is not disruptive and has a stabilizing effect, at least in mouse. However, that does not explain the observed disparity between human and mouse. As mentioned, the most notable difference among the amino acids adjacent to Ser178 in the two structures is Arg167 in human, which is Lys167 in mouse. These residues belong to the loop region from 162 to 167 and, therefore, are expected to be loosely structured. However, Figure 6B shows that murine Lys167 is strongly tethered in between Asp163 and Asp170 during the simulations, while the bulkier side chain of human Arg167 is more mobile. Consequently, the associated loop 162–167 is less rigid in human than in mouse. Therefore, we speculate that human residue 178 is more exposed to the solvent and to the electrostatic fluctuations arising from the conformational changes the neighboring charged residues (Arg166, Arg167, Asp163 and Asp170), while murine residue 178 faces a more compact pocket. This arrangement would then favor the more hydrophobic leucine over serine, in mouse more than in human. In summary, FEP simulations indicate that p.Ser178Leu has a stabilizing effect in mouse, but not in human.

4. Discussion

Pathogenic variants of human *TBC1D24* are associated with a spectrum of skeletal and neurological disorders including deafness, seizures, onychodystrophy, osteodystrophy and intellectual disability [5]. There is decisive data supporting an association of deafness with variants of human TBC1D24 (Figure 1A). In this study, we report recessive variants of *TBC1D24* c.641G > A p.(Arg214His) and c.965 + 1G > A segregating in a non-consanguineous Pakistani family. In affected individuals of this family, the donor splice-site mutation of exon 2 (c.965 + 1G > A) is novel and present in trans to c.641G > A p.(Arg214His). Bakhchane and colleagues reported that individuals with *TBC1D24* compound heterozygous p.Arg214His/p.Val445Glyfs*33 and p.Arg214His/p.Glu153Lys exhibited non-syndromic deafness *DFNB86* [43]. Surprisingly, in two affected members of family PKDF1429 (Figure 1) a compound heterozygous genotype resulted in deafness with seizure, while for the same compound heterozygous genotype the other two siblings in this family have non-syndromic deafness *DFNB86*. A common phenomenon for variants of *TBC1D24* is that phenotype varies depending upon the second pathogenic variant in trans. For example, compound heterozygosity for p.Glu153Lys and p.Arg214His resulted in *DFNB86* non-syndromic deafness [43], whereas p.Glu153Lys with p.Ala39Val or p.Glu153Lys with p.Thr182Serfs*6 in trans cause seizure without deafness [50,51].

The distinctly different functions of TBC and TLDc domains have been individually studied in orthologues, but not in TBC1D24, which is the only protein that has both of these domains. The TBC domain is a GTPase activator and TLDc domain is neuro-protective against oxidative stress [16,17]. Surprisingly, there is no genotype-phenotype correlation yet with variant location, either with the location in the *TBC1D24* gene or in one or the other of the two domains of the TBC1D24 protein as illustrated in Figure 1A [52]. Perhaps the pleiotropy, associated with different variants of *TBC1D24*, results from a composite of disabled binding motifs for an array of interacting protein partners of TBC1D24. To date, the reported binding partners of TBC1D24 include ARF6 (ADP-ribosylation factor) [53,54] and ephrinB2 [55].

A second non-mutually exclusive possibility to explain the great variety of phenotypes associated with variants of TBC1D24 is a variable contribution to compensation among individuals resulting from their different genetic backgrounds [56,57]. For example, the *TBC1D24*-associated phenotype may be influenced by common polymorphic variants of one or more of the 26 other TBC-containing proteins [58] or variants of one of the other four TLDc-containing proteins in the mammalian genome [16,17].

To determine if the inner ear cell-type-specific expression is the same in human and mouse, we performed immunohistochemistry on human temporal bones. TBC1D24 protein localized in human SGN just as we and others have reported in mouse SGN [10,12,13]. However, TBC1D24 protein was not reliably detected in mouse hair cells but was detected in human inner and outer hair cells of five different temporal bones (Figure 3B). These data suggest that one possible cause of deafness in human from variants of *TBC1D24* is a necessary function of human TBC1D24 in the sensory epithelium of the inner ear. In mouse, TBC1D24 is not detected in hair cells by RNAscope probes and is at a background level in RNAseq data, comparable with the level of CLDN11, which is known to be expressed in basal cells of the stria vascularis, but not in hair cells of early postnatal mouse inner ear (Figure S1). We also cannot rule out the possibility that human TBC1D24 may also have a necessary function in the spiral ganglion neurons as well.

Using CRISPR/Cas9 gene editing, we engineered in mouse the same deafness-causing variants as in human *TBC1D24*. Unexpectedly, *Tbc1d24* mutant mice have normal auditory functions even though they have biallelic recessive or dominant missense mutations orthologous to either of two variants associated with human non-syndromic deafness, *DFNB86* and *DFNA65* (Table 1). There is precedent for animal models not recapitulating a human inherited pathology. For example, a variety of engineered mouse models of Huntington disease (HD) do not reproduce the severe constellation of neuropathology cascades, observed in HD patients or features of HD postmortem brains [59,60].

Table 1. *TBC1D24* variants and associated phenotypes.

Variant	Genotype	Human Phenotype	Mouse Phenotype
p.Ser178Leu	p.Ser178Leu/p.Ser178Leu	not reported	normal hearing, no seizures
	p.Ser178Leu/+	progressive hearing loss [11,12]	normal hearing, no seizures
p.Asp70Tyr	p.Asp70Tyr/p.Asp70Tyr	congenital profound hearing loss [10]	normal hearing, no seizures
	p.Asp70Tyr/+	no clinical phenotype	normal hearing, no seizures
p.His336Glnfs*12	p.His336Glnfs*12/ p.His336Glnfs*12	not reported	embryonic lethality
	p.His336Glnfs*12/ p.Asp11Gly	seizures with deafness [20]	not reported
	p.His336Glnfs*12/ c.1206 + 5G > A	DOORS syndrome [20]	not reported
	p.His336Glnfs*12/ p.Ser324Thrfs*3	not reported	seizures, postnatal death ~P20, normal hearing

In mouse, homozygosity for the p.His336Glnfs*12 allele results in embryonic lethality, while compound heterozygosity of p.His336Glnfs*12 with p.Ser324Thrfs*3 produces postnatal death at about P20 due to seizures. Given that heterozygous p.Ser324Thrfs*3 mice do not show seizure and otherwise appear to be phenotypically wild type [13], we conclude that the phenotype of the p.His336Glnfs*12 allele in compound heterozygosity with p.Ser324Thrfs*3 is pathogenic. These results indicate that the p.His336Glnfs*12 variant in mouse is pathogenic but does not result in a hearing loss. In addition to our results, a heterozygous $Tbc1d24^{tm1b(EUCOMM)Hmgu}$ mutant mouse has normal hearing [36] and in our laboratory the homozygote for $Tbc1d24^{tm1b(EUCOMM)Hmgu}$ obtained from the KOMP repository at the Baylor College of Medicine is also an embryonic lethal.

Since TBC1D24 is localized in human and mouse spiral ganglion neurons (Figures 2 and 3B), we evaluated ABR wave 1 latency and amplitude (Figure 4A,C). However, there was no significant difference among three genotypes. In mouse, homozygotes for *Tbc1d24* p.Asp70Tyr variant have normal hearing despite deafness associated with homozygosity for p.Asp70Tyr in human. In the mouse cochlea, *Tbc1d24* mRNA and TBC1D24 protein were detected only in the spiral ganglion neurons (Figure 2A,B). This result is different from the localization of human TBC1D24, which was detected in both organ of Corti and spiral ganglion neurons (Figure 3B). Perhaps in the mouse, expression of TBC1D24 protein in spiral ganglion neurons is not necessary for normal hearing. While TBC1D24 is not expressed in mouse hair cells, it is an open question as to whether TBC1D24 has a necessary function in human spiral ganglion neurons, hair cells or both. To answer this question, in future studies we will introduce in the presence of a homozygous null allele of the endogenous mouse *Tbc1d24* gene, a human wild type BAC transgene or a mutant *TBC1D24*. Would such mice, expressing only functional human *TBC1D24*, show detectable TBC1D24 mRNA and protein in hair cells and would the human TBC1D24 be necessary for hearing in mice? In a study of Parkinson disease (PD) in mouse models, a mutant α-synuclein encoded by human *SNCA* expressed from a human transgene resulted in a human-like PD-associated phenotype in mice homozygous for a null allele of the endogenous mouse *Snca* gene [61].

The genetic background in humans and mice may have a significant impact on variants of human *TBC1D24*, mouse *Tbc1d24*, or both. For example, there may be a modifier variant in the human genome that enhances the deafness phenotype of biallelic pathogenic variants of *TBC1D24*. We engineered *Tbc1d24* mutant mice using only a C57BL/6J background. The phenotype of a variant in a mouse gene can change substantially, depending upon genetic background [62]. We have yet to explore the possibility that the recessive variant p.Asp70Tyr and the dominant variant p.Ser178Leu in mouse may result in deafness when placed in the context of a different genetic background. The genotype-phenotype relationship of human TBC1D24 variants associated with seizures are recapitulated in variants of mouse *Tbc1d24* [13], unlike deafness. Does the genetic background of the B6 strain provide functional compensation for a disabled TBC1D24 protein? Might there be a strain-specific modifier in the background of a different mouse inbred strain that would suppress the non-penetrance of deafness in a B6 background? Compensation for the loss of TBC1D24 in mouse may be provided by a paralog in the mouse genome or compensation by a gene involved in the same network or signaling pathway [63]. For example, a dominant variant of *METTL13* (*DFNM1*) completely suppresses recessive non-syndromic deafness *DFNB26*, associated with a variant of *GAB2* with both genes functioning in the HGF/MET signaling pathway [64–66].

Another non-mutually exclusive possibility to explain the divergent outcomes of the same variant of human *TBC1D24* and mouse *Tbc1d24* is that some variants are damaging in human but only in combination with other wild type substitutions in TBC1D24 protein that have become fixed during human evolution. From molecular dynamic simulations, we provide data indicating that p.Ser178Leu, a dominant variant with a pathogenic leucine at residue 178, destabilizes human TBC1D24 protein; but surprisingly the same substitution stabilizes mouse TBC1D24, despite the considerable sequence identity between human and mouse TBC domains.

In summary, we report a novel pathogenic splice-site variant of *TBC1D24* segregating in a Pakistani family, and describe several mouse models of human *TBC1D24* associated with DFNB86, DFNA65 and syndromic deafness. We propose various possible explanations for the differences in phenotypes despite the same variant in mouse *Tbc1d24* and human *TBC1D24*, and provide experimental data from molecular dynamics to support one of many possible explanations for this species-specific outcome. Nevertheless, a comprehensive understanding as to how human *TBC1D24* variants cause DFNB86 deafness, as well as a panoply of other allele-associated abnormalities remains to be explored. Future studies will focus on the networks and protein complexes in which TBC1D24 functions in the auditory system and brain.

Supplementary Materials: The following are available online at http://www.mdpi.com/2073-4425/11/10/1122/s1, Figure S1: Single cell RNA-sequencing of inner and outer hair cells. Figure S2: ABR thresholds of *Tbc1d24* mice. Figure S3: Sequence alignment of human and mouse TBC domain of TBC1D24 protein obtained using Clustal Omega. Figure S4: Structural model of the human TBC (hTBC) domain of human TBC1D24 (hTBC1D24). Figure S5: Representation of the Molecular Dynamics setup. Table S1: Observed difference in the structures of hTBC and mTBC. Table S2: Free energy differences (ΔG) from the FEP simulations.

Author Contributions: Conceptualization, R.T., T.B.F., I.A.B.; methodology, R.T., T.B.F.; validation, R.T., I.A.L., C.F.-F., C.A., R.F., A.A.K., M.S., S.G., A.I.; formal analysis, R.T., I.A.L., C.F.-F., M.H.; investigation, R.T., T.B.F.; data curation, R.T., T.B.F., I.A.B.; writing—original draft preparation, R.T., T.B.F.; writing—review and editing, R.T., I.A.L., C.F.-F., R.F., C.A., A.A.K., M.S., R.J.M., S.G., M.H., L.D., A.I., I.A.B., S.R., T.B.F.; supervision, T.B.F.; funding acquisition, T.B.F., S.R., A.I., M.H. All authors have read and agreed to this version of the manuscript.

Funding: This work is supported by the Intramural Research Program of the NIDCD/NIH to T.B.F. (DC000039), to M.H. (DC000088), to R.J.M. for the GCBC (DC000086), to TSF (DC000080) and to L.D., NEI (EY000458-13) and the Extramural Research Program of NIDCD to A.I. (U24 DC 015910).

Acknowledgments: We thank the participants in this study. We are grateful to the advice from Ronald Petralia, Mhamed Grati, Tracy Fitzgerald, Elizabeth Wilson and Barbara Zwiesler. This work utilized the computational resources of the NIH HPC Biowulf cluster (http://hpc.nih.gov).

Conflicts of Interest: The authors declare no conflict of interest.

References

1. Barbi, M.; Binda, S.; Caroppo, S.; Ambrosetti, U.; Corbetta, C.; Sergi, P. A wider role for congenital cytomegalovirus infection in sensorineural hearing loss. *Pediatr. Infect. Dis. J.* **2003**, *22*, 39–42. [CrossRef]
2. Brock, P.R.; Knight, K.R.; Freyer, D.R.; Campbell, K.C.; Steyger, P.S.; Blakley, B.W.; Rassekh, S.R.; Chang, K.W.; Fligor, B.J.; Rajput, K.; et al. Platinum-induced ototoxicity in children: A consensus review on mechanisms, predisposition, and protection, including a new International Society of Pediatric Oncology Boston ototoxicity scale. *J. Clin. Oncol.* **2012**, *30*, 2408–2417. [CrossRef]

3. Hilgert, N.; Smith, R.J.; Van Camp, G. Function and expression pattern of nonsyndromic deafness genes. *Curr. Mol. Med.* **2009**, *9*, 546–564. [CrossRef]
4. Griffith, A.J.; Friedman, T.B. *Hereditary Hearing Loss*, 18th ed.; Wackym, P.A., Snow, J.B., Eds.; People's Medical Publishing House-USA: Shelton, CT, USA, 2016.
5. Rehman, A.U.; Friedman, T.B.; Griffith, A.J. Unresolved questions regarding human hereditary deafness. *Oral. Dis.* **2017**, *23*, 551–558. [CrossRef]
6. Toriello, H.V.; Smith, S.D. *Hereditary Hearing Loss and ITS Syndromes*; Oxford University Press: Oxford, UK, 2013.
7. Liu, X.Z.; Walsh, J.; Tamagawa, Y.; Kitamura, K.; Nishizawa, M.; Steel, K.P.; Brown, S.D. Autosomal dominant non-syndromic deafness caused by a mutation in the myosin VIIA gene. *Nat. Genet.* **1997**, *17*, 268–269. [CrossRef]
8. Weil, D.; Blanchard, S.; Kaplan, J.; Guilford, P.; Gibson, F.; Walsh, J.; Mburu, P.; Varela, A.; Levilliers, J.; Weston, M.D.; et al. Defective myosin VIIA gene responsible for Usher syndrome type 1B. *Nature* **1995**, *374*, 60–61. [CrossRef]
9. Weil, D.; Küssel, P.; Blanchard, S.; Lévy, G.; Levi-Acobas, F.; Drira, M.; Ayadi, H.; Petit, C. The autosomal recessive isolated deafness, DFNB2, and the Usher 1B syndrome are allelic defects of the myosin-VIIA gene. *Nat. Genet.* **1997**, *16*, 191–193. [CrossRef]
10. Rehman, A.U.; Santos-Cortez, R.L.; Morell, R.J.; Drummond, M.C.; Ito, T.; Lee, K.; Khan, A.A.; Basra, M.A.; Wasif, N.; Ayub, M.; et al. Mutations in TBC1D24, a gene associated with epilepsy, also cause nonsyndromic deafness DFNB86. *Am. J. Hum. Genet.* **2014**, *94*, 144–152. [CrossRef]
11. Azaiez, H.; Booth, K.T.; Bu, F.; Huygen, P.; Shibata, S.B.; Shearer, A.E.; Kolbe, D.; Meyer, N.; Black-Ziegelbein, E.A.; Smith, R.J. TBC1D24 mutation causes autosomal-dominant nonsyndromic hearing loss. *Hum. Mutat.* **2014**, *35*, 819–823. [CrossRef]
12. Zhang, L.; Hu, L.; Chai, Y.; Pang, X.; Yang, T.; Wu, H. A dominant mutation in the stereocilia-expressing gene TBC1D24 is a probable cause for nonsyndromic hearing impairment. *Hum. Mutat.* **2014**, *35*, 814–818. [CrossRef]
13. Tona, R.; Chen, W.; Nakano, Y.; Reyes, L.D.; Petralia, R.S.; Wang, Y.X.; Starost, M.F.; Wafa, T.T.; Morell, R.J.; Cravedi, K.D.; et al. The phenotypic landscape of a Tbc1d24 mutant mouse includes convulsive seizures resembling human early infantile epileptic encephalopathy. *Hum. Mol. Genet.* **2019**, *28*, 1530–1547. [CrossRef]
14. Fukuda, M. TBC proteins: GAPs for mammalian small GTPase Rab? *Biosci. Rep.* **2011**, *31*, 159–168. [CrossRef]
15. Pan, X.; Eathiraj, S.; Munson, M.; Lambright, D.G. TBC-domain GAPs for Rab GTPases accelerate GTP hydrolysis by a dual-finger mechanism. *Nature* **2006**, *442*, 303–306. [CrossRef]
16. Finelli, M.J.; Sanchez-Pulido, L.; Liu, K.X.; Davies, K.E.; Oliver, P.L. The Evolutionarily Conserved Tre2/Bub2/Cdc16 (TBC), Lysin Motif (LysM), Domain Catalytic (TLDc) Domain Is Neuroprotective against Oxidative Stress. *J. Biol. Chem.* **2016**, *291*, 2751–2763. [CrossRef]
17. Finelli, M.J.; Oliver, P.L. TLDc proteins: New players in the oxidative stress response and neurological disease. *Mamm. Genome* **2017**, *28*, 395–406. [CrossRef]
18. Guven, A.; Tolun, A. TBC1D24 truncating mutation resulting in severe neurodegeneration. *J. Med. Genet.* **2013**, *50*, 199–202. [CrossRef]
19. Campeau, P.M.; Kasperaviciute, D.; Lu, J.T.; Burrage, L.C.; Kim, C.; Hori, M.; Powell, B.R.; Stewart, F.; Félix, T.M.; van den Ende, J.; et al. The genetic basis of DOORS syndrome: An exome-sequencing study. *Lancet Neurol.* **2014**, *13*, 44–58. [CrossRef]
20. Stražišar, B.G.; Neubauer, D.; Paro Panjan, D.; Writzl, K. Early-onset epileptic encephalopathy with hearing loss in two siblings with TBC1D24 recessive mutations. *Eur. J. Paediatr. Neurol.* **2015**, *19*, 251–256. [CrossRef]
21. Li, H.; Durbin, R. Fast and accurate short read alignment with Burrows-Wheeler transform. *Bioinformatics* **2009**, *25*, 1754–1760. [CrossRef]
22. Varshney, G.K.; Pei, W.; LaFave, M.C.; Idol, J.; Xu, L.; Gallardo, V.; Carrington, B.; Bishop, K.; Jones, M.; Li, M.; et al. High-throughput gene targeting and phenotyping in zebrafish using CRISPR/Cas9. *Genome Res.* **2015**, *25*, 1030–1042. [CrossRef]
23. Richardson, C.D.; Ray, G.J.; DeWitt, M.A.; Curie, G.L.; Corn, J.E. Enhancing homology-directed genome editing by catalytically active and inactive CRISPR-Cas9 using asymmetric donor DNA. *Nat. Biotechnol.* **2016**, *34*, 339–344. [CrossRef]

24. Wang, H.; Yang, H.; Shivalila, C.S.; Dawlaty, M.M.; Cheng, A.W.; Zhang, F.; Jaenisch, R. One-step generation of mice carrying mutations in multiple genes by CRISPR/Cas-mediated genome engineering. *Cell* **2013**, *153*, 910–918. [CrossRef]
25. Johnson, K.R.; Erway, L.C.; Cook, S.A.; Willott, J.F.; Zheng, Q.Y. A major gene affecting age-related hearing loss in C57BL/6J mice. *Hear. Res.* **1997**, *114*, 83–92. [CrossRef]
26. Keithley, E.M.; Canto, C.; Zheng, Q.Y.; Fischel-Ghodsian, N.; Johnson, K.R. Age-related hearing loss and the ahl locus in mice. *Hear. Res.* **2004**, *188*, 21–28. [CrossRef]
27. Morozko, E.L.; Nishio, A.; Ingham, N.J.; Chandra, R.; Fitzgerald, T.; Martelletti, E.; Borck, G.; Wilson, E.; Riordan, G.P.; Wangemann, P.; et al. ILDR1 null mice, a model of human deafness DFNB42, show structural aberrations of tricellular tight junctions and degeneration of auditory hair cells. *Hum. Mol. Genet.* **2015**, *24*, 609–624. [CrossRef]
28. Lopez, I.A.; Ishiyama, G.; Hosokawa, S.; Hosokawa, K.; Acuna, D.; Linthicum, F.H.; Ishiyama, A. Immunohistochemical techniques for the human inner ear. *Histochem. Cell Biol.* **2016**, *146*, 367–387. [CrossRef]
29. Kolla, L.; Kelly, M.C.; Mann, Z.F.; Anaya-Rocha, A.; Ellis, K.; Lemons, A.; Palermo, A.T.; So, K.S.; Mays, J.C.; Orvis, J.; et al. Characterization of the development of the mouse cochlear epithelium at the single cell level. *Nat. Commun.* **2020**, *11*, 2389. [CrossRef]
30. Zimmermann, L.; Stephens, A.; Nam, S.Z.; Rau, D.; Kübler, J.; Lozajic, M.; Gabler, F.; Söding, J.; Lupas, A.N.; Alva, V. A Completely Reimplemented MPI Bioinformatics Toolkit with a New HHpred Server at its Core. *J. Mol. Biol.* **2018**, *430*, 2237–2243. [CrossRef]
31. Fischer, B.; Lüthy, K.; Paesmans, J.; De Koninck, C.; Maes, I.; Swerts, J.; Kuenen, S.; Uytterhoeven, V.; Verstreken, P.; Versées, W. Skywalker-TBC1D24 has a lipid-binding pocket mutated in epilepsy and required for synaptic function. *Nat. Struct. Mol. Biol.* **2016**, *23*, 965–973. [CrossRef]
32. Berman, H.M.; Westbrook, J.; Feng, Z.; Gilliland, G.; Bhat, T.N.; Weissig, H.; Shindyalov, I.N.; Bourne, P.E. The Protein Data Bank. *Nucleic Acids Res.* **2000**, *28*, 235–242. [CrossRef]
33. Ashkenazy, H.; Abadi, S.; Martz, E.; Chay, O.; Mayrose, I.; Pupko, T.; Ben-Tal, N. ConSurf 2016: An improved methodology to estimate and visualize evolutionary conservation in macromolecules. *Nucleic Acids Res.* **2016**, *44*, W344–W350. [CrossRef]
34. Wallner, B.; Elofsson, A. Can correct protein models be identified? *Protein Sci.* **2003**, *12*, 1073–1086. [CrossRef]
35. Sali, A.; Blundell, T.L. Comparative protein modelling by satisfaction of spatial restraints. *J. Mol. Biol.* **1993**, *234*, 779–815. [CrossRef] [PubMed]
36. Finelli, M.J.; Aprile, D.; Castroflorio, E.; Jeans, A.; Moschetta, M.; Chessum, L.; Degiacomi, M.T.; Grasegger, J.; Lupien-Meilleur, A.; Bassett, A.; et al. The epilepsy-associated protein TBC1D24 is required for normal development, survival and vesicle trafficking in mammalian neurons. *Hum. Mol. Genet.* **2019**, *28*, 584–597. [CrossRef]
37. Jo, S.; Kim, T.; Iyer, V.G.; Im, W. CHARMM-GUI: A web-based graphical user interface for CHARMM. *J. Comput. Chem.* **2008**, *29*, 1859–1865. [CrossRef]
38. Morozenko, A.; Leontyev, I.V.; Stuchebrukhov, A.A. Dipole Moment and Binding Energy of Water in Proteins from Crystallographic Analysis. *J. Chem. Theory Comput.* **2014**, *10*, 4618–4623. [CrossRef]
39. Bennett, C.H. Efficient estimation of free energy differences from Monte Carlo data. *J. Comp. Phys.* **1976**, *22*, 245–268. [CrossRef]
40. Van Der Spoel, D.; Lindahl, E.; Hess, B.; Groenhof, G.; Mark, A.E.; Berendsen, H.J. GROMACS: Fast, flexible, and free. *J. Comput. Chem.* **2005**, *26*, 1701–1718. [CrossRef]
41. Best, R.B.; Zhu, X.; Shim, J.; Lopes, P.E.; Mittal, J.; Feig, M.; Mackerell, A.D., Jr. Optimization of the additive CHARMM all-atom protein force field targeting improved sampling of the backbone φ, ψ and side-chain $\chi(1)$ and $\chi(2)$ dihedral angles. *J. Chem. Theory Comput.* **2012**, *8*, 3257–3273. [CrossRef]
42. Klauda, J.B.; Venable, R.M.; Freites, J.A.; O'Connor, J.W.; Tobias, D.J.; Mondragon-Ramirez, C.; Vorobyov, I.; MacKerell, A.D., Jr.; Pastor, R.W. Update of the CHARMM all-atom additive force field for lipids: Validation on six lipid types. *J. Phys. Chem. B* **2010**, *114*, 7830–7843. [CrossRef]
43. Bakhchane, A.; Charif, M.; Salime, S.; Boulouiz, R.; Nahili, H.; Roky, R.; Lenaers, G.; Barakat, A. Recessive TBC1D24 Mutations Are Frequent in Moroccan Non-Syndromic Hearing Loss Pedigrees. *PLoS ONE* **2015**, *10*, e0138272. [CrossRef]

44. Gow, A.; Davies, C.; Southwood, C.M.; Frolenkov, G.; Chrustowski, M.; Ng, L.; Yamauchi, D.; Marcus, D.C.; Kachar, B. Deafness in Claudin 11-null mice reveals the critical contribution of basal cell tight junctions to stria vascularis function. *J. Neurosci.* **2004**, *24*, 7051–7062. [CrossRef]
45. Kitajiri, S.; Miyamoto, T.; Mineharu, A.; Sonoda, N.; Furuse, K.; Hata, M.; Sasaki, H.; Mori, Y.; Kubota, T.; Ito, J.; et al. Compartmentalization established by claudin-11-based tight junctions in stria vascularis is required for hearing through generation of endocochlear potential. *J. Cell Sci.* **2004**, *117*, 5087–5096. [CrossRef]
46. Kitajiri, S.I.; Furuse, M.; Morita, K.; Saishin-Kiuchi, Y.; Kido, H.; Ito, J.; Tsukita, S. Expression patterns of claudins, tight junction adhesion molecules, in the inner ear. *Hear. Res.* **2004**, *187*, 25–34. [CrossRef]
47. Liu, W.; Schrott-Fischer, A.; Glueckert, R.; Benav, H.; Rask-Andersen, H. The Human "Cochlear Battery"—Claudin-11 Barrier and Ion Transport Proteins in the Lateral Wall of the Cochlea. *Front. Mol. Neurosci.* **2017**, *10*, 239. [CrossRef]
48. Melcher, J.R.; Kiang, N.Y. Generators of the brainstem auditory evoked potential in cat. III: Identified cell populations. *Hear. Res.* **1996**, *93*, 52–71. [CrossRef]
49. Eilers, M.; Patel, A.B.; Liu, W.; Smith, S.O. Comparison of helix interactions in membrane and soluble α-bundle proteins. *Biophys. J.* **2002**, *82*, 2720–2736. [CrossRef]
50. Ngoh, A.; Bras, J.; Guerreiro, R.; McTague, A.; Ng, J.; Meyer, E.; Chong, W.K.; Boyd, S.; MacLellan, L.; Kirkpatrick, M.; et al. TBC1D24 Mutations in a Sibship with Multifocal Polymyoclonus. *Tremor Other Hyperkinet Mov. (N. Y.)* **2017**, *7*, 452. [CrossRef]
51. Ragona, F.; Castellotti, B.; Salis, B.; Magri, S.; DiFrancesco, J.C.; Nardocci, N.; Franceschetti, S.; Gellera, C.; Granata, T. Alternating Hemiplegia and Epilepsia Partialis Continua: A new phenotype for a novel compound TBC1D24 mutation. *Seizure* **2017**, *47*, 71–73. [CrossRef]
52. Balestrini, S.; Milh, M.; Castiglioni, C.; Lüthy, K.; Finelli, M.J.; Verstreken, P.; Cardon, A.; Stražišar, B.G.; Holder, J.L., Jr.; Lesca, G.; et al. TBC1D24 genotype-phenotype correlation: Epilepsies and other neurologic features. *Neurology* **2016**, *87*, 77–85. [CrossRef]
53. Falace, A.; Buhler, E.; Fadda, M.; Watrin, F.; Lippiello, P.; Pallesi-Pocachard, E.; Baldelli, P.; Benfenati, F.; Zara, F.; Represa, A.; et al. TBC1D24 regulates neuronal migration and maturation through modulation of the ARF6-dependent pathway. *Proc. Natl. Acad. Sci. USA* **2014**, *111*, 2337–2342. [CrossRef]
54. Falace, A.; Filipello, F.; La Padula, V.; Vanni, N.; Madia, F.; De Pietri Tonelli, D.; de Falco, F.A.; Striano, P.; Dagna Bricarelli, F.; Minetti, C.; et al. TBC1D24, an ARF6-interacting protein, is mutated in familial infantile myoclonic epilepsy. *Am. J. Hum. Genet.* **2010**, *87*, 365–370. [CrossRef]
55. Yoon, J.; Hwang, Y.S.; Lee, M.; Sun, J.; Cho, H.J.; Knapik, L.; Daar, I.O. TBC1d24-ephrinB2 interaction regulates contact inhibition of locomotion in neural crest cell migration. *Nat. Commun.* **2018**, *9*, 3491. [CrossRef]
56. Bunton-Stasyshyn, R.K.A.; Wells, S.; Teboul, L. When all is not lost: Considering genetic compensation in laboratory animals. *Lab. Anim. (N. Y.)* **2019**, *48*, 282–284. [CrossRef]
57. Sittig, L.J.; Carbonetto, P.; Engel, K.A.; Krauss, K.S.; Barrios-Camacho, C.M.; Palmer, A.A. Genetic Background Limits Generalizability of Genotype-Phenotype Relationships. *Neuron* **2016**, *91*, 1253–1259. [CrossRef]
58. Frasa, M.A.; Koessmeier, K.T.; Ahmadian, M.R.; Braga, V.M. Illuminating the functional and structural repertoire of human TBC/RABGAPs. *Nat. Rev. Mol. Cell Biol.* **2012**, *13*, 67–73. [CrossRef]
59. DiFiglia, M. An early start to Huntington's disease. *Science* **2020**, *369*, 771–772. [CrossRef]
60. Vonsattel, J.P. Huntington disease models and human neuropathology: Similarities and differences. *Acta Neuropathol.* **2008**, *115*, 55–69. [CrossRef]
61. Kuo, Y.M.; Li, Z.; Jiao, Y.; Gaborit, N.; Pani, A.K.; Orrison, B.M.; Bruneau, B.G.; Giasson, B.I.; Smeyne, R.J.; Gershon, M.D.; et al. Extensive enteric nervous system abnormalities in mice transgenic for artificial chromosomes containing Parkinson disease-associated α-synuclein gene mutations precede central nervous system changes. *Hum. Mol. Genet.* **2010**, *19*, 1633–1650. [CrossRef]
62. Tian, C.; Gagnon, L.H.; Longo-Guess, C.; Korstanje, R.; Sheehan, S.M.; Ohlemiller, K.K.; Schrader, A.D.; Lett, J.M.; Johnson, K.R. Hearing loss without overt metabolic acidosis in ATP6V1B1 deficient MRL mice, a new genetic model for non-syndromic deafness with enlarged vestibular aqueducts. *Hum. Mol. Genet.* **2017**, *26*, 3722–3735. [CrossRef]
63. Peng, J. Gene redundancy and gene compensation: An updated view. *J. Genet. Genom.* **2019**, *46*, 329–333. [CrossRef]

64. Morell, R.J.; Olszewski, R.; Tona, R.; Leitess, S.; Wafa, T.T.; Taukulis, I.; Schultz, J.M.; Thomason, E.J.; Richards, K.; Whitley, B.N.; et al. Noncoding Microdeletion in Mouse Hgf Disrupts Neural Crest Migration into the Stria Vascularis, Reduces the Endocochlear Potential, and Suggests the Neuropathology for Human Nonsyndromic Deafness DFNB39. *J. Neurosci.* **2020**, *40*, 2976–2992. [CrossRef]
65. Riazuddin, S.; Castelein, C.M.; Ahmed, Z.M.; Lalwani, A.K.; Mastroianni, M.A.; Naz, S.; Smith, T.N.; Liburd, N.A.; Friedman, T.B.; Griffith, A.J.; et al. Dominant modifier DFNM1 suppresses recessive deafness DFNB26. *Nat. Genet.* **2000**, *26*, 431–434. [CrossRef]
66. Yousaf, R.; Ahmed, Z.M.; Giese, A.P.; Morell, R.J.; Lagziel, A.; Dabdoub, A.; Wilcox, E.R.; Riazuddin, S.; Friedman, T.B.; Riazuddin, S. Modifier variant of METTL13 suppresses human GAB1-associated profound deafness. *J. Clin. Investig.* **2018**, *128*, 1509–1522. [CrossRef]

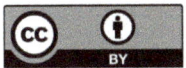
© 2020 by the authors. Licensee MDPI, Basel, Switzerland. This article is an open access article distributed under the terms and conditions of the Creative Commons Attribution (CC BY) license (http://creativecommons.org/licenses/by/4.0/).

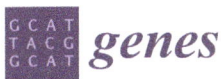

Review

Molecular Mechanisms and Biological Functions of Autophagy for Genetics of Hearing Impairment

Ken Hayashi [1,2,3,*]**, Yuna Suzuki** [2]**, Chisato Fujimoto** [4] **and Sho Kanzaki** [3]

1. Department of Otolaryngology, Kamio Memorial Hospital, Tokyo 101-0063, Japan
2. Department of Biochemistry, Nihon University, Tokyo 173-0032, Japan; meyu18003@g.nihon-u.ac.jp
3. Department of Otolaryngology-Head and Neck Surgery, Keio University, Tokyo 160-8582, Japan; skan@keio.jp
4. Department of Otolaryngology-Head and Neck Surgery, The University of Tokyo, Tokyo 113-8655, Japan; cfujimoto-tky@umin.ac.jp
* Correspondence: kenhayashi0811@icloud.com; Tel.: +81-3-3252-3351

Received: 29 September 2020; Accepted: 5 November 2020; Published: 11 November 2020

Abstract: The etiology of hearing impairment following cochlear damage can be caused by many factors, including congenital or acquired onset, ototoxic drugs, noise exposure, and aging. Regardless of the many different etiologies, a common pathologic change is auditory cell death. It may be difficult to explain hearing impairment only from the aspect of cell death including apoptosis, necrosis, or necroptosis because the level of hearing loss varies widely. Therefore, we focused on autophagy as an intracellular phenomenon functionally competing with cell death. Autophagy is a dynamic lysosomal degradation and recycling system in the eukaryotic cell, mandatory for controlling the balance between cell survival and cell death induced by cellular stress, and maintaining homeostasis of postmitotic cells, including hair cells (HCs) and spiral ganglion neurons (SGNs) in the inner ear. Autophagy is considered a candidate for the auditory cell fate decision factor, whereas autophagy deficiency could be one of major causes of hearing impairment. In this paper, we review the molecular mechanisms and biologic functions of autophagy in the auditory system and discuss the latest research concerning autophagy-related genes and sensorineural hearing loss to gain insight into the role of autophagic mechanisms in inner-ear disorders.

Keywords: classical degradative autophagy; genetics of hearing impairment; autophagy- and lysosomal function-related genes; congenital disorder

1. Introduction

Cells are continuously exposed to various stresses, including both extracellular oxidative stress as well as intracellular endoplasmic reticulum (ER) stress. There is a positive feed-forward loop between oxidative stress and ER stress in cells. Oxidative stress occurs when the proper balance between antioxidants and reactive oxygen species (ROS) is lost. A higher production of ROS may change DNA structure, resulting in cell death, including apoptosis, necrosis, and necroptosis or cellular senescence. ER stress activates the signaling pathway of the unfolded protein response (UPR) triggered in response to the accumulation of unfolded or misfolded proteins in the ER. In cases where ER stress cannot be reversed, cellular functions deteriorate, often leading to cell death. Various stressors can disturb the intracellular redox balance, accumulating protein aggregation, and misfolding or unfolding proteins, leading to conformational disease. Inner-ear diseases may have aspects of conformational disease. Based on this concept, considerable research has been conducted on apoptosis and antioxidants in inner-ear diseases [1–6]. However, in the case of patients with hearing loss, the hearing levels and patterns are often diverse and not permanent. As a result, it may be difficult to explain hearing loss only from the aspect of cell death, apoptosis, necroptosis, or necrosis at the cellular level. Therefore, we focused on autophagy as a cellular phenomenon functionally competing against cell death for auditory cell fate decision. The lysosomal degradation pathway of autophagy (referred to as macroautophagy) plays an important role in adaptation to cellular stress, clearance of autophagic cargo (damaged organelles, intracellular pathogens, or protein aggregates), cellular development and differentiation, and mitigation of genomic damage. Crosstalk occurs among apoptosis, necroptosis, and autophagy [7]. Since the autophagic process controls auditory cell fate, protecting against hearing impairment, autophagy-related genes could potentially hold the key to the genetics of hearing impairment. To the best of our knowledge, there is no review article describing the effects of the autophagy process on the genetics of hearing impairment and autophagy–lysosomal function-related genes for hearing impairment. In this article, the first part describes the mechanisms and biologic functions of autophagy as a decision factor in auditory cell fate and the role of autophagy in the auditory system (or hearing), while the second part focuses on the relationship between autophagy (elongation and completion steps)- and lysosomal function (fusion step)-related genes and hearing loss, congenital disorder of autophagy with hearing loss, and the effect of autophagy for genetics of hearing loss.

2. The Mechanisms and Biologic Functions of Autophagy

Autophagy plays fundamental roles in cellular homeostasis and exerts a major impact on cells as the fate decision factor under various physiological and pathologic conditions [8]. Since Professor Ohsumi won the Nobel Prize in 2016 for his seminal research on autophagy, many inner-ear researchers have placed autophagy as the central target of their research. Today, the relationship between autophagy and inner-ear disease is a hot spot in inner-ear research.

2.1. Autophagy Gene-Dependent Pathways for the Formation of Autophagosome

As shown in Figure 1, classical degradative autophagy (macroautophagy) involves the delivery of cytoplasmic cargo to the lysosome for degradation. All autophagy-related genes (*ATGs*) are required for efficiently-sealed autophagosome formation and proceeding to fusion with lysosomes. The subsequent elongation and closure of the isolation membrane (phagophore) is mediated by two ubiquitin-like *ATG* conjugation systems, *ATG5–ATG12* and *LC3* (light chain 3)-PE, in mammals. These *ATG* conjugation systems are important for driving the biogenesis of the autophagosomal membrane [9].

The ubiquitin-like protein ATG12 is conjugated to ATG5 by ATG7. ATG16L1 and ATG12–ATG5 form a complex. This ATG16L1 complex specifically localizes to the isolation membrane (phagophore) and then dissociates from it for the completion of autophagosome formation. LC3 is processed at its C terminus by Atg4 and then becomes LC3-I. LC3-I is subsequently conjugated with phosphatidylethanolamine (PE) to become LC3-II by ATG7 (E1-like) and ATG3 (E2-like) and recruited to autophagosomes, forming with the support of WD-repeat protein interacting with phosphoinositide (WIPI) proteins. LC3-II enables autophagosomes to bind p62 for ubiquitinated cargo [10].

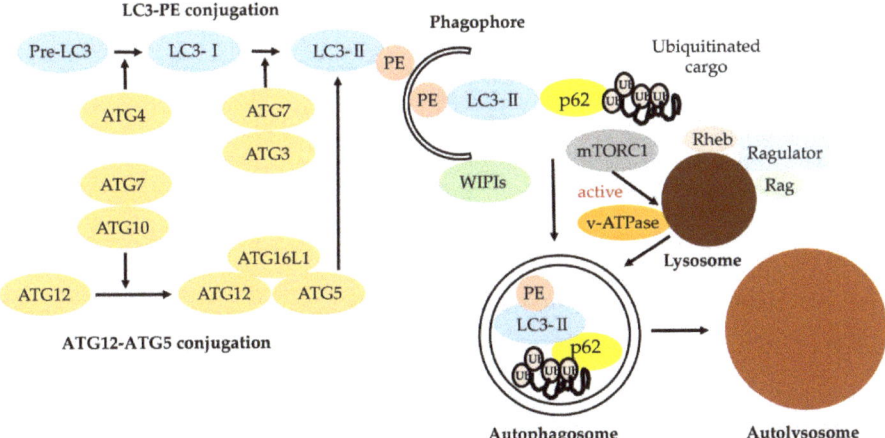

Figure 1. Classical degradative autophagy (macroautophagy). The autophagy-related gene (ATG) conjugation systems (LC3-PE and ATG12–ATG5) are important for degrading the inner autophagosomal membrane. Phagophore elongation involves two ubiquitin-like conjugation systems (LC3-PE and ATG12–ATG5 conjugation). ATG7 and ATG10 operate sequentially to catalyze the formation of ATG12–ATG5:ATG16L1 complexes. ATG4, ATG7, and ATG3 cooperate to cleave the precursors of LC3-like proteins into their mature forms, followed by conjugation to phosphatidylethanolamine (PE) and recruitment to autophagosomes forming with the support of WD-repeat protein interacting with phosphoinositide (WIPI) proteins. LC3 and LC3 homologs enable autophagosomes with the ability to bind autophagic substrates including p62 for ubiquitinated cargo [10]. The mammalian target of rapamycin (mTOR)C1 amino-acid-sensing pathway. V-ATPase triggers the guanine nucleotide exchange factor activity of Rag small GTP-binding protein in an amino-acid-dependent manner, which is followed by the recruitment of mTOR to lysosomal membranes. Upon its localization to the lysosome, mTORC1 kinase is activated by the small GTP-binding protein Rheb, which receives input from growth factor signaling. The lysosome is responsible for recycling amino acids and cellular components via degradation of proteins and other macromolecules, although acidification of the lysosomal lumen is dispensable for mTORC1 signaling.

2.2. Autophagy Regulation by Lysosome through mTORC1 and v-ATPase

The inactivation of mTORC1 (mechanistic or mammalian target of rapamycin complex1) is one of the main inducers of autophagy. Multiple cues, including cellular amino acid levels or oxidative stress, modulate mTORC1 activity. Importantly, the recruitment to the lysosomal lumen and activation of mTORC1 requires lysosomes and vacuolar H^+-ATPase (V-ATPase) (Figure 1). The V-ATPases are electrogenically-conserved proton pumps that acidify multiple intracellular organelles and extracellular compartments and are implicated as critical components of cellular signal transduction pathways including the wingless-related integration site (Wnt), Notch, and the mechanistic or mammalian target of rapamycin (mTOR) signaling. These three molecule-signaling cascades are linked to cell-growth regulation, coordinating downstream pathways involved in aging control. Due to these dependencies, complete loss of V-ATPase activity results in embryonic lethality in mammals. Partial loss is related to multiple disease states, including neurodegeneration or cancer [11]. The lysosome provides the key indication of cell metabolic state including autophagy, enhancing cellular clearance based on lysosomal mTOR-V-ATPase signaling [12,13].

3. The Role of Autophagy in Auditory System (or Hearing)

3.1. Otic Epithelium

A previous study [14] indicated that ATG5, beclin-1(ATG6), and LC3B (ATG8) are expressed during early development of the chicken inner ear, and that the otic epithelium has intense lysosomal activity and numerous autophagic vesicles, especially at neuroblast exit zones. Autophagy is an active process during early inner-ear development, providing the energy required for the generation of neuronal otic precursors via the clearing of dead neuroepithelial cells; autophagic activity is necessary for the otoconial biogenesis in inner-ear development.

3.2. Hair Cells, Spiral Ganglion Cells, and Brain Stem Nuclei

There were few reports on the relationship between autophagy and hearing loss before Professor Yoshinori Ohsumi's Nobel Prize-winning work of 2016. Since this time, the number of reports has dramatically increased. Most inner-ear research has focused on the function of autophagy as constituting an important mechanism for the recycling of cytoplasmic materials and in fine cleaning and rejuvenating extranuclear compartments, especially in non-diving cells (or postmitotic cells) as typified by neurons [15]. In the auditory pathway, hair cells (HCs) in the cochlea convert sound information into electrical signals, then carry these signals to the central nervous system (CNS) via chemical synapses on the spiral ganglion (SG) neurons dendrites [16,17]. The central afferents of these SG neurons converge to form the auditory nerve, connecting to the cochlear nuclei in the brainstem [18].

A previous study [19] confirmed the expression of the autophagy machinery genes (*BECN1, ATG4g, ATG5,* and *ATG9a*) by qRT-PCR in the E18.5 mouse cochlea and the expression of *BECN1, ATG4g* and *ATG5* in the brain-stem nuclei. Autophagy was also confirmed to be abundant in spiral ganglion neurons by the expression of LC3B. The most important aspect of this study is that inner-ear autophagy flux was revealed to be developmentally regulated and is lower at perinatal stages than in the adult mouse. Another study [20] indicated that the deletion of *ATG5* results in the degeneration of hair cells (HCs) and profound congenital hearing loss. In this study, basal autophagy flux was detected in both the inner and outer hair cells, whereas autophagosome formation was suppressed in the *ATG5*-deficient HCs. Aggregates containing ubiquitin and p62 also accumulated. This suggests that *ATG5* deficiency results in congenital profound hearing loss due to the degeneration rather than maldevelopment of auditory HCs and that *ATG5* in cochlear HCs is essential for the maintenance of the morphology of these cells and acquiring normal hearing acuity. These in vivo studies suggested that autophagy plays a crucial role in the development, maintenance of morphology, and functional maturation of the auditory system, and that abnormality of the autophagy machinery genes may cause both congenital and acquired sensorineural hearing loss.

3.3. Synapse Ribbon

Glutamatergic ribbon-type synapses (cochlear ribbon synapses) are composed of molecular machinery transducing mechano-electric components on the apical side of inner hair cells (IHCs), connecting IHCs and spiral ganglion neurons (SGNs). Although ribbon synapses are immature at birth, they mature, morphologically and functionally, between IHCs and SGNs with hearing onset during development, coordinating with SGN (type 1) myelination, spontaneous activity, and synaptic pruning. A recent study [21] indicated that autophagy plays an essential role in the development and maturation of cochlear ribbon synapses in mice. According to this report, autophagy in IHCs was highly activated in the early stage of hearing development (P1 to P15) and then decreased at P28 to P30. In contrast, deficiency of autophagy before hearing onset impaired the pruning and refinement of ribbon synapses in IHCs and the impairment of autophagy flux results in the exocytosis of cochlear IHCs in postnatal mice. They proposed that in postnatal mice, the remodeling process of ribbon synapses in cochlear IHCs during development may be mainly controlled by autophagy, and that deficiency of autophagy at the early stage of hearing development may induce auditory disorders via impairment of cochlear ribbon synapses.

3.4. Auditory Neurons

The SGNs of the cochlea transmit all auditory information to the brain. In a recent study using single-cell RNA sequencing [22], four types of SG neurons, including three novel subclasses of type I neurons (Ia, Ib, and Ic neurons) and the type II neurons that exist at birth, were identified, and a comprehensive genetic framework that constructs their potential synaptic communication patterns was provided. The authors also found that many inhibitory modulators of *TGFβ* signaling (Smad6, Smad7, Nog, Nbl1, Smad9, and Smurf2) were particularly enriched in the type II neurons, whereas all SG neurons expressed the molecules essential for activating this cascade, despite the specific role of this signaling only in type I neurons. The striking aspect here is that autophagy is a regulator of *TGFβ* [23] and links Smad signaling [24]. Autophagy should regulate the function of SG neurons (type I and II) and play a key role for the neuronal development of SG neurons. A study [25] described that the autophagy protein *ATG7* is required for membrane trafficking and turnover in the axons, and impairment of axonal autophagy as a possible mechanism for axonopathy related to neurodegeneration. A recent study indicated that the initial stages of SGN and nerve fiber degeneration in the mouse cochlear cause the impairment of autophagy flux, while restoring autophagy–lysosomal pathway disruption by the translocation of TFEB (transcription factor EB) liking autophagy to lysosomal biogenesis into nuclear via inhibiting mTOR (mammalian target of rapamycin) cascade mitigated SGN and nerve fiber degradation [26]. These results suggested that the lysosome function via TFEB in autophagy–lysosome fusion step plays an essential role for restoring SGN and nerve fiber degradation.

4. Autophagy- and Lysosomal-Function-Related Genes and Hearing Loss

4.1. Autophagy-Related Genes Essential for Autophagosome Formation

4.1.1. ATG5 Gene

As shown in Figure 1, the formation of the autophagosome requires the action of two evolutionarily-conserved ubiquitin-like conjugation systems (ATG5–ATG12 and LC3-PE), both of which require the *ATG5* gene [27,28]. *ATG5* is a key player for autophagic vesicle formation [29]. Knocking down in vitro or knocking out *ATG5* in vivo could result in downregulation or total inhibition of autophagy, suggesting that *ATG5* plays a central role in autophagy regulation. Thus, *ATG5* is one of the most commonly-targeted genes in autophagy gene-editing assays. *ATG5* also functions in the immune system, regulating innate and adaptive immune responses and is associated with autoimmune diseases, including SLE and autoinflammatory diseases, such as Crohn's disease (Table 1). Inner-ear researchers [20] indicated that deletion of autophagy-related 5 (*ATG5*) resulted in hair cell (HC) degeneration and profound congenital hearing loss, generating mice deficient in *ATG5*. They indicated that both the morphology and mechanotransduction of *ATG5*-deficient auditory HCs were normal at P5, although polyubiquitinated proteins and p62 had already accumulated. However, at P14, polyubiquitinated protein aggregates and p62 progressively accumulated in auditory HCs of mice deficient in *ATG5*, as well as HC degeneration and profound hearing loss. They concluded that the cause of hearing loss in auditory HCs in mice deficient in *ATG5* is associated with degeneration of auditory HCs rather than maldevelopment. Hence, polyubiquitinated protein aggregates and p62 accumulation may play an important role in the progression of damage.

Table 1. Characteristics of autophagy- and lysosome- related genes inducing sensorineural hearing loss.

Gene	Gene Locus	Encoding	Genetic Defects	Related Disease	Affected Process of Autophagy
Atg5	6q21	ATG protein	Deletion	Autoinflammatory disease Autoimmune disease	Autophagosome formation
miRNA96	7q32.2	DFNA50 (OMIM #613074)	Point mutations	Sensorineural hearing loss	Autophagosome formation
WDR45	Xp11.23	WD repeat protein	Uncovered mutations	BPAN	Autophagosome formation
GBA	1q21	(Lyso)glucosylceramide	Missense mutations Point mutations Deletions Insertions Splicing aberrations Various rearrangements	Gaucher disease Type 1 (GD1) Type 2 (GD2) Type 3 (GD3)	Lysosome biogenesis
GLA	Xq22.1	lysosomal α-galactosidase A	Missense mutations Nonsense mutations Splicing mutations Deletions Insertions	Fabry disease	Lysosome biogenesis
GAA	17q25.3	lysosomal α-glucosidase	Nonsense mutations Multiple exon deletion	Pompe disease	Lysosome biogenesis
NPC1	18q11.2	NPC protein	Missense mutations Point mutation Duplication mutation Splicing mutation Frame deletion	Niemann–Pick type C	Lysosome biogenesis
NPC2	14q24.3	NPC protein	Missense mutations of homozygous state	Niemann–Pick type C	Lysosome biogenesis
IDUA	4p16.3	alpha-L-iduronidase	Missense mutations Nonsense mutation Deletion	Mucopolysaccharidoses	Lysosome biogenesis

WD repeat: tryptophan-aspartic acid (WD) residues; BRAN: Beta-propeller protein-associated neurodegeneration; DDOD: Dominant deafness-onychodystrophy.

4.1.2. miRNA 96 Gene

miRNA 96 is a member of the miRNA183 family (miRNA-183, miRNA-96, and miRNA-182) that is coordinately expressed from a single genetic locus in vertebrates. In the human genome, the miRNA-183 family cluster is located on chromosome 7q32 with a 4.5 kb region, including a locus that has been linked to autosomal-dominant non-syndromic hearing loss (NSHL) (*DFNA50*, OMIM #613074). As shown in Table 1, initially, two mutations in the seed region of miRNA-96 were detected in two Spanish families with autosomal-dominant progressive NSHL. Both mutations (+13 G > A and +14 C > A) affect the nucleolar targeting signals (NTSs) that are fully conserved among vertebrates (from fish to humans) and segregated with hearing loss in the affected families [30]. The description of novel causative variants within the *miRNA96* gene may be useful for clarifying the pathogenic mechanisms underlying the DFNA50-associated phenotype. Inner-ear researchers [31] detected the +57 T > C mutation as the third mutation of the *miRNA96* gene in humans that contributes quantitative defects in miRNA-96 related to the pathogenesis of sensorineural hearing loss, independent from additional qualitative defects (i.e., changes in the actual mature miRNA-96 sequence). The family carrying the +57 T > C mutation on hearing is characterized by late onset (between 25 and 40 years) and a slow progression of hearing impairment. Researchers indicated that autophagy is modulated dose-dependently by *miRNA96* through regulation of *mTOR* and *ATG7* required for the efficient formation of autophagosomes and suggested that the inhibition of mTOR by upregulation of *miRNA-96* may promote autophagy in prostate cancer, which is involved in maintaining a dynamic balance of *miRNA 96* in hypoxia [32]. Mutations of miRNA96 could make autophagy impaired through the activation of *mTOR* and the downregulation of *ATG7* in the cochlea, leading to sensorineural hearing loss.

4.2. Lysosomal-Function-Related Genes Essential for the Autophagy–Lysosome Pathway

The autophagy–lysosome pathway is an important mechanism for regulating the homeostasis of intracellular long-lived proteins and organelles [33,34]. Lysosomes release metabolites and ions that serve as a signaling hub for metabolic sensing and longevity, linking the functions of the lysosome to various pathways for intracellular metabolism and nutrient homeostasis [35]. The intraluminal pH of the lysosome is usually sustained in the low acidic range (4.2–5.3) for regulating many functions of lysosomes with the vacuolar-type ATPase (V-ATPase) acting as an ATP-dependent proton pump [36].

Based on these physiological characteristics, V-ATPases has been found to be deeply involved in the initiation of deafness [37]. In particular, dominant deafness-onychodystrophy (DDOD) syndrome caused by de novo mutation c.1516 C > N (p.Arg506X) in ATP6V1B2 is a rare disorder with chief complaints of severe deafness, onychodystrophy, and brachydactyly (Table 1) [38]. This group's latest research [39] indicated four interesting results: (1) atp6v1b2 knockdown zebrafish had developmental defects in multiple organs and systems; (2) Atp6v1b2 c.1516 C > N knock-in mice led to cognitive disorders, based on the impaired hippocampal CA1 region from the pathology; (3) the normal hearing thresholds of Atp6v1b2 c.1516 C > N in 24-week-old knock-in mice, suggested that a compensation mechanism exists in the auditory system; and (4) V-ATPases assembly still occurred in Atp6v1b2 c.1516 C > N. However, the interaction between the E and B2 subunits was weaker than in the wild type (WT). They confirmed that the defectiveness of Atp6v1b2 leads to CNS impairments and extends the phenotype range of DDOD syndrome. ATP6V1B2 encodes the B2 subunit in V-ATPases, a multisubunit protein complex consisting of a soluble V1 subcomplex (responsible for hydrolyzing ATP) and a membrane-bound V0 subcomplex (involved in H+ translocation) expressed in almost all eukaryotes. Mutations in this gene theoretically result in lysosomal dysfunction or lysosomal damage. Consequently, autophagy dysfunction is caused by suppressing the degradation of autophagosomes in lysosomes, finally leading to cell death or aging. After this, these situations lead to distal renal tubular acidosis (dRTA, MIM: 602722), a rare disease characterized by metabolic acidosis and sensorineural hearing loss [40]. A recent genome-wide association study suggested that the ATP6V1B2 rs1106634 A allele increases the lifetime risk of depression and hippocampal cognitive deficits [41]. An abnormal rise in lysosomal pH, therefore, can have far-ranging effects on lysosomal digestion, strongly inhibiting hydrolases with the most acidic pH optima, but also potentially elevating activities of other hydrolases with pH optima closer to neutral. New reports implicate altered V-ATPase activity and lysosomal pH dysregulation in cellular aging [42], longevity [43], and adult-onset neurodegenerative diseases, including forms of Parkinson's disease and Alzheimer's disease [44]. Hence, the gene analysis of V-ATPase in the auditory–brain pathway may be a key to resolving the relationship between hearing loss and cognitive dysfunction.

Lysosomal storage diseases (LSDs) are inherited metabolic disorders caused by defects in lysosomal proteins or lysosomal-related proteins, which lead to lysosomal dysfunction resulting in accumulation of undegraded substrate. LSD-associated genes encode different lysosomal proteins, including lysosomal enzymes and lysosomal membrane proteins [45]. Mutations in genes encoding lysosomal hydrolases, accessory proteins, membrane transport, or trafficking proteins may cause LSDs in vivo. LSDs are inherited in an autosomal recessive or, in some types, in an X-linked manner. As listed in Table 1, hearing loss has been found in several LSDs including Gaucher disease (caused by more than 400 mutations in the *GBA* gene (locus 1q21), encoding for the lysoglucosylceramide-degrading enzyme β-glucocerebrosidase (EC 3.2.1.45)) [46], Fabry disease (X-linked glycosphingolipidosis caused by deficiency of the lysosomal α-galactosidase A (EC 3.2.1.22), encoded by the *GLA* gene (Xq22.1)) [47],

Pompe disease (a deficiency in the lysosomal α-glucosidase (EC 3.2.1.3) encoded by the *GAA* gene (17q25.3)) [48], Niemann–Pick type C (NPC) (mutations in *NPC1* (18q11.2) and *NPC2* (14q24.3) genes, intralysosomal cholesterol, and sphingolipid accumulation) [49], and mucopolysaccharidoses (mutations in the *IDUA* gene providing instructions for producing an enzyme (α-L-iduronidase), which is involved in the breakdown of glycosaminoglycans (GAGs)) [50]. LSDs are caused by disruptions in the lysosomal network and intralysosomal accumulation of substrates in certain cell types. However, many aspects of the molecular pathology of the cochlea due to LSDs remain unclear. According to the recent study [51], it will be interesting to shed light on whether the endosomal sorting complex required for transport (ESCRT)-dependent membrane sealing is involved in mammalian LSDs caused by different genetic defects and whether lysophagy—one of selective autophagy and ESCRT repair—acts in concert during the development of lysosomal storage [52].

5. Congenital Disorder of Autophagy with Hearing Loss

β-Propeller Protein-Associated Neurodegeneration (BPAN): Mutations in the WDR45 Gene

Some congenital disorders of autophagy with an emerging phenotype of inborn errors of metabolism involve hearing impairment as one of the associated symptoms (Table 1) [53]. Recently, two groups independently reported mutations in the *WDR45* gene as the genetic cause of β-propeller protein-associated neurodegeneration (BPAN), a disease that had been previously labeled using the term 'static encephalopathy of childhood with neurodegeneration in adulthood (SENDA) syndrome' [54]. This disease is characterized by the onset of dystonia, Parkinsonism, and progressive cognitive decline with visual and auditory disabilities in early adulthood or adolescence. *WDR45*, also known as *WIPI4*, is located on the X-chromosome and is one of the four mammalian homologs of the core autophagy gene *epg-6* in *Caenorhabditis elegans* [55]. *WDR45* encodes a WD repeat protein, a superfamily of proteins with a conserved core of 40 amino acids terminating in tryptophan–aspartic acid (WD) residues. WD40 proteins fold into similar β-propeller structures that function as protein–protein autophagy or protein–DNA interaction platforms and mediate molecular signaling cascades mainly through the smaller top surface [56]. Based on these properties, WD-repeat proteins consist of components with many essential biologic functions and pathways including autophagy. Importantly, *WDR45*, the WD-repeat protein mutated in BPAN, interacts with autophagy-related proteins *ATG2* and *ATG9* to regulate crucial steps for autophagosome formation and elongation [57]. Therefore, depletion of *WDR45* in mammalian cells could lead to the accumulation of early autophagic vesicles or immature autophagosomes [58]. According to a recent report [59], conditional CNS-specific *WDR45* knockout mice (Nes-WDR45fl/Y) show swollen axons and accumulation of autophagy substrates p62 and ubiquitin as the characteristics of axonal pathology. Neither neurodegeneration nor iron deposition are prominent phenotypes. However, at the behavioral level, Nes-WDR45fl/Y mice displayed subtle deficits of coordinated motor skills, poor memory, and learning impairment. These situations indicated deficits in neuronal circuit formation or neurotransmission. Another aspect of the pathogenesis of BPAN should be the role of autophagy in iron metabolism, which is called ferritinophagy as selective autophagy. The bioavailability of intracellular iron is critically regulated by the delivery of ferritin to autophagosomes and the degradation in lysosomes, allowing release of iron into the cytoplasm [60,61]. These recent studies showed that hearing impairment in BPAN may be related to the accumulation of p62 and ubiquitin in neural cells of central auditory pathway or ferritinophagy impairment.

6. The Effect of Autophagy for Genetics of Hearing Loss

6.1. Genetics of Sensorineural Hearing Loss (DFNA5 and DFNB59) and Autophagy

DFNA5 was first identified in a Dutch family as a gene causing autosomal dominant hearing loss (HL). In almost all cases, the *DFNA5* mRNA transcript skips exon 8, leading to a frameshift and a premature truncation of the protein [62]. DFNA5-associated HL is characterized by non-syndromic HL with no other symptoms. A recent study [63] indicated that gasdermin-E (GSDME), which was originally identified as *DFNA5* (deafness gene, autosomal dominant 5) [64], could transform caspase-3-mediated apoptosis induced by chemotherapy drugs, etc., into pyroptosis, an inflammatory form of programmed cell death. GSDME was specifically cleaved by caspase-3-mediating cleavage of autophagy-associated protein beclin-1, inactivating autophagy and promoting apoptosis. Beclin-1 is a dual regulator for both autophagy and apoptosis and a substrate of caspase-3 with two cleavage sites at positions 124 and 149 [65]. The N-terminal domain of GSDME, as the functional characteristic, displays an apoptosis-inducing activity while the C-terminal domain functions as an apoptosis-inhibiting regulator by shielding the N-terminal domain [66]. A specific form of autosomal dominant progressive sensorineural hearing loss due to DFNA5 may cause the disruption of balance among apoptosis, pyroptosis, and autophagy in sensory hair cells.

DFNB59 was the first reported human gene leading to nonsyndromic deafness due to neuronal defect through the auditory pathway neurons [67]. Nonsense mutations in the *PJVK* gene encoding protein PJVK, which is present in hair cells supporting cells and spiral ganglion cells, resulted in autosomal recessive nonsyndromic deafness in humans at the DFNB59 locus on chromosome 2q31.2 [68,69]. A recent study indicated that the *DFNB59* form of deafness is a pexophagy disorder [70]. Pexophagy means that peroxisomes are degraded by lysosomes through autophagic pathways as a selective autophagy (Figure 2) [71]. Peroxisome membrane proteins are ubiquitinated by PEX2, the E3 ubiquitin ligase, for inducing pexophagy. Ubiquitinated peroxisome membrane proteins are removed from peroxisomes by the AAA-type ATPase PEX1–PEX6–PEX26 and the deubiquitinase USP30 for preventing pexophagy. The expression of PEX3 on peroxisome membranes also increases for inducing pexophagy. Ubiquitinated peroxisomes are bound to autophagosomes through interacting with the autophagic adapter proteins (cargo receptors), NBR1 and p62, and facilitating its binding to LC3-II. Peroxisomes are also sequestered into autophagosomes when PEX14 interacts with LC3-II rather than PEX5. Peroxisomes are dynamic organelles whose metabolism, size, abundance, and phenotype can change in response to alterations in nutritional and other environmental conditions. Peroxisomes are routinely turned over by pexophagy for the quality control of organelles, referred to as peroxisome dynamics, for several processes of peroxisome biogenesis. *PJVK* also has another function—triggering pyroptosis when pexophagy is induced by oxidative stress [72–75]. DFNB59 could play an essential role in oxidative-stress-induced peroxisome biogenesis and pexophagy in auditory hair cells [70]. Hence, autosomal-recessive non-syndromic hearing loss caused by *DFNB59* mutations may be affected by the impairment of pexophagy in sensory hair cells in terms of progressive hearing loss.

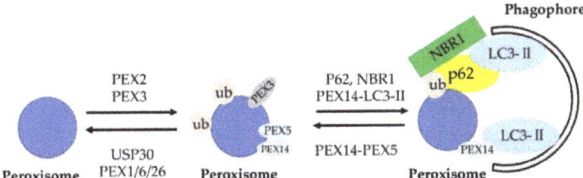

Figure 2. Schematic of molecular mechanisms of pexophagy. Peroxisome membrane proteins are ubiquitinated by the E3 ubiquitin ligase, *PEX2*, to designate peroxisomes for pexophagy. Opposing the action of PEX2 on peroxisomes is the deubiquitinating enzyme USP30. Ubiquitinated peroxisome membrane proteins are removed from peroxisomes by the AAA-type ATPase (*PEX1–PEX6–PEX26*) and the deubiquitinase USP30 to prevent pexophagy. Increasing the expression of *PEX3* on peroxisome membranes may also designate them for pexophagy. Ubiquitinated peroxisomes are targeted to autophagosomes through interactions with the autophagy receptors NBR1 and p62, which facilitate sequestration within autophagosomes through binding with LC3-II. Peroxisomes are also targeted and sequestered within autophagosomes when LC3-II out-competes *PEX5* for binding to *PEX14*. Import-competent peroxisomes deter pexophagy through *PEX14–PEX5*-binding, whereas import-incompetency frees *PEX14* allowing it to bind LC3-II and facilitate pexophagy [71].

6.2. Presbycusis Accelerated by Connexin 26 Partial Loss and Autophagy through Nrf2/Keap1 Pathway

Mutations in the gap junction protein β-2 (*GJB2*) gene encoding connexin 26 (*Cx26*) are the most common cause of sensorineural hearing impairment [76–79]. In several populations, the truncating variant 35delG involved in the prevalent *GJB2* mutation results in a complete loss of function of *Cx26* protein whose structure has been solved with a 3.5 Å resolution. A recent study indicated that the partial loss of *Cx26* results in accelerated presbycusis (age-related hearing loss (ARHL)) caused by redox imbalance and dysregulation of the nuclear factor (erythroid-derived-2)-like 2 (Nrf2) pathway [80]. It was confirmed that the hearing level more rapidly worsened in *Gjb2+/−* mice than control mice using auditory brainstem responses (ABRs) and distortion product otoacoustic emission (DPOAE) thresholds. Levels of oxidative stress increased in the cochlear duct of the auditory phenotype of *Gjb2+/−* mice and, as a result, apoptosis was induced, the release of glutathione from connexin hemichannels was reduced, nutrient delivery to the sensory epithelium via cochlear gap junctions was decreased, and the expression of target genes of Nrf2 was deregulated. Conversely, *Gjb2−/−* mice failed to express acquired deafness although levels of oxidative stress increased in the cochlea [81]. This research group also indicated that two NRF2 target genes (*PRKCE* and *TGFβ1*) (p-value $< 4 \times 10^{-2}$) were detected in a large cohort of 4091 individuals with hearing phenotype (including 1076 presbycusis patients and 1290 healthy matched controls from Europe, Caucasus, and Central Asia) by a genome-wide association study. In this study, the authors suggested from the both basic research and clinical study that: (1) it is important for hearing maintenance to normally run the Nrf2 pathway and (2) dysfunction of the Nrf2 pathway may result in human presbycusis. As shown in Figure 3, Nrf2 is a transcription factor in response to gene expression of antioxidant proteins [82]. The common Nrf2-binding motif known as the antioxidant response element (ARE) should be activated for inducing Nrf2 target genes [83]. In auditory cells under oxidative stress, an autophagic pathway is maintained by a Kelch-like ECH-associated protein 1 (Keap1)–Nrf2 feedback loop through p62, a protein encoded by the sequestosome 1 gene (SQSTM1) [84]. Kelch-like ECH-associated protein 1 (Keap1) is an adaptor protein of cullin-3-based ubiquitin ligase. The N-terminally lying Neh2 domain of Nrf2 contains two Keap1-binding motifs, DLG and ETGE. Interactions between these two binding motifs and Keap1 compose a key regulatory site for Nrf2 activity through the formation of a two-site-binding hinge-and-latch mechanism, although this two-site binding is necessary for ubiquitinated Nrf2 [85,86]. ETGE tightly binds to Keap1, whereas DLGex binds more weakly than ETGE. Here, this binding plays a role as a fine-tuner of the ubiquitination of Nrf2 [87]. Nrf2-repressor function was lost by chemical modification of specific cysteine sensors of KEAP1 by oxidative stressor, and then Nrf2 was released from the Keap1 interaction and translocated into the nucleus to induce the expression of Nrf2-target gene [88,89]. The Keap1–Nrf2 system functions as a major oxidative stress response pathway in auditory cells. *p62/SQSTM1* is a stress-inducible protein with multifunctional domains including an LC3-interacting region (LIR), a Keap1-interacting region (KIR), and a ubiquitin-associated (UBA) domain [90], regulating the activation and stabilization of Nrf2 by inhibiting the ability of Keap1 to hold Nrf2. It also functions as an adaptor protein between selective autophagy and ubiquitin signaling [91,92]. This means that the Keap1–Nrf2 pathway and selective autophagy could be mediated by *p62/SQSTM1*. Taken together, p62-mediated selective autophagy may regulate presbycusis accelerated by *Cx26* partial loss through Nrf2/Keap1 pathway in cochlea.

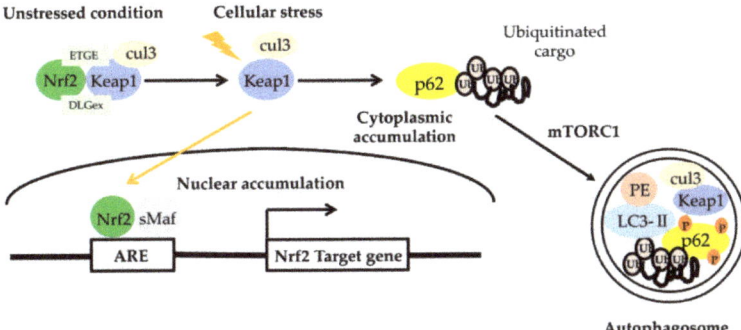

Figure 3. The role of the p62– Kelch-like ECH-associated protein 1 (Keap1)–nuclear factor (erythroid-derived-2)-like 2 (Nrf2) axis. Upon selective autophagy, oligomerized p62 undergoes phosphorylation at Ser residues (S407, S403) (shown as 'P') and increases the binding affinity of p62 to ubiquitin, followed by sequestration of polyubiquitinated cargos. Then, mTORC1 phosphorylates S349 of p62 and increases the binding affinity of p62 to Keap1, resulting in the escape of Nrf2 from the Keap1 interaction. Free Nrf2 enables the activation of various target genes. Keap1 is degraded together with the polyubiquitinated cargo-binding to p62 into autophagosome. ARE, antioxidant response element [82].

7. Conclusions

In this review article, we summarized the effects of the autophagy process on the genetics of hearing impairment and autophagy–lysosomal function-related genes for hearing impairment (Figure 4). Sensorineural hearing loss (SNHL) may be caused by both environmental and hereditary factors. Approximately 60% of cases are due to genetics. We described how three important deafness genes (*DFNA5, DFNA59* and *connexin26*) linked with autophagy are sensitive to oxidative stress, inducing SNHL, or age-related hearing loss (ARHL), and that autophagy deficiency caused by autophagy- and lysosomal-function-related genes can induce hearing impairment. Taken together, autophagy may play crucial roles in the genetics of hearing loss. However, this remains speculative, as few genes related to the autophagy process as a gene-causing autosomal dominant hearing loss have been detected to date. Exploring genes related to the autophagy–lysosome pathway will provide new insight into the genetics of hearing impairment in the near future. In conclusion, investigating the autophagy–lysosomal-function-related genes will open new doors for the therapeutic targets of sensorineural hearing loss. Furthermore, we hope that in the near future, new investigations into the genetic variants of autophagy- and lysosomal-function-related genes will be conducted based on the American College of Medical Genetics (ACMG) guidelines.

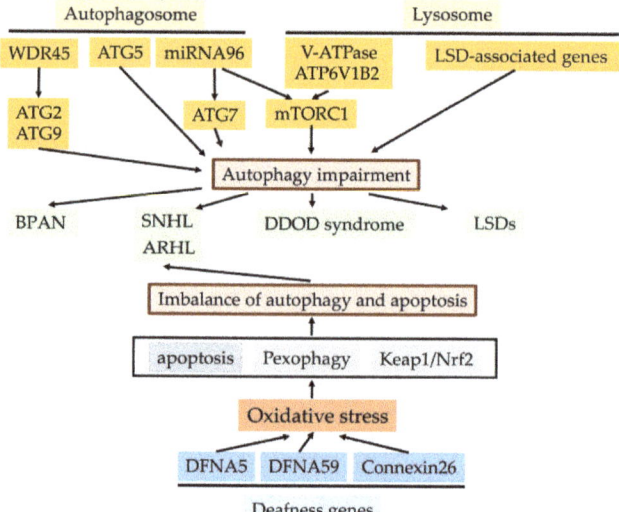

Figure 4. The effects of the autophagy process for genetics of hearing impairment and autophagy- and lysosomal-function-related genes for hearing impairment. Genetic-defect-linked autophagy- and lysosomal-related genes, including mutation or deletion result in sensorineural hearing loss or hereditary disorders with sensorineural hearing loss (BRAN, DDOD syndrome, and LSDs). Mutations of three deafness genes (DFNA5, DFNA59, and connexin26) linked with autophagy induce oxidative stress in the cochlea and the resulting imbalance of autophagy and apoptosis in sensory hair cells due to depressed pexophagy or Keap1/Nrf2, causing the progression of SNHL or ARHL (Cx26 partial loss). BRAN, β-propeller protein-associated neurodegeneration; SNHL, sensorineural hearing loss; ARHL, age-related hearing loss; DDOD syndrome, dominant deafness–onychodystrophy; LSDS, lysosomal storage diseases.

Author Contributions: Conceptualization, K.H., Y.S., C.F., and S.K.; writing—original draft preparation, K.H.; writing—review and editing, K.H., Y.S., C.F., and S.K.; supervision, C.F. and S.K.; project administration, K.H.; funding acquisition, K.H. All authors have read and agree to the published version of the manuscript.

Funding: This research was funded by Japan Society for the Promotion of Science (JSPS) KAKENHI, Grant Number 19K09899 for K.H.

Conflicts of Interest: The authors declare no conflict of interest.

References

1. Fujimoto, C.; Yamasoba, T. Mitochondria-Targeted Antioxidants for Treatment of Hearing Loss: A Systematic Review. *Antioxidants* **2019**, *8*, 109. [CrossRef]
2. Wong, A.C.; Ryan, A.F. Mechanisms of sensorineural cell damage, death and survival in the cochlea. *Front. Aging Neurosci.* **2015**, *7*, 58. [CrossRef]
3. Morrill, S.; He, D.Z.Z. Apoptosis in inner ear sensory hair cells. *J. Otol.* **2017**, *12*, 151–164. [CrossRef]
4. Dirain, C.O.; Vasquez, T.K.; Antonelli, P.J. Prevention of Chlorhexidine Ototoxicity with Poloxamer in Rats. *Otol. Neurotol.* **2018**, *39*, e738–e742. [CrossRef]
5. Jadidian, A.; Antonelli, P.J.; Ojano-Dirain, C.P. Evaluation of apoptotic markers in HEI-OC1 cells treated with gentamicin with and without the mitochondria-targeted antioxidant mitoquinone. *Otol. Neurotol.* **2015**, *36*, 526–530. [CrossRef] [PubMed]
6. Jankauskas, S.S.; Plotnikov, E.Y.; Morosanova, M.A.; Pevzner, I.B.; Zorova, L.D.; Skulachev, V.P.; Zorov, D.B. Mitochondria-targeted antioxidant SkQR1 ameliorates gentamycin-induced renal failure and hearing loss. *Biochemistry* **2012**, *77*, 66–70. [CrossRef] [PubMed]

7. Ouyang, L.; Shi, Z.; Zhao, S.; Wang, F.T.; Zhou, T.T.; Liu, B.; Bao, J.K. Programmed cell death pathways in cancer: A review of apoptosis, autophagy and programmed necrosis. *Cell Prolif.* **2012**, *45*, 487–498. [CrossRef] [PubMed]
8. Choi, A.M.; Ryter, S.W.; Levine, B. Autophagy in human health and disease. *N. Engl. J. Med.* **2013**, *368*, 651–662. [CrossRef] [PubMed]
9. Tsuboyama, K.; Koyama-Honda, I.; Sakamaki, Y.; Koike, M.; Morishita, H.; Mizushima, N. The ATG conjugation systems are important for degradation of the inner autophagosomal membrane. *Science* **2016**, *354*, 1036–1041. [CrossRef] [PubMed]
10. Galluzzi, L.; Green, D.R. Autophagy-Independent Functions of the Autophagy Machinery. *Cell* **2019**, *177*, 1682–1699. [CrossRef]
11. Sun-Wada, G.H.; Wada, Y. Role of vacuolar-type proton ATPase in signal transduction. *Biochim. Biophys. Acta* **2015**, *1847*, 1166–1172. [CrossRef] [PubMed]
12. Zoncu, R.; Bar-Peled, L.; Efeyan, A.; Wang, S.; Sancak, Y.; Sabatini, D.M. mTORC1 senses lysosomal amino acids through an inside-out mechanism that requires the vacuolar H(+)-ATPase. *Science* **2011**, *334*, 678–683. [CrossRef] [PubMed]
13. Abu-Remaileh, M.; Wyant, G.A.; Kim, C.; Laqtom, N.N.; Abbasi, M.; Chan, S.H.; Freinkman, E.; Sabatini, D.M. Lysosomal metabolomics reveals V-ATPase- and mTOR-dependent regulation of amino acid efflux from lysosomes. *Science* **2017**, *358*, 807–813. [CrossRef] [PubMed]
14. Aburto, M.R.; Sánchez-Calderón, H.; Hurlé, J.M.; Varela-Nieto, I.; Magariños, M. Early otic development depends on autophagy for apoptotic cell clearance and neural differentiation. *Cell Death Dis.* **2012**, *3*, e394. [CrossRef] [PubMed]
15. Maiuri, M.; Kroemer, G. Autophagy in stress and disease. *Cell Death Differ.* **2015**, *22*, 365–366. [CrossRef] [PubMed]
16. Nayagam, B.A.; Muniak, M.A.; Ryugo, D.K. The spiral ganglion: Connecting the peripheral and central auditory systems. *Hear. Res.* **2011**, *278*, 2–20. [CrossRef]
17. Reijntjes, D.O.J.; Pyott, S.J. The afferent signaling complex: Regulation of type I spiral ganglion neuron responses in the auditory periphery. *Hear. Res.* **2016**, *336*, 1–16. [CrossRef]
18. MacLeod, K.M.; Carr, C.E. Beyond timing in the auditory brainstem: Intensity coding in the avian cochlear nucleus angularis. *Prog. Brain Res.* **2007**, *165*, 123–133.
19. de Iriarte Rodríguez, R.; Pulido, S.; Rodríguez-de la Rosa, L.; Magariños, M.; Varela-Nieto, I. Age-regulated function of autophagy in the mouse inner ear. *Hear. Res.* **2015**, *330*, 39–50. [CrossRef]
20. Fujimoto, C.; Iwasaki, S.; Urata, S.; Morishita, H.; Sakamaki, Y.; Fujioka, M.; Kondo, K.; Mizushima, N.; Yamasoba, T. Autophagy is essential for hearing in mice. *Cell Death Dis.* **2017**, *8*, 2780. [CrossRef]
21. Xiong, W.; Wei, W.; Qi, Y.; Du, Z.; Qu, T.; Liu, K.; Gong, S. Autophagy is Required for Remodeling in Postnatal Developing Ribbon Synapses of Cochlear Inner Hair Cells. *Neuroscience* **2020**, *431*, 1–16. [CrossRef] [PubMed]
22. Petitpré, C.; Wu, H.; Sharma, A.; Tokarska, A.; Fontanet, P.; Wang, Y.; Helmbacher, F.; Yackle, K.; Silberberg, G.; Hadjab, S.; et al. Neuronal heterogeneity and stereotyped connectivity in the auditory afferent system. *Nat. Commun.* **2018**, *9*, 3691. [CrossRef] [PubMed]
23. Ghavami, S.; Cunnington, R.H.; Gupta, S.; Yeganeh, B.; Filomeno, K.L.; Freed, D.H.; Chen, S.; Klonisch, T.; Halayko, A.J.; Ambrose, E.; et al. Autophagy is a regulator of TGF-β1-induced fibrogenesis in primary human atrial myofibroblasts. *Cell Death Dis.* **2015**, *6*, e1696. [CrossRef]
24. Pang, M.; Wang, H.; Rao, P.; Zhao, Y.; Xie, J.; Cao, Q.; Wang, Y.; Wang, Y.M.; Lee, V.W.; Alexander, S.I.; et al. Autophagy links β-catenin and Smad signaling to promote epithelial-mesenchymal transition via upregulation of integrin linked kinase. *Int. J. Biochem. Cell Biol.* **2016**, *76*, 123–134. [CrossRef]
25. Komatsu, M.; Wang, Q.J.; Holstein, G.R.; Friedrich, V.L., Jr.; Iwata, J.; Kominami, E.; Chait, B.T.; Tanaka, K.; Yue, Z. Essential role for autophagy protein Atg7 in the maintenance of axonal homeostasis and the prevention of axonal degeneration. *Proc. Natl. Acad. Sci. USA* **2007**, *104*, 14489–14494. [CrossRef]
26. Ye, B.; Wang, Q.; Hu, H.; Shen, Y.; Fan, C.; Chen, P.; Ma, Y.; Wu, H.; Xiang, M. Restoring autophagic flux attenuates cochlear spiral ganglion neuron degeneration by promoting TFEB nuclear translocation via inhibiting MTOR. *Autophagy* **2019**, *15*, 998–1016. [CrossRef]
27. Mizushima, N.; Yamamoto, A.; Hatano, M.; Kobayashi, Y.; Kabeya, Y.; Suzuki, K.; Tokuhisa, T.; Ohsumi, Y.; Yoshimori, T. Dissection of autophagosome formation using Apg5-deficient mouse embryonic stem cells. *J. Cell. Biol.* **2001**, *152*, 657–668. [CrossRef]

28. Mizushima, N.; Ohsumi, Y.; Yoshimori, T. Autophagosome formation in mammalian cells. *Cell Struct. Funct.* **2002**, *27*, 421–429. [CrossRef]
29. Ye, X.; Zhou, X.J.; Zhang, H. Exploring the Role of Autophagy-Related Gene 5 (ATG5) Yields Important Insights Into Autophagy in Autoimmune/Autoinflammatory Diseases. *Front. Immunol.* **2018**, *9*, 2334. [CrossRef]
30. Mencía, A.; Modamio-Høybjør, S.; Redshaw, N.; Morín, M.; Mayo-Merino, F.; Olavarrieta, L.; Aguirre, L.A.; del Castillo, I.; Steel, K.P.; Dalmay, T.; et al. Mutations in the seed region of human miR-96 are responsible for nonsyndromic progressive hearing loss. *Nat. Genet.* **2009**, *41*, 609–613.
31. Soldà, G.; Robusto, M.; Primignani, P.; Castorina, P.; Benzoni, E.; Cesarani, A.; Ambrosetti, U.; Asselta, R.; Duga, S. A novel mutation within the MIR96 gene causes non-syndromic inherited hearing loss in an Italian family by altering pre-miRNA processing. *Hum. Mol. Genet.* **2012**, *21*, 577–585. [CrossRef] [PubMed]
32. Ma, Y.; Yang, H.Z.; Dong, B.J.; Zou, H.B.; Zhou, Y.; Kong, X.M.; Huang, Y.R. Biphasic regulation of autophagy by miR-96 in prostate cancer cells under hypoxia. *Oncotarget* **2014**, *5*, 9169–9182. [CrossRef] [PubMed]
33. de Duve, C. The lysosome turns fifty. *Nat. Cell. Biol.* **2005**, *7*, 847–849. [CrossRef] [PubMed]
34. Shintani, T.; Klionsky, D.J. Autophagy in health and disease: A double-edged sword. *Science* **2004**, *306*, 990–995. [CrossRef] [PubMed]
35. Colacurcio, D.J.; Nixon, R.A. Disorders of lysosomal acidification-The emerging role of v-ATPase in aging and neurodegenerative disease. *Ageing Res. Rev.* **2016**, *32*, 75–88. [CrossRef]
36. Mindell, J.A. Lysosomal acidification mechanisms. *Annu. Rev. Physiol.* **2012**, *74*, 69–86. [CrossRef]
37. Escobar, L.I.; Simian, C.; Treard, C.; Hayek, D.; Salvador, C.; Guerra, N.; Matos, M.; Medeiros, M.; Enciso, S.; Camargo, M.D.; et al. Mutations in ATP6V1B1 and ATP6V0A4 genes cause recessive distal renal tubular acidosis in Mexican families. *Mol. Genet. Genom. Med.* **2016**, *4*, 303–311. [CrossRef]
38. Menendez, I.; Carranza, C.; Herrera, M.; Marroquin, N.; Foster, J., 2nd; Cengiz, F.B.; Bademci, G.; Tekin, M. Dominant deafness-onychodystrophy syndrome caused by an ATP6V1B2mutation. *Clin. Case Rep.* **2017**, *5*, 376–379. [CrossRef]
39. Zhao, W.; Gao, X.; Qiu, S.; Gao, B.; Gao, S.; Zhang, X.; Kang, D.; Han, W.; Dai, P.; Yuan, Y. A subunit of V-ATPases, ATP6V1B2, underlies the pathology of intellectual disability. *Ebiomedicine* **2019**, *45*, 408–421. [CrossRef]
40. Palazzo, V.; Provenzano, A.; Becherucci, F.; Sansavini, G.; Mazzinghi, B.; Orlandini, V.; Giunti, L.; Roperto, R.M.; Pantaleo, M.; Artuso, R.; et al. The genetic and clinical spectrum of a large cohort of patients with distalrenal tubular acidosis. *Kidney Int.* **2017**, *91*, 1243–1255. [CrossRef]
41. Gonda, X.; Eszlari, N.; Anderson, I.M.; Deakin, J.F.; Bagdy, G.; Juhasz, G. Association of ATP6V1B2 rs1106634 with lifetime risk of depression and hippocampal neurocognitive deficits: Possible novel mechanisms in the etiopathology of depression. *Transl. Psychiatry* **2016**, *6*, e945. [CrossRef] [PubMed]
42. Hughes, A.L.; Gottschling, D.E. An early age increase in vacuolar pH limits mitochondrial function and lifespan in yeast. *Nature* **2012**, *492*, 261–265. [CrossRef] [PubMed]
43. Molin, M.; Demir, A.B. Linking Peroxiredoxin and Vacuolar-ATPase Functions in Calorie Restriction-Mediated Life Span Extension. *Int. J. Cell Biol.* **2014**, *2014*, 913071. [CrossRef] [PubMed]
44. Dubos, A.; Castells-Nobau, A.; Meziane, H.; Oortveld, M.A.; Houbaert, X.; Iacono, G.; Martin, C.; Mittelhaeuser, C.; Lalanne, V.; Kramer, J.M.; et al. Conditional depletion of intellectual disability and Parkinsonism candidate gene ATP6AP2 in fly and mouse induces cognitive impairment and neurodegeneration. *Mol. Genet.* **2015**, *24*, 6736–6755. [CrossRef] [PubMed]
45. Ferreira, C.R.; Gahl, W.A. Lysosomal storage diseases. *Tranlational Sci. Rare Dis.* **2017**, *2*, 1–71. [CrossRef] [PubMed]
46. Bamiou, D.E.; Campbell, P.; Liasis, A.; Page, J.; Sirimanna, T.; Boyd, S.; Vellodi, A.; Harris, C. Audiometric abnormalities in children with Gaucher disease type 3. *Neuropediatry* **2001**, *32*, 136–141. [CrossRef] [PubMed]
47. Keilmann, A.; Hajioff, D.; Ramaswami, U. FOS Investigators. Ear symptoms in children with Fabry disease: Data from the Fabry Outcome Survey. *J. Inherit. Metab Dis.* **2009**, *32*, 739. [CrossRef] [PubMed]
48. van Capelle, C.I.; Goedegebure, A.; Homans, N.C.; Hoeve, H.L.; Reuser, A.J.; van der Ploeg, A.T. Hearing loss in Pompe disease revisited: Results from a study of 24 children. *J. Inherit. Metab. Dis.* **2010**, *33*, 597–602. [CrossRef] [PubMed]
49. King, K.A.; Gordon-Salant, S.; Yanjanin, N.; Zalewski, C.; Houser, A.; Porter, F.D.; Brewer, C.C. Auditory phenotype of Niemann-Pick disease, type C1. *Ear Hear.* **2014**, *35*, 110–117. [CrossRef] [PubMed]

50. Schachern, P.A.; Cureoglu, S.; Tsuprun, V.; Paparella, M.M.; Whitley, C.B. Age-related functional and histopathological changes of the ear in the MPS I mouse. *Int. J. Pediatr. Otorhinolaryngol.* **2007**, *71*, 197–203. [CrossRef] [PubMed]
51. Skowyra, M.L.; Schlesinger, P.H.; Naismith, T.V.; Hanson, P.I. Triggered recruitment of ESCRT machinery promotes endolysosomal repair. *Science* **2018**, *360*, 6384. [CrossRef] [PubMed]
52. Marques, A.R.A.; Saftig, P. Lysosomal storage disorders—Challenges, concepts and avenues for therapy: Beyond rare diseases. *J. Cell Sci.* **2019**, *132*, 1–14. [CrossRef] [PubMed]
53. Ebrahimi-Fakhari, D.; Saffari, A.; Wahlster, L.; Lu, J.; Byrne, S.; Hoffmann, G.F.; Jungbluth, H.; Sahin, M. Congenital disorders of autophagy: An emerging novel class of inborn errors of neuro-metabolism. *Brain* **2016**, *139*, 317–337. [CrossRef] [PubMed]
54. Haack, T.B.; Hogarth, P.; Kruer, M.C.; Gregory, A.; Wieland, T.; Schwarzmayr, T. Exome sequencing reveals de novo WDR45 mutations causing a phenotypically distinct, X-linked dominant form of NBIA. *Am. J. Hum. Genet.* **2012**, *91*, 1144–1149. [CrossRef] [PubMed]
55. Proikas-Cezanne, T.; Waddell, S.; Gaugel, A.; Frickey, T.; Lupas, A.; Nordheim, A. WIPI-1alpha (WIPI49), a member of the novel 7-bladed WIPI protein family, is aberrantly expressed in human cancer and is linked to starvation-induced autophagy. *Oncogene* **2004**, *23*, 9314–9325. [CrossRef] [PubMed]
56. Stirnimann, C.U.; Petsalaki, E.; Russell, R.B.; Muller, C.W. WD40 proteins propel cellular networks. *Trends Biochem. Sci.* **2010**, *35*, 565–574. [CrossRef] [PubMed]
57. Behrends, C.; Sowa, M.E.; Gygi, S.P.; Harper, J.W. Network organization of the human autophagy system. *Nature* **2010**, *466*, 68–76. [CrossRef]
58. Lu, Q.; Yang, P.; Huang, X.; Hu, W.; Guo, B.; Wu, F. TheWD40 repeat PtdIns (3) P-binding protein EPG-6 regulates progression of omegasomes to autophagosomes. *Dev. Cell* **2011**, *21*, 343–357. [CrossRef]
59. Zhao, Y.G.; Sun, L.; Miao, G.; Ji, C.; Zhao, H.; Sun, H.; Miao, L.; Yoshii, S.R.; Mizushima, N.; Wang, X.; et al. The autophagy gene Wdr45/Wipi4 regulates learning and memory function and axonal homeostasis. *Autophagy* **2015**, *11*, 881–890. [CrossRef]
60. Asano, T.; Komatsu, M.; Yamaguchi-Iwai, Y.; Ishikawa, F.; Mizushima, N.; Iwai, K. Distinct mechanisms of ferritin delivery to lysosomes in iron- depleted and iron-replete cells. *Mol. Cell Biol.* **2011**, *31*, 2040–2052. [CrossRef]
61. Mancias, J.D.; Wang, X.; Gygi, S.P.; Harper, J.W.; Kimmelman, A.C. Quantitative proteomics identifies NCOA4 as the cargo receptor mediating ferritinophagy. *Nature* **2014**, *509*, 105–109. [CrossRef] [PubMed]
62. De Beeck, K.O.; Van Camp, G.; Thys, S.; Cools, N.; Callebaut, I.; Vrijens, K.; Van Laer, L. The DFNA5 gene, responsible for hearing loss and involved in cancer, encodes a novel apoptosis-inducing protein. *Eur. J. Hum. Genet.* **2011**, *19*, 965–973. [CrossRef] [PubMed]
63. Wang, Y.; Gao, W.; Shi, X.; Ding, J.; Liu, W.; He, H.; Wang, K.; Shao, F. Chemotherapy drugs induce pyroptosis through caspase-3 cleavage of a gasdermin. *Nature* **2017**, *547*, 99–103. [CrossRef]
64. Van Laer, L.; Huizing, E.H.; Verstreken, M.; van Zuijlen, D.; Wauters, J.G.; Bossuyt, P.J.; Van de Heyning, P.; McGuirt, W.T.; Smith, R.J.; Willems, P.J.; et al. Nonsyndromic hearing impairment is associated with a mutation in DFNA5. *Nat. Genet.* **1998**, *20*, 194–197. [CrossRef]
65. Zhu, Y.; Zhao, L.; Liu, L.; Gao, P.; Tian, W.; Wang, X.; Jin, H.; Xu, H.; Chen, Q. Beclin 1 cleavage by caspase-3 inactivates autophagy and promotes apoptosis. *Protein Cell* **2010**, *1*, 468–477. [CrossRef]
66. Rogers, C.; Fernandes-Alnemri, T.; Mayes, L.; Alnemri, D.; Cingolani, G.; Alnemri, E.S. Cleavage of DFNA5 by caspase-3 during apoptosis mediates progression to secondary necrotic/pyroptotic cell death. *Nat. Commun.* **2017**, *8*, 14128. [CrossRef]
67. Collin, R.W.; Kalay, E.; Oostrik, J.; Caylan, R.; Wollnik, B.; Arslan, S.; den Hollander, A.I.; Birinci, Y.; Lichtner, P.; Strom, T.M.; et al. Involvement of DFNB59 mutations in autosomal recessive nonsyndromic hearing impairment. *Hum. Mutat.* **2007**, *28*, 718–723. [CrossRef]
68. Mujtaba, G.; Bukhari, I.; Fatima, A.; Naz, S. A p.C343S missense mutation in PJVK causes progressive hearing loss. *Gene* **2012**, *504*, 98–101. [CrossRef]
69. Delmaghani, S.; del Castillo, F.J.; Michel, V.; Leibovici, M.; Aghaie, A.; Ron, U.; Van Laer, L.; Ben-Tal, N.; Van Camp, G.; Weil, D.; et al. Mutations in the gene encoding pejvakin, a newly identified protein of the afferent auditory pathway, cause DFNB59 auditory neuropathy. *Nat. Genet.* **2006**, *38*, 770–778. [CrossRef]
70. Defourny, J.; Aghaie, A.; Perfettini, I.; Avan, P.; Delmaghani, S.; Petit, C. Pejvakin-mediated pexophagy protects auditory hair cells against noise-induced damage. *Proc. Natl. Acad. Sci. USA* **2019**, *116*, 8010–8017. [CrossRef]

71. Germain, K.; Kim, P.K. Pexophagy: A Model for Selective Autophagy. *Int. J. Mol. Sci.* **2020**, *21*, 578. [CrossRef] [PubMed]
72. Shi, J.; Zhao, Y.; Wang, K.; Shi, X.; Wang, Y.; Huang, H.; Zhuang, Y.; Cai, T.; Wang, F.; Shao, F. Cleavage of GSDMD by inflammatory caspases determines pyroptotic cell death. *Nature* **2015**, *526*, 660–665. [CrossRef] [PubMed]
73. Kayagaki, N.; Stowe, I.B.; Lee, B.L.; O'Rourke, K.; Anderson, K.; Warming, S.; Cuellar, T.; Haley, B.; Roose-Girma, M.; Phung, Q.T.; et al. Caspase-11 cleaves gasdermin D for non-canonical inflammasome signalling. *Nature* **2015**, *526*, 666–671. [CrossRef]
74. Ding, J.; Wang, K.; Liu, W.; She, Y.; Sun, Q.; Shi, J.; Sun, H.; Wang, D.C.; Shao, F. Pore-forming activity and structural autoinhibition of the gasdermin family. *Nature* **2016**, *535*, 111–116. [CrossRef] [PubMed]
75. Karmakar, M.; Minns, M.; Greenberg, E.N.; Diaz-Aponte, J.; Pestonjamasp, K.; Johnson, J.L.; Rathkey, J.K.; Abbott, D.W.; Wang, K.; Shao, F.; et al. N-GSDMD trafficking to neutrophil organelles facilitates IL-1β release independently of plasma membrane pores and pyroptosis. *Nat. Commun.* **2020**, *11*, 2212. [CrossRef]
76. Kelsell, D.P.; Dunlop, J.; Stevens, H.P.; Lench, N.J.; Liang, J.N.; Parry, G.; Mueller, R.F.; Leigh, I.M. Connexin 26 mutations in hereditary non-syndromic sensorineural deafness. *Nature* **1997**, *387*, 80–88. [CrossRef]
77. Kenna, M.A.; Feldman, H.A.; Neault, M.W.; Frangulov, A.; Wu, B.L.; Fligor, B.; Rehm, H.L. Audiologic phenotype and progression in GJB2 (Connexin 26) hearing loss. *Arch. Otolaryngol.-Head Neck Surg.* **2010**, *136*, 81–87. [CrossRef]
78. Snoeckx, R.L.; Huygen, P.L.; Feldmann, D.; Marlin, S.; Denoyelle, F.; Waligora, J.; Mueller-Malesinska, M.; Pollak, A.; Ploski, R.; Murgia, A.; et al. GJB2 mutations and degree of hearing loss: A multicenter study. *Am. J. Hum. Genet.* **2005**, *77*, 945–957. [CrossRef]
79. Font, M.A.; Feliubadaló, L.; Estivill, X.; Nunes, V.; Golomb, E.; Kreiss, Y.; Pras, E.; Bisceglia, L.; d'Adamo, A.P.; Zelante, L.; et al. International Cystinuria Consortium. Functional analysis of mutations in SLC7A9, and genotype-phenotype correlation in non-Type I cystinuria. *Hum. Mol. Genet.* **2001**, *10*, 305–316. [CrossRef]
80. Fetoni, A.R.; Zorzi, V.; Paciello, F.; Ziraldo, G.; Peres, C.; Raspa, M.; Scavizzi, F.; Salvatore, A.M.; Crispino, G.; Tognola, G.; et al. Cx26 partial loss causes accelerated presbycusis by redox imbalance and dysregulation of Nfr2 pathway. *Redox Biol.* **2018**, *19*, 301–317. [CrossRef]
81. Johnson, S.L.; Ceriani, F.; Houston, O.; Polishchuk, R.; Polishchuk, E.; Crispino, G.; Zorzi, V.; Mammano, F.; Marcotti, W. Connexin-Mediated Signaling in Nonsensory Cells Is Crucial for the Development of Sensory Inner Hair Cells in the Mouse Cochlea. *Neuroscience* **2017**, *37*, 258–268. [CrossRef] [PubMed]
82. Mitsuishi, Y.; Motohashi, H.; Yamamoto, M. The Keap1-Nrf2 system in cancers: Stress response and anabolic metabolism. *Front. Oncol.* **2012**, *2*, 200. [CrossRef] [PubMed]
83. Katsuragi, Y.; Ichimura, Y.; Komatsu, M. p62/SQSTM1 functions as a signaling hub and an autophagy adaptor. *FEBS J.* **2015**, *282*, 4672–4678. [CrossRef] [PubMed]
84. Hayashi, K.; Dan, K.; Goto, F.; Tsuchihashi, N.; Nomura, Y.; Fujioka, M.; Kanzaki, S.; Ogawa, K. The autophagy pathway maintained signaling crosstalk with the Keap1-Nrf2 system through p62 in auditory cells under oxidative stress. *Cell Signal.* **2015**, *27*, 382–393. [CrossRef]
85. McMahon, M.; Thomas, N.; Itoh, K.; Yamamoto, M.; Hayes, J.D. Dimerization of substrate adaptors can facilitate cullin-mediated ubiquitylation of proteins by a "tethering" mechanism: A two-site interaction model for the Nrf2-Keap1 complex. *J. Biol. Chem.* **2006**, *281*, 24756–24768. [CrossRef]
86. Fukutomi, T.; Takagi, K.; Mizushima, T.; Ohuchi, N.; Yamamoto, M. Kinetic, thermodynamic, and structural characterizations of the association between Nrf2-DLGex degron and Keap1. *Mol. Cell Biol.* **2014**, *34*, 832–846. [CrossRef]
87. Kageyama, S.; Saito, T.; Obata, M.; Koide, R.H.; Ichimura, Y.; Komatsu, M. Negative Regulation of the Keap1-Nrf2 Pathway by a p62/Sqstm1 Splicing Variant. *Mol. Cell Biol.* **2018**, *38*, e00642-17. [CrossRef]
88. Zhang, D.D.; Hannink, M. Distinct cysteine residues in Keap1 are required for Keap1-dependent ubiquitination of Nrf2 and for stabilization of Nrf2 by chemopreventive agents and oxidative stress. *Mol. Cell Biol.* **2003**, *23*, 8137–8151. [CrossRef]
89. Kobayashi, M.; Li, L.; Iwamoto, N.; Nakajima-Takagi, Y.; Kaneko, H.; Nakayama, Y.; Eguchi, M.; Wada, Y.; Kumagai, Y.; Yamamoto, M. The antioxidant defense system Keap1-Nrf2 comprises a multiple sensing mechanism for responding to a wide range of chemical compounds. *Mol. Cell Biol.* **2009**, *29*, 493–502. [CrossRef]

90. Komatsu, M.; Kurokawa, H.; Waguri, S.; Taguchi, K.; Kobayashi, A.; Ichimura, Y.; Sou, Y.S.; Ueno, I.; Sakamoto, A.; Tong, K.I.; et al. The selective autophagy substrate p62 activates the stress responsive transcription factor Nrf2 through inactivation of Keap1. *Nat. Cell Biol.* **2010**, *12*, 213–223. [CrossRef]
91. Johansen, T.; Lamark, T. Selective autophagy mediated by autophagic adapter proteins. *Autophagy* **2011**, *7*, 279–296. [CrossRef] [PubMed]
92. Ichimura, Y.; Kominami, E.; Tanaka, K.; Komatsu, M. Selective turnover of p62/A170/SQSTM1 by autophagy. *Autophagy* **2008**, *4*, 1063–1066. [CrossRef] [PubMed]

Publisher's Note: MDPI stays neutral with regard to jurisdictional claims in published maps and institutional affiliations.

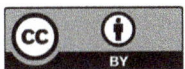 © 2020 by the authors. Licensee MDPI, Basel, Switzerland. This article is an open access article distributed under the terms and conditions of the Creative Commons Attribution (CC BY) license (http://creativecommons.org/licenses/by/4.0/).

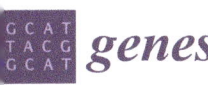

Article

Peripheral Anomalies in USH2A Cause Central Auditory Anomalies in a Mouse Model of Usher Syndrome and CAPD

Peter A. Perrino [1,*], Dianne F. Newbury [2] and R. Holly Fitch [1]

1 Department of Psychological Science/Behavioral Neuroscience, University of Connecticut, Storrs, CT 06269, USA; roslyn.h.fitch@uconn.edu
2 Faculty of Health and Life Sciences, Oxford Brookes University, Oxford OX3 0BP, UK; diannenewbury@brookes.ac.uk
* Correspondence: peter.perrino@uconn.edu; Tel.: +1-(860)-486-3910

Citation: Perrino, P.A.; Newbury, D.F.; Fitch, R.H. Peripheral Anomalies in USH2A Cause Central Auditory Anomalies in a Mouse Model of Usher Syndrome and CAPD. *Genes* **2021**, *12*, 151. https://doi.org/10.3390/genes12020151

Academic Editors: Ignacio del Castillo and Hannie Kremer
Received: 8 November 2020
Accepted: 21 January 2021
Published: 24 January 2021

Publisher's Note: MDPI stays neutral with regard to jurisdictional claims in published maps and institutional affiliations.

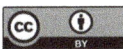

Copyright: © 2021 by the authors. Licensee MDPI, Basel, Switzerland. This article is an open access article distributed under the terms and conditions of the Creative Commons Attribution (CC BY) license (https://creativecommons.org/licenses/by/4.0/).

Abstract: Central auditory processing disorder (CAPD) is associated with difficulties hearing and processing acoustic information, as well as subsequent impacts on the development of higher-order cognitive processes (i.e., attention and language). Yet CAPD also lacks clear and consistent diagnostic criteria, with widespread clinical disagreement on this matter. As such, identification of biological markers for CAPD would be useful. A recent genome association study identified a potential CAPD risk gene, *USH2A*. In a homozygous state, this gene is associated with Usher syndrome type 2 (USH2), a recessive disorder resulting in bilateral, high-frequency hearing loss due to atypical cochlear hair cell development. However, children with heterozygous *USH2A* mutations have also been found to show unexpected low-frequency hearing loss and reduced early vocabulary, contradicting assumptions that the heterozygous (carrier) state is "phenotype free". Parallel evidence has confirmed that heterozygous *Ush2a* mutations in a transgenic mouse model also cause low-frequency hearing loss (Perrino et al., 2020). Importantly, these auditory processing anomalies were still evident after covariance for hearing loss, suggesting a CAPD profile. Since usherin anomalies occur in the peripheral cochlea and *not* central auditory structures, these findings point to upstream developmental feedback effects of peripheral sensory loss on high-level processing characteristic of CAPD. In this study, we aimed to expand upon the mouse behavioral battery used in Perrino et al. (2020) by evaluating central auditory brain structures, including the superior olivary complex (SOC) and medial geniculate nucleus (MGN), in heterozygous and homozygous *Ush2a* mice. We found that heterozygous *Ush2a* mice had significantly larger SOC volumes while homozygous *Ush2a* had significantly smaller SOC volumes. Heterozygous mutations did not affect the MGN; however, homozygous *Ush2a* mutations resulted in a significant shift towards more smaller neurons. These findings suggest that alterations in cochlear development due to *USH2A* variation can secondarily impact the development of brain regions important for auditory processing ability.

Keywords: central auditory processing disorder; Usher syndrome type 2; USH2A; superior olivary complex; medial geniculate nucleus

1. Introduction

Individuals diagnosed with central auditory processing disorder (CAPD) experience difficulties with multiple mechanisms that subserve acoustic information processing. These include, but are not limited to, sound localization, temporal discrimination, discrimination between two or more competing auditory stimuli, auditory pattern recognition and dichotic listening [1,2]. Moreover, affected individuals have difficulties with speech processing that include attending to verbal input (i.e., oral instruction) and comprehending complex sentences [3]. As a result, affected children often experience poor academic performance and reduced quality of life [4,5].

Nonetheless, there is ongoing debate within the audiology community as to the definition of—and diagnostic criteria for—CAPD. This includes whether CAPD should be considered a DSM-defined disorder. According to the American Speech and Hearing Association (ASHA), individuals clinically diagnosed with any of the aforementioned auditory impairments have clinically defined CAPD [1]. However, multiple other audiology groups (i.e., the American Academy of Audiology (2010) [6], the British Society of Audiology (2011) [4] and the Canadian Interorganizational Steering Group for Speech-Language Pathology and Audiology (2012) [7]) adopt different standards. The discrepancies across organizations include differences in phenotypic description, ascribed causal mechanisms and classification of co-morbidities (see [2] for a review). These disparities contribute to controversy in recognizing CAPD, with varied results in the attribution of symptoms to other disorders. For instance, Dawes and Bishop (2010) [8] reported that 52% of children diagnosed with CAPD could also fit a diagnosis of dyslexia, specific language impairment, or both. Children with CAPD have also been shown to meet behavioral profiles for attention deficit disorder [9,10], suggesting CAPD may resemble a more general cognitive disorder rather than an auditory perception disorder.

The lack of a clear causal genetic, peripheral or neurologic mechanism adds another layer of difficulty to defining CAPD. Ongoing research is crucial to determining whether CAPD is the result of poor auditory processing and/or integration with higher-order cognitive processes, subclinical hearing impairments that affect cochlear development, comorbid cognitive disorders (as discussed above), or a combination of factors. Additionally, genetic contributions to CAPD remain understudied [11]. Brewer et al. (2016) [12] reported that auditory processing skills (i.e., temporal processing and pitch discrimination) subserving the perception of spoken language are heritable. As such, it is possible that auditory processing difficulties seen in individuals with CAPD arise from genetic variants and/or mutations.

One promising CAPD-risk gene is *USH2A*, which is clinically associated with Usher syndrome type 2 (USH2; [13]). Individuals with USH2 experience bilateral hearing loss at high frequencies and retinitis pigmentosa beginning at puberty [14,15]. USH2 results from homozygous loss-of-function of *USH2A*, with heterozygous individuals considered to be unaffected carriers [16,17]. The *USH2A* protein is expressed primarily in the cochlea and retina but not in the brain, meaning that USH2 is considered a peripheral disorder [18]. Usherin plays a critical role in cochlear hair cell maturation and acts to connect developing stereocilia with kinocilium via a transient lateral ankle link that helps guide developing hair cells into their proper orientation [19,20]. Lui et al. (2007) [19] reported that the outer hair cells of the basal cochlea were missing in mice with a homozygous knockout of *Ush2a* (the rodent homolog of *USH2A*), consistent with high-frequency hearing loss in individuals with USH2.

While it is well established that homozygous mutations of *USH2A* cause UHS2, little is known about how heterozygous mutations affect hearing ability or auditory processing. Historically, heterozygous mutations of *USH2A* have been considered nonpathogenic, with such individuals classified as "unaffected carriers" of USH2. Yet several studies report low-frequency hearing loss or sensorineural abnormalities in USH2 carriers [20–23]. As a result of abnormalities reported in USH2 carriers, researchers have recently become interested in how heterozygous mutations of *USH2A* might contribute to auditory processing ability, including disorders like CAPD.

To study the relationship between heterozygous *USH2A* mutations, CAPD and language outcomes, Perrino et al. (2020) [24] sought to combine human whole genome sequencing with mouse model behavioral phenotyping. Specifically, we conducted genome sequencing of a family with individuals affected by a severe expressive language disorder, as well as phenotypic characteristics of CAPD (i.e., difficulties understanding oral instructions). Affected family members were found to have a heterozygous stop-gain mutation in the *USH2A* gene (NP_996816:p.Gln4541*), suggesting that the heterozygous *USH2A* mutation might have caused the auditory processing deficits in affected family members. To further test this hypothesis, we evaluated *Ush2a* heterozygous (HT) mice on a battery of rapid auditory processing tasks. We found that HT mice had low-frequency hearing impairments, which subsequently contributed to higher-order auditory processing difficulties that persisted even when hearing deficits were covaried out. Importantly, simultaneous testing showed that *Ush2a* KO mice were affected by significant high-frequency auditory processing impairments, a defining characteristic of USH2. These low-level hearing deficits in homozygous mice also contributed to higher-order auditory processing difficulties reflective of central mechanisms. Human genome-wide association studies (GWAS) also suggest that heterozygous *USH2A* mutations contribute to a CAPD phenotype. Specifically, though the same stop-gain mutation that was reported in our discovery family was not present in the UK10K dataset [25], children with pathogenic heterozygous *USH2A* variants nonetheless showed low-frequency hearing impairments (i.e., increased low-frequency hearing thresholds (+1.2 dB HL at 500 Hz)), as well as reductions in vocabulary, when compared to children without an *USH2A* mutation [24]. These results were highly novel in identifying heterozygous *USH2A* mutations as a CAPD risk, with impacts on low-frequency hearing as well as higher-order auditory processing abilities necessary for typical language and communication development.

This current study builds upon Perrino et al. (2020) [24]. Here, using *postmortem* brains from the behaviorally evaluated mice, we analyzed the neuroanatomical consequences of *Ush2a* genetic variations. We hypothesized that, despite the lack of *Ush2a* expression in the CNS, anatomical anomalies may be evident in the overall volume, neuron size and/or neuronal population in brain structures that subserve central auditory processing (i.e., the medial geniculate nucleus (MGN) and superior olivary complex (SOC)) in both heterozygous and knockout subjects. We predicted differing anatomical anomalies between heterozygous (HT) and homozygous (KO) subjects, given that HT mutations affect low-frequency processing and KO mutations affect high-frequency processing. Results from volumetric analysis showed a significant increase in right SOC volume for *Ush2a* HT mice, coupled with a significant decrease in right SOC volume for *Ush2a* KO mice. Within the right MGN, we found a significant shift towards more smaller neurons in *Ush2a* KO mice, while HT mice were unaffected. Together, our results suggest that altered cochlear development impacts higher-order auditory processing at both a functional and structural level, but differently so in *Ush2a* HT and KO subjects. These anomalies could account for complex auditory and speech processing impairments observed in some individuals with CAPD, as well as those with Usher syndrome type 2.

2. Materials and Methods

2.1. Subject Generation

Six homozygous *Ush2a* male subjects (F1 generation) were rederived on an 129S4/SvJaeJ background strain at the Center for Mouse Genome Modification (previously known as the Gene Targeting and Transgenic Facility) at UConn Health via genetic material obtained from Dr. Jun Yang (University of Utah; [19]). These six male *Ush2a* KO mice were crossed with six wildtype (WT) control mice (29S4/SvJaeJ; stock number 009104) obtained from the Jackson Laboratory (Bar Harbor, ME) to generate an all heterozygous (HT) F2 generation. To generate experimental (F3) subjects, HT × HT breeding pairs from the F2 generation were established, resulting in litters containing all three genotypes (homozygous, heterozygous and wildtype). Following weaning (postnatal day (P) 21), ear punches were collected from each subject and used for genotyping via PCR (DNA primer information can be found in [19]). After puberty (P40), subjects from the F3 generation were randomly selected and used for behavioral testing and histological assessment. Additionally, at this time, experimental subjects were single housed in standard Plexiglass mouse chambers (12 h/12 h light–dark cycle) with food and water available *ad libitum*. The subjects used here, as well as the breeding information, are the same as used in Perrino et al. (2020) [24].

2.2. Behavioral Testing

Beginning at P65, subjects were assessed on a battery of auditory processing tasks aimed to evaluate the subject's ability to process and discriminate complex acoustic information relevant to communication ability (see [26] for review). For a complete description of the behavioral battery each subject underwent, see [24]. In short, acoustic processing ability was assessed using a modified prepulse inhibition (PPI) paradigm in which the subject's acoustic startle response was measured following the presentation of a loud (105 dB, 50 ms) startle eliciting stimulus (SES; 1000–10,000 Hz broadband burst) ("uncued" trials). During each testing session, acoustic cues were pseudorandomly presented before the SES—the subject's acoustic startle response during "cued" trials was measured. If the subject was able to detect the acoustic cue—the goal of each auditory processing task—their acoustic startle response should have been reduced (or attenuated) as the cue informs the subject that the SES is about to occur. The difference in startle response during "uncued" and "cued" trials can be calculated as an "attenuation score"—a ratio of [average "cued" startle response/average "uncued" startle response] × 100. The lower the attenuation score, the better the subject's performance in detecting the cue. Subjects with an attenuation score of 100% were deemed to have not detected the cue, as their "uncued" and "cued" startle responses were similar.

Each subject underwent a variety of acoustic processing tasks, each designed to assess a different aspect of acoustic processing ability. Subjects were first evaluated on a normal single tone (NST) task that used a simple pure tone cue to assess baseline hearing ability, typical acoustic startle response (i.e., motor ability), and prepulse inhibition. Attenuation scores for the NST task were used as a covariate for subsequent auditory processing tasks to eliminate individual differences. More complex auditory processing tasks were used to evaluate spectral, temporal, or both spectral and temporal (spectro-temporal) aspects of auditory processing ability. For example, embedded tone (EBT) consisted of a pure tone background and an auditory cue that was different than the pure tone background and varied in duration. Pitch discrimination (PD) consisted of a pure tone background and an acoustic cue that had a fixed duration but varied in frequency. Additionally, each task was presented in both a sub-ultrasonic and an ultrasonic frequency range. The use of multiple auditory processing tasks, combined with the use of multiple frequency ranges, allows for the detailed evaluation of how *USH2A* mutations affect different aspects of acoustic processing ability. See [24] for a description of each task used.

2.3. Histology

Following the completion of behavioral testing (P150) and after being weighed, subjects were anesthetized using ketamine (100 mg/kg) and xylazine (15 mg/kg) and transcardially perfused using a 0.9% saline solution followed by 10% formalin. The brains were postfixed in 10% formalin following extraction. Each brain was serially and coronally sectioned (60 μm) using a Leica VT1000 S vibratome (Leica Biosystems Inc., Buffalo Grove, IL, USA). Olfactory bulbs were removed using a surgical blade and the flat surface that remained was glued to the vibratome stage—slicing began at the cerebellum and progressed towards the frontal cortex (posterior → anterior). Every coronal section of the brain was mounted to a gelatin-subbed glass slide until the cerebellum was completely sectioned. This methodology was performed to ensure the complete sectioning of the superior olivary complex. Sectioning continued past the cerebellum and every second section was mounted on a gelatin-subbed glass slide. All slides were subjected to cresyl violet to stain for Nissl bodies. Slides were then cover-slipped with DPX mounting medium.

2.4. Stereological Measurements

Brain tissue underwent stereological analysis via Stereo Investigator (MBF Biosciences, Williston, VT, USA) using a Zeiss Axio Imager A2 microscope (Carl Zeiss, Thornwood, NY, USA). Superior olivary complex (Figure 1A) and medial geniculate nucleus (Figure 1B) volumes were estimated using the Cavalieri Estimator probe, neuron population was estimated using the Optical Fractionator probe (Figure 1C), and the Nucleator probe was used to measure neuronal cell area (Figure 1D). Measurements within the SOC were performed at a sampling frequency of every section (across eight total sections), while measurements within the MGN were performed with a sampling frequency of every second section (across six total sections). Contours to define each region and to provide volumetric estimates were determined via stereotaxic atlas [27] and drawn at 2.5× magnification. All other stereological measurements (i.e., neuron population and neural cell area) were evaluated at 100× magnification. A sampling grid of 150 µm × 150 µm and a 30 µm × 30 µm counting frame was selected for the SOC, while a sampling grid of 225 µm × 225 µm and a 25 µm × 25 µm counting frame was selected for the MGN. Neurons were defined as having one distinct nucleolus within the nucleus—glial cells or other cell types within the brain were not counted (Figure 1C).

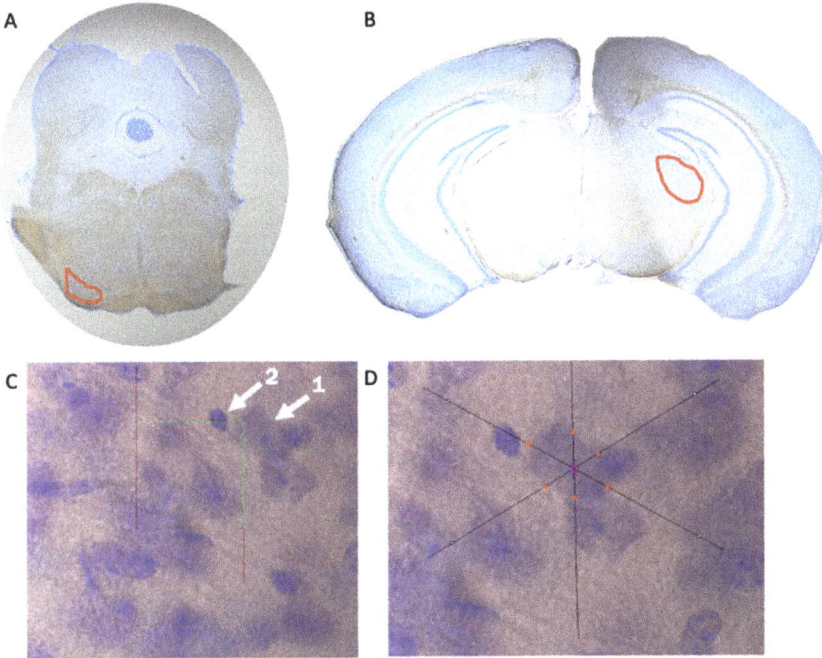

Figure 1. Stereological Measurements. Visual representation of the superior olivary complex (SOC) (**A**) and medial geniculate nucleus (MGN) (**B**) taken at 2.5× magnification to determine volume of brain region. (**C**) The Optical Fractionator probe of Stereo Investigator was used to determine neuron population. Arrow 1 indicates a neuron that was counted due to the presence of a clearly defined nucleolus, while Arrow 2 indicates a cell that was not counted. (**D**) The Nucleator probe was used to determine neuron size (area). Optical Fractionator and Nucleator probes were used at 100× magnification.

2.5. Statistical Analysis

Genotype differences for the volume of each region (i.e., SOC and MGN), neuron population within each region, and average neuronal cell area within each region, were analyzed using univariate ANOVAs. Additionally, univariate ANOVAs were performed between each Genotype to determine how heterozygous *Ush2a* mutations differed from homozygous mutations—a necessary analysis for determining how each mutation contributes to the behavioral differences between HT and KO subjects (low-frequency vs. high-frequency auditory processing). To evaluate how *Ush2a* mutations affect neuronal cell size (area) distribution, the Kolmogorov–Smirnov (K–S) test was conducted on the cumulative percent distribution for each Genotype. Analyses were conducted for the left and right hemispheres, as well as both together (i.e., total SOC or total MGN). All univariate ANOVAs and correlational analyses were conducted via the car package [28] in R (v3.4.4; [29]). A total of 21 subjects were used in the histological assessment of the SOC

(WT, n = 7 (one subject dropped due to poor tissue integrity); HT, n = 7; KO, n = 7) and 22 subjects for the histological assessment of the MGN (WT, n = 8; HT, n = 7; KO, n = 7).

2.6. Ethics

All animal procedures were approved by the University of Connecticut's Institute for Animal Care and Use Committee (IACUC; Protocol No. A18-050) and followed the Guide for the Care and Use of Laboratory Animals [30]. This study was designed to comply with ARRIVE guidelines [31].

3. Results

3.1. SOC Volumetric Analysis

A univariate ANOVA comparing SOC volume revealed a main effect of Genotype in the right SOC [right: $F(2, 18) = 4.034$, $p < 0.05$], reflecting a volumetric increase in HT subjects relative to WTs, coupled with a volumetric decrease in KO subjects (HT vs. KO; $F(1, 12) = 9.558$, $p < 0.05$). There was no significant Genotype effect in the left SOC [$F(2, 18) = 0.568$, $p > 0.05$], nor for the total SOC [$F(2, 18) = 1.874$, $p > 0.05$] (Figure 2A).

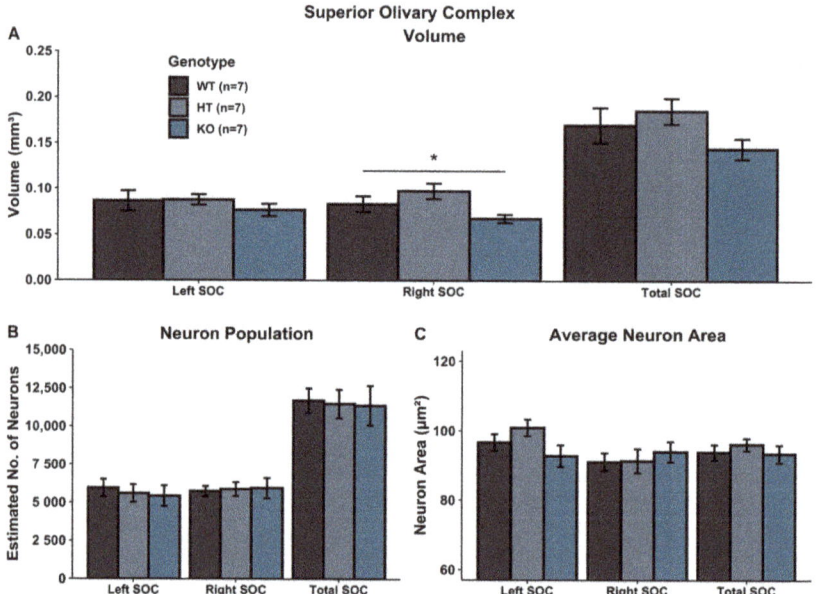

Figure 2. Histological assessment in SOC. (**A**) Volumetric analysis of left, right and total (left + right) SOC. Heterozygous *Ush2a* mutations increased the volume of the right SOC while homozygous *Ush2a* mutations reduced the volume of the right SOC. (**B**,**C**) There were no significant genotype differences in neuron population (**B**) or average neuron area (**C**). * $p < 0.05$.

3.2. MGN Volumetric Analysis

A univariate ANOVA comparing MGN volume revealed no main effect of genotype in either hemisphere (left: $F(2, 19) = 0.468$, $p > 0.05$; right: $F(2, 19) = 0.0598$, $p > 0.05$; total: $F(2, 19) = 0.232$, $p > 0.05$) (Figure 3A).

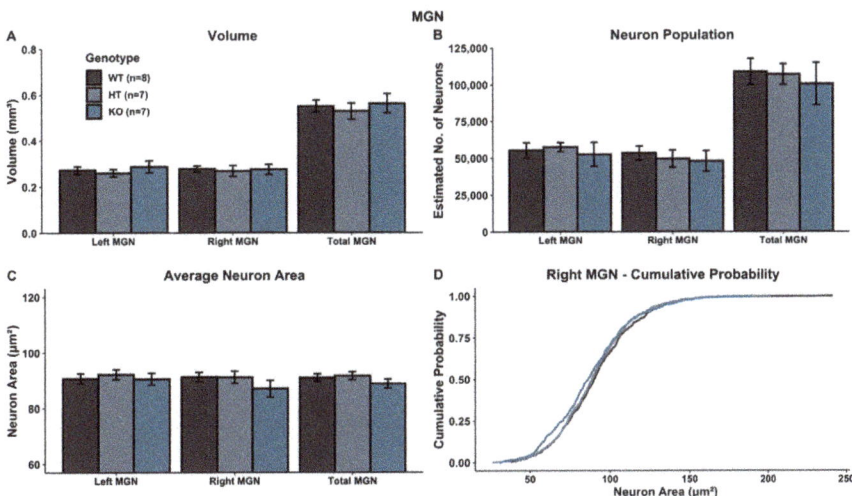

Figure 3. Histological assessment in MGN. (**A–C**) There were no significant genotype differences when evaluating volume (**A**), neuron population (**B**) or neuron area (**C**). (**D**) Comparison of cumulative percent distribution of neuronal cell size (area) revealed a significant shift towards fewer larger neurons and more smaller neurons in the right MGN in *Ush2a* homozygous (KO) mice.

3.3. SOC Cellular Analysis

There was no significant Genotype effect when evaluating neuron population within the SOC (left SOC: $F(2, 18) = 0.183$, $p > 0.05$; right SOC: $F(2, 18) = 0.040$, $p > 0.05$; total SOC: $F(2, 18) = 0.028$, $p > 0.05$) (Figure 2B). Additionally, there was no Genotype effect on average neuron size (area) in the SOC (left SOC: $F(2, 18) = 2.3048$, $p > 0.05$; right SOC: $F(2, 18) = 0.290$, $p > 0.05$; total SOC: $F(2, 18) = 0.437$, $p > 0.05$) (Figure 2C).

3.4. MGN Cellular Analysis

There was no significant Genotype effect on neuron population within the MGN (left MGN: $F(2, 19) = 0.174$, $p > 0.05$; right MGN: $F(2, 19) = 0.174$, $p > 0.05$; total MGN: $F(2, 19) = 0.168$, $p > 0.05$) (Figure 3B), nor for average neuron size (area) within the MGN (left MGN: $F(2, 19) = 0.219$, $p > 0.05$; right MGN: $F(2, 19) = 1.039$, $p > 0.05$; total MGN: $F(2, 19) = 0.965$, $p > 0.05$) (Figure 3C). Additionally, in the left MGN, no significant K–S statistics for the cumulative distribution of cell size were seen (left MGN (WT vs. HT): $p > 0.05$; left MGN (WT vs. KO): $p > 0.05$; left MGN (HT vs. KO): $p > 0.05$). However, within the right MGN, WT and KO subjects were significantly different (right MGN (WT vs. KO): $p < 0.05$), with a shift towards more smaller neurons in KO subjects. WT vs. HT subjects did not yield a significant K–S statistic (right MGN (WT vs. HT): $p > 0.05$), nor did HT vs. KO subjects (right MGN (HT vs. KO): $p > 0.05$) (Figure 3D). No effects were seen for the overall MGN (total MGN (WT vs. HT): $p > 0.05$; total MGN (WT vs. KO): $p > 0.05$; total MGN (HT vs. KO): $p > 0.05$).

4. Discussion

The current study was designed to neuroanatomically evaluate the central auditory consequences of heterozygous and homozygous mutations in an *Ush2a* mouse model. The study was based on human clinical evidence that homozygous mutations of *USH2A* result in Usher syndrome type 2 [13], as well as recent evidence that heterozygous *USH2A* mutations may be a genetic risk factor for CAPD [24]. Since anomalies in auditory processing represent core features of both CAPD and USH2 (though with very different functional profiles; [3,14]), central auditory structures of the superior olivary complex and medial geniculate nucleus were evaluated. Results showed that heterozygous *Ush2a* mutations resulted in an increase in right SOC volume, while homozygous *Ush2a* mutations resulted in a decrease in right SOC volume, as well as a shift towards fewer large and more small neurons in the right MGN. To the best of our knowledge, these results are the first to report neuroanatomical anomalies in a mouse model of either CAPD or Usher syndrome type 2. The results are particularly exciting given a lack of usherin expression in the brain [18], which suggests substantial developmental effects of peripheral auditory anomalies on the central auditory system.

Neuroanatomical Differences between HT and KO Subjects

The two structures evaluated in this study, SOC and MGN, both play an important role in the central auditory system (see [32] for review). The SOC is one of the first stops for ascending auditory information, primarily mediating sound localization via the convergence of binaural sensory input [33,34]. To our knowledge, there are not significant processing differences between right and left SOC, both of which receive input from ipsilateral and contralateral cochlea [35]. Here, we report that the right SOC is smaller in KO subjects, and larger in HT subjects. In considering possible mechanisms for these anomalies, Liu et al. (2007) [19] reported that mice with a homozygous *Ush2a* deletion had an absence of outer hair cells in the basal cochlea, an area primarily responsible for the detection of high-frequency auditory information. This cochlear abnormality could have contributed to the observed reductions in right SOC volume, since regions that respond to high-frequency auditory information are presumably receiving anomalous/degraded sensory input. The notion that anomalous brain development may result from altered or absent sensory input is well established and has been studied in multiple sensory modalities, including the auditory system [36–41]. These SOC reductions in KO subjects may have further contributed to the high-frequency processing impairments reported by Perrino et al. (2020) [24]. The increase in SOC volume in subjects with heterozygous *Ush2a* mutations was surprising. However, there is ample evidence that atypical structural increases in the CNS can cause functional impairments (e.g., macrocephaly). Future studies are needed to (1) evaluate cochlear development and organization in heterozygous *Ush2a* mutant mice, and (2) determine how non-neuronal cell types (i.e., glial cells) might contribute to the volumetric differences reported here. It is possible that changes in glial morphology within the SOC in HT and/or KO mice contributed to the observed behavioral phenotypes. Nonetheless, the increase in right SOC volume in HT subjects provides evidence that altered sensory input can impact CNS development, as well as evidence that underlying neurologic anomalies may exist in CAPD.

In addition to the SOC, we assessed the MGN, a thalamic nucleus responsible for auditory processing. The MGN has been shown to be affected in other language- and communication-neurodevelopmental disorders; for example, Galaburda et al. (1994) [42] reported a shift towards more smaller MGN neurons in the brains of individuals with dyslexia. These initial findings of atypical MGN morphology led to further studies with animal models using induced mutations of dyslexia-risk genes and induced neuronal migration abnormalities. Both models showed anomalous MGN anatomy [43–45]. Importantly, atypical MGN development has been shown to impact auditory processing ability [46–48], which is a fundamental skill necessary for language development, as well as a good predictor of later language outcomes [49]. Within the autism spectrum disorders (ASD) population, for example, reductions in MGN volume [50] and altered thalamocortical connectivity [51] have been reported, and similar MGN anomalies have been observed in genetic mouse models of ASD [52], a disorder frequently characterized by anomalous language development and language impairments. Our findings that homozygous *Ush2a* mutations shift the cell size distribution towards fewer large and more small neurons in the right MGN further substantiate the potential role of MGN in language functions [53].

Finally, it is important to note that effects were observed explicitly in the right SOC and right MGN in both HT and KO mice. Given overwhelming evidence of left hemisphere lateralization for language and underlying auditory temporal processing [54–56], these results may seem puzzling. However, it is important to note that recent mouse research has shown evidence of left hemisphere lateralization in A1 specifically for processing of ultrasonic vocalizations and other spectro-temporal acoustic information, while right A1 may play a stronger role in frequency-based processing [57]. Although lateralization of MGN was not observed in this study, it is nonetheless possible that feedback effects of altered frequency-specific input could have selective effects on the projecting pathways to right A1, including the right SOC and MGN.

5. Conclusions

The goal of the current study was to provide a histological follow-up to Perrino et al. (2020) [24] by evaluating the consequences of heterozygous and homozygous *USH2A* mutations on central auditory structures in a transgenic mouse model. We report that *Ush2a* HT mice, a putative mouse model for CAPD, exhibited significantly increased right SOC volumes. Conversely, *Ush2a* KO mice—a well-accepted mouse model for USH2—exhibited significantly decreased right SOC volumes, and a shift towards smaller right MGN neurons. These neuroanatomical abnormalities may contribute to the low-frequency auditory processing impairments seen in HT mice, as well as associated language and communication impairments seen in individuals with pathogenic, heterozygous *USH2A* variants. Subcortical anomalies may also contribute to the high-frequency auditory processing impairments seen in KO mice, corresponding to clinical USH2 symptoms. Importantly, given evidence of usherin expression in the cochlea but not the brain, our results indicate: (1) an upstream impact of altered cochlear function on the central auditory system and (2) that the impacts differ for heterozygous and homozygous *Ush2a* mutations, commensurate with different hearing profiles. Future studies will be important in assessing additional central auditory structures in these mouse models (e.g., inferior colliculus, A1). Taken together, our findings strongly advocate for early genetic screening as a tool for detecting hearing and auditory processing disorders that may impact subsequent language development, and add to evidence from Perrino et al. (2020) [24] that *USH2A* carriers are not "phenotype-free".

Author Contributions: P.A.P. was responsible for histological methodology and experimental design, statistical analysis and drafting the manuscript. D.F.N. was a key contributor to the conception and design of experiments. R.H.F. was responsible for experimental design, manuscript editing and obtaining funding for this project. All authors have read and agreed to the published version of the manuscript.

Funding: This work was supported by funding from the University of Connecticut Murine Behavioral Neurogenetics Facility, the Connecticut Institute for Brain and Cognitive Sciences (IBACS), and Science of Learning & Art of Communication (NSF Grant DGE-1747486). Any opinions, findings, and conclusions or recommendations expressed in this material are those of the author(s) and do not necessarily reflect the views of the National Science Foundation.

Institutional Review Board Statement: The study was conducted according to the guidelines of the Declaration of Helsinki, and approved by the University of Connecticut's Institutional Animal Care and Use Committee (IACUC) (Protocol No. A18-050; Approval Date 27 February 2020).

Informed Consent Statement: Not applicable.

Data Availability Statement: The data presented in this study are available on request from the corresponding author.

Acknowledgments: We would like to thank Jun Yang at the University of Utah for generously sharing the original *Ush2a* KO breeding pairs, as well as the Center for Mouse Genome Modification at UConn Health for their rederivation services. Additionally, we would like to thank Kirantheja Daggula for his role in sectioning *Ush2a* experimental mice.

Conflicts of Interest: The authors declare no conflict of interest.

References

1. American Speech-Language-Hearing Association. *(Central) Auditory Processing Disorders*; American Speech-Language-Hearing Association: Rockville, MD, USA, 2005.
2. Heine, C.; O'Halloran, R. Central Auditory Processing Disorder: A systematic search and evaluation of clinical practice guidelines. *J. Eval. Clin. Pr.* **2015**, *21*, 988–994. [CrossRef] [PubMed]
3. Moore, D.R.; Rosen, S.; Bamiou, D.-E.; Campbell, N.G.; Sirimanna, T. Evolving concepts of developmental auditory processing disorder (APD): A British Society of Audiology APD special interest group 'white paper'. *Int. J. Audiol.* **2013**, *52*, 3–13. [CrossRef] [PubMed]
4. British Society of Audiology. Position Statement on Auditory Processing Disorder. 2011. Available online: https://www.thebsa.org.uk/wp-content/uploads/2011/04/OD104-39-Position-Statement-APD-2011-1.pdf (accessed on 14 April 2020).
5. Dawes, P.; Bishop, D. Auditory processing disorder in relation to developmental disorders of language, communication and attention: A review and critique. *Int. J. Lang. Commun. Disord.* **2009**, *44*, 440–465. [CrossRef] [PubMed]
6. American Academy of Audiology. American Academy of Audiology Clinical Practice Guidelines. Guidelines for the Diagnosis, Treatment and Management of Children and Adults with Central Auditory Processing Disorder. 2010. Available online: https://audiology-web.s3.amazonaws.com/migrated/CAPD%20Guidelines%208-2010.pdf_539952af956c79.73897613.pdf (accessed on 16 April 2020).
7. Canadian Introorganizational Steering Group for Speech-language Pathology and Audiology. The Canadian Guidelines on Auditory Processing Disorder in Children and Adults: Assessment and Intervention. 2012. Available online: https://www.acslpa.ca/wp-content/uploads/2019/05/Canadian-Guidelines-on-Auditory-Processing-Disorder-in-Children-and-Adults-English-Final-2012-V-2.pdf (accessed on 16 April 2020).
8. Dawes, P.; Bishop, D.V. Psychometric profile of children with auditory processing disorder and children with dyslexia. *Arch. Dis. Child.* **2010**, *95*, 432–436. [CrossRef]
9. Cook, J.R.; Mausbach, T.; Burd, L.; Gascon, G.G.; Slotnick, H.B.; Patterson, B.; Johnson, R.D.; Hankey, B.; Reynolds, B.W. A preliminary study of the relationship between central auditory processing disorder and attention deficit disorder. *J. Psychiatry Neurosci.* **1993**, *18*, 130.
10. Gascon, G.G.; Johnson, R.; Burd, L. Central auditory processing and attention deficit disorders. *J. Child Neurol.* **1986**, *1*, 27–33. [CrossRef]
11. Witton, C. Childhood auditory processing disorder as a developmental disorder: The case for a multi-professional approach to diagnosis and management. *Int. J. Audiol.* **2010**, *49*, 83–87. [CrossRef]
12. Brewer, C.C.; Zalewski, C.K.; King, K.A.; Zobay, O.; Riley, A.; Ferguson, M.A.; Bird, J.E.; McCabe, M.M.; Hood, L.J.; Drayna, D.; et al. Heritability of non-speech auditory processing skills. *Eur. J. Hum. Genet.* **2016**, *24*, 1137–1144. [CrossRef]
13. Eudy, J.D.; Weston, M.D.; Yao, S.; Hoover, D.M.; Rehm, H.L.; Ma-Edmonds, M.; Yan, D.; Ahmad, I.; Cheng, J.J.; Ayuso, C.; et al. Mutation of a gene encoding a protein with extracellular matrix motifs in Usher syndrome type IIa. *Science* **1998**, *280*, 1753–1757. [CrossRef]
14. Boughman, J.A.; Vernon, M.; Shaver, K.A. Usher syndrome: Definition and estimate of prevalence from two high-risk populations. *J. Chronic. Dis.* **1983**, *36*, 595–603. [CrossRef]
15. Keats, B.J.; Corey, D.P. The usher syndromes. *Am. J. Med. Genet.* **1999**, *89*, 158–166. [CrossRef]
16. Weston, M.D.; Luijendijk, M.W.J.; Humphrey, K.D.; Möller, C.; Kimberling, W.J. Mutations in the VLGR1 gene implicate G-protein signaling in the pathogenesis of Usher syndrome type II. *Am. J. Hum. Genet.* **2004**, *74*, 357–366. [CrossRef] [PubMed]
17. Ebermann, I.; Scholl, H.P.N.; Charbel Issa, P.; Becirovic, E.; Lamprecht, J.; Jurklies, B.; Millán, J.M.; Aller, E.; Mitter, D.; Bolz, H. A novel gene for Usher syndrome type 2: Mutations in the long isoform of whirlin are associated with retinitis pigmentosa and sensorineural hearing loss. *Hum. Genet.* **2007**, *121*, 203–211. [CrossRef] [PubMed]
18. Pearsall, N.; Bhattacharya, G.; Wisecarver, J.; Adams, J.; Cosgrove, D.; Kimberling, W. Usherin expression is highly conserved in mouse and human tissues. *Hear Res.* **2002**, *174*, 55–63. [CrossRef]
19. Liu, X.; Bulgakov, O.V.; Darrow, K.N.; Pawlyk, B.; Adamian, M.; Liberman, M.C.; Li, T. Usherin is required for maintenance of retinal photoreceptors and normal development of cochlear hair cells. *Proc. Natl. Acad. Sci. USA* **2007**, *104*, 4413–4418. [CrossRef] [PubMed]
20. De Haas, E.B.H.; Van Lith, G.H.M.; Rijnders, J.; Rümke, A.M.L.; Volmer, C.H. Usher's syndrome. *Doc. Ophthalmol.* **1970**, *28*, 166–190. [CrossRef]
21. Kloepfer, H.W.; Laguaite, J.K.; Mclaurin, J.W. The hereditary syndrome of congenital deafness and retinitis pigmentosa. *Laryngoscope* **1966**, *76*, 850–862. [CrossRef]
22. Sondheimer, S.; Fishman, G.A.; Young, R.S.; Vasquez, V.A. Dark adaptation testing in heterozygotes of Usher's syndrome. *Br. J. Ophthalmol.* **1979**, *63*, 547–550. [CrossRef]
23. van Aarem, A.; Cremers, C.W.; Pinckers, A.J.; Huygen, P.L.; Hombergen, G.C.; Kimberling, B.J. The Usher syndrome type 2A: Clinical findings in obligate carriers. *Int. J. Pediatr. Otorhinolaryngol.* **1995**, *31*, 159–174. [CrossRef]
24. Perrino, P.A.; Talbot, L.; Kirkland, R.; Hill, A.; Rendall, A.R.; Mountford, H.S.; Taylor, J.; Buscarello, A.N.; Lahiri, N.; Saggar, A.; et al. Multi-level evidence of an allelic hierarchy of USH2A variants in hearing, auditory processing and speech/language outcomes. *Commun. Biol.* **2020**, *3*, 1–14. [CrossRef]

25. Walter, K.; Min, J.L.; Huang, J.; Crooks, L.; Memari, Y.; McCarthy, S.; Perry, J.R.B.; Xu, C.; Futema, M.; Lawson, D.; et al. The UK10K project identifies rare variants in health and disease. *Nature* **2015**, *526*, 82–90. [CrossRef] [PubMed]
26. Fitch, R.H.; Threlkeld, S.W.; McClure, M.M.; Peiffer, A.M. Use of a modified prepulse inhibition paradigm to assess complex auditory discrimination in rodents. *Brain Res. Bull.* **2008**, *76*, 1–7. [CrossRef] [PubMed]
27. Paxinos, G.; Franklin, K.B.J. *Paxinos and Franklin's the Mouse Brain in Stereotaxic Coordinates*; Academic Press: Cambridge, MA, USA, 2019; ISBN 978-0-12-816158-6.
28. Fox, J.; Weisberg, S. *An R Companion to Applied Regression*, 3rd ed.; Sage: Newcastle upon Tyne, UK, 2019.
29. R Core Team. *R: A Language and Environment for Statistical Computing*; R Foundationfor Statistical Computing: Vienna, Austria, 2013.
30. Council, N.R. *Guide for the Care and Use of Laboratory Animals*, 8th ed.; National Academies Press: Washington, DC, USA, 2010; ISBN 978-0-309-15400-0.
31. du Sert, N.P.; Hurst, V.; Ahluwalia, A.; Alam, S.; Avey, M.T.; Baker, M.; Browne, W.J.; Clark, A.; Cuthill, I.C.; Dirnagl, U.; et al. The ARRIVE guidelines 2.0: Updated guidelines for reporting animal research. *PLoS Biol.* **2020**, *18*, e3000410. [CrossRef] [PubMed]
32. Pannese, A.; Grandjean, D.; Frühholz, S. Subcortical processing in auditory communication. *Hear Res.* **2015**, *328*, 67–77. [CrossRef] [PubMed]
33. Jenkins, W.M.; Masterton, R.B. Sound localization: Effects of unilateral lesions in central auditory system. *J. Neurophysiol.* **1982**, *47*, 987–1016. [CrossRef]
34. Masterton, B.; Diamond, I.T.; Harrison, J.M.; Beecher, M.D. Medial Superior Olive and Sound Localization. *Science* **1967**, *155*, 1696–1697. [CrossRef]
35. Moore, J.K. Organization of the human superior olivary complex. *Microsc. Res. Tech.* **2000**, *51*, 403–412. [CrossRef]
36. Kitzes, L.M.; Semple, M.N. Single-unit responses in the inferior colliculus: Effects of neonatal unilateral cochlear ablation. *J. Neurophysiol.* **1985**, *53*, 1483–1500. [CrossRef]
37. Kral, A.; Hartmann, R.; Tillein, J.; Heid, S.; Klinke, R. Congenital auditory deprivation reduces synaptic activity within the auditory cortex in a layer-specific manner. *Cereb. Cortex* **2000**, *10*, 714–726. [CrossRef]
38. Moore, D.R.; Russell, F.A.; Cathcart, N.C. Lateral superior olive projections to the inferior colliculus in normal and unilaterally deafened ferrets. *J. Comp. Neurol.* **1995**, *357*, 204–216. [CrossRef]
39. de Villers-Sidani, E.; Merzenich, M.M. Lifelong plasticity in the rat auditory cortex: Basic mechanisms and role of sensory experience. *Prog. Brain Res.* **2011**, *191*, 119–131. [CrossRef] [PubMed]
40. Kilgard, M.P.; Pandya, P.K.; Vazquez, J.; Gehi, A.; Schreiner, C.E.; Merzenich, M.M. Sensory input directs spatial and temporal plasticity in primary auditory cortex. *J. Neurophysiol.* **2001**, *86*, 326–338. [CrossRef] [PubMed]
41. Shrestha, B.R.; Chia, C.; Wu, L.; Kujawa, S.G.; Liberman, M.C.; Goodrich, L.V. Sensory Neuron Diversity in the Inner Ear Is Shaped by Activity. *Cell* **2018**, *174*, 1229–1246.e17. [CrossRef] [PubMed]
42. Galaburda, A.M.; Menard, M.T.; Rosen, G.D. Evidence for aberrant auditory anatomy in developmental dyslexia. *Proc. Natl. Acad. Sci. USA* **1994**, *91*, 8010–8013. [CrossRef] [PubMed]
43. Herman, A.E.; Galaburda, A.M.; Fitch, R.H.; Carter, A.R.; Rosen, G.D. Cerebral microgyria, thalamic cell size and auditory temporal processing in male and female rats. *Cereb. Cortex* **1997**, *7*, 453–464. [CrossRef]
44. Rosen, G.D.; Herman, A.E.; Galaburda, A.M. Sex Differences in the Effects of Early Neocortical Injury on Neuronal Size Distribution of the Medial Geniculate Nucleus in the Rat Are Mediated by Perinatal Gonadal Steroids. *Cereb. Cortex* **1999**, *9*, 27–34. [CrossRef]
45. Szalkowski, C.E.; Booker, A.B.; Truong, D.T.; Threlkeld, S.W.; Rosen, G.D.; Fitch, R.H. Knockdown of the Candidate Dyslexia Susceptibility Gene Homolog Dyx1c1 in Rodents: Effects on Auditory Processing, Visual Attention, and Cortical and Thalamic Anatomy. *Dev. Neurosci.* **2013**, *35*, 50–68. [CrossRef]
46. Cohen-Mimran, R.; Sapir, S. Auditory temporal processing deficits in children with reading disabilities. *Dyslexia* **2007**, *13*, 175–192. [CrossRef]
47. Fitch, R.H.; Tallal, P. Neural Mechanisms of Language-Based Learning Impairments: Insights from Human Populations and Animal Models. *Behav. Cogn. Neurosci. Rev.* **2003**, *2*, 155–178. [CrossRef]
48. Vandermosten, M.; Boets, B.; Luts, H.; Poelmans, H.; Wouters, J.; Ghesquière, P. Impairments in speech and nonspeech sound categorization in children with dyslexia are driven by temporal processing difficulties. *Res. Dev. Disabil.* **2011**, *32*, 593–603. [CrossRef]
49. Benasich, A.A.; Thomas, J.J.; Choudhury, N.; Leppänen, P.H.T. The importance of rapid auditory processing abilities to early language development: Evidence from converging methodologies. *Dev. Psychobiol.* **2002**, *40*, 278–292. [CrossRef] [PubMed]
50. Tsatsanis, K.D.; Rourke, B.P.; Klin, A.; Volkmar, F.R.; Cicchetti, D.; Schultz, R.T. Reduced thalamic volume in high-functioning individuals with autism. *Biol. Psychiatry* **2003**, *53*, 121–129. [CrossRef]
51. Müller, R.-A.; Chugani, D.C.; Behen, M.E.; Rothermel, R.D.; Muzik, O.; Chakraborty, P.K.; Chugani, H.T. Impairment of dentato-thalamo-cortical pathway in autistic men: Language activation data from positron emission tomography. *Neurosci. Lett.* **1998**, *245*, 1–4. [CrossRef]
52. Truong, D.T.; Rendall, A.R.; Castelluccio, B.C.; Eigsti, I.-M.; Fitch, R.H. Auditory processing and morphological anomalies in medial geniculate nucleus of Cntnap2 mutant mice. *Behav. Neurosci.* **2015**, *129*, 731–743. [CrossRef] [PubMed]

53. Levy, S.E.; Giarelli, E.; Lee, L.-C.; Schieve, L.A.; Kirby, R.S.; Cunniff, C.; Nicholas, J.; Reaven, J.; Rice, C.E. Autism spectrum disorder and co-occurring developmental, psychiatric, and medical conditions among children in multiple populations of the United States. *J. Dev. Behav. Pediatr.* **2010**, *31*, 267–275. [CrossRef] [PubMed]
54. Chi, J.G.; Dooling, E.C.; Gilles, F.H. Left-right asymmetries of the temporal speech areas of the human fetus. *Arch Neurol.* **1977**, *34*, 346–348. [CrossRef]
55. Szaflarski, J.P.; Rajagopal, A.; Altaye, M.; Byars, A.W.; Jacola, L.; Schmithorst, V.J.; Schapiro, M.B.; Plante, E.; Holland, S.K. Left-Handedness and Language Lateralization in Children. *Brain Res.* **2012**, *1433C*, 85–97. [CrossRef]
56. Sininger, Y.S.; Bhatara, A. Laterality of Basic Auditory Perception. *Laterality* **2012**, *17*, 129–149. [CrossRef]
57. Levy, R.B.; Marquarding, T.; Reid, A.P.; Pun, C.M.; Renier, N.; Oviedo, H.V. Circuit asymmetries underlie functional lateralization in the mouse auditory cortex. *Nat. Commun.* **2019**, *10*, 2783. [CrossRef]

MDPI
St. Alban-Anlage 66
4052 Basel
Switzerland
Tel. +41 61 683 77 34
Fax +41 61 302 89 18
www.mdpi.com

Genes Editorial Office
E-mail: genes@mdpi.com
www.mdpi.com/journal/genes

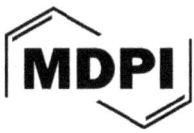

www.ingramcontent.com/pod-product-compliance
Lightning Source LLC
LaVergne TN
LVHW070203100526
838202LV00015B/1990